Clinical Microbiolo and Inf ti Diseas

SECOND EDITION

AN ILLUSTRATE

THE SANDERS
Learning P
Orm

To my late great Chief, Mr Glen Buckle, who inspired me to study Microbiology; to my patients, especially in Bangladesh, who inspired me to study Infectious Diseases; and to my students and colleagues, who inspire me still.

Commissioning Editor: Timothy Horne
Project Development Manager: Lulu Stader
Project Manager: Frances Affleck
Design Direction: Erik Bigland

Clinical

SECOND EDITION

Microbiology and Infectious Diseases

AN ILLUSTRATED COLOUR TEXT

W. John Spicer

MB.BS (Melbourne) FRACP FRCPA FACSHP FASM DTM&H (Sydney) Dip.Bact (London)

Senior Consultant in Infectious Diseases, The Alfred Hospital, and Austin Health
Senior Consultant in Microbiology, The Alfred Hospital
Associate Professor of Microbiology and Medicine, Monash University
Consultant Microbiologist, Dorevitch Pathology

Melbourne, Australia

Illustrated by Peter Lamb and Robert Britton

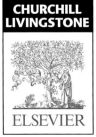

CHURCHILL
LIVINGSTONE

ELSEVIER

EDINBURGH   LONDON   NEW YORK   OXFORD   PHILADELPHIA   ST LOUIS   SYDNEY   TORONTO   2008

CHURCHILL
LIVINGSTONE
ELSEVIER

An Imprint of Elsevier Limited

© Harcourt Publishers Limited 2000
© Elsevier Limited 2008

The right of Professor W. John Spicer to be identified as author of this
work has been asserted by him in accordance with the Copyright, Designs
and Patents Act 1988.

First edition 2000
Second edition 2008

ISBN (10) 0-443-10303-8
ISBN (13) 978-0-443-10303-2

British Library Cataloguing in Publication Data
A catalogue record for this book is available from the British Library

Library of Congress Cataloging in Publication Data
A catalog record for this book is available from the Library of Congress

ELSEVIER   your source for books,
journals and multimedia
in the health sciences

www.elsevierhealth.com

Working together to grow
libraries in developing countries

www.elsevier.com | www.bookaid.org | www.sabre.org

ELSEVIER   BOOK AID International   Sabre Foundation

The
publisher's
policy is to use
**paper manufactured
from sustainable forests**

Printed in China

Preface to the second edition

While a three-legged table or chair can be very satisfactory, most prefer the conventional four legs, so I am delighted that the major change from the first edition is the addition of virology and viral infections to the original threesome of clinical bacteriology, mycology and parasitology. This has been achieved both by thirteen new explicit chapters within the five major parts of the book, and also by incorporating relevant information on viruses throughout the text. Prions and prion diseases are also described.

Revision of the entire first edition text including all tables and figures has included new knowledge, new organisms (and old ones with new names), new diseases, new tests and new antimicrobials.

A new table of abbreviations and a list of further reading of larger, or more specialised, books have been added.

The index has been expanded, the few typographic mistakes in the text removed, and no new errors added, I trust.

Some of these improvements come from comments by readers of the first edition, and I look forward to further helpful feedback through the publishers or directly to me at PO Box 450, Canterbury, 3126, Victoria, Australia (nice stamps for my grandniece, please) or by email to spicerwj@ozemail.com.au.

2007   W. J. S.

Preface to the first edition

All medical students, and all nurses, general practitioners and medical specialists seeing patients, need to understand the basics of microbiology and infections. Infection cannot be understood without knowing some microbiology; and infection is one of the major mechanisms causing disease and can affect every body tissue and organ.

This book aims to present – clearly, concisely and memorably – the clinically relevant basic facts and processes in the twin disciplines of microbiology and infectious diseases. The range of the book is wide, including fungi and parasites as well as bacteria and their consequent infections.

The organisation of any book on microbiology and infectious diseases depends particularly on one question – to present the twins integrated in each chapter, or separately? If all infections were like tetanus or anthrax, where one organism causes only one disease which is in turn caused only by that organism, the integrated approach would be obvious and easy. But life, apparently, was not meant to be easy. Consider the amazing Group A streptococcus (S. pyogenes, p. 36–37), causing numerous diseases by numerous mechanisms in numerous organs; or the versatile 'golden staph' (S. aureus, p. 34–35), causing infections ranging from a trivial pimple through cellulitis to serious deep abscesses and bone infections, to endocarditis and overwhelming septicaemia with septic shock.

Conversely, many common disease presentations such as pneumonia, urinary infections and gut infections have more than one possible causative organism. So I have chosen, after an introductory section on general characteristics of the organisms and a second section on their attack on us and our intrinsic defences, to present the third section on specific organisms in more detail (microbiology), and then the fourth section on clinical infections in each body organ system and some special categories, with extensive cross-references between the third and fourth sections. The fifth and final section is on the extrinsic defences we have invented, such as vaccines, asepsis and antisepsis, and antimicrobials.

The format of the book is exciting, being specifically designed to help both initial learning and revision. Each subject is presented in an 'easy learning' module complete on a single or double page spread, with numerous coloured photographs, coloured graphics, integrated tables, and a 'key point' summary in the bottom right hand corner, useful both for initial orientation and for revision.

In a book of this size it is obviously impossible to give extended detail, or cover all organisms and diseases, yet I have intentionally included rarer and 'tropical' infections. Every GP and Emergency Department clinician must be able to recognise the rare meningococcal bacteraemia or meningitis, which they may never have seen before, yet the patient's life depends on early recognition and emergency treatment by the first doctor to see them. Similarly, any GP or other 'front line' doctor in a temperate industrialised country may be confronted by a sick patient with malaria or typhoid fever in a returned traveller or immigrant, needing early recognition and urgent relevant investigation and treatment. I aimed to make this book useful in both industrialised and developing countries.

I have enjoyed writing this book, and I hope you enjoy and profit from reading it. I will be interested to hear your opinions and suggestions.

2000   W. J. S.

Acknowledgements

While many of the slides and images illustrating this book came from my own collection of the last 40 years, I am indebted to many colleagues for filling gaps with particular slides I needed. My own staff in the Departments of Infectious Diseases and Microbiology, Alfred Hospital, were always wonderfully helpful, especially Associate Professor Denis Spelman and Dr Andrew Fuller, also Drs Ashley Watson, Sally Roberts, Adam Jenney and numerous other registrars and residents in the ID Unit; Mr Grant Perry, Ms Clare Franklin, Mrs Jenni Williams and the late Mr Glen Buckle in Microbiology; and Ms Glenys Harrington in Infection Control. I am very grateful to all the patients who gave permission to be photographed, and to Alfred Hospital and Monash University Departments and individual colleagues who willingly provided particular slides from their patients in Melbourne or overseas: in the Departments of Radiology and Nuclear Medicine, Associate Professors Nina Sacharias and Victor Kalff, and Drs Chris O'Donnell and Stephen Booth; in the Department of Anatomical Pathology, Professor John Dowling, the late Associate Professor Brian Essex and Drs Shant Khan, S K Tang, the late Ross Anderson and Mr John Hall; in Monash Microbiology, Drs Geoff Cross, Ian Denham, Mrs Lyn Howden and Mrs Jan Savage. Individually, Professors Hugh Taylor, Suzanne Garland, John Murtagh and Dan Sexton (Duke University, USA), Associate Professors Geoff Hogg, John Kelly, Hector McLean and Alison Street, and Drs David Abell, Barry Elliott, Reuben Glass, Tony Hall, Robin Hooper, the late Don Jacobs, David Looke (Brisbane), Fiona McCurragh, Hugh Newton-John, Jo Sabto, Jack Swann, Hugo Standish, the late Brian Smith, Richard Stawell, Peter Thompson, Jonathan Tversky, John Waterston, Robert West and Bob Zacharin, and also Ms Karen Flett and Mr Guy Brown. If I have unknowingly been provided with previously published slides, I apologize in advance. Several slides from the former Fairfield Hospital and the Royal Victorian Eye and Ear Hospital Slide Libraries were used with permission, and my thanks to Ms Caroline Hedt, Mr Gavin Hawkins and Mr Cam Harvey in the Alfred Visual Communications Department who were always helpful in duplicating slides, with which the Monash University Department at Alfred also assisted at times. For the second edition I am particularly indebted to Drs Andrew Fuller, Mike Catton and John Marshall and Professor Catriona McLean for most of the new digital images, and for additional images from Dr Philip du Cros, Dr Reuben Glass, Prof Stephen Kent and his son Tom.

In Churchill Livingstone, now part of Elsevier, I received particular help, expert advice, and unfailing courtesy from Mr Jim Killgore, Ms Frances Affleck and Mr Timothy Horne, with much help behind the scenes from Dr Jane Ward, Leslie Smillie, Dr Laurence Errington and Dr Susan Boobis, and from Peter Lamb and Robert Britton who transformed my line drawings, examples and directions to the excellent figures you see. Dr Lulu Stader has been an excellent editorial colleague in Scotland and I have much enjoyed our 12 months working together though so far apart.

Finally I thank my wife Heather and my family, who are almost as pleased as I am to see such a beautiful book emerge again!

Contents

Preface to the second edition **v**

Preface to the first edition **v**

Acknowledgements **vi**

Microbial names changed from the first edition **ix**

Abbreviations **ix**

Microbes 2

Characteristics of bacteria **2**

Characteristics of fungi **6**

Characteristics of protozoa **10**

Characteristics of multicellular parasites **12**

Characteristics of viruses **14**

Microbial attack and control by intrinsic defences 20

Uneasy peace: host–microbial relationships **20**

Attackers: normal flora and pathogens **22**

Attack begins: attack and first-line defences **24**

Attack continues: non-specific second-line defences **26**

Attack contained: specific immune defences **28**

Defences disordered or evaded **30**

Defences disturbed: general host responses **32**

Specific pathogens 34

Bacteria 34

Staphylococci **34**

Streptococci and enterococci **36**

Gram-positive rods: *Corynebacterium, Listeria, Bacillus* **38**

Clostridia **40**

Neisseria, Moraxella, Kingella and *Acinetobacter* **42**

Haemophilus, Bordetella and *Legionella* **44**

Enterobacteriaceae **46**

Vibrio, Campylobacter, Helicobacter, Aeromonas, Plesiomonas **50**

Pseudomonads and rare Gram-negative rods **52**

Bacteroides, Fusobacterium and other anaerobes **54**

Zoonotic bacteria **56**

Spirochaetes: treponemes, borreliae, leptospires **58**

Mycobacteria **60**

Actinomyces, Nocardia and rare Gram-positive bacilli **62**

Mycoplasma and *Ureaplasma* **63**

Chlamydia and *Chlamydophila* **64**

Rickettsiae and bartonellae **66**

Fungi 68

Aspergillus and *Candida* **68**

Cryptococcus and *Histoplasma* **70**

Blastomyces, Coccidioides, Paracoccidioides **72**

Fungi infecting skin and adjacent tissues **74**

Fungi causing invasive zygomycosis (mucormycosis) **76**

Arthropods 77

Arthropods **77**

Parasites 78

Sporozoa: *Plasmodium, Toxoplasma, Cryptosporidium* **78**

Amoebae: *Entamoeba, Naegleria, Acanthamoeba* **80**

Intestinal and vaginal flagellates and ciliates **81**

Blood and tissue flagellates **82**

Intestinal nematodes (worms) **84**

Tissue nematodes (worms) **86**

Cestodes (tapeworms) **88**

Trematodes (flukes) **90**

Viruses 92

Microbial attack succeeds: clinical infection 94

Acute meningitis **94**

Acute encephalitis and polio **96**

Chronic diffuse non-viral CNS infections **98**

Chronic diffuse viral and prion CNS diseases **100**

CNS abscesses and other focal infections **102**

Nervous system: tropical and rare infections **104**

Otitis, mastoiditis and sinusitis **106**

Superficial ocular infections **108**

Tropical ocular infections **110**

Deep eye infections **112**

Stomatitis **113**

Dental and periodontal infections **114**

Viral respiratory infections **116**

Throat infections **118**

Epiglottitis, diphtheria and Ludwig's angina **120**

Tropical and rare oro-facial infections **122**

Laryngitis, tracheitis and pertussis **123**

Bronchial infections **124**

Pneumonia I: in the normal host **126**

Pneumonia II: in the abnormal host **128**

Lung abscess and empyaema **130**

Tuberculosis and atypical mycobacterial infections **132**

Tropical or rare respiratory infections **134**

Suppurative thrombophlebitis/lymphangitis/lymphadenitis **136**

Myocarditis, pericarditis and rheumatic fever **138**

Infective endocarditis **140**

Bacteraemia, septicaemia and fungaemia **142**

Viral systemic infections of the young **144**

Viral systemic infections of all ages **146**

HIV and AIDS **149**

Tropical systemic infections **152**

Rarer systemic infections **154**

Pyrexia of unknown origin (PUO) **156**

Diarrhoeal disease I: general features **158**

Diarrhoeal disease II: bacteria and viruses **160**

Diarrhoeal disease III: protozoa and worms **162**

Peritonitis and intra-abdominal abscesses **164**

Biliary infections **166**

Hepatic non-viral infections **168**

Viral hepatitis **170**

Tropical and rare abdominal infections **173**

Urinary tract infections: cystitis and pyelonephritis **174**

Renal and perinephric abscesses/prostatitis **176**

Tropical and rare urinary infections **178**

Urethritis **180**

Cervical infections **182**

Salpingitis and pelvic inflammatory disease **184**

Epididymitis, orchitis and balanitis **186**

Vaginitis and vulvo-vaginitis **187**

Tropical and rare sexually transmitted diseases **188**

Streptococcal skin and soft tissue infections **190**

Staphylococcal skin and soft tissue infections **192**

Gas-forming and gangrenous infections **194**

Wound, bite and burn infections **196**

Fungal infections of the skin, hair or nails **198**

Viral infections of skin, mucosa and soft tissues **200**

Tropical and rare bacterial skin and soft tissue infections **202**

Tropical and rare fungal and parasitic skin and soft tissue infections **204**

Osteomyelitis **206**

Special, tropical or rare bone infections **208**

Joint infections **210**

Zoonoses **212**

Maternal, fetal and neonatal infections **214**

Travellers and recent immigrants **216**

Hospital-acquired infections **218**

Infections in compromised patients **220**

Infections in General Practice patients **222**

Infections in elderly patients **223**

Microbe control by extrinsic defences 224

Sterilisation and disinfection **224**

Antimicrobials: general properties **226**

Antimicrobials: specific antibacterials **228**

Antimicrobials: special antimicrobials **232**

Antimicrobials: antiviral drugs **234**

Vaccines and immunisation **236**

Clinician and laboratory: microbial detection and identification **238**

Clinician and laboratory: antibody response and guiding therapy **240**

Further reading 242

Index 243

Microbial names changed from the first edition:

OLD NAME

Actinobacillus actinomycetemcomitans
Branhamella catarrhalis
Borrelia burgdorferi
Calymmatobacterium granulomatis
Chlamydia pneumoniae
Flavobacterium spp.
Opisthorchis sinensis
Pneumocystis carinii
Pseudomonas pseudomallei
Pseudomonas mallei
Pseudomonas cepacia
Rochalimaea henselae
Rochalimaea quintana
Xanthomonas maltophilia

NEW NAME

Haemophilus actinomycetemcomitans
Moraxella catarrhalis
Borrelia burgdorferi group now includes two other species.
Klebsiella granulomatis
Chlamydophila pneumoniae
Chryseobacterium spp.
Clonorchis sinensis
Pneumocystis jirovecii
Burkholderia pseudomallei
Burkholderia mallei
Burkholderia cepacia
Bartonella henselae
Bartonella quintana
Stenotrophomonas maltophilia

Abbreviations

Abbreviation	Meaning
AFB	Acid-Fast Bacilli (usually mycobacteria)
AGN	Acute Glomerulo-Nephritis
AIDS	Acquired Immune Deficiency Syndrome
ASOT	Anti-Streptolysin O Titre (Test)
BCG	Bacillus Calmette-Guérin
CD4	Cluster of Differentiation (T-cell receptors)
CMI	Cell-Mediated Immunity
CMV	CytoMegaloVirus
CT	Computed Tomography (Scan)
DFA	Direct Fluorescent Antibody (Test)
DGM	Dark Ground Microscopy
DIC	Disseminated Intravascular Coagulation
DNA	De-oxyribo Nucleic Acid
EBV	Epstein-Barr Virus
EIA	Enzyme Immuno-Assay
ELISA	Enzyme-Linked Immuno-Sorbent Assay
FTA	Fluorescent Treponemal Antibody (test)
GLC	Gas-Liquid Chromatography
GNR/B/C	Gram Negative Rod/Bacillus/Coccus
GPR/C	Gram Positive Rod/Coccus
HACEK	Rare causes of endocarditis
HAV, HBV,	Hepatitis A Virus, Hepatitis B Virus,
HCV, HDV,	Hepatitis C Virus, Hepatitis D Virus,
HEV, HGV	Hepatitis E Virus, Hepatitis G Virus
HIV	Human Immunodeficiency Virus
HPF	High Powered Field (in microscopy)
HSV, HZV	Herpes Simplex Virus, H. Zoster Virus
IFA	Indirect Fluorescent Antibody (test)
IgA, E, G, M	Immunoglobulin A, E, G, M
IL-1	Interleukin-1 (cytokine from macrophages)
LFTs	Liver Function Tests
LPS	LipoPolySaccharide (endotoxin)
MAC	*Mycobacterium avium* Complex
MRI	Magnetic Resonance Imaging
NAD	No Abnormality Detected
NGU/NSU	Non-Gonococcal/Non-Specific Urethritis
NK	Natural Killer (Cells)
PCR	Polymerase Chain Reaction (Test)
PMEC	Pseudo-Membranous Entero-Colitis
PPD	Purified Protein Derivative (of *Myco. TB*)
RNA	Ribo Nucleic Acid
RPR	Rapid Plasma Reagin (test for syphilis)
SOL	Space Occupying Lesion (in body organ)
(S)SSS	(Staphylococcal) Scalded Skin Syndrome
STD/I	Sexually Transmitted Disease/Infection
TNF	Tumour Necrosis Factor
TPHA/TPPA	*T. pallidum* Haem/Particle Agglutination
TSS/TSST	Toxic Shock Syndrome (Toxin)
UTI	Urinary Tract Infection
VDRL	Venereal Disease Research Lab. (test)
VZV	Varicella-Zoster Virus
XR	XRay

Characteristics of bacteria (1)

Nomenclature

All living things, hence all bacteria, have two names, firstly their generic (genus) name, e.g. *Staphylococcus*, then their specific (species) name, e.g. *aureus*. The generic name is often abbreviated to the initial letter(s), e.g. *S. aureus*.

Special additions to this universal scheme may include:

- a third name to distinguish several varieties within one species, e.g. *Acinetobacter calcoaceticus* var *anitratus* (!)
- a common, non-scientific, historical name, e.g. pneumococcus for *Streptococcus pneumoniae*, gonococcus for *Neisseria gonorrhoeae*, meningococcus for *Neisseria meningitidis*
- a serological group name, e.g. *Streptococcus pyogenes* is also called 'the group A streptococcus'
- a toxin profile name, e.g. *Clostridium perfringens* type A.

Classification

Increasing knowledge of the properties of bacteria, fungi, protozoa and algae has necessitated revision of the simple division of living things into two kingdoms: plants and animals. One classification has two super-kingdoms: procaryotes (bacteria and blue-green algae) and eucaryotes.

Eucaryotes include four kingdoms, Protista (Protozoa and Algae), Fungi, Animalia and Plantae. Viruses are not included because they do not have the essential characteristics of living organisms (capable of independent replication or survival).

Bacteria are fundamentally different from all other living things in being *procaryotes*, distinguished by:

- DNA in a double-stranded loop, not within a nuclear membrane
- small ribosomes free in the cytoplasm; there is no endoplasmic reticulum
- the absence of mitochondria or other membrane-enclosed organelles
- a complex peptidoglycan-protein cell wall (absent in *Mycoplasma*).

Bacteria are classified by several criteria (see Table 1):

- shape
- stain
- ability to grow with or without oxygen
- size

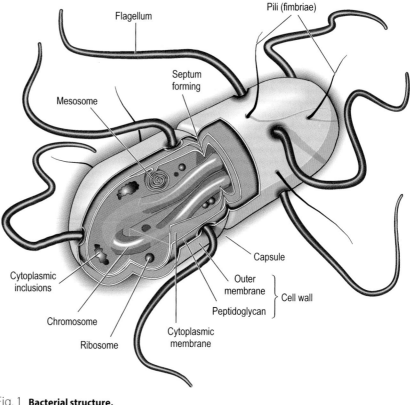

Fig. 1 **Bacterial structure.**

Labels: Flagellum · Pili (fimbriae) · Septum forming · Mesosome · Cytoplasmic inclusions · Chromosome · Ribosome · Cytoplasmic membrane · Capsule · Outer membrane · Peptidoglycan · Cell wall

Criteria	Groups	Examples
Shape	Cocci (spherical)	*Staphylococcus, Neisseria*
	Bacilli (rods)	*Bacillus, Listeria, Salmonella*
	Spirilla (curved or spiral rods)	*Vibrio, Campylobacter*
Stain	Gram stain positive	*Staphylococcus, Streptococcus, Bacillus*
	Gram stain negative	*Haemophilus, Escherichia, Salmonella*
	Acid-fast stains	*Mycobacterium*
	Special stains for specialised structures	*Clostridia* spores
Gas requirements	Strict aerobes	*Pseudomonas aeruginosa*
	Facultative anaerobes	*Escherichia coli*
	Strict anaerobes	*Clostridium* spp.
	Capnophiles (need high CO_2)	*Neisseria* spp.
Specialised features	Spores	*Clostridium* spp.
	Enzymes	Coagulase-producing staphylococci
	Antibiotic resistance	Meticillin-resistant *Staphylococcus aureus* (MRSA)
	Antigens	*Streptococcus* (Lancefield groups), *Chlamydia*
Nucleic acids	DNA probes	Enterotoxic *Escherichia coli*; rapid detection of meningococcus infection
	DNA amplification	*Mycobacterium leprae*

Table 1 **Major criteria for classifying medically important bacteria**

- growth characteristics
- DNA content (G + C content) and homology.

The Gram stain is the most important staining procedure in medical microbiology. Gram-positive organisms retain the purple of crystal violet after iodine fixation and alcohol washing, whereas Gram-negative organisms lose the colour with alcohol and need counterstaining with a pink dye. Special stains are needed for organisms with unusual cell walls, e.g. acid-fast stains for mycobacteria.

Although staining and growth characteristics have formed the basis of diagnostic microbiology, the availability of techniques such as DNA probes and amplification, and polyclonal and monoclonal antibodies have greatly increased the speed, range and sensitivity of diagnostic testing.

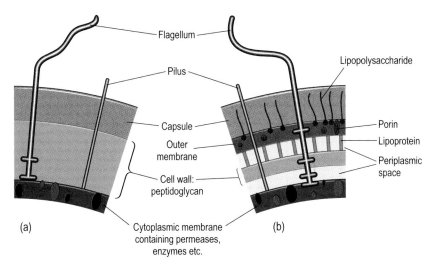

Fig. 2   **Structure of Gram-positive (a) and Gram-negative (b) bacteria.**

Size and structure (Fig. 1)

Pathogenic bacteria vary widely in size: from *Mycoplasma* spp. (0.2–0.8µm = micrometre diameter) to enteric Gram-negative rods (0.5–6.0µm). Gram-positive and Gram-negative bacteria differ in their cell wall composition but have typical procaryote internal structure.

Cell membrane

The cell (cytoplasmic) membrane is made of protein and phospholipids, but (except in *Mycoplasma*) not the sterols that are found in eucaryotes. It is the osmotic barrier between cell and environment, and its essential functions include electron transport, enzyme systems (as in eucaryotic mitochondria), solute transport and cell product transport.

Cell wall (Fig. 2)

The cell wall has numerous functions reflected in its structure:

- protects by its rigidity the cell membrane from osmotic or mechanical rupture
- contains numerous characteristic antigens, important both in bacterial virulence and endotoxins, and in host antibody formation
- provides a firm base for pili (fimbriae) and flagella.

Gram-positive cells

The cell wall of Gram-positive organisms (Fig. 2a) consists mainly of many layers of *peptidoglycan* (murein), a complex polymer of long glycan (sugar) chains of alternating *N*-acetylglucosamine and *N*-acetyl muramic acid with short penta-peptide side chains cross-linked to each other by peptide bonds between the lysine of one and the D-alanine of the other, giving a rigid polar wall (Fig. 1,

p. 226). Other polymers in the wall include teichoic acids and chains of glycerol or ribitol linked by phospho-diester bonds.

Gram-negative cells

The cell wall of Gram-negative organisms (Fig. 2b) consists of a thinner layer of the same *peptidoglycan* but the cross-linking is between D-amino pimelic acid and D-alanine. This peptidoglycan layer is in a *periplasmic space* between the inner cytoplasmic membrane and a unique bi-layered phospholipid *outer membrane*, with lipoprotein on the inner surface binding to the peptidoglycan, and a special *lipopolysaccharide* (LPS) on the outer.

The three components of LPS are the lipid (lipid A, the active component of endotoxin, very important in causing septic shock, p. 32), a core polysaccharide and a variable carbohydrate chain, which is the distinctive O antigen detected serologically. Its hydrophobicity gives some antibiotic and bile salt resistance.

Mycobacteria

The cell wall of mycobacteria (p. 60) and other acid-fast organisms contains characteristic *waxes*, complex long-chain

hydrocarbons with sugars. This almost impervious coat prevents stains being removed by acid and gives resistance to desiccation and many disinfectants and antibiotics. It also slows the entry of nutrients.

Capsule

A capsule protects the cell wall of many bacteria, particularly in adverse conditions; this mucoid polysaccharide layer may be lost in laboratory cultures. In infections, it resists phagocytosis by white blood cells and aids adherence to tissues, catheters and prostheses.

Pili

Pili (fimbriae) are hair-like in appearance and are of at least two types:

- *Sex pili* are specialised structures that enable DNA transfer by conjugation (literally, 'joined with')
- *Common pili* are shorter and aid attachment to host cells, are anti-phagocytic and by rapid changes in their antigenic protein (pilin) avoid host antibody response.

Flagella

Flagella are much longer than pili and give motility to bacteria, which may be *monotrichous* (one flagellum at one or both ends), *lophotrichous* (many flagella at one or both ends), or *peritrichous* ('covered with hair'). Coherent counter-clockwise flagellar rotation, because of the counter-clockwise helical pitch of the flagellar protein, gives a straight swimming motion, as in chemotaxis toward an attractant, while clockwise rotation gives tumbling motility, seen particularly with repellents.

Spores

Spores, formed especially by *Clostridium* spp. and *Bacillus* spp., are concentrated bacterial DNA surrounded by an extremely tough protective coat. The cell is metabolically inert and survives drying, heat and most chemical agents for months, years or more.

Characteristics of bacteria (1)

- The first name of a bacterium is its genus, and the second its species.
- Bacteria were initially classified by their shape, Gram stain and oxygen requirements, supplemented by biochemical and serological characters. Genetics is now being used to establish fundamental relationships.
- Bacteria are procaryotes with free circular DNA, ribosomes, no mitochondria and a peptidoglycan cell wall.
- Bacterial structure includes:
  - internal structure: nuclear material, ribosomes, cell membrane
  - cell wall: peptidoglycan (plus periplasmic space and outer membrane in Gram-negative bacteria)
  - external structures: capsule, pili, flagella.
- Spores are metabolically inert in a protective coat.

Characteristics of bacteria (2)

Energy, nutrition and growth

Energy sources and processes

Bacteria use three sources for their energy requirements: chemical reactions (*chemotrophy*), light (*phototrophy*) or the host cell (*paratrophy*). If the energy-yielding reactions use organic compounds they are termed organotrophy; those using inorganic compounds are termed lithotrophy. So energy derived from light using organic hydrogen donors would be described as photo-organotrophy (in some anaerobic bacteria).

Nutrition

Bacteria show a wide variety of nutritional requirements. *Autotrophs* can live in an entirely inorganic environment; they are free living and rarely are of medical importance. *Heterotrophs* need an exogenous supply of one or more essential metabolites. Most bacteria of medical importance come into this group and they vary from those with great synthetic capacity (e.g. *Escherichia coli*) to those pathogens that require exogenous supplies of growth factors such as vitamins to grow (e.g. some streptococci). Finally, some of the parasitic and pathogenic species can only survive intracellularly (*paratrophy or auxotrophy*); they possess DNA and RNA, but only a limited range of independent metabolic activity.

Growth

The doubling time or the generation time is the time between bacterial divisions (by binary fission) and ranges from about 20 minutes for *E. coli* and similar bacteria provided with rich nutrients like laboratory media, to 24 hours for tubercle bacilli. *Balanced growth* occurs when all necessary nutrients are supplied, while *unbalanced growth* is more usual in nature where changing environments and unbalanced nutritional supplies will occur. The phases in the growth of bacteria introduced into a nutrient-rich environment are shown in Fig. 1. Cells in log phase are most virulent.

Metabolism

This is best considered in three stages:

- **Intermediary metabolism**: the utilisation of a carbon source, e.g. glucose, to provide energy and small molecules such as pyruvate.
- **Biosynthetic pathways**: to build these small molecules with nitrogen, sulphur and other minerals into amino acids, purines, pyrimidines, polysaccharides and lipids.
- **Genetic instructions**: to build these into macromolecules and bacterial organelles ready for cell division.

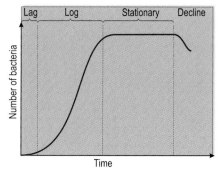

Fig. 1 **The phases of a bacterial growth curve.**

Intermediary metabolism

Bacteria have adapted to use a vast range of substances as energy sources and are capable of widely differing metabolic activities. Glucose is used by almost all bacteria and the interlinking of pathways is common to all regardless of their metabolic capacity (Fig. 2). Two central metabolic pathways are:

- *Embden-Meyerhof-Parnas glycolytic pathway (EMP)*, which converts glucose to pyruvate with the formation of ATP as an energy source.
- *Tricarboxylic acid (Krebs) cycle* then uses pyruvate and ATP both to provide further energy and to form intermediate substances for amino acid and fatty acid biosynthesis.

Additional pathways are used by various bacteria, including:

- *Pentose phosphate cycle* to utilise pentoses (instead of hexoses like glucose) to provide energy for ATP and NADPH formation, and carbon compounds for nucleotide (purine and pyrimidine) synthesis.
- *Entner-Doudoroff anaerobic pathway* to convert glucose to pyruvate via 6-phosphogluconic acid instead of by the aerobic EMP pathway. It is also used by pseudomonads, important in hospital infections, to metabolise gluconate and related compounds extracellularly, using enzymes in their cell membrane and thus avoiding energy use on hexose transport.
- *Conversion of 4-carbon to 3-carbon compounds*, e.g. malate to pyruvate, and acetoacetate to pyruvate via phosphoenolpyruvate.

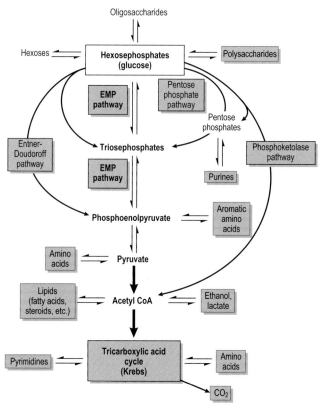

Fig. 2 **Intermediary metabolism and major biosynthetic pathways.**

■ *Phosphoketolase pathway*, fermenting glucose or pentoses to pyruvate, lactate, acetate or ethanol when some enzymes of the EMP glycolytic pathway are lacking.

■ *Pyruvate metabolism* to lactate, succinate, propionate, acetone, acetate, acetoin, butanol and ethanol.

Biosynthetic pathways

Purine synthesis

Purines are synthesised from ribose 5-phosphate produced in the pentose phosphate cycle or the phosphoketolase pathway.

Pyrimidine synthesis for RNA

The amino group of glutamine plus CO_2 and aspartate form carbamyl aspartic acid, which loses water to become dihydro-orotic acid, the precursor for the pyrimidines, uridine and cytidine.

Amino acid synthesis

The essential feature of each amino acid is its carbon skeleton; biosyntheses occur from four intermediates of metabolism (Fig. 3) into four families.

Utilisation of complex substrates

Bacteria can use many large molecules as substrates, decomposing them by oxidation, reduction and by specific enzymatic attack to recycle carbon and nitrogen and produce energy. Bacteria have a greater range of such processes than fungi and both perform chemical feats impossible for plants and animals.

Bacteria and fungi can use not only nitrate but also nitrite, ammonia and even nitrogen to provide their nitrogen needs. Some (chemolithoautotrophic) bacteria even reverse this process, forming nitrogen from nitrate.

Genetics

The *genome* (genetic material) of bacteria is DNA contained in one long continuous ('circular') chromosome, tightly supercoiled by the enzyme DNA gyrase. The chromosome consists of 3000 to 6000 *genes*, which are specific DNA sequences coding by *codons* of three nucleotide base pairs to messenger RNA for specific amino acids to form polypeptides. A few genes are structural, coding for ribosomal and transfer RNA. There are no introns (sequences between genes) as in eucaryotes. The full expression of the genome is the *genotype* but what is apparent – the *phenotype* – is often less, because of latent, unexpressed qualities.

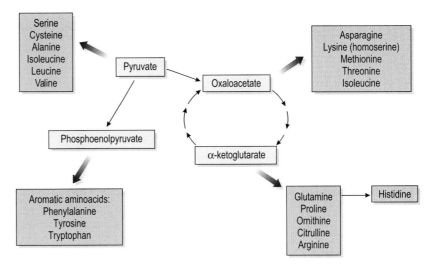

Fig. 3 **Biosynthesis of amino acids.**

Genetic changes in bacteria

As bacteria are haploid, there is no genetic exchange by meiosis and zygote formation as in eucaryotes. Genetic change comes only by random mutations or from one of three types of gene exchange. The random mutation rate is about 1 in 10^7 to 10^8 cell divisions and can lead, for example, to changes in colony colour, loss of a biochemical activity, or resistance to an antibiotic. The result of some donor bacterial genome (exogenote) entering an intact recipient is a merozygote leading to *recombination* of donor and recipient genes.

The three types of gene exchange are:

■ *Transformation*: the transfer of a free fragment of DNA from one bacterium to another of the same genus, e.g. occurring in *Strep. pneumoniae*, *H. influenzae*.

■ *Transduction*: a fragment of bacterial DNA is carried by a bacteriophage (a virus which infects bacteria) from one bacterium to another.

■ *Conjugation*: transfer in bacteria carrying transmission plasmids, the fertility (F) factor. F⁺ bacteria join to F⁻ bacteria and transfer part of the donor cell's chromosome, about 1% per minute (interrupting this process at different times enables mapping of the donor chromosome).

Many bacteria contain plasmids, smaller circular bits of DNA containing 1000 to 25 000 base pairs. Plasmids carry much important genetic information, including antibiotic resistance. They can also become incorporated into the chromosome as transposons.

Characteristics of bacteria (2)

■ Bacterial energy comes from one of three sources: light, chemical reactions (most pathogens) or a host cell.

■ Most pathogenic bacteria are heterotrophs, needing an external source for some essential metabolites.

■ The doubling time (time between cell divisions) for most pathogens is about 20 minutes but is 24 hours for *M. tuberculosis*.

■ Bacteria stimulated to grow enter balanced growth with an initial lag phase, then exponential growth and, finally, the stationary phase when some essential nutrient is exhausted.

■ Bacterial intermediary metabolism varies widely but is founded on two pathways basic to most living things: the EMP glycolytic path from glucose to pyruvate and the Krebs TCA cycle.

■ Bacteria have powerful and varied catabolic pathways that break down macromolecules and are especially important in recycling carbon and nitrogen.

■ The bacterial genome is in a single tightly coiled chromosome without a nuclear membrane, coding by three nucleotide pairs via mRNA to amino acids.

■ Genetic change occurs by mutation, by translocation of fragments of free DNA, by transduction through a bacteriophage, or by conjugation, a form of sexual transfer of DNA involving small free pieces of DNA called plasmids.

Characteristics of fungi (1)

Nomenclature

Fungi, like bacteria, are named by the binomial Linnaean system with a generic name (capitalised and in italics) and a specific name (not capitalised, in italics). However all fungi reproduce asexually, giving the anamorphic state, and most also reproduce sexually giving the teliomorphic state. Unfortunately many pairs of these were described and named before it was realised that they were different forms of the one fungus, e.g. *Cryptococcus neoformans* (anamorph) = *Filobasidiella neoformans* (teliomorph). The name of the tissue form (anamorph) is used by clinicians.

Fungi can be normal inhabitants of the mouth and intestinal tract. In predisposing conditions, e.g. pregnancy, diabetes, immunodeficiency, therapy with broad-spectrum antibiotics, the fungi can proliferate and cause disease, e.g. thrush or even endocarditis.

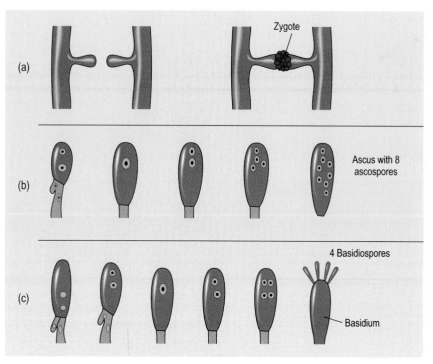

Fig. 1 **Classification by reproductive structures. (a)** Zygote formation in *Zygomycota*, e.g. *Mucor* species. **(b)** Ascus formation in *Ascomycotina*, e.g. *Trichophyton* species. **(c)** Basidium formation in *Basidiomycotina*, e.g. *Cryptococcus neoformans*.

Classification

The kingdom Fungi is divided into two phyla:

- *Zygomycota*, which quickly produce a diploid zygote sexually and sporangiophores asexually. Examples are *Rhizopus*, *Mucor* and other species producing zygomycosis (Fig. 1a and p. 76).
- *Dikaryomycota*, in which the haploid nuclei do not fuse quickly, giving a prolonged dikaryotic sexual cycle.

Phylum *Dikaryomycota* has two subphyla: *Ascomycotina* and *Basidiomycotina*. In the subphylum Ascomycotina, which includes most fungi causing ringworm, this cycle occurs entirely within a sac (an ascus), producing ascospores (Fig. 1b). In the subphylum Basidiomycotina, which includes *Cryptococcus* spp., this begins in a bag (a basidium) and ends with maturation on the outside of the basidium, producing basidiospores (Fig. 1c).

Fungi for which a sexual form is not yet recognised and which, therefore, cannot be fully classified are called Fungi imperfecti. These include many pathogens: *Candida*, *Torulopsis* and *Epidermophyton* spp.

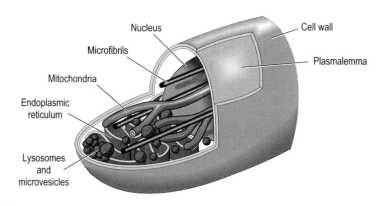

Fig. 2 **Structure of fungal cells.**

Structure

Fungi, being eucaryotes, have a structure (Fig. 2) differing considerably from procaryotic bacteria (see p. 2–3). Fungi have *a nucleus* containing their chromosomal DNA and an RNA-rich nucleolus within a nuclear membrane.

The cytoplasm contains not only ribosomes but also *mitochondria, lysosomes and microvesicles, microtubules, Golgi apparatus and a double-membraned endoplasmic reticulum*. Surrounding the above structures (the cytosol) is the cell membrane or *plasmalemma*, which contains not only lipids and glycoproteins but also ergosterol. Bacteria (except for *Mycoplasma*) do not contain sterols, and mammalian cells contain cholesterol rather than ergosterol, which is, therefore, a site of attack by antifungal drugs.

Outside the plasmalemma is a rigid cell wall containing a polymer of N-acetylglucosamine, *chitin*, on which are layers of polypeptides with complex polysaccharides including mannans and glucans. Some fungi, e.g. *Cryptococcus* spp., have a further layer, a polysaccharide *capsule*. The cell wall and capsule have multiple functions, including protection, transport and virulence, and are involved in invoking the host response.

Morphology

There are two major morphological forms of fungi (Fig. 3), small round yeasts, and long filaments called hyphae. Both have sexual and asexual forms.

Yeasts
Yeasts are round, unicellular and multiply by budding or by fission. Some yeasts form long buds called pseudo-hyphae ('germ tubes', used to identify *Candida albicans*) but not true hyphae.

Filamentous fungi
Filamentous fungi form hyphae, long tubes which may have cross-walls called septa, or simply be multinucleate (coenocytic). A collection of hyphae is called a mycelium, which may be vegetative, growing on a nutrient surface, or extending upwards as an aerial mycelium producing conidia ('spores') which spread very easily, contaminating a laboratory if culture plates are carelessly opened! The morphology of conidia is important in classifying fungi.

Dimorphic fungi
Dimorphic fungi exist in both forms. Many pathogenic fungi are dimorphic, usually the yeast form occurring in tissues and the filamentous (mould) form in the environment or on culture at 25°C. *Candida albicans* is an exception, forming mycelium in tissues.

Diagnosis of fungal infection

Yeasts and fungi grow on ordinary media but are mostly slow growing, and cultures need to be examined over 2–3 weeks. A glucose or blood agar is often used at acid pH to inhibit bacterial growth.

Identification of fungi is mainly made from morphology (Fig. 4a), and yeasts may be detected in stained films during routine examination of swabs etc. Special stains are usually needed for filamentous fungi. Antibodies (Fig. 4b) and DNA probes can also be used.

Clinical classification
Fungi are sometimes grouped by the clinical syndromes they cause:

- superficial and cutaneous mycoses (p. 74–75), e.g. 'athlete's foot' caused by *Trichophyton* spp.
- subcutaneous mycoses, e.g. sporotrichosis, ulcerative lesions caused by *Sporothrix* spp.
- systemic/deep mycoses (p. 70–73), e.g. histoplasmosis, a pulmonary or generalised disease caused by *Histoplasma capsulatum*.

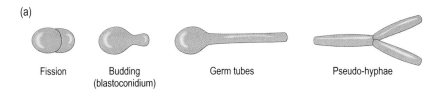
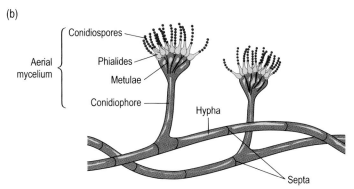

Fig. 3 **Morphology of fungi. (a)** Yeasts, e.g. Candida; **(b)** filamentous moulds, e.g. Aspergillus.

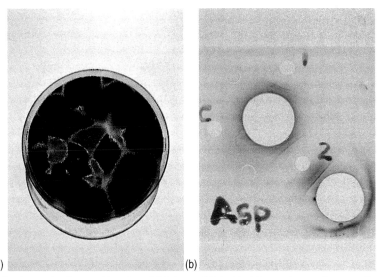

(a)　　(b)

Fig. 4 **Diagnosis of *Aspergillus niger*. (a)** Colonies; **(b)** double diffusion plate test for aspergillus precipitins (antibodies). (Reproduced with permission from Inglis T J J. 1999 Colour Guide Microbiology, 2nd edn. Churchill Livingstone, Edinburgh.)

Characteristics of fungi (1)

- Nomenclature is confused because, historically, sexual and asexual forms were separately named.
- Classification depends on the sexual reproductive mode and structures.
- Structure is eucaryotic and therefore, unlike the procaryotic bacteria, fungi have a nucleus with a nuclear membrane and the cytoplasm contains mitochondria, Golgi apparatus, lysosomes and an endoplasmic reticulum.
- Morphology is either small round yeasts, or filamentous moulds with a mycelium of hyphae. Many fungi are dimorphic, with a yeast form in tissues and an environmental mycelial form.

Characteristics of fungi (2)

Reproduction

Asexual reproduction is most commonly seen when haploid cells divide by mitosis to form spores, the chromosome number being unchanged. There is, by definition, no sexual mating prior to this sporulation. It is the only type of reproduction seen to date in some human fungal pathogens, which are therefore called Fungi imperfecti, sexual reproduction being considered the perfect state.

Sexual reproduction produces spores by mating when two haploid cells fuse to become diploid and then divide by meiosis. Many fungi need two colonies of the opposite mating type for sexual mating to occur (heterothallic fungi), while others need only one colony (homothallic). Spore formation occurs either within a sac called an ascus or partly on the surface of a bag called a basidium (see p. 6). The characteristic appearance of the spore-bearing structure and the spore is used in classification and hence identification of pathogens (Fig. 1).

Pathogenicity

Fungal pathogenicity describes the pathogen's attack mechanisms, whereas resistance describes the host's defence mechanisms. It is essential to distinguish between:

- *primary pathogens*, i.e. fungi such as *Cryptococcus* spp. that can infect normal hosts
- *opportunistic fungi*, i.e. those only able to infect abnormal hosts with impaired defences resulting from, for example, antibiotics, cytotoxics, x-ray 'therapy', steroids and other immunosuppressant drugs, endocrine disease such as diabetes mellitus, or AIDS.

Although less is known about fungal than bacterial pathogenicity, the following mechanisms are recognised:

- mycotoxins
- hypersensitivity
- invasive infection.

Mycotoxins

Unlike bacteria, fungi are not known to produce any endotoxins. Some make exotoxins, i.e. elaborated outside the fungus. These are also only made outside the human body. There are three major groups causing mycotoxicoses:

- *Aflatoxins*, made by *Aspergillus flavus*, causing turkey X disease, and human disease via coumarin anticoagulant action. Aflatoxins are also carcinogenic.
- *Ergot alkaloids*, made by *Claviceps purpurea* infecting rye, causing St Anthony's fire or ergotism, with smooth muscle contraction, peripheral vasoconstriction and then gangrene. Ergot alkaloids are used with care in obstetrics to contract uterine smooth muscle.
- *Psychotropics*, such as psilocybin and the derivative LSD.

Hypersensitivity

Hypersensitivity results from repeated exposure to fungal spores and consequent immunoglobulin or sensitised lymphocyte production. There is no toxin production or tissue invasion. Inhalation of spores (e.g. of *Aspergillus*) causes allergic rhinitis, asthma and alveolitis, i.e. hypersensitivity pneumonitis (p. 134).

Invasive infection

Colonisation is the continuing presence of the organism without disease, whereas infection means tissue invasion and damage (p. 20). Anatomically, fungal infection causes superficial, cutaneous, subcutaneous or systemic mycoses (p. 68–76). Tissue damage in infection can occur by at least six mechanisms (Fig. 2):

(a) direct invasion leads to distortion (e.g. fungus balls formed from *Aspergillus*, Fig. 3) hence tissue destruction and ill-understood toxic effects
(b) obstruction leads to secondary bacterial infection and further tissue damage
(c) blood vessel wall invasion causes thrombosis, obstruction, ischaemia and infarction of tissues, e.g. with *Aspergillus* spp. and Zygomycetes (Phycomycetes) such as *Mucor*
(d) embolism to distant vessels occurs, e.g. in endocarditis
(e) intracellular persistence and even multiplication in macrophages and neutrophils by some fungi, e.g. *Histoplasma*, being resistant to lysosomal enzymes
(f) capsule formation can occur in species such as *Cryptococcus*; this protects the fungus and may damage tissues.

Host resistance

All four lines of defence (p. 25–29) are of some but variable importance against fungi:

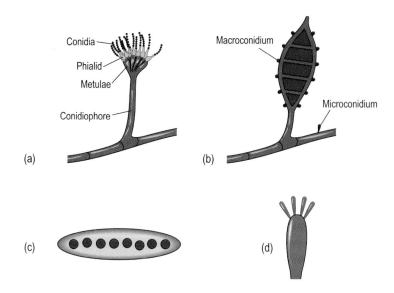

Fig. 1 **Fungal reproductive structures. (a)** Asexual fruiting structure. **(b)** Macroconidium and microconidium. **(c)** Ascospores in ascus. **(d)** Basidiospores on a basidium.

Labels in figure: Conidia, Phialid, Metulae, Conidiophore (a); Macroconidium, Microconidium (b); (c); (d)

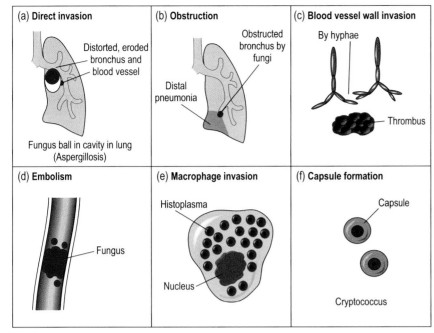

Fig. 2 **Six mechanisms of tissue damage in fungal infection.**

1. Intact skin and mucous membranes plus the associated chemical and bacterial factors are primary barriers. Normal bacterial flora compete with fungi for nutrients, the balance being upset by antibiotics.
2. Non-specific inflammatory reactions occur, though neutrophil phagocytosis and macrophage activity is often less against fungal than bacterial infection.
3. Antibodies and complement can kill *Aspergillus* and *Candida* spp., though many antibodies are not protective.
4. Cell-mediated immunity is the most important defence, and its loss, in diseases such as AIDS, causes a multitude of serious and often fatal fungal infections.

Ecology

The ecology of fungi include their *reservoirs* in the environment, animals and humans, hence the *sources* of infection.

Environmental reservoirs
These are the natural habitat of many fungi, e.g. free living in soil or air. These reservoirs are the usual source of most human pathogenic fungi, infection occur-ring after inhalation or implantation. Geophilic ('soil loving') dermatophytes (p. 74–75) live in the soil.

Some fungi have particular ecological niches, for example:

- *Cryptococcus neoformans*: soil and buildings contaminated with pigeon droppings; their high urea content is a fungal nutrient
- *Sporothrix schenckii*: rose thorns and rotting vegetation
- *Histoplasma capsulatum*: soil contaminated with bat, starling or chicken droppings.

In addition, some have particular geographic distribution:

- *Blastomyces dermatitidis* is limited to North America and a few foci in Africa
- *Coccidioides immitis* is limited to hot dry areas in south-west USA, Central and South America
- *Paracoccidioides brasiliensis* is limited to Central and South America.

Animals
Zoophilic ('animal-loving') dermatophytes obviously live on (and infect) animals, such as cats, dogs and horses, and, at times, humans.

Humans
Two yeasts are commonly found as part of our normal flora: *Candida albicans* on skin and mucous membranes, and *Pityrosporum ovale* on skin rich in nutrient lipids from sebaceous glands. Thirdly, dermatophytes are sometimes found in the absence of symptoms, probably as colonisation (p. 20–21).

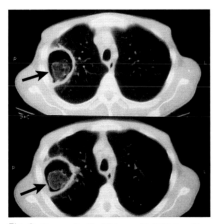

Fig. 3 **Fungus ball within cavity (CT chest).**

Characteristics of fungi (2)

- All fungi reproduce asexually with haploid cells dividing by mitosis to form spores.
- Fungi imperfecti, in which only asexual replication is known, include some human pathogens.
- Sexual reproduction by meiosis is the basis for definitive classification and naming.
- Primary pathogens are fungi able to infect normal hosts.
- Opportunist pathogens are only able to infect abnormal hosts with impaired defences.
- Fungi cause disease by mycotoxins, hypersensitivity or invasive infection with tissue damage.
- Cell-mediated immunity is the most important defence.
- Reservoirs and sources of infection are frequently the environment, sometimes animals, and commonly ourselves (*Candida* spp.).

Characteristics of protozoa

Nomenclature and classification

Protozoa are unicellular eucaryotic organisms that were initially classified in the kingdom Animalia but are now usually considered in the kingdom Protista along with Algae. There are three phyla of medical importance:

- Sarcomastigophora, containing the amoebae such as *Entamoeba histolytica* and the flagellates such as *Giardia* and *Trypanosoma*. Division is by binary fission, and locomotion by pseudopodia (amoebae) or whip-like flagellar movement (p. 80–83).
- Ciliophora, the ciliates, such as *Balantidium coli*, which divide by binary fission or by conjugation with nuclear exchange. Locomotion is by co-ordinated movement of the rows of hair-like cilia (p. 81).
- Apicomplexa, containing the Sporozoa such as *Plasmodium* and the Coccidia such as *Toxoplasma*. Their more complicated life cycles are described on pages 78–79.

Structure

All protozoa are unicellular (Fig. 1). All have a trophozoite form with one or more nuclei containing nucleoli or karyosomes and bounded by a nuclear membrane, and the usual eucaryotic cytoplasmic organelles including mitochondria, ribosomes and endoplasmic reticulum. Vacuoles are often prominent and specialised structures such as sucking discs (*Giardia*) or a mouth-like cytosome (*Balantidium*) are found in the larger, more complex protozoa. Trophozoites have a cell membrane but no cell wall. Most intestinal protozoa also develop cysts that are more resistant than the fragile trophozoites to drying, cold or other environmental stresses.

Reproduction

Amoebae replicate either by simple binary fission of the trophozoite or by formation of trophozoites within the multinucleate cyst. Flagellates and ciliates multiply by longitudinal binary fission.

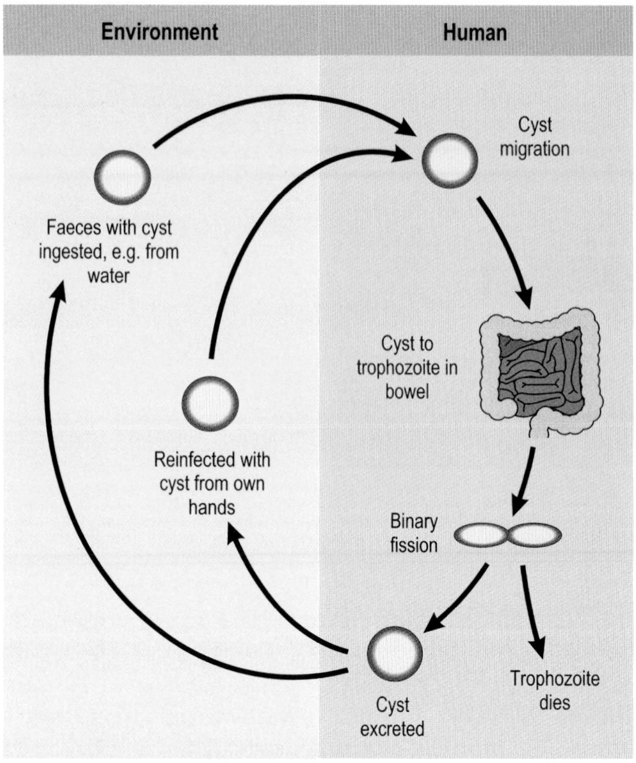

Fig. 1 **Typical life cycle of a simple protozoon.**

Sporozoa and coccidia have complex asexual and sexual life cycles, which are described on pages 78–79. Hosts and generations classically alternate, e.g. the malarial asexual cycle (schizogony) in humans alternates with the sexual cycle (gametogeny) in mosquitoes.

Pathogenicity and host defences

Pathogenicity

The pathogenicity of protozoa is not well understood and varies between genera. Details for particular organisms are given on pages 78–83. In general, however, protozoa:

- have fewer pathogenic mechanisms than bacteria
- have several surface attachment mechanisms (e.g. *Giardia*)
- are less invasive than bacteria
- have few known cytotoxins; *E. histolytica* means 'tissue lysis', and this species is an exception

- avoid host defences by several ingenious mechanisms, e.g. trypanosomes frequently alter their surface antigens, making antibody formation or vaccine development extremely difficult, while leishmaniae produce a superoxide dismutase that protects them from macrophage superoxide so well that they actually live within the macrophage!

Host defences

Host defences are similarly less well defined and variable, but in general:

- chronic rather than acute disease and inflammation are associated with protozoan infection; again *E. histolytica* is an exception, causing acute amoebic dysentery
- eosinophils, so characteristic of metazoan infections (p. 12–13), are few or absent
- both antibody formation and cell-mediated immunity (p. 28–29) are stimulated but are relatively ineffective.

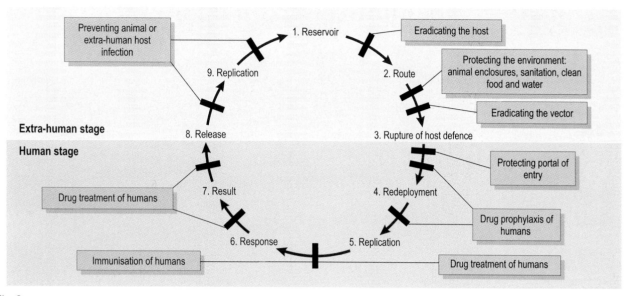

Fig. 2 **Achieving control by interrupting the life cycle** (see also Fig. 2, p. 20).

Ecology: reservoirs and sources of infection (Table 1)

Geographic distribution

Protozoal diseases are most common in poor and tropical communities, but this is principally because of poor control measures.

Reservoirs

Reservoirs can be:

- animal, e.g. for *Toxoplasma* and *Cryptosporidium*
- human, e.g. *Entamoeba* and *Giardia*
- soil contaminated with faeces.

Spread

Spread can occur by:

- ingestion, either directly faecal–oral (or ano–oral) or by contaminated water, unwashed food (particularly fruit and vegetables) or uncooked meat
- direct contact, either sexual or through the nose (*Naegleria fowleri*)
- injection, usually by an insect vector, or, rarely, by needle or blood transfusion.

Control

Theoretically, control can be achieved by interrupting the life cycle (Fig. 2) at any point. The practical difficulties are noted in the discussion of the individual species.

Table 1 **Protozoal infections**

Protozoa	Source	Spread by	Syndromes
Intestinal and genital			
Entamoeba histolytica	Human faeces	Water, fruit, vegetables	Diarrhoeal, dysentery, dissemination
Giardia lamblia	Human faeces	As above	Diarrhoeal, malabsorption
Dientamoeba fragilis	Human pinworm eggs	As above	Diarrhoeal, discomfort (abdominal)
Balantidium coli	Pig faeces	Water and food	Diarrhoea, dysentery
Cryptosporidium spp.	Human, calf, sheep	Food and water, sex.	Diarrhoea, dehydration, debility
Trichomonas vaginalis	Genital tract	Sexual contact	Vaginitis, urethritis
Blood and tissue protozoa			
Naegleria fowleri	Free-living	Water	Meningitis, keratitis
Toxoplasma gondii	Cat faeces, beef, lamb, pork	Fingers, undercooked meat	Congenital, systemic, latent
Sarcocystis hominis	Dog faeces, beef	As above	Diarrhoea, discomfort
Leishmania spp.	Canines, rodents	Sandfly vector	Cutaneous, visceral
Trypanosoma gambiense	Human	Tse-tse fly	Encephalitis
Trypanosoma rhodesiense	Cattle	Tse-tse fly	Encephalitis
Trypanosoma cruzi	Human	Reduviid bugs	Cardiomyopathy, megacolon
Plasmodium spp.	Human	Mosquito	Systemic

Characteristics of protozoa

- Protozoa include intestinal and genital parasites, e.g. *Entamoeba histolytica* and *Trichomonas vaginalis*, and blood and tissue parasites, e.g. *Toxoplasma gondii* and malarial parasites.

- Protozoa are unicellular with eucaryote cellular structures. They all have a fragile trophozoite stage and most have a resistant cyst form.

- All are so small that they are invisible without a microscope.

- All have life cycles outside the human host, and most can multiply in humans. Infection is by ingestion, by inhalation, by insect bite or by intercourse.

- Their life cycles vary from direct passage of trophozoite during coitus (*Trichomonas*) or passage of cysts in faeces and subsequent ingestion (Entamoeba and other intestinal protozoa) to complex alternation of generations in different hosts (malaria).

- Eosinophilia is not found in protozoal infections (unlike Metazoan infections, p. 12–13)

- Protective immunity is poorly developed in most protozoan infections, which are very common and may be multiple.

- Drug prophylaxis and therapy are often unsatisfactory.

Characteristics of multicellular parasites

Nomenclature and classification

It is sensible but scarcely scientific to include some of these medically important parasites in microbiology – only the eggs of 25cm roundworms and 6m tapeworms are microscopic! A general overview of these varied and important parasites is given here, with details on pages 77 and 84–91.

The sub-kingdom **Metazoa** of the kingdom Animalia contains the **helminths** (worms) in two phyla:

- **Nematoda** are roundworms with round cylindrical bodies. Some are intestinal parasites, e.g. hookworms and thread (pin) worms, while others are blood and tissue parasites, such as filarial and guinea worms.
- **Platyhelminthes** are flatworms ('plate like') and are divided into Trematoda, comprising the leaf-like flukes such as schistosomes, and Cestoda, which are the ribbon-like tapeworms such as the beef and pork tapeworms.

A third phylum of medical importance in the Metazoa is the **Arthropoda** ('jointed limbs') comprising invertebrates with segmented bodies, paired jointed limbs, a hard exoskeleton of chitin and well-developed respiratory and digestive systems (p. 77). It includes:

- **Crustacea**, including crabs, shrimps and copepods, some of which are intermediate hosts in the life cycles of some helminths (p. 86, 90–91).
- **Arachnida**, including mites and ticks (vectors for some microbial diseases) plus venomous animals such as spiders and scorpions. All adult arachnids have eight legs, but no wings or antennae.
- **Insecta** comprising mosquitoes, bugs, fleas and lice (vectors for further important microbial diseases) plus venomous stinging animals such as bees and wasps. All insects have six legs, antennae and wings.

Structure

All the above are multicellular eucaryotes: their cells have nuclei, nucleoli, nuclear membranes, mitochondria, ribosomes, endoplasmic reticulum and other specialised structures within a cell membrane and cell wall. Their multicellular structure is variable and complex:

Nematodes (roundworms) are cylindrical, have complete digestive systems and separate sexes.

Trematodes (flukes) are flat, leaf-shaped worms with an oral muscular sucker and an incomplete digestive system. Schistosomes have separate sexes but other trematodes are hermaphrodites (see below).

Cestodes (tapeworms) are ribbon-like and may reach enormous size. The head (scolex) usually has characteristic hooklets and suckers, and the body is divided into segments (proglottids). There is no digestive system, nutrients being absorbed through the soft body wall from the host gut. Cestodes are also hermaphrodites, each proglottid having male and female sexual organs.

Reproduction

Some parasites have very complex life cycles; a knowledge of the life cycle is essential for understanding the method of infec-

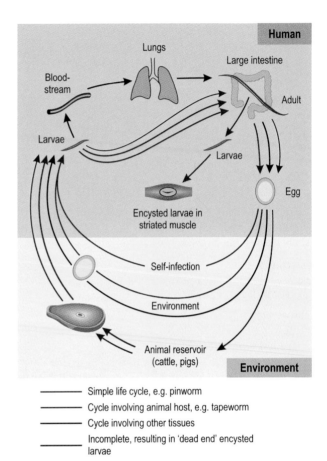

Fig. 1 **Levels of complexity in the life cycles of multicellular parasites.**

tion and the prevention of disease. In the simplest life cycle, seen in pinworm and whipworm infections, eggs are ingested, hatch to larvae in the gut and develop to adult worms that produce eggs that embryonate outside the body (Fig. 1). Similarly, ingested encysted larvae in meat or on vegetables develop in the gut into tapeworms or *Fasciolopsis*. In more complex cycles, larvae may pass through the lungs before migrating to the adult's niche in gut (e.g. roundworm, hookworm) or blood vessels (schistosomes). Lastly, helminths ingested, or injected by insects, migrate through tissues to live in the lungs, liver, skin, muscles or lymphatics.

The part of the life cycle outside the human body also increases in complexity, from simple eggs, to skin-penetrating larvae, to the development of infectious larvae in insects or other animals, and finally to alternation of generations when schistosomes have asexual reproduction in snails and sexual reproduction in humans. Individual life cycles are discussed below (p. 84–91).

Pathogenicity and resistance

Pathogenicity

As with protozoa, the pathogenicity of many multicellular parasites is variable and poorly understood (see p. 84–91 for particular organisms). In general, however, these parasites:

- have fewer known pathogenic mechanisms than bacteria
- have several surface attachment mechanisms (e.g. tapeworms)

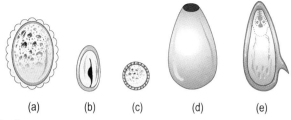

Fig. 2 **Eggs of helminths. (a)** Roundworm; **(b)** pinworm; **(c)** tapeworm; **(d)** intestinal fluke; **(e)** blood fluke.

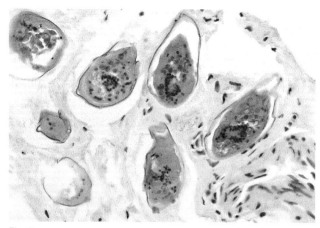

Fig. 3 **Bladder biopsy showing *Schistosoma haematobium* eggs.**

- are often less invasive than bacteria, living only in gut
- have few known cytotoxins
- avoid host defences by several ingenious mechanisms, e.g. schistosomes cover themselves with host plasma proteins, hence are antigenically invisible to host defences
- show marked but largely unexplained tissue tropism.

Resistance
Host defences are similarly less well defined and variable but, in general, metazoan infection results in:

- chronic disease and chronic inflammation more often than acute
- raised levels of eosinophils (which is characteristic of metazoan infections) occurring in response to parasite surface polysaccharides and glycoproteins. Concomitant increased IgE production with the eosinophilia assists killing of parasites
- stimulated antibody formation and cell-mediated immunity (see p. 28–29), although these are relatively ineffective.

Ecology: reservoirs and sources of infection (Table 1)

Geographic distribution
Metozoan diseases, like protozoan, are commonest in poor and tropical communities, but again this is principally because of poor control measures.

Reservoirs
Reservoirs include:

- animal, e.g. *Taenia* or *Echinococcus* spp.
- human, e.g. pinworm, whipworm
- soil contaminated with faeces, e.g. roundworm.

All trematodes have at least one *intermediate* host as well as the reservoir host (p. 90–91).

Spread
Spread can be by ingestion, either directly faecal–oral or by contaminated water, unwashed food (particularly fruit and vegetables) or uncooked meat; by direct contact, through the skin; or by injection by an insect vector.

Diagnosis

Most of the helminths encountered in developed countries are intestinal parasites, and diagnosis usually depends on detection of the parasites or their eggs in faeces (Fig. 2). Eosinophilia is often used as an indicator of infection. Biopsy may be necessary for tissue parasites (Fig. 3).

Control

Control, as with protozoa, can be by attack on:

- the host(s)
- the vector or route of spread
- the human infection, by immunisation (in theory) or by drug prophylaxis or treatment.

Table 1 **Features of infection involving multicellular parasites**

Group	Examples	Special features
Nematodes		
Intestinal	Pinworm, roundworm	Spread from faeces via food, water
Tissue/blood	Filariae, guinea worm	Spread via food or insect bites or by skin-penetrating larvae
Animal nematodes	Dog and cat ascaris	Human is an accidental host so life cycle is not completed; disease is caused by migrating larvae
Trematodes	Liver fluke	Spread from faeces via infected food from the intermediate host
Cestodes	Beef tapeworm	Humans ingest encysted larvae or eggs from the intermediate host
Arachnida	Mites, ticks, spiders	Venomous bites, or acting as vectors for microbial disease
Crustacea	Crabs, shrimps	Intermediate hosts for helminths
Insecta	Mosquitoes, fleas	Venomous bites, or acting as disease vectors

Multicellular parasites

- Multicellular parasites include nematodes (roundworms), trematodes (flukes), cestodes (tapeworms) and arthropods.
- All are metazoa, with eucaryote cellular structures.
- All are large, being visible without a microscope.
- All have life cycles outside the human host and most cannot multiply in humans. Infection is by ingestion, by skin penetration or by insect bite.
- Life cycles vary from simple embryonation outside humans, to complex alternation of generations in different hosts.
- Eosinophilia is found in almost all helminth infections.
- Protective immunity is poorly developed in most helminth infections, which are very common and often multiple.
- Drug prophylaxis and therapy are often unsatisfactory.

Characteristics of viruses (1)

A. The virus particle

Basic properties

- Viruses are *not living*, as they lack two essential properties of life – they cannot *replicate* independently, and they cannot *survive* long-term independently, needing a bigger living organism for both functions, as they contain no ribosomes, so unaided cannot synthesise protein.
- They are *much smaller* than bacteria: human viral pathogens are usually 20 to 300 nanometres (nm) in diameter, compared to about 1000nm for coccal bacteria like staphylococci. Fungi and protozoa are of course much bigger again.
- Their *structure is simple*: a nucleocapsid consisting of a central *genome* of either DNA or RNA, and a protein shell called the *capsid*. Many viruses also have an outer *envelope*.

Structure and composition

Structure

- The virus particle is called a **virion**, and consists (Fig. 1) of the **nucleocapsid** with two components – the single- or double-stranded, linear, circular or segmented DNA or RNA **genome**, with a surrounding protein shell called the **capsid**. Viruses contain either DNA or RNA, never both like living organisms and cells.
- The capsid's repeating protein units form structural units called **capsomeres**: these are usually arranged with either **helical** or **icosahedral** (**20-sided**) **symmetry**, the exceptions including pox viruses with **complex** symmetry (Fig. 1b). Small icosahedral viruses appear spherical on electron microscopy.
- The nucleocapsid of some human viruses is 'naked', but all helical and many icosahedral are sheathed by a large **envelope** with an inner structural protein layer, an outer lipid layer, and projecting spikes of glycoprotein (Fig. 1c-d).

Composition

- **Viral nucleic acids** are usually double-stranded (DS) DNA or single-stranded (SS) RNA. The RNA can be either positive-strand (+) which functions as messenger RNA (mRNA), or negative strand (–) RNA which functions as a template for the production

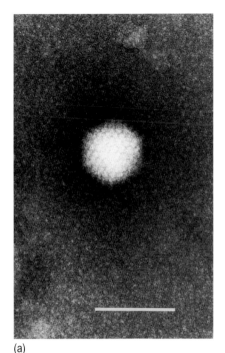
(a)

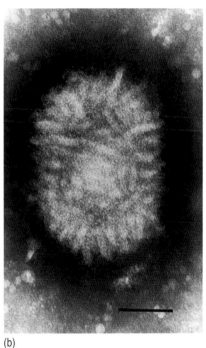
(b)

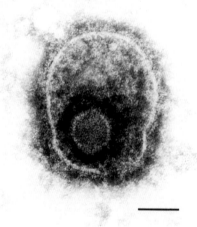
(c)

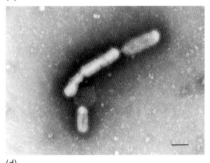
(d)

Fig. 1 **Virus structure. (a)** Naked icosahedral (Parvo-, picorna-, papova-, reo- and adenoviruses). **(b)** Complex symmetry (poxviruses). **(c)** Enveloped icosahedral (herpesviruses). **(d)** Enveloped helical (orthomyxoviruses, paramyxoviruses).

of mRNA. There may be a single strand of RNA as in paramyxoviruses, two copies in retroviruses, or definite fragments in reoviruses and orthomyxoviruses. DNA is usually linear, but is circular in hepadnaviruses and papovaviruses.

- **Viral proteins and viral enzymes.** Viral proteins are either structural or non-structural:
  - *Structural proteins* are essential components, either of the capsid, or basic core proteins to 'package' the nucleic acid, or envelope glycoproteins.
  - *Non-structural proteins* are usually enzymes to produce virus components, for example RNA-dependent transcriptase in negative-strand RNA viruses to produce mRNA, or DNA-

dependent RNA polymerase in poxviruses, or a polymerase complex in hepadnaviruses, or reverse transcriptase in retroviruses.

- **Viral envelopes** are lipoprotein, composed of an inner structural virus-derived protein and an outer host-cell-derived lipid layer. In addition there are often projecting spikes of glycoprotein, which are important as viral attachment proteins (VAPs) to host cells or erythrocytes (haemagglutinins), as neuraminidases (influenza virus), as receptors, or as antigens which stimulate protective immunity.

Atypical viral-like agents

There are four types:

- **Defective viruses** such as Hepatitis D have viral protein but defective nucleic

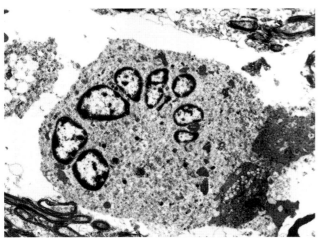

Fig. 2   **Multi-nucleated giant cell.**

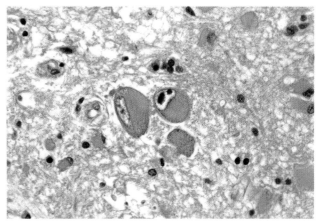

Fig. 3   **Classical inclusion bodies in CMV encephalitis.**

acid (by mutation or deletion), so cannot replicate without a helper virus, in this case Hepatitis B.

- **Pseudovirions** have the viral DNA replaced by host-cell DNA which has fragmented and been incorporated into the viral capsid. They can infect but of course cannot replicate.
- **Viroids** are only a single small molecule of RNA, with no capsid or envelope. How they replicate is unclear. They can infect plants, but apparently not humans.
- **Prions** are made of a single glycoprotein with no detectable nucleic acid, yet replicate! The protein is encoded by a host cell gene, not a viral gene. The increase in numbers of prions in infected nervous tissue is apparently due to a post-translational modification in the conformation of the normal alpha-helical form (PrPc, prion protein cellular) to the abnormal beta-pleated sheet form (PrPsc, prion protein scrapie); these abnormal forms then recruit further normal forms and change their configuration. They cause the transmissible spongiform encephalopathies including scrapie in sheep and Creutzfeldt–Jakob disease in humans (p. 100–101).

- *Latent,* with no apparent effect on the cell, but may re-activate, e.g. herpes.
- *Productive,* which may give chronic carriage or disease e.g. hepatitis B.
- *Transforming* producing tumours e.g. EBV lymphomas.

Host cell morphological effects due to viral infection can be:

1. *No* morphological change, in abortive or latent infection.
2. *Multi-nucleated cells* by fusion (Fig. 2) due to herpes- or paramyxovirus infection.
3. *Cytopathic effects (CPE)* including rounding or darkening of the cell, or *inclusion bodies* in the nucleus (owl's eye inclusions from CMV, Fig. 3), or in the cytoplasm (Negri bodies in rabies), or actual *cell death* from inhibition of cellular (but not viral) protein synthesis.
4. *Haemagglutination,* by viral surface haemagglutinins adhering to red blood cells.
5. *Transformation* to malignant cells e.g. by papillomaviruses, EBV, Hepatitis B or C viruses.

Host cell pathologic mechanisms (pathogenesis) are:

1. *Virus-induced inhibition of macromolecular synthesis* (see Replication, p. 16–17) causing cell death. This is the commonest and most important mechanism.
2. *Virus-induced immunologic attack i.e. immunopathogenesis.* This can be by:
   - Immune attack by cytotoxic T cells on viral antigens in the cell membrane, e.g. on hepatocytes in hepatitis B, and in hepatitis C, and on vascular endothelium in the rash of measles.
   - Immune-complexes of virus-antibody-complement depositing in tissues, e.g. causing arthritis in hepatitis B, rubella, and parvovirus B19 infections.
3. *Virus-induced cytokines from infected cells stimulating other cells,* e.g. Rotavirus infected enterocytes produce cytokines which stimulate enteric neurons, causing fluid and electrolyte loss into the bowel, with consequent diarrhoea.
4. *Virus envelope glycoprotein damage to other cells,* e.g. vascular endothelial cells by Ebola virus.

B. The virus and the host cell (1)

The infected cell

Three major types of viral infection occur:

1. *Abortive,* with no replication, no visible host cell effects, no disease.
2. *Cytolytic,* with cell death and virus dissemination, then disease, then death or recovery of the host.
3. *Persistent,* which is of three further sub-types:

Viral characteristics (1)

- Viruses can only replicate inside a host cell, and cannot survive long-term outside a host cell.
- Viruses consist of a central *genome* of either RNA or DNA, and a protein *capsid* shell (together forming the nucleocapsid). Many viruses also have an outer *envelope*.
- The genome is usually double-stranded DNA, or single-stranded RNA, which may be positive or negative polarity, linear or circular, one piece or segmented.
- Viral proteins are either structural, or non-structural (usually enzymes)
- Viral envelopes are lipoprotein, often with glycoprotein spikes.
- Viral infection of the host cell may be abortive, cytolytic or persistent (latent, productive or transforming to tumours).
- Cell morphologic changes include giant-cell formation, cytopathic effects, inclusion bodies, haemagglutination or malignant transformation.
- Cell pathologic mechanisms include arrest of macro-molecular synthesis causing cell death, immunologic attack, cytokine production and envelope damage to other cells.

Characteristics of viruses (2)

B. The virus and the host cell (2)

This section describes the steps in Replication, and should be read with the next section, 'Genetics', and the previous section on 'The Infected Cell'.

Replication

Growth curve

This describes the number of virus particles in a host cell from the time of infection. Often one virion infects, and after a *latent period* of about 10 hours 100 virus progeny (the '*burst size*') are released! Surprisingly the virus disappears on cell entry, for up to 5 hours during the *eclipse period*, and then during the *rise period* the nucleic acid content and then the number of new virus particles rise exponentially. The details follow.

Growth cycle

Events during the growth cycle may be understood in three stages (Fig. 1).

1. Early stage of recognition, attachment, penetration and uncoating

Recognition and *attachment* are due to interaction between each type of virus and a specific receptor on the human cell. The virus may have an identifiable structure such as the spikes on adeno-viruses, and the haemagglutinin of influenza virus, while numerous receptors are known on human cells, such as the CD4 molecule on T cells for HIV, and sialic acid on glycoproteins for influenza virus.

Penetration or *entry* is either by uptake into a phagosome, or by fusion of viral and host cell membranes.

Uncoating in the cell cytoplasm is by cell enzymes from lysosomes, which remove the virus protein coat and so make the viral genome accessible for the next stage.

2. Central stage of mRNA synthesis, protein synthesis and genome replication

This can be considered in four steps: firstly of *mRNA synthesis* by transcription (unnecessary for positive-sense single strand RNA viruses where by definition their RNA *is* the mRNA), and *early protein (enzyme) synthesis*, then *genome replication* to produce new viral nucleic acid, and *late protein synthesis*.

a. mRNA synthesis. The method of transcription to form the mRNA depends on the genome, arranged by the Baltimore classification into six groups, shown in Table 1.

b. Early protein synthesis is by translation of the above mRNA using host cell ribosomes in the cytoplasm to make viral protein. If the viral genome is a single nucleic acid molecule, one large polyprotein is produced and then cleaved by enzymes into a number of smaller proteins. If the viral genome consists of several nucleic acid molecules, several mRNAs are made, each translated into one protein. These early proteins are usually enzymes and regulatory molecules for the next stage.

c. Genome replication. Like mRNA synthesis, this depends on the type of genome, so is complicated (Table 1).

d. Late protein synthesis by translation of viral mRNA produces the capsid structural proteins.

3. Final stage of assembly and release (with or without envelopment)

Assembly of progeny virus particles occurs in the cytoplasm, or in the nucleus (in herpes-, adeno- and papillomaviruses) or at the cell membrane of the host cell. The viral genome is assembled with the capsid proteins and viral enzymes into new viral progeny.

Release of unenveloped virus usually occurs through the host cell wall by rupture ('lysis'), causing cell death.

Enveloped viruses undergo a further step, by incorporating host cell nuclear or plasma membrane components and inserted viral proteins and glycoproteins to form the envelope prior to release.

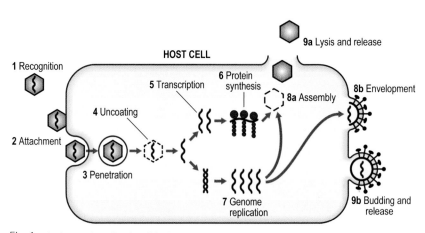

Fig. 1 **Viral growth cycle, simplified.**

Table 1	mRNA synthesis and genome replication from six types of viral genome	
Genome	**mRNA synthesis**	**Genome replication**
DS DNA (All DNA viruses except Parvovirus, therefore all adenoviruses, papovaviruses including papillomaviruses, BK and JC virus, hepadnaviruses, herpesviruses and poxviruses)	Transcribed using host-cell or viral polymerase to form mRNA	DS DNA is the template for new progeny virus DNA in the nucleus (except for pox virus, in the cytoplasm). These new progeny virus DNA molecules act as templates for more genomes for new virus particles, and also for transcription of late virus mRNA. Hepatitis B virus is unique because of its circular incompletely double-stranded DNA, so it needs a DNA polymerase to fill the gap and make a complete DS molecule. The polymerase also has reverse transcriptase activity, which from an RNA template synthesises an RNA/DNA intermediate which is then converted to DS DNA
SS DNA (Parvovirus)	'Hairpin' loops at both ends provide DS DNA intermediate for synthesis of mRNA by cellular RNA polymerase, in the cell nucleus	Makes both positive and negative strand DNA, later packaging one or the other into new separate virus particles
DS RNA (Reoviruses including Rotavirus)	Synthesise mRNA from the 10 or 11 fragments of DS RNA using viral RNA polymerase	Use a transcriptase to produce a complementary RNA strand from mRNA, thus producing the double stranded segments of the genome.
SS RNA (Positive polarity, e.g. picornaviruses including rhino- and enteroviruses, astro-, calici-, corona-, toga- and flaviviruses)	The RNA genome is itself the mRNA	Use an RNA polymerase to produce a complementary (–) strand to form a replicative DS RNA, and new (+) progeny are synthesised off this (–) template using the polymerase. The (+) progeny function as templates for more replicative forms, and as genomes for new virus particles, and as viral mRNA for protein synthesis.
SS RNA (Negative polarity, e.g. ortho- and paramyxoviruses, Deltavirus, bunya-, rhabdo-, arena- and filoviruses)	Transcribed using a virion RNA polymerase to provide mRNA	Produce a complementary (+) strand to form a template for the synthesis of new (–) viral progeny genomes
SS RNA (Retroviruses, e.g. HIV, HTLV 1, 2, and 4)	First use a viral reverse transcriptase to convert their positive-sense SS RNA into a negative-sense SS DNA, then a positive sense DNA. The + and – SS DNA then align into DS DNA which is integrated into the host genome. Then this viral DNA is transcribed by host polymerase into RNA.	Use the RNA both for new genomes and as mRNA for translation into viral proteins

Release is usually by budding, and does not necessarily cause cell death, so infectious enveloped virus can be shed for a long time.

Unusual events

Unusual events can occur during the above replication:

■ *Economy*, to use limited nucleic acid (NA) to best advantage has two major forms:
  1. *Overlapping genes* code for more than one protein from the same stretch of NA, either by reading the same sequence in different frames, or by starting and ending at different places.
  2. *Splicing* of mRNA, when *noncoding* sequences called introns are removed from precursor mRNA leaving only the coding sequences, the exons. This allows different proteins to be encoded, by a shift in reading frame. When splicing removes *coding* sequences, smaller

proteins can be made from the same reading frames.

■ *Lysogeny* is a special form of persistent infection, when viral DNA is integrated into host cell DNA. It is particularly important medically when the host cell is a bacterium infected by a virus called a bacteriophage which is integrated as a prophage. This 'lysogenic conversion' gives the bacterium new properties, particularly exotoxin

production in diphtheria, botulism, cholera and scarlet fever. If the DNA is damaged, the viral DNA may be released from the host DNA, and intact infectious virus be released.

■ *Mutation or deletions* of the nucleic acid can cause a Defective virus, described on pages 14–15.

■ *Interactions* with host cells or other viruses are described in the Genetics section, below.

Viral characteristics (2)

The *usual* growth cycle can be understood in three stages:

■ early, of recognition, attachment (fusion), penetration (entry) and uncoating in the cytoplasm

■ central, of mRNA synthesis, protein synthesis, and genome replication (by six different methods depending on type of nucleic acid)

■ final, of assembly and release (± enveloping).

Unusual events can occur:

■ economy, by overlapping or splicing

■ lysogeny, with viral DNA integrated into host cell DNA

■ mutation or deletion of nucleic acid to give a defective virus

■ interactions occur with host cells or other viruses

Characteristics of viruses (3)

B. The virus and the host cell (3)

Genetics

There are three important considerations here:

1. Mutations

The RNA or DNA of the usual 'wild type' of virus may mutate by two major mechanisms:

- *by base substitution* of one base for another, by mistake or by a mutagen (physical or chemical). This mutation is called a *missense* mutation if a different amino acid is coded, or a *nonsense* mutation if no amino acid is coded, stopping protein synthesis, and thus usually a lethal mutation.
- *by frameshift*, when one or more base pairs are deleted or added, thus shifting the reading frame, and so leading to the wrong amino acids and hence an inactive protein.

Mutations are recognised by their effects:

- *a lethal* mutation stops replication
- *a plaque mutant* alters the appearance in tissue culture
- *a host range mutant* alters the cells which can be infected
- *an attenuated mutant* is less virulent and becomes a vaccine candidate if the mutation is stable
- *a conditional mutant* can only survive under particular conditions, e.g. a particular temperature. A temperature-sensitive influenza mutant has been used as a vaccine, multiplying in the cooler upper airways with few symptoms yet antibody production, but not able to multiply in the warmer lungs to cause pneumonia.

2. Interactions

Four major interactions can occur between host and virus, or between two viruses infecting the same cell (Fig. 1).

- *Recombination* is the exchange of *genes* between two chromosomes of DNA viruses, by crossing over of regions with significant base homology. It may not occur in RNA viruses.
- *Re-assortment* is the exchange of *segments of genome* in viruses with segmented genomes, like the RNA influ-

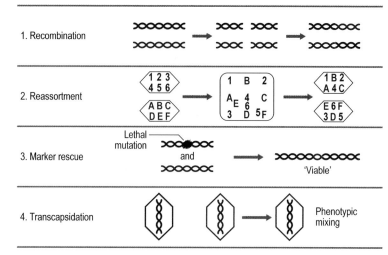

enza viruses, giving major antigenic changes, therefore a non-immune population and so influenza epidemics.

- *Complementation* occurs when one genome has by mutation a non-functional protein and hence is a defective virus, which is complemented by a functional protein from the other 'helper' virus. Hepatitis B provides its surface antigen to Hepatitis D which cannot make its own outer protein. If the mutation is otherwise lethal, the second virus provides *marker rescue*, which can be used to map viral genomes.
- *Phenotypic mixing* occurs when virus with genome X acquires *capsid protein Y* from virus Y, called *transcapsidation*. The progeny will however have capsid protein X from the X genome. A *pseudotype* occurs when virus A has the *envelope* of virus B.

3. Therapy and vaccines

- *Gene therapy* can use a defective retrovirus to which has been added a human gene to infect humans with a congenital defect of that gene. Retroviruses are particularly suitable vectors because a DNA copy of their RNA genome becomes integrated into the human genome, yet cannot replicate because some viral genes have been removed.
- *Recombinant vaccines* are being developed which use as a vector the vaccinia virus made defective by excising

Fig. 1 **Genetic exchanges.**

some genes, to carry the genes from another virus which encode an antibody-stimulating antigen.

C. The virus and the human host

Step 1. Initiation of infection

The initiation of microbial infection requires, in sequence:

- **R**eservoir and *source* of infection,
- **R**oute of transmission, and
- **R**upture of the non-specific surface defences of the body, providing a portal of entry (Fig. 1, p. 24). Details are in p. 24–25.

Step 2. Host defences

A summary follows, so p. 20–33 should be read for full details.

1. First line: This is the skin and mucous membranes, see p. 25.
2. Second line: These are non-specific, i.e. not depending on a specific microbe, and include general *Cellular Factors* such as natural killer (NK) cells, and phagocytosis by white cells, and *Humoral factors* such as complement, proteins and protein systems, discussed on p. 26–27. In addition there are humoral factors specially for viral infections, including:
   - Interferon alpha from leucocytes, and interferon beta from fibroblasts (interferon gamma from T cells is

active in non-viral as well as viral infections). These are host-species-specific but active against most viruses in one host, are induced by viruses and nucleic acids, and inhibit virus replication by preventing both virus transcription and viral protein synthesis. Synthetic interferons are used in the therapy of virus infections including hepatitis B and C (p. 170–172). Interferons are an example of *cytokines*, meaning 'cell activators', which are proteins produced by numerous cells including lymphocytes, neutrophils, monocytes and macrophages (p. 29). Other cytokines include interleukins and tumour necrosis factor. They are mediators or signals which activate and control cellular immune responses, and other body functions including cell differentiation, tissue repair and CNS signalling. They often interact sequentially.

- Defensins, alpha from intestinal crypt cells, and beta from respiratory mucosa, which interfere with the binding of HIV to a cell receptor, thus blocking entry and infection (defensins are also active against bacteria).
- Apolipoprotein B RNA-Editing Enzyme (APOBEC3G) which inactivates mRNA and retroviral DNA in HIV, reducing infectivity.

3. Third line: This is *Antibody production* by B lymphocytes (plasma cells). Antibodies are specific, i.e., produced after contact with a specific microbe, including viruses. They act directly on the virus by neutralising virus infectivity, and also act indirectly in Cell Mediated Immunity with T cells by Antibody-dependent Cell-mediated Cytotoxicity (ADCC, see below). Antibodies are particularly important in protective immunity against subsequent viral attack (p. 28–29).

4. Fourth line: *Cell Mediated Immunity.* This depends on T (thymus-dependent) lymphocytes of two main types, CD4-positive Helper T cells and CD8-positive Cytotoxic T cells. They lyse virus-infected cells by two major mechanisms:
- Non-antibody-dependent cytotoxicity by Cytotoxic T cells, mainly CD8-positive (and also by two other cells in non-immune hosts, NK cells, see above, and Lymphokine Activated Killer cells).
- Antibody-Dependent Cell-mediated Cytotoxicity (ADCC). Virus-infected

cells with anti-viral IgG bound to virus on the cell surface are lysed when T cells with IgG receptors form a cell-IgG antibody-T cell complex.

Step 3. Immune evasion of host defences

Mechanisms used by bacteria, fungi and parasites are described on page 31. Viruses evade host defences in three major ways:

1. *Cytokine decoys*: some viruses encode proteins called cytokine decoys which bind to immune mediators such as interleukin-1 (IL-1, by vaccinia virus), which blocks the mediator interaction with our immune cells, thus impairing host defence.
2. *Virokines*, which are viral virulence factors. They act in several ways:
   - HIV and CMV can reduce the expression of Class I MHC proteins, so cytotoxic T cells can't kill the virus-infected cells
   - HSV virokine inhibits complement
   - HIV, EBV, and adenoviruses synthesise RNAs which block an initiation factor which reduces interferon blocking of viral replication.
3. *Multiple serotypes (by multiple antigens)*. Antibodies are *serotype*-specific, so the usually protective effect of antibody after recovery from a previous infection is not protective against infection by a different serotype – rhinoviruses and influenza viruses are well-known examples. Fortunately measles, rubella, varicella-zoster and rabies

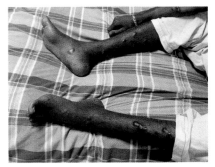

Fig. 2 **Kaposi's sarcoma, showing vascular tumours of both legs due to HumanHerpesVirus 8 (HHV 8).**

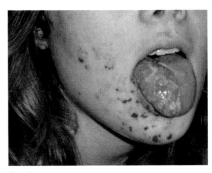

Fig. 3 **Mandibular Herpes zoster, showing vesicles on face and tongue.**

have only one serotype, and polio only three, so vaccines are feasible and effective.

Step 4. Clinical viral infection

Viral infection of the body's tissues and organs is described in Section 4, Microbial attack succeeds, p. 94–223. Examples are in Figs 2 and 3.

Viral characteristics (3)

Viral genetics

- mutations occur mainly by *base substitution* or *frameshift*. Their effects may be lethal, or a plaque mutant, a host-range mutant, an attenuated mutant, or a conditional mutant.

- interactions include *recombination* by the exchange of genes between two chromosomes of a DNA virus, *re-assortment* of genome segments, *complementation* where one helper virus supplies a missing protein to a defective virus, or *phenotype mixing* where a virus has its own genome but a capsid from another virus.

- therapy and vaccines: *Gene therapy* uses a defective retrovirus to deliver a missing human gene to a human with a congenital defect of that gene. *Recombinant vaccines* use a defective vaccinia virus to deliver antibody-stimulating genes.

The virus and the human host

Step 1. The initiation of infection: This requires a Reservoir (+/– a source), a Route of transmission, and a Rupture of the first line of defence through a portal of entry.

Step 2. Host defences. These are the First Line of Skin and Mucous Membranes; the Second Line of Non-Specific Defences including NK cells, other white cells, and humoral factors including complement, interferons and defensins; the Third Line of Antibodies, and the Fourth Line of Cell Mediated Immunity.

Step 3. Immune evasion of host defences is specifically by cytokine decoys, virokines and multiple serotypes.

Step 4. Clinical Infection ensues if the virus overcomes host defences.

Uneasy peace: host–microbial relationships

Microbes and hosts live in an uneasy peace between microbial attack and host defence. Some microbes within the normal human microflora can become pathogenic if the state of the host changes. Other microbes are present in the environment and can infect a host if the host defences are penetrated. In this and the following six sections the relationship between microbes and humans in health and disease is described in sequence; first, the terminology and principles involved.

Contamination, colonisation and infection

It is important to distinguish between the above three concepts though the practical distinction is not so simple!

Contamination is the transient presence of microbes, pathogenic or non-pathogenic, on our skin or other body surfaces, without any injury or invasion of our tissues.

Colonisation is the continuing presence of such microbes, usually for weeks, months or even years, again without injury or invasion of our tissues.

Infection is injury to or invasion and damage of our tissues by microbes. Tissue invasion is usual in microbial attack, but cholera is an example of severe injury and disease from a bacterial toxin without any significant tissue invasion.

The microbes which can infect us fall into one of four groups (Fig. 1):

- Normal flora inhabit the surfaces of the body although these can be both external, the skin, hair and nails, and internal, the mucous membranes of our digestive tract, the respiratory tract down to the larynx, the terminal urethra and the vagina.
- Aggressive pathogens or primary pathogens are those microbes which can cause disease in normal hosts, i.e. those with normal defence mechanisms.
- Opportunistic pathogens (p. 23) are those microbes which do not cause disease in normal hosts but do so in those with impaired defences (Fig. 1).
- Latent pathogens (p. 23).

Microbial attack and host defence

Nine steps can be distinguished in the development of infection (Fig. 2):

1. The **Reservoir** or source of the infecting organism (p. 24).

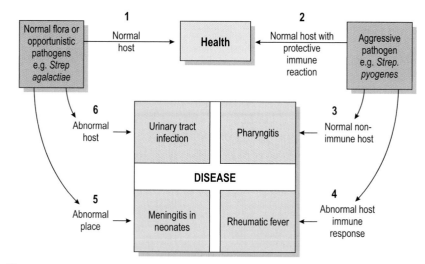

Fig. 1 **Six major microbiological principles illustrated by streptococcal interaction with host defences.**

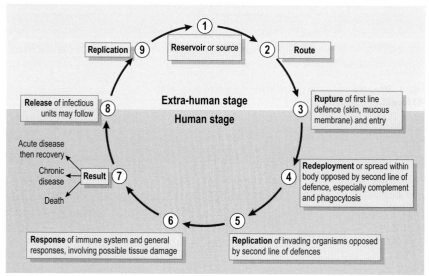

Fig. 2 **The nine steps in the development of infection.**

2. The **Route** by which the organisms spread externally to reach us.
3. The **Rupture** of our first line of defence, the skin or mucous membrane, i.e. entry into the body.
4. The **Redeployment** of the invading microbes, i.e. spread within the body, opposed by our second line of defence, complement and phagocytosis (p. 26–27).
5. The **Replication** of the invading microbes (p. 26–27), again opposed by our second line of defence.
6. The **Response** of our immune system and our general responses to infection with tissue damage (p. 26–29).
7. The **Result** of successful microbial attack, i.e. clinical disease (p. 94–223), opposed also by our external defences.
8. The **Release** of infectious units into the environment may follow step 7,

especially for protozoan cysts and multicellular parasites (p. 78–91) with extra-human life cycles.
9. **Replication**, in Step 1.

Hopefully the body's external defences can deal with the infection and the result is Recovery rather than Recumbency (chronic disease) or Rigor mortis.

Pathogenicity, virulence and invasiveness

Pathogenicity is the ability to cause disease. It therefore includes virulence and toxins, microbial factors determining adherence, invasiveness (the ability to enter and spread in the body), the ease and speed of microbial replication, and their ability to impede host defences. See also Viral pathogenesis, p. 19.

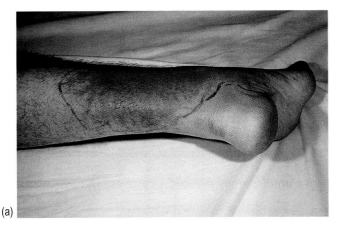

(a)

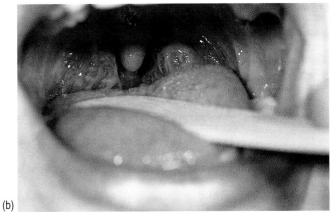

(b)

Fig. 3 *Strep. pyogenes* **can cause both (a) erysipelas (local spread) or (b) tonsillitis (direct invasion).**

Table 1 **Some important microbial toxins**

Toxin and organism	Result	Mechanism
Anthrax toxins		
B. anthracis		
Oedema factor	Oedema	Adenylate cyclase
Lethal factor	Pulmonary oedema	Cytotoxin
Botulinum toxin		
C. botulinum	Neurotoxicity	Neuromuscular block
Cholera toxin		
Vibrio cholerae	Diarrhoea	Adenylate cyclase, CAMP activation
Clostridial toxins		
C. difficile	Diarrhoea	Membrane permeability
C. perfringens		
alpha toxin	Necrosis	Phospholipase C
beta toxin	Oedema	Capillary leakage
delta toxin	Haemolysis	Haemolysin
kappa toxin	Spread, necrosis	Collagenase
mu toxin	Spread, necrosis	Hyaluronidase
Diphtheria toxin		
C. diphtheriae	Cytotoxicity	ADP ribosylation of elongation factor 2
Enterotoxin		
E. coli and enteric bacilli	Diarrhoea	As cholera toxin
(Also cytotoxin)	Haemorrhage	As shigella toxin
Shigella toxin	Haemorrhagic enteritis	60S ribosome inactivation

See also Staphylococci (p. 34–35) and Streptococci (p. 36–37).

- antibody production: impedins are antibody-degrading enzymes
- cell-mediated immunity: impeded by mechanisms such as surface disguise (p. 31).

In addition to these microbial factors in pathogenesis, an abnormal host response may cause further damage (p. 30).

Interplay of factors

The interplay between the virulence of the microbe (normal flora, opportunist or aggressive pathogen), the invasion of the host, the host defences and the host response is illustrated by the streptococci, showing six major microbiological principles (Fig. 1).

Disease and microbial species

While sometimes one species of organism only causes one disease and that disease is only caused by one species (e.g. anthrax, tetanus), very frequently one species causes numerous diseases, e.g. *Strep. pyogenes* (Fig. 3); similarly, one disease, e.g. impetigo, can be caused by different organisms.

Two related concepts are the **infective dose**, which is the number of microbes necessary to cause infection, and the **period of infectivity**, which is the time during which a source, usually human, is disseminating organisms and hence is potentially able to cause infections in others.

Virulence factors

Virulence factors are the microbial factors essential for the development of infection and disease.

Toxins are usually protein exotoxins, though many Gram-negative organisms have a very important complex lipopolysaccharide endotoxin. The more important are in Table 1.

Adhesins determine adhesiveness to cells and are usually found on fibrillae, fimbriae or pili, the fine hair-like structures on the outside of many bacteria. They are known to be important in streptococci and staphylococci, in *Neisseria* spp., *E. coli*, *Pseudomonas* spp. and *Shigella* spp., and have been found in many other bacteria, in *Candida albicans* and in some protozoa and viruses.

Impedins (as the name suggests) impede host defence mechanisms (p. 24–29) and act against:

- anatomical barriers: impedins include bacteriocins and factors for direct skin penetration and mucosal invasion, and connective tissue-disrupting enzymes
- serum factors: impedins can act against complement ('serum resistance') and fibrinolysins
- phagocytosis: impedins include protective capsules, blocking of the oxidative burst, stopping phagosome-lysosome fusion and resisting lysosomal enzymes.

> ### Host–microbial relationships
>
> - Contamination is transient, colonisation is more permanent but produces no tissue damage, while infection entails tissue damage.
>
> - Normal flora live on our skin and mucous membranes and cause no disease in normal hosts. Aggressive or primary pathogens cause disease in normal hosts, while opportunist pathogens only cause disease in hosts with impaired defences.
>
> - Microbial virulence factors in pathogenicity include toxins, adhesins and impedins.
>
> - Infection depends on the balance between virulence, invasiveness, host defences and host response.
>
> - Various microbial species cause more than one disease and many diseases can be caused by more than one microbial species.

Attackers: normal flora and pathogens

Definition

Pathogenic ('disease-causing') microbes are of three types, opportunist pathogens (including much of our normal flora), latent pathogens, or aggressive ('primary' or 'true') pathogens. First it is necessary to understand our normal flora.

Normal flora

Microbes that are adapted to life on our skin and the mucous membranes lining the surface of the respiratory, digestive, urinary and genital systems (which are in continuity with the skin and actually or potentially in contact with our exterior environment) are called our normal flora and have a typical spectrum in each body region (Table 1):

- flora of the small bowel, as expected, is intermediate between that of the mouth and colon
- vaginal flora resembles a mixture of the skin and colonic flora
- nose, conjunctiva and external ear have similar flora
- *Staph. aureus*, *Staph. epidermidis* and *Streptococcus* spp. are widespread
- *Escherichia coli* and other aerobic Gram-negative rods and *Enterococcus* spp. are far outnumbered in the gut by anaerobic rods (*Bacteroides* and *Fusobacterium* spp.) and anaerobic cocci (peptostreptococci, peptococci and veillonellae).
- *Candida albicans* is frequently found in the mouth, colon, vagina and skin.

Useful roles of normal flora
Protection from invading microbes
Normal flora form part of our first line of defence (p. 25). There are at least two mechanisms: first their simple physical presence, often in large numbers (Fig. 1) and well established in their niche with necessary nutrients, and, secondly, the antimicrobial protein bacteriocins and antibiotics which some produce. When part of our bacterial flora is removed by antibiotics intended as therapy, we may instead suffer from overgrowth of resistant normal flora such as *Candida albicans* or *Clostridium difficile*, causing thrush or enterocolitis, respectively.

Immune stimulation
Our bacterial normal flora in particular stimulates production of the surface antibody IgA in our mucous membranes, presumably protecting us from invasion of deeper tissues by normal flora or by similar exogenous species.

Human nutrition and metabolism
Normal flora in the gut, including *E. coli* and *Bacteroides* spp. (some now called *Prevotella* spp.) synthesise vitamin K, and make enzymes which deconjugate bile salts and sex hormones after excretion from the liver so they can be reabsorbed in the so-called enterohepatic loop.

Harmful roles of normal flora
The normal flora also have several less desirable attributes.

Table 1 **Normal flora in different regions of the body**

Organism	Skin	Conjunctiva	Nose	Mouth/oropharynx	Small bowel	Colon	Vagina
Staph. aureus	+	±	+	±	±	±	–
Staph. epidermidis	+++	++	+++	–	–	±	±
Streptococci	±	±	±	+++	–	+	±
Enterococci	–	–	–	–	–	+	+
Diphtheroids	++	–	–	–	–	–	+
Lactobacilli	–	–	–	–	++	++	+++
Haemophilus spp.	–	±	±	±	–	–	–
Moraxella spp.	–	±	±				
Neisseria spp.	–	±	±	±	+	–	–
E. coli	±	±	–	±	+	+++	±
Klebsiella spp.	±	±	–	±	+	++	±
Other aerobic GNR[a]	±	–	+[c]	±	±	±	±
Bacteroides and *Fusobacterium* spp.	±	–	–	+++	+	+++	±
Veillonella spp.	–	–	–	+++	–	±	+
Clostridium spp.	–	–	–	–	+	+++	+
Peptococcus and *Peptostreptococcus* spp.	±	–	–	±	++	+++	+
Mycobacteria spp.	±	–	–	–	+	±	±
Mycoplasma spp.	–	–	–	–	–	–	±
Treponemes	–	–	–	++	–	±	–
Candida albicans	±	–	–	+	–	±	+
Other fungi	+++[b]	–	–	–	–	±	±

+++, almost always present; ++, usual; +, frequent; ±, occasional or rare.
[a] GNR, Gram-negative rods.
[b] *Pityrosporum* spp.
[c] *Pseudomonas aeruginosa* frequent in external ear.

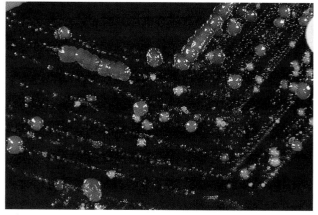

Fig. 1 **Oral flora colonies on horse blood agar.**

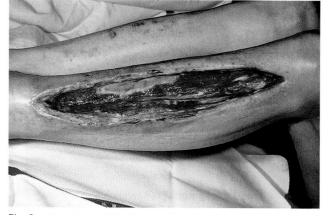

Fig. 2 **Infected wound.** *Staph. aureus* from the skin is the commonest cause.

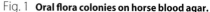

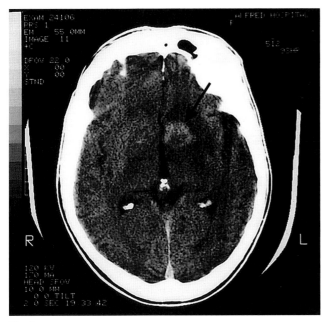

Fig. 3 **Toxoplasmosis: brain cyst (light) and oedema (dark).**

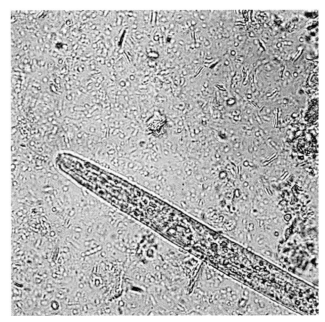

Fig. 4 *Strongyloides stercoralis* **larva.**

Opportunist pathogens – see below

Possible source of carcinogens

While controversial, it is known that enzymes from the gut flora, including sulphatases, can modify ingested chemicals to known carcinogens. Whether this is actually important in the production of colonic or bladder carcinoma is as yet unknown.

Opportunist pathogens

Opportunist pathogens are microbes which do not cause disease in normal hosts but take the opportunity to become pathogenic when the host defences are impaired. The normal flora are an obvious source of such organisms: they occur in large numbers adjacent to our tissues, well placed to invade and infect if our host defences become impaired. For example, when patients become neutropenic through disease or anti-cancer 'chemotherapy', they are frequently infected by their own gut, skin or respiratory flora unless precautions are taken. Similarly, a surgical wound can give entry of the patient's skin flora into their deeper tissues, causing a surgical wound infection (Fig. 2). Other opportunists come from hospital and natural environments, and sometimes from other people, e.g. from the skin or throat of hospital staff to immunocompromised patients.

Latent pathogens

Pathogenic organisms which are *not* normal flora can become resident and lie dormant in a host with normal defences, either after inapparent subclinical infection or after clinical infection with apparent recovery. Months, years or even decades later they cause clinical disease, especially when host defences become impaired ('compromised') by disease, drugs or other cause (p. 220–221).

Latent pathogens include:

- bacteria, particularly intracellular ones, causing brucellosis, listeriosis, melioidosis, nocardiosis, salmonellosis (especially

S. typhi), tuberculosis and other mycobacterial infections such as that caused by the *M. avium* complex (MAC).
- fungi: *Candida*, *Pneumocystis jirovecii* (formerly *carinii*), *Cryptococcus neoformans* and *Histoplasma capsulatum*.
- protozoa, particularly those with persistent cyst forms, as in amoebiasis (*E. histolytica*), cryptosporidiosis (*C. parvum*) or toxoplasmosis (*T. gondii*) (Fig. 3)
- helminths (worms), particularly those with a life cycle wholly in humans, e.g. strongyloidiasis from *S. stercoralis* (Fig. 4)
- viruses, particularly HSV, CMV and EBV.

All these infections occur in AIDS patients with severe immune impairment. Details of these pathogens and diseases are found on the relevant pages (including p. 149–151).

Aggressive pathogens

These cause disease in normal hosts – see especially pages 34–93.

Normal flora and pathogens

- Normal flora are important in:
  - protection from invading microbes
  - immune stimulation
  - human nutrition and metabolism
  - opportunist infection
  - possible production of carcinogens
  - opportunist pathogens infect when host defences are impaired.

- Latent pathogens
  - lie dormant in a normal host but cause clinical disease when host defences are compromised
  - often are intracellular bacteria, tissue fungi, protozoa with cyst forms, or helminths with life cycles only involving humans
  - cause disease that is more acute, more severe and more life-threatening in the immunocompromised host than in normal hosts.

- Aggressive pathogens (= primary pathogens)
  - cause disease in normal hosts.

Attack begins: attack and first-line defences

The initiation of microbial infection requires firstly a Reservoir or source of infection, secondly a Route of transmission and thirdly Rupture of the non-specific surface defences of the body, providing a portal of entry.

Reservoirs and sources

Epidemiology is the study of the behaviour of diseases in the community rather than in individual patients. It includes the study of the reservoirs and sources of human diseases (Fig. 1). Strictly speaking, **a reservoir is the organism's usual residence**, where it resides, replenishes and replicates. **The source is the site from which spread immediately occurs to the host**, directly or indirectly. For example, the soil is the reservoir of eggs or cysts of many parasites, while soil-contaminated vegetables are the source of human infection with the parasite. Sometimes the reservoir and the source are the same site, e.g. nasopharyngeal carriage of streptococci and staphylococci.

Epidemiological information can be used statistically to generate **incidence rates** (number acquiring a disease in a certain period, divided by total population) and **prevalence rates** (number of people having a disease at a specific time divided by total population). These figures can give indications of populations at-risk, e.g. using age-adjusted data the high incidence of shigellosis among children under 5 years is highlighted in what is a relatively rare disease in the population as a whole. Epidemiology can also indicate possible causes of disease and possible means of prevention, e.g. diseases transmitted by insect vectors or by food.

Reservoirs

Reservoirs can be almost anywhere on our planet, including:

- soil: for many parasitic infections (p. 78–89)
- water or other fluids: even disinfectants! (p. 225)
- inanimate objects: often important in hospital-acquired infections (p. 218)
- animals: infections from this source are called zoonoses (p. 212–213)
- people: spread their normal flora (harmless to themselves) to those with impaired defences; people called carriers may be colonised with aggressive pathogens against which they have protection by their own antibodies or immunisation, but which cause disease in those not so protected. Note below four other categories of people who can be temporary sources rather than permanent reservoirs.

Sources

Sources of infections are also extremely varied, but can be divided into three groups:

- Inanimate objects include water and food, particularly fruit and vegetables for many parasitic and bacterial diseases. Industrial or hospital equipment may also be a temporary or immediate source as well as a permanent reservoir.
- Animals may be a source, e.g. some snails, crustacea or fish act as intermediate hosts between humans and another animal reservoir in many cestode infections (p. 88–89). Uncooked or undercooked meat or fish is another source, e.g. clostridial or staphylococcal food poisoning

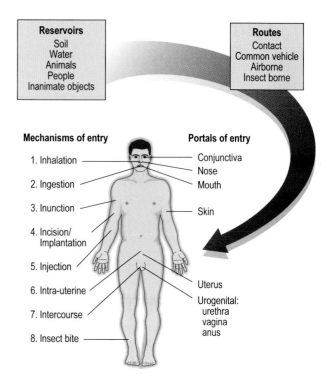

Fig. 1 **Reservoirs, routes and entry of disease.**

- People are the third important source: those **Infected** with an obvious illness; those **Incubating** an illness without developed symptoms; those with **Inapparent** or subclinical infection; or those **Improving**, i.e. convalescing but still infectious to others. They may, therefore, be patients, family members, hospital and health-care staff, or daily or casual contacts, and only those obviously infected will be easily identifiable as a potential source.

Route of transmission

There are four major ways in which microbes can move from a reservoir or source to a host:

- Contact can be either *direct* ('person-to-person') such as a boil or a skin infection transmitting directly by touch, or *indirect* via some object. (Droplet infection is sometimes illogically classified as a contact infection.)
- Common vehicle transmission occurs when some object touches first the reservoir or source and then the hosts. This common vehicle infects many; replication of the microbe may occur in the food or liquid vehicle. Common vehicle transmission is really a special form of indirect contact, differentiated for epidemic investigations. Food and water are the commonest common vehicles, but batches of blood products, intravenous or dialysis fluids, or drugs may also be contaminated common vehicles.
- Airborne transmission occurs either in *droplets* larger than 5nm, which only travel about 1 metre, or by *droplet nuclei* less than 5nm, or skin squames or dust, which can be carried for kilometres.
- Vector-borne transmission usually involves insects (vector means carrier). They may be passive vectors ('flying pins') like houseflies, simply carrying salmonellae externally from

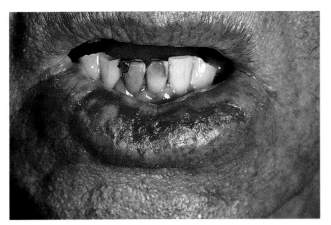

Fig. 2 **Candidiasis of the lips caused by lip licking allowing breakage of the skin barrier.**

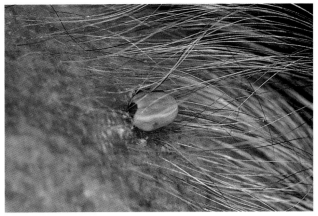

Fig. 3 **Ixodes tick.**

a reservoir to us, or be harbouring the organism internally without change of the organism (as *Yersinia pestis* within a plague flea), or be an active, essential part of the biological life cycle of the organism, as mosquitoes are in malaria.

Ruptured defences: entry

Once bacteria have been carried to the human body by one of the above four routes of transmission, how do they enter? The four major *portals of entry* are:

- mouth and gastrointestinal tract
- respiratory tract
- skin (by four different mechanisms) (Figs 1 and 2)
- genital tract.

The eye and placenta are less common.

Table 1 Pathogens using differing portals of entry

Portal	Disease	Pathogen example
Skin		
Direct invasion	Abscesses	*Staph. aureus*
Injection	Hepatitis	Hepatitis B and C
Wounds	Tetanus	*Clostridium tetani*
Bites	Plague	*Yersinia pestis*
Nose	Pneumonia	*Strep. pneumoniae*
Conjunctiva	Trachoma	*Chlamydia trachomatis*
Mouth	Cholera	*Vibrio cholerae*
	Salmonellosis	*Salmonella* spp.
	Diphtheria	*Corynebacterium diphtheriae*
Urethra	Gonorrhoea	*Neisseria gonorrhoeae*
	Urinary tract infection (UTI)	*Escherichia coli*
Vagina	Vaginitis	*Trichomonas vaginalis*
	Gonorrhoea	*Neisseria gonorrhoeae*
Placenta	Syphilis	*Treponema pallidum*

Table 2 Chemical protection of body surfaces

Organ/system	Origin	Protective chemicals
Skin	Sebaceous glands	Fatty acids
	Sweat	Fatty acids
Mucous membrane	Secretions	Mucus, lysozyme
Gut	Salivary glands	Thiocyanate
	Parietal cells (stomach)	Hydrochloric acid
	Hepatocytes	Bile acids
	Crypt cells	Alpha defensins
	Normal flora	Fatty acids (short chain)
Lung	A cells	Surfactant
	Mucosa	Beta defensins

Exogenous infection ('arising from outside') therefore can occur by eight **mechanisms** (Fig. 1):

- Inhalation: usually of airborne infection, but in hospital it may be direct contact into the respiratory tract
- Ingestion: by eating or drinking something contaminated by contact or common vehicle
- Inunction: literally rubbing on, hence by direct or indirect contact to skin or conjunctiva
- Incision ± implantation: by traumatic or surgical wounds, or organ transplant
- Injection by needle (e.g. illicit drug use) or by transfusion
- Intra-uterine: by transplacental spread from the mother
- Intercourse: in sexually transmitted diseases arising from some variety of sexual intercourse. While this is microbiologically only another form of direct contact, the pathogens and portals have sufficient special characteristics to be listed separately
- Insect bite: in vector-borne transmission (Fig. 3).

Table 1 lists examples of pathogens linked to specific portals of entry.

Endogenous infection ('arising from within') occurs when our normal flora become opportunist pathogens (p. 23).

The first line of defences: skin and mucous membranes

The skin and mucous membranes enclose the body forming a physical barrier to infection; additional physical factors such as ciliary and mucus movement over the mucosal surfaces also contribute. The normal flora on these surfaces reduce the ability of pathogens to survive by competing for nutrients and by producing antimicrobial chemicals (Table 2 and p. 22).

> *Initiation of disease: attack*
>
> - Permanent reservoirs of infection are soil, water, inanimate objects, animals and people.
> - Immediate sources of infection are usually inanimate objects (including food and water), animals and people.
> - Routes of transmission are direct and indirect contact, common vehicle, airborne and vector-borne.
> - Exogenous infection enters by rupture of body defences and occurs by inhalation, ingestion, inunction, incision/implantation, injection, intra-uterine spread, intercourse, or insect bites.
> - Endogenous infection occurs when our normal flora become pathogenic.

Attack continues: non-specific second-line defences

The non-specific defences form part of the body's normal constitution so do not need prior contact with a particular microbe, i.e. they are constitutive or innate.

By contrast, the specific defences (p. 28–29) form the immune response, and are inducible, i.e. are only present after being induced by the presence of a particular microbial species.

The non-specific defences include:

- normal flora (p. 22)
- physicochemical factors (p. 25)
  - skin
  - mucosal membranes with cilia and mucous secretions
- cellular factors (phagocytic cells)
  - neutrophils
  - macrophages
  - natural killer cells
- humoral factors in blood, mucosal secretions and cerebrospinal fluid
  - complement
  - opsonins
  - enzymes
  - interferons (p. 19).

These innate defences are most useful in providing protection against pyogenic organisms, fungi, multicellular parasites and some viruses.

Second line of defence – cellular factors

Phagocytosis

Phagocytosis ('the eating of cells') is the process by which neutrophils, and tissue macrophages derived from monocytes, find, engulf and kill microbes (Table 1). Neutrophils, particularly, phagocytose extracellular bacteria, while macrophages are most active against intracellular bacteria, protozoa and viruses. Eosinophils are involved in metazoan parasitic infections.

The first steps in phagocytosis are (Fig. 1):

- **Chemotaxis**. The attraction of neutrophils by chemicals, some made by bacteria, others by the host's complement cascade.
- **Adhesion**. This is facilitated by C3b from the complement system, by pattern recognition molecules including Toll-like Receptors (TLRs) on macrophages (p. 29) (and by specific antibodies if they exist at this time).
- **Ingestion**. This occurs when membrane activation leads to pseudopodia forming around the organism and its inclusion into a vacuole called a phagosome.

1. Chemotaxis

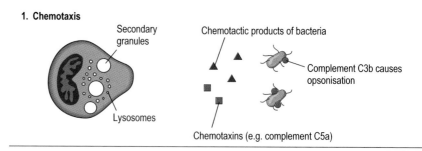

2. Adhesion

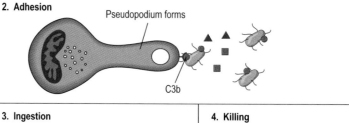

3. Ingestion

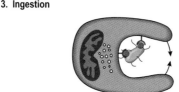

4. Killing

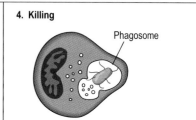

(a) Oxidative burst (oxygen dependent killing)
(b) Oxygen independent killing
(c) Death and degranulation

Fig. 1 **The steps in phagocytosis.**

Table 1 **Cellular defences**		
Phagocytic cell	**Origin**	**Antimicrobial mechanism**
Neutrophil	Bone marrow	Margination, diapedesis, and chemotaxis, then phagocytosis, degranulation, O_2-dependent killing (H_2O_2), O_2-independent killing, e.g. by lactoferrin, lysozyme
Eosinophil	Bone marrow	O_2-independent especially anti-parasitic
Monocyte	Bone marrow	As neutrophils except for degranulation (in addition, inducible activity, see p. 29)
Macrophage	Blood monocyte	As monocytes, major inducible activities

Opsonins are cofactors that coat microbes and enhance the ability of neutrophils to engulf them. Opsonins include complement C3b, C-reactive protein Mannan Binding Lectin (MBL), a serum protein, and antibodies. The last enable the specific immune system to activate the innate system.

Within the phagosome the microbe is **killed and degraded** by the following mechanisms initiated by fusion of the phagocyte granules with the phagosome:

- **Oxygen-dependent killing (oxidative burst)**. Active oxygen molecules – superoxide anion, hydrogen peroxide, 'singlet' activated oxygen and hydroxyl free radicals – are formed from O_2 and NADPH in the presence of cytochrome b_{245}. The active oxygen molecules kill microbes.
- **Oxygen-independent killing after phagosome-lysosome fusion with degranulation**. Lysosomes are primary granules within neutrophils that contain myeloperoxidase, lysozyme and cationic proteins which damage bacterial membranes and lead to microbial killing and digestion. In addition, the secondary 'specific' secretory granules, containing lactoferrin and lysozyme, discharge these inside the phagosome, helping bacterial killing and digestion.
- **Degradation**. Once microbes are killed, they are degraded by hydrolytic enzymes and the products released from the neutrophils. When the granule contents are released outside the phagocyte, they can lead to tissue damage.

Natural killer cells

These are special lymphocytes which recognise virus-infected cells and release a cytolysin which kills the host cell before it can release further virus.

Second line of defence – humoral factors

Complement

The complement system is a group of about 20 serum proteins which respond to a stimulus such as invading microbes by a cascade of serial chemical reactions where the product of one reaction is the enzyme catalysing the next. There are three major parts in the complement system, the classical pathway, found first and important in antibody action (the third line of defence, p. 28–29), the alternative pathway (Fig. 2), is important in the second line of defence with phagocytes and the recently discovered Lectin pathway (Fig. 2, p. 29).

The major actions of complement are:

- assisting phagocytosis by facilitating adherence, stimulating mast cells to release chemotaxins, stimulating chemotaxis directly, stimulating the respiratory burst
- increasing vascular permeability
- lysing organisms.

These occur by a complex series of reactions which are much simplified here. Even the nomenclature is complex (Table 2).

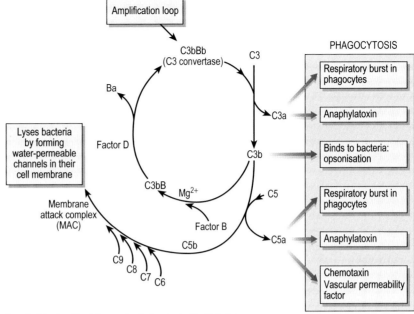

Anaphylatoxin: stimulates mast cells to release chemotaxins and vascular permeability mediators
Chemotaxin: assists chemotaxis of phagocytes
Vascular permeability factor: assists phagocyte movement from the capillaries into tissues

Fig. 2 **The alternative complement pathway and phagocytosis.**

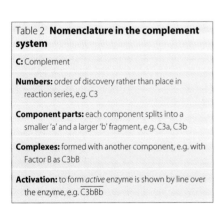

Table 2 **Nomenclature in the complement system**
C: Complement
Numbers: order of discovery rather than place in reaction series, e.g. C3
Component parts: each component splits into a smaller 'a' and a larger 'b' fragment, e.g. C3a, C3b
Complexes: formed with another component, e.g. with Factor B as C3bB
Activation: to form *active* enzyme is shown by line over the enzyme, e.g. C3bBb

Further components

In addition to the major components of phagocytosis and complement activation, the non-specific tissue defences include:

- simple chemicals and ions (Table 3)
- some individual proteins (Table 3)
- some complicated protein systems.
- specific antiviral substances (p. 18–19). The individual proteins include:
- Acute phase proteins. These include C-reactive protein (CRP) which binds to numerous bacteria and activates the classical complement pathway independently of antibody, causing binding of C3b to the bacterial cell and hence opsonisation and phagocytosis.

- Lysozyme. This is an important enzyme that is widely distributed in the body. It is a muramidase which breaks the peptidoglycan in bacterial cell walls.

Coagulation, fibrinolysin and kallikrein systems.

These complicated protein systems play only a small role in controlling most infections but become very important in overwhelming infections when excess activation of these systems contributes to shock and death (p. 32–33).

Non-specific defences

- The first line of defences are skin and mucous membranes.
- Second-line defences are provided by integrated phagocytosis and complement (alternative pathway) with some additional chemical factors.
- Phagocytosis is principally by neutrophils for most common bacterial infections and by macrophages for intracellular bacteria, protozoa and viruses.
- Complement acts by assisting phagocytosis (adherence, chemotaxis and respiratory burst), by increasing vascular permeability and hence the supply of neutrophils to infected tissues, and by lysing bacteria.
- Additional chemical factors include lysozyme, acute phase proteins such as CRP, and interferons.

Table 3 **Chemical humoral mediators**		
Substance	**Origin**	**Antimicrobial mechanism**
Simple chemicals		
Hydrogen ion	Phagocytes	Low pH is antimicrobial
Reduced oxygen	Phagocytes	Directly antimicrobial
Chloride ion	Tissue fluid	Combination with H_2O_2
Fatty acids	Metabolites	Antimicrobial at low pH
Individual proteins		
Acute-phase proteins:		
C-reactive protein	Liver cells	Activates complement
α1-antitrypsin	Liver cells	Inhibits proteases
Fibronectin	Macrophages, fibroblasts	Opsonin for staphylococci
Interferons	Infected cells	Virus entry and virus multiplication impeded
Lactoferrin	Neutrophils	Binds iron needed for microbial growth
Lysozyme	Macrophages, neutrophils, secretions (e.g. tears, saliva)	Murein degradation
Myeloperoxidase	Neutrophils	Combines with H_2O_2 and Cl
Transferrin	Liver cells	Binds iron needed for microbial growth

Attack contained: specific (immune) third- and fourth-line defences

Microbes have many mechanisms for successfully overcoming or avoiding our first and second lines of defence (p. 25–27); evidence of such success is the ability to infect again, or to actually enter our cells. So our third and fourth lines of defence are integrated with the initial innate defences, are slower to develop but particularly effective against microbes experienced previously (antibody formation against specific microbes), or intracellular microbes (cell-mediated immunity, CMI). Developing only after exposure to a microbe, they are called the **acquired immune response**.

Serologic immunity by antibodies – the third line

This specific response is adroitly achieved with an antibody molecule that couples phagocytosis, complement activation and specific microbial recognition. So each antibody molecule has three particular regions: two constant for activating phagocytes and complement, and one variable recognition site to bind a specific microbe.

How can we have the myriad different antibodies needed for recognition of all the different microbes we meet in life? The answer is in our lymphocytes. These are of two types, **B-cells**, bone-marrow-derived and antibody producing, and **T-cells**, which are thymus processed, help B cells to make antibody and are especially important in cell-mediated immunity.

It used to be thought that B-cells used each new antigen ('any substance causing antibody to be generated') as a template to make the corresponding antibody. It is now known that each B-cell is programmed to make one single antibody and no other, and has about 100 000 copies on its surface as receptors. When a microbe invading tissues meets a B-cell with an antibody which fits a microbial surface antigen, the B-cell is stimulated to proliferate and differentiate to plasma cells, which make more antibody. Thus a huge clone of the one **effector cell** selected is produced (as predicted by the clonal selection theory of Burnet and Fenner), resulting in an increased amount of antibody against the invader. This takes some days and is the **primary response**.

In addition, a smaller number of B-cells persist as **memory cells**, ready to proliferate and produce large amounts of antibody if an invader returns. This explains the amplified **secondary response** of antibody production in a second infection (Fig. 1).

Immunisation

Immunisation (or vaccination) is based on the ability of B-cells to produce memory cells. The B-cells are primed by a harmless antigen (live-attenuated or killed) to produce memory cells ready to proliferate and differentiate when stimulated by a microbial antigen, thus producing large amounts of antibody in a short time (p. 236–237).

How do antibodies work?

In summary, antibodies activate the classical complement pathway that then activates phagocytosis, either directly or indirectly via the mast cell. This is shown in Fig. 2 (see also Fig. 2, p. 27).

Antibody has two further benefits:

- Immunoglobulin E (see below) can bind directly to mast cells, and subsequent antigen binding *directly* triggers release

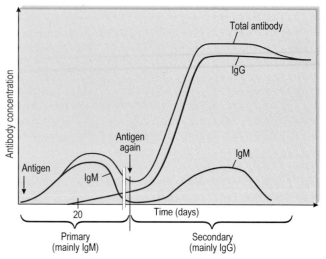

Fig. 1 **Primary and secondary antibody responses.**

of the mediators (VPF, chemotaxins, MAC) without needing complement activation.
- Antibody binding carries 'the bonus of multivalency', meaning that while a single molecule of antibody may be insufficient to cause phagocytosis of a C3b-coated microbe, the attraction forces of multiple bonds is geometric, so three antibodies bound closely on a microbe can have 1000 times the attraction to a phagocyte. This is called high avidity multiple binding.

How does antibody structure give these functions?

There are five major classes of antibodies, called IgG, IgM, IgA, IgE and IgD. All except IgM have a similar structure (Fig. 3). Two identical heavy peptide chains are flanked by two identical light chains and all are linked by disulphide bonds. This is conventionally shown in a Y shape, but in reality it is considerably folded to expose three hypervariable regions in each adjacent light and heavy chain, which form the antigen-recognising area. This area can vary enormously allowing for specific recognition of innumerable antigens.

The C-terminal ends of the heavy chains by contrast are constant, being responsible for complement activation, and hence activation of phagocytosis, and binding to cell surface Fc receptors (the base of the Y is the Fc region).

Why do we have different classes of antibody?

The five major classes of antibodies have diverse functions:

- IgM is formed early in infection (primary response) and is composed of five Y-shaped molecules. It activates complement very efficiently.
- IgG is the major immunoglobulin in blood and tissues, is found particularly in the secondary response (Fig. 1), activates complement, binds to phagocytes and also acts with NK (natural killer) cells.
- IgA is present particularly at mucous membranes, often as a dimer with an extra 'secretory' component. It is exceptional in *not* activating complement or binding to Fc receptors, and probably acts by preventing microbial attachment to mucous membranes.

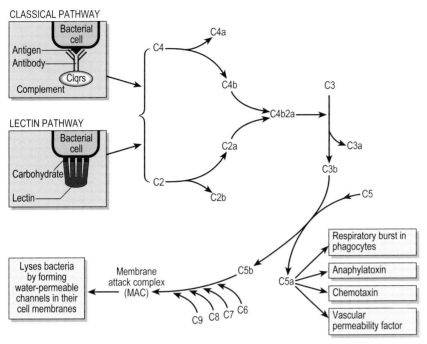

Fig. 2 **Activation of the classical complement pathway by antibody, and activation of the lectin pathway by carbohydrate *without* antibody.**

- IgD is a minor Ig, probably a membrane antigen receptor.
- IgE binds to mast cells and basophils, releasing histamine and other vasoactive mediators in the inflammatory response. It is particularly important in parasitic infections. In excess it causes the symptoms of hay fever and other allergies.

Cell-mediated immunity (CMI) – the fourth line

CMI is particularly aimed at intracellular microbes and again consists of the three components – lymphocytes, specific chemical messengers and phagocytes – but differs in that:

- the lymphocytes are T-cells, not B-cells

- the chemicals are called cytokines (meaning 'cell activators') and are made not only by the T-cells (lymphokines), but also by macrophages (monokines), neutrophils and other cells. Their aim is other cells, not antigen.
- the phagocyte is the macrophage (and its predecessor, the blood monocyte). Recently-discovered Toll-like receptors (TLRs) on macrophages and dendritic cells not only innately recognise various components of pathogens (e.g. staphylococcal lipoteichoic acid; p. 34–35), but also induce cytokines and activate antigen-specific immune responses.

There are different types (subsets) of T cells, distinguished by their function and their surface markers (e.g. CD8, CD4). The important types are:

- cytotoxic T-cells *(CD8, T8)* which recognise antigen plus class I MHC (see below) in virus-infected cells, killing the cell before it releases infective virus; they also release gamma-interferon, making nearby cells resistant to infection
- suppressor T-cells *(also CD8, T8)* that decrease (downregulate) the activity of other T-cells and B-cells
- helper/inducer T-cells *(CD4, T4)* which help other T-cells to become cytotoxic, help B-cells make antibody and help macrophages kill intracellular microbes.

How does a T-helper cell help a macrophage kill a microbe within the macrophage? It must be able to do three things – recognise the macrophage, recognise that it contains microbes, and then activate the macrophage to kill the intracellular microbes. To achieve this, the T-cell recognises not one but always a pair of substances on macrophages containing intracellular microbes. First it recognises the macrophage by molecules belonging to class II of the major histocompatibility complex (MHC); these are tissue type markers originally discovered through their role in rejection of incompatible tissue or organ transplants. Secondly, it recognises adjacent antigenic fragments of the microbes which the macrophage has processed onto its surface. Thirdly the T-helper cell releases gamma-interferon and activates the macrophage and other cells so that they can kill the intracellular parasites.

In addition, T-cells help the proliferation and differentiation of B-cells by production of B-cell stimulating factor (BSF-1), B-cell growth factor (BCGF-II), B-cell differentiation factors (BCDF-mu and BCDF-gamma), and other lymphokines.

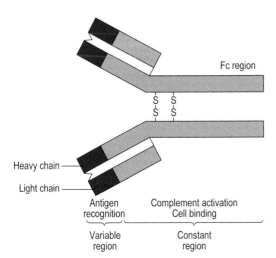

Fig. 3 **Stylised antibody molecule.**

> ### *Specific (immune) defences*
>
> - Antibodies link phagocytosis, complement activation and specific microbial recognition.
> - Antibody activates the classical complement pathway.
> - Antibody plus complement activates phagocytosis, both directly, and via mast cell activation.
> - Antibody specific for one antigen is made by B-cell lymphocytes (each making only one antibody); when stimulated, this cell proliferates and differentiates to a clone of identical selected plasma cells (effector cells).
> - Some lymphocytes persist (memory cells) ready for a more rapid secondary response to any subsequent invasion; this forms the basis for immunisation.
> - T helper cells recognise antigen and class II MHC on the surface of macrophages containing intracellular microbes, release gamma interferon and activate the macrophage to kill the microbes.
> - Soluble cytokines from T-cells stimulate B-cell proliferation and differentiation.

Defences disordered: immune disorders; defences evaded

Immune disorders

The immune system developed to protect the organism against infection and, probably, malignancy. Shifts to a too active state (hypersensitivity) or to a weakened state (immunodeficiency) can have devastating effects, both direct from the disordered immune response, and indirect from the vulnerability to infection this allows.

Hypersensitivity

Hypersensitivity can occur by five basic mechanisms (see Fig. 1).

'Innate' hypersensitivity has been used to describe a sixth, non-immune type of exaggerated response, such as septic shock in Gram-negative septicaemia (p. 32 and 142–143).

Immunodeficiency

When the immune system fails, a major consequence is an increased risk of infection (other alterations in immune function occur in hypersensitivity, autoimmune disease and malignancy). Immunodeficiency can be either a **primary** event caused by congenital or genetic abnormalities, or it can be **secondary** to a wide range of systemic insults including disease or medical treatment. Secondary immunodeficiency has become more common with the widespread use of drugs such as corticosteroids, cytotoxic agents, anti-cancer chemotherapy, and immunosuppressive drugs, or treatments such as x-ray therapy and organ and bone marrow transplantation. Immunocompromised patients, whether from disease such as AIDS or treatment, are vulnerable not only to serious attacks of the infections seen in normal hosts but also to unusual pathogens rare in normal hosts, and to opportunistic infections by normally harmless microbes (see p. 220–221).

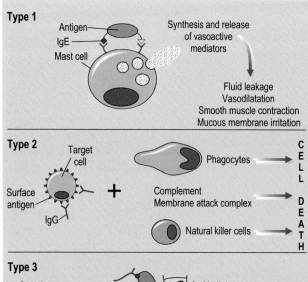

Type 1 Anaphylactic hypersensitivity and atopic allergy. Here antigen reacts with IgE antibody and mast cells to cause release of vasoactive mediators such as preformed histamine, eosinophil and neutrophil chemotaxins, and platelet-activating factor from the granules, and newly synthesised leukotrienes and prostaglandins. These cause fluid leakage, vasodilatation, smooth muscle contraction and mucous membrane irritation. The result is hay fever or extrinsic asthma, depending on the site. This is also the mechanism seen in anaphylaxis to penicillins, cephalosporins and other antibiotics.

Type 2 Antibody-dependent cytotoxicity. Surface antigen reacts with IgG antibody causing cell death. Cell death may occur because coating the cell with IgG (with or without C3b) increases adherence of phagocytes (this is called opsonisation), or because activation of complement to C9 causes cell lysis by the membrane-attack complex, or because of antibody-dependent cell-mediated cytotoxicity (ADCC), a direct non-specific method without phagocytosis, by phagocytes or natural killer (NK) cells. Type 2 mechanisms are not common in microbiology and infectious diseases, but do occur in *Mycoplasma pneumoniae* pneumonia with cold agglutinins, in virus infections, and in some drug reactions. They are very important in other areas of medicine, including Rh and ABO blood group incompatibility, organ transplants, and autoimmune diseases.

Type 3 Immune-complex mediated hypersensitivity. This involves the reaction of antigen with antibody (either in excess) causing tissue damage through excess activation of complement and neutrophil chemotaxis with release of vasoactive mediators, tissue-damaging enzymes and platelet-activating factor causing tissue damage and microthrombi. If excess antibody is circulating, this reaction occurs near the entry site of antigen, while in antigen excess circulating soluble complexes form and often deposit in filtering tissues like kidney or choroid plexus. Examples include farmer's lung from thermophilic actinomycetes, allergic broncho-pulmonary aspergillosis, filariasis causing elephantiasis, streptococcal glomerulonephritis, malarial nephrotic syndrome, serum sickness, and reactions to chemotherapy such as erythema nodosum leprosum (ENL) in leprosy, and the Herxheimer reaction in syphilis.

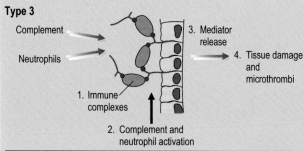

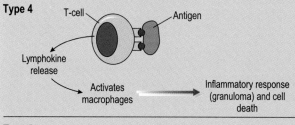

Type 4 Cell-mediated hypersensitivity. Antigen reacts with class II MHC and primed T-cells. This causes lymphokine release that in turn causes macrophage and lymphocyte infiltration, and target cell death by the action of the killer T-cells. Note this is simply an exaggerated normal CMI response. Persisting antigen stimulation leads to chronic granuloma formation in the tissue. Type 4 is also called **delayed-type hypersensitivity** for, being cell-mediated, it takes several days to develop while the other four types are more immediate. Clinically it causes redness and swelling as in the Mantoux reaction. Other examples are the rash in smallpox and measles, and much of the pathogenesis in TB (caseation), borderline leprosy, fungal diseases including candidiasis and histoplasmosis, and parasitic diseases including leishmaniasis and schistosomiasis.

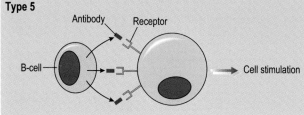

Type 5 Stimulatory hypersensitivity. This occurs when antibody reacts with surface receptors causing cell stimulation, such as that resulting in excess thyroid hormone production in thyrotoxicosis.

Fig. 1 **Types of hypersensitivity reaction.**

The defect can occur at any point in the immune system and will give rise to a distinct spectrum of disease (Table 1).

Diagnosis

Diagnostic tests in **hypersensitivity** diseases depend on the type.

Type 1 (anaphylactic) is investigated by intradermal scratch tests that provoke the release of histamine and other mediators causing an immediate wheal (oedema) and flare (erythema).

Type 2 (antibody-dependent cytotoxicity) is usually investigated with haemagglutination tests to predict and avoid Rh and ABO incompatibility. Tissue typing of the MHC antigens is used to avoid incompatible tissue transplants.

Type 3 (immune complex formation) is detected in tissues by immunofluorescence with anti-C3 and conjugated anti-immunoglobulins.

Type 4 (cell-mediated) is investigated by biopsy if necessary.

Diagnostic tests in **immune deficiency diseases** depend on the defect suspected by the clinical presentation.

Complement components can be measured and in vitro function quantified.

B-cell function is assessed by measuring immunoglobulin levels, naturally occurring antibodies like A and B isoagglutinins, and antibody response (if any) to killed vaccines.

T-cell function is assessed by skin tests to tuberculin, *Candida*, or mumps antigen, or by the reactivity of monocytes to phytohaemagglutinin. The numbers in each T-cell subset can be measured, and this test is widely available because of the management needs in AIDS.

Evading host defences

The clinical picture of infectious illness results from the interaction of microbial factors and host factors, both the non-specific defences and the immune system.

For a pathogen to survive successfully it must reach the site where it is best adapted to survive, and there it must avoid the host defences and multiply.

Adherence. The ability of pathogens to adhere to specific tissues assists them in overcoming the non-specific defence mechanisms, including desquamation of epithelial cells and ciliary action. Specific adhesin membrane proteins bind to host cell membrane components. Some strains of bacteria show preference for particular surfaces, e.g. group A β-haemolytic streptococci from throat culture adhere better to oral epithelial cells than to skin. Many adhesins are associated

with fimbriae or pili and this is often a determinant of virulence.

Adherence to prosthetic surfaces. The use of prosthetic devices has allowed different organisms to become pathogenic, e.g. infection of synthetic intravascular devices with coagulase-negative staphylococci is a major cause of bacteraemia in hospital patients.

Capsules. The formation of a slippery mucoid capsule, e.g. in *Klebsiella pneumoniae*, prevents opsonisation, presents a relatively non-immunogenic surface and may make antibody or complement that does bind inaccessible to phagocytic cell receptors. All three properties assist in avoiding phagocytosis.

Evasion of respiratory burst. Some intracellular pathogens, e.g. *Leishmania donovani*, enter cells by binding to complement receptors and so do not activate NADPH oxidase as the Fc receptor would normally do.

Survival within the phagosome. Intracellular organisms can avoid non-oxidative killing by:

- inhibiting fusion of phagosome and lysosome (*Toxoplasma gondii*)
- rupturing the phagolysosome so the microbe can multiply in the cytoplasm (*Shigella flexneri*)
- withstanding inactivation, and replicating in the phagolysosome (*Mycobacteria* spp.)

Bacterial cell wall. Surface proteins, for example the M protein in Gram-positive bacteria, can bind to molecules such as complement and prevent them activating host defences. In Gram-negative bacteria outer membrane proteins can block antibody- and complement-mediated lysis (e.g. in *Campylobacter fetus*) as can the lipopolysaccharide.

Antigenic variation. By varying the structure and antigenic composition of

surface molecules, pathogens can avoid antibodies and appear to be a constantly 'new' infection, e.g. *Neisseria gonorrhoeae* varies its pilin protein. *Trypanosoma brucei* has a variable surface glycoprotein (VSG) that limits complement activation; during infection, waves of new parasites are produced every few days, each with a new variant VSG.

Nutrient supply. Although microbial methods of ensuring sufficient nutrients are not directly related to avoidance of the immune system, they do assist the survival of the pathogen. Iron-scavenging mechanisms using secreted iron chelators called siderophores occur in *Escherichia coli* infections.

Damaging the host

Pathogens damage the host in three ways:

- direct tissue injury (mechanical or chemical) or by subverting the cellular machinery so it becomes non-viable
- toxicity: exo- and endotoxins damage the host locally and at sites distant to the site of microbial growth
- immunopathogenic injuries result when the pathogen causes the host immune system to damage the host.

Table 1 **Some major immunodeficiency diseases**		
Defective component	**Clinical disease**	**Defect/result**
Phagocyte	Chronic granulomatous disease	Cytochrome b-245
	Myeloperoxidase deficiency	*Candida* survives
	'Lazy leucocyte' syndrome	Chemotaxis impaired
Complement	Deficiency of C1, 2, 3 or 4	(SLE common)
	Deficiency of C5, 6, 7 or 8	Disseminated Neisserial infection
	Hereditary angio-oedema	C1-inhibitor defect
B-cells	X-linked hypogammaglobulinaemia (Bruton's)	Immunoglobulins absent
	Common, acquired hypogammaglobulinaemia	Low B-cells, poor B & T function
T-cells	DiGeorge syndrome (congenital thymic aplasia)	Absent T-cells, absent CMI (cell-mediated immunity)
	Chronic mucocutaneous candidiasis	MIF deficiency
Combined B- and T-cells	Severe Combined Immunodeficiency Disease (SCID)	T- & B-cell defect, adenosine deaminase defect

---

> **Immune disorders/evading host defences**
>
> - Hypersensitivity reactions occur when an overactive immune system causes injury; it can involve five mechanisms.
> - Immunodeficiency can occur as a result of a primary genetic or congenital abnormality or secondarily from systemic disease or medical treatment.
> - Any component of the immune system can be defective in immunodeficiency.
> - Pathogens have evolved mechanisms to evade each level of the immune response.
> - Pathogens damage the host directly by destroying cells, through toxins and by initiating immunopathogenic mechanisms.

Defences disturbed: general host responses

Fever

Fever is an elevated body temperature, of 37.4°C (99°F) or higher. It is almost always present in any significant bacterial infection but is less frequent and less severe in viral, fungal and parasitic infections. Four questions arise. How is fever produced? Is it useful? Is it harmful? How is it treated?

Production of fever

In the production of fever, five substances are important (Fig. 1):

- endotoxin: the lipopolysaccharide of the Gram-negative cell wall; it is composed of a long carbohydrate chain, a core polysaccharide and the active component lipid A, a unique glycophospholipid of disaccharide, short-chain fatty acids and phosphate groups (p. 46–47)
- peptidoglycan (murein) in the cell walls of Gram-positive bacteria, which lack endotoxin
- cytokines: interleukin-1 (IL-1) and tumour necrosis factor (TNF) from macrophages (p. 29)
- acute phase reactants including prostaglandins.

Endotoxin from Gram-negative bacteria, and cell wall peptidoglycan from Gram-positive bacteria are called **exogenous pyrogens** because when infection occurs they stimulate macrophages to release the **endogenous pyrogens** IL-1 and TNF. These stimulate the acute phase response, and the resultant prostaglandins stimulate the thermoregulatory centre in the hypothalamus to reset the body's thermostat higher, thus producing fever (Fig. 1).

Is fever useful?

Perhaps the greatest use of fever is as an alerting mechanism, so that the host (or its parents!) knows it is infected and ill. In only two infections, syphilis and leishmaniasis, is there evidence that fever harms the organism directly.

Is fever harmful?

Stimulation of the thermoregulatory centre initially results in attempted heat conservation by vasoconstriction, headache and shivering, seen clinically as a *rigor*. When the fever continues, there is vasodilatation and sweating to lose heat. These are uncomfortable but not intrinsically harmful, unless fluid loss or the accompanying metabolic changes (see below) are excessive or long-continued. Temperatures above 40°C can permanently affect the brain or other organ functions. Temperatures above 43°C usually kill.

Treatment of fever

Treatment of fever follows from the above: treatment of the infection, and fluids, nutrition and prostaglandin inhibitors such as aspirin for symptom control.

Shock

Shock, characterised by hypotension and decreased tissue perfusion, is a serious, often fatal consequence of severe sepsis, i.e. systemic infection. It is commonest in bacterial infections, infrequent in fungal infection and occurs in a few specific viral infections. It is best studied in Gram-negative infections (endotoxic shock); shock in Gram-positive infections probably shares some final pathways with endotoxic shock, though it is probably initiated by exotoxins in sepsis caused by *Staph. aureus* [e.g. pyrogenic toxin C, enterotoxin F (TSST-1, Fig. 2)], *Strep. pyogenes* (e.g. streptolysins, proteases) and *Strep. pneumoniae* (pneumolysin, purpura-producing principle, neuraminidase). Yet another mechanism, myocarditis, is the major cause of shock in meningococcal sepsis.

It is ironic that in severe Gram-negative infections endotoxic shock is a consequence of excessive, uncontrolled normal defence mechanisms (see p. 26–29 and Fig. 3).

Endotoxin in small amounts leads to:

- complement activation and acute inflammation
- macrophage and neutrophil activation and phagocytosis
- minor degrees of fibrinolysis and kinin activation.

All of these are beneficial defences to the host. However, endotoxin in large amounts leads to:

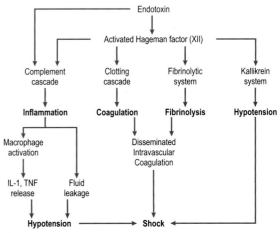

Fig. 2 **Staphylococcal toxic shock – ankle.**

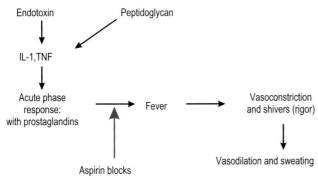

Fig. 1 **Mechanism of fever.**

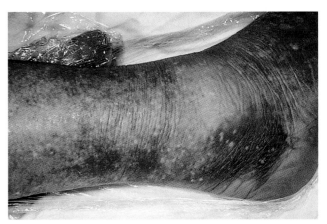

Fig. 3 **Endotoxic shock.**

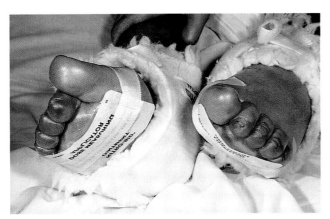

Fig. 4 **DIC with infarcts (death of tissue) on toes.**

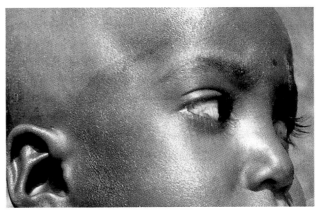

Fig. 5 **Vitamin A deficiency in malnutrition leads to Bitot's spots (xerosis conjunctivae).**

- excessive complement activation and capillary leakage, and hypercoagulation with excess consumption (and therefore lack) of platelets and coagulation factors, hence clotting and bleeding
- excessive macrophage activation and release of IL-1 and TNF, hence hypotension
- excessive fibrinolysis, which with hypercoagulation leads to disseminated intravascular coagulation (DIC) (Fig. 4)
- excessive kinin activation and hence hypotension (Fig. 3).

The end results are severe shock, organ underperfusion and organ failure (cardiac, pulmonary, renal, cerebral) and death.

Treatment of shock attempts to prevent or reverse the pathological mechanisms. It includes early diagnosis and treatment of the causative infection, reversal of clotting abnormalities and excess fibrinolysis, and maintenance of blood pressure and organ function. Anti-endotoxin antibody is available but its place is not established owing to doubtful efficacy and great expense.

Metabolic changes

Changes in energy/carbohydrate, protein, fat and mineral metabolism with infection depend on the severity and duration of infection; the site of infection is also important if it diminishes food intake or increases loss of protein.

Energy/carbohydrate metabolism is increased, with glucose mobilisation from liver glycogen and other carbohydrate stores, from body fat and, in extreme situations, by gluconeogenesis (making new glucose) from body protein. Thus there is increased urinary nitrogen from amino acid destruction, and increased serum insulin, growth hormone and corticosteroids.

Protein metabolism is affected not only by the above protein breakdown (gluconeogenesis), but also by diminished albumin and transferrin synthesis. Conversely, there is use of some of the liberated amino acids in the production of some new proteins for host defence, including complement C3, C-reactive protein and fibrinogen, carrier proteins like haptoglobin and caeruloplasmin, and enzyme inhibitors like α_1-antitrypsin.

Fat metabolism is altered by both defective lipid clearance from plasma, and defective lipid uptake into storage; hence there are increased levels of serum lipids, especially triglycerides.

Mineral metabolism alters. Serum copper increases as it is bound to caeruloplasmin, which also increases. Oxidising ferrous iron for haemopoiesis increases but serum iron falls because it complexes with lactoferrin from neutrophils and is taken up by the liver; this may help to protect the host because iron is important for the pathogenicity of some bacteria. Serum zinc decreases with uptake into lymphoid cells, important in some key enzymes.

Cytokine control. The mediators of most of these changes are the now-familiar IL-1 and TNF (also called cachectin, 'substance causing wasting').

IL-1 increases carbohydrate metabolism and acute-phase protein production, decreases hepatic albumen and transferrin synthesis, depletes fat stores, and moves iron and zinc into tissues from serum.

TNF induces IL-1 production, causes anorexia and weight loss, and has most of the above activities of IL-1.

The consequence of these changes is frequently malnutrition.

Malnutrition

There is a vicious circle that occurs in which infection leads to malnutrition, which in turn leads to impaired host defences and then to further infections. In addition, malnutrition is already a problem in poor communities where contaminated food and water are more likely to result in further infections (Fig. 5 and p. 78–91).

We have seen above how infection leads to malnutrition through fever, anorexia, diarrhoea, increased nutritional requirements and increased catabolism. In turn, malnutrition leads to impaired host defence through skin diseases such as pellagra, or by decreased gastric and gut secretions: both impair the first-line of defence. Decreased complement activity and impaired T-cell activity, also resulting from malnutrition, impair the 2nd and 3rd lines of defence, which impair the 4th line of defence. By contrast, immunoglobulin synthesis and phagocytosis are usually normal.

> ### General host responses to infection
>
> - Fever is produced by the sequential action of microbial cell wall components (especially endotoxin), IL-1 and TNF and, finally, prostaglandins on the hypothalamic thermoregulatory centre.
> - Fever is a useful alerting mechanism, has an effect on few pathogens but affects the host adversely if high or long continued.
> - Shock is also usually endotoxin-induced, causing excessive activation of the complement, coagulation, fibrinolytic and kinin systems, resulting in hypotension, disseminated intravascular coagulation, decreased tissue perfusion and death if severe.
> - Metabolic changes are predominantly adverse, and affect energy, carbohydrate, protein, fat and mineral metabolism.
> - Infection leads to malnutrition, impaired host defences and further infections. In addition, malnutrition frequently co-exists with socioeconomic factors which increase infection.

Staphylococci

Staphylococci are ancient, common, versatile and important human pathogens: some of the osteomyelitis in Egyptian mummies is almost certainly staphylococcal. The microscopic grape-like clusters were described by Robert Koch in 1878, and grown by Louis Pasteur in 1880, who rightly said 'osteomyelitis is a boil in bone marrow'.

Classification and description

Staphylococcus is by far the most important genus in the family of Gram-positive cocci called Micrococcaceae. Two other genera in the family, *Stomatococcus* and *Micrococcus*, very rarely cause human infections.

Staphylococcus aureus, which produces the enzyme coagulase and usually has golden-yellow colonies, is the major human pathogen. It is pyogenic (pus-producing), causing abscesses in skin and most other organs, leading to bacteraemia and endocarditis, and also produces many toxins (Table 2). It has four special characteristics:

- virulence: causing severe disease in normal hosts
- difference: causing different disease in different sites, by different mechanisms, and involving different strains
- persistence: both in the environment, and on humans, who are frequently asymptomatic carriers
- resistance: to many antibiotics that were previously effective.

The rest of the genus are coagulase-negative staphylococci (CNS), and the most important are S. *epidermidis* (formerly S. *albus* because colonies are usually white), and S. *saprophyticus*.

Cell structure and function

Staphylococci have the typical bacterial procaryotic internal structure and Gram-positive cell walls (Fig. 1). In addition to the usual peptidoglycan (murein), S. *aureus* has two special components in the cell wall:

- **Protein A** is unique to S. *aureus*. It is linked to the peptidoglycan with an outer end that surprisingly binds to the Fc receptor of IgG, protecting the microbe from opsonisation. This property is used in some serological tests for other organisms, to carry an antibody against them.
- **Teichoic acids** are polyribitol glycerophosphates found in all staphylococci and are involved in complement activation and attachment to mucosal surfaces as they bind to fibro-

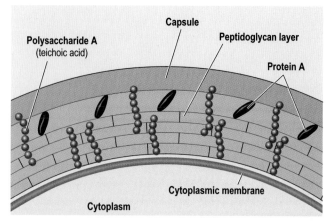

Fig. 1 **Staphylococcal structure.**

nectin. Anti-teichoic acid antibodies are a research test for systemic staphylococcal infections.

Other components include:

- **Capsules** are rare in culture but more common in infected tissue. The capsule protects from complement, antibodies and phagocytes
- **Slime layers** are found in some coagulase-negative staphylococci, which assist adherence to synthetic catheters, grafts, and prostheses while hindering chemotaxis and phagocytosis.

Confirmatory tests

Microscopy shows Gram-positive cocci about 1µm (1 micrometre = 1000 nanometres) in diameter, classically in clusters (Fig. 2) but often singly or in small groups in clinical specimens (Fig. 3).

Culture on blood agar shows large smooth colonies after 24 hours; these are usually golden-yellow surrounded by haemolysis for S. *aureus*, and pale yellow or white for others, but colony colour is not constant enough for speciation. Selective media may also be used, e.g. 7.5% sodium chloride in the blood agar suppresses other genera as staphylococci are unusually salt tolerant, ± meticillin if seeking meticillin-resistant S. *aureus* (MRSA, see below). Meticillin has been standard in laboratory use, now replaced by oxacillin or cefoxitin.

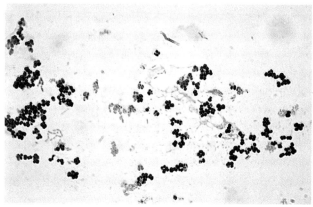

Fig. 2 **Staphylococci in grape-like clusters.**

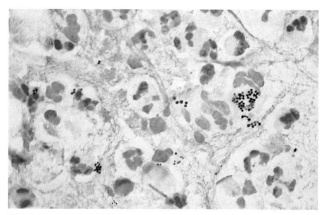

Fig. 3 **Staphylococci singly and in small groups.**

Table 1 Clinical laboratory identification

	Haemolysis blood agar	Coagulase and DNAase	Mannitol fermentation	Novobiocin
S. aureus	+	+	+	Sensitive
S. epidermidis	+/−	−	−	Sensitive
S. saprophyticus	−	−	−	Resistant

Table 3 Clinical syndromes

Organism	Pathogenic mechanism	Clinical syndrome
S. aureus	Tissue destruction	Abscess, e.g. skin, joint, bone, brain, lung, etc.
	Blood spread	Bacteraemia, endocarditis
	Toxin	Scalded skin, toxic shock, food poisoning
S. epidermidis	Adhesion (slime?)	Infected prosthesis or catheter
S. saprophyticus	Adhesion	Urinary tract infection

Table 2 Virulence factors

Type	Virulence factors	Action
Toxins	Cytotoxins (5), alpha to epsilon (haemolysins) (epsilon = leucocidin)	Lyse neutrophils, RBC, other cells
		Inhibit phagocytosis
	Exfoliatin (epidermolytic toxin) A & B	Separates skin granulosum cells
	Toxic shock syndrome toxin-1 (TSST-1) (= enterotoxin F, exotoxin C)	Stimulates IL-1 release
	Enterotoxins (6), A to F	Stimulate vomiting and peristalsis
Enzymes	Coagulase (bound form, and free)	Protects by fibrin formation
	Catalase	Protects by destroying H_2O_2 in WBC
	Fibrinolysin (staphylokinase)	Dissolves fibrin
	Hyaluronidase (spreading factor)	Hydrolyses hyaluronic acid in CT
	Lipases	Allow survival in sebaceous glands
	Nuclease	Degrades DNA
	β-Lactamases (penicillinases, cephalosporinases)	Destroy β-lactam antibiotics
Structure	Cell wall, capsules	Decrease chemotaxis, opsonisation and phagocytosis
	Slime	Facilitates adhesion to synthetics

Biochemical tests and resistance to novobiocin distinguish between species (Table 1). Additional specialised tests are used for confirmation, or for other coagulase-negative strains.

Further tests are used to distinguish between different strains, especially of S. aureus in hospital cross-infection studies. Antibiotic sensitivity patterns may be of some help, or further biochemical tests. Phage typing (susceptibility to lysis by standard panels of bacteriophages), PFGE (pulse field gel electrophoresis) or DNA typing are specialised techniques.

Pathogenesis and virulence

S. epidermidis and related species are members of the normal skin flora, and opportunist pathogens in hosts with impaired defences. They particularly infect by attaching to foreign, synthetic materials like intravascular catheters or joint prostheses, often assisted by slime production. They lack most of the toxins and enzymes of S. aureus

S. saprophyticus has special adherence factors for urinary tract epithelium.

S. aureus, by contrast, has many virulence factors. These are toxins, enzymes and the actual structure of the organism (Table 2). Its success as a pathogen also results from its lack of antigenicity and the consequent lack of protective antibodies.

Clinical syndromes

Staphylococcal infection presents with a wide range of syndromes affecting many tissues (Table 3 and p. 94–223) and caused by three mechanisms:

- local destruction (abscess, Fig. 4)
- blood spread
- toxin production.

Chemotherapy

Penicillinase-resistant penicillins such as oxacillin and flucloxacillin are used for serious infections. First- or second-generation cephalosporins such as cephalothin, cephalexin and cefuroxime are usually safe in patients who are hypersensitive to penicillins. Vancomycin is usually effective for meticillin-resistant staphylococci. Erythromycin and its newer relatives are used in milder infections.

Control

Control is both important and difficult in hospitals, for staphylococci persist for months in dust, curtains and linen, and human carriage is often permanent. Reservoirs, routes of spread and ruptures of skin and mucous membranes differ, so different measures are appropriate in different circumstances; these include cleaning, hand disinfection, air-control, decrease in direct and indirect contact, and portal protection by aseptic or no-touch technique for all invasive procedures.

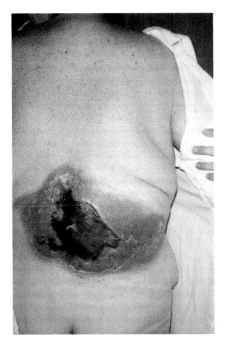

Fig. 4 **Huge abscess (carbuncle) on back with yellow pus, necrosis, ulceration and local spread.**

Staphylococci

- Staphylococci are Gram-positive cocci. They are important pathogens, particularly the coagulase-positive S. aureus.
- Coagulase-negative staphylococci include S. epidermidis, important in infecting prostheses and catheters, and S. saprophyticus, a cause of urinary infections.
- S. aureus is a virulent primary pathogen causing many different infections in many different tissues by three major mechanisms: by abscess formation, by blood spread (bacteraemia and endocarditis) and by toxins.
- Cell structure includes the usual Gram-positive cell wall plus protein A and teichoic acid.
- Virulence factors include many enzymes, toxins and the bacterial structure.
- Management includes antibiotics (testing for susceptibility) and minimising infection by cleansing techniques, control of air and contact, and aseptic procedures.

Streptococci and enterococci

Classification and description

Streptococci and enterococci have certain <u>characteristics</u> that contribute to their ability to cause disease:

- the ability to live as normal flora on our skin and mucosal surfaces, mainly in the nasopharynx, gut and vagina
- *Strep. pyogenes* and *Strep. pneumoniae* are aggressive pathogens with numerous **virulence factors**, which give the ability to adhere, invade and damage tissues.
- other strains are 'opportunistic pathogens': normal flora that can become pathogenic in abnormal sites or in abnormal hosts
- infection is followed by spread locally, to distant organs and to other people.

The <u>description</u> of these organisms is:

- Gram-positive cocci (GPC), usually in chains, sometimes in pairs (Fig. 1a, b)
- non-motile, non-sporing and may be capsulated (Fig. 1c)

- facultatively anaerobic
- nutritionally fastidious, needing blood or other rich media, with some important strains growing only in pyridoxal-rich media
- catalase negative, unlike staphylococci.

The <u>classification</u> of streptococci is confusing, as three separate criteria are used:

- **biochemical** into species
- **serological** into Lancefield groups based on specific polysaccharide antigens in the cell wall
- **haemolytic** by the lysis seen when cultured on sheep blood agar: beta means a clear zone; alpha, a green zone (viridans means 'making green' in Latin) and gamma means no haemolysis (see Table 1 and Fig. 2).

Enterococci are now placed in a separate genus because of different characteristics, including resistance to bile, 6.5% NaCl and antibiotics.

Streptococci that are **obligate** anaerobes are also placed in a separate genus, *Peptostreptococcus* (see p. 55).

Cell structure and function

Streptococci have a complex cell wall (Fig. 3). The biological principle that structure relates to function is illustrated by the components:

- pneumococcal capsule gives resistance to phagocytosis

- lipoteichoic acid on pili helps adhesion to host cells
- type-specific M-Protein in group A gives virulence
- Lancefield group-specific carbohydrate protects peptidoglycan
- linear peptidoglycan with cross-linking gives rigidity.

Confirmatory tests

Clinical specimens (throat swabs, pus, sputum, etc.) are examined by:

- Gram stain
- culture on sheep blood agar shows small colonies, usually glistening, mucoid if encapsulated, and with haemolysis as in Table 1
- biochemical tests (Table 2), and Grouping
- serology for the development of serum antibodies, i.e. antistreptolysin O titre (ASOT) or antiDNAase B (Table 3).

Pathogenesis and virulence

Virulence factors (Table 3) are found in the aggressive pathogens *Strep. pyogenes* and *Strep. pneumoniae* and are related to surface antigens and extracellular products. Some appear to help the spread of disease, but it is not yet possible to link every individual toxin with particular clinical infections.

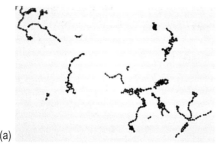

(a)

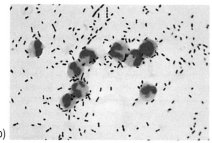

(b)

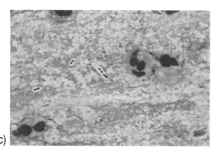

(c)

Fig. 1 **Gram stain showing *Strep. pyogenes* in chains (a) and *Strep. pneumoniae* in pairs (b) and encapsulated (c).**

Table 1 **Classification and normal habitat**			
Species (biochemical)	**Serologic Lancefield group**	**Haemolysis on sheep blood agar**	**Normal flora (nf) or asymptomatic carriage (ac)**
Strep. pyogenes	A	Beta	Throat, nose (ac)
Strep. agalactiae	B	Beta (alpha, gamma)	Vagina, gut (nf)
E. faecalis	D	Gamma (alpha)	Gut, perineum (nf)
Strep. bovis, equinus	D	Gamma (alpha)	Gut, perineum (nf)
Strep. pneumoniae	Ungroupable	Alpha	Nasopharynx (ac)
Strep. viridans group (*Strep. sanguis, salivarius, mitis, 'milleri', mutans*)	Ungroupable	Alpha (gamma)	Mouth (nf)

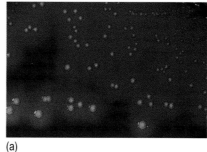

(a)

(b)

Fig. 2 **Haemolysis by (a) *Strep. pyogenes* (beta) and (b) *Strep. pneumoniae* (alpha).**

Table 2 Identification of streptococci and enterococci

Organism	Group	Susceptibility to: Bacitracin	Susceptibility to: Optochin	CAMP[a,b] test	Hydrolysis of: Hippurate[b]	Hydrolysis of: Aesculin	Growth in: Bile	Growth in: 6.5% NaCl
Strep. pyogenes	A	S	R	–	–	–	–	–
Strep. agalactiae	B	R(S)	R	+	+	–	–	+(–)
Enterococci	D	R	R	–	– (+)	+	+	+
Strep. bovis, equinus	D	R	R	–	–	+	+	–
Strep. pneumoniae	–	R	S	–	–	–	–	–

S, sensitive; R, resistant; +, present; –, absent.
[a]Extracellular protein giving synergistic haemolysis with β-haemolysin of *Staph. aureus*.
[b]Now largely replaced by commercial latex or co-agglutination tests. ( ) less common.

Table 3 Virulence factors of *Strep. pneumoniae* and *pyogenes*

Virulence factor	Actions
Strep. pneumoniae	
Capsular 'C' polysaccharides (the most important)	Inhibit phagocytosis and opsonisation
Pneumolysin	Beta haemolytic, dermotoxic
Neuraminidase	Splits membrane glycoproteins, may aid invasion and spread
Purpura-producing principle	Active in animals, may be in humans
Strep. pyogenes	
Structural components	
Capsule (if present)	Not a virulence factor
M-protein	Anti-phagocytic, anti-complementary (i.e. blocks action of complement)
Lipoteichoic acid	Adheres to epithelial cells
Toxins and enzymes	
Streptolysin O (oxygen labile)	Lyses red cells, white cells, tissue cells and platelets, releasing cell enzymes
Streptolysin S (oxygen stable)	Action as for streptolysin O
DNAase, type B	Depolymerises DNA in pus
Streptokinases	Lyse clots, help bacterial spread
Hyaluronidases	Solubilise collagen in tissues, may help bacterial spread
Erythrogenic toxins	Mediate rash in scarlet fever

Table 4 Streptococcal organisms and associated clinical syndromes

Organism	Direct invasion and inflammation	Local spread	Distant spread	Distant toxin effects	Immune mechanisms
Strep. pyogenes	Throat, wound and burn infections Puerperal sepsis	Erysipelas	Septicaemia	Scarlet fever	Rheumatic fever Glomerulonephritis
Strep. agalactiae	Neonatal pneumonia Puerperal sepsis	Abscess	Neonatal meningitis		
Enterococci	Urinary tract infection	Abscess	Endocarditis Septicaemia		
Strep. pneumoniae	Bronchitis	Pneumonia	Septicaemia Meningitis		
Strep. viridans	Caries		Endocarditis Bacteraemia		

Clinical syndromes

Disease is caused by:

- direct invasion and inflammation
- local spread
- distant spread
- distant toxin effects, e.g. scarlet fever
- immune mechanisms, e.g. rheumatic fever.

There is therefore a wide range of clinical syndromes associated with streptococcal infections (see Table 4):

- *Strep. pyogenes*: throat infections, wound and burn infections, puerperal sepsis, scarlet fever, rheumatic fever, glomerulonephritis, septicaemia etc.
- *Strep. agalactiae*: neonatal pneumonia and meningitis, puerperal sepsis
- enterococci: urinary tract and wound infections, endocarditis, septicaemia
- *Strep. pneumoniae*: bronchitis, pneumonia, bacteraemia, meningitis
- *Strep. viridans* group: caries, endocarditis, bacteraemia.

Chemotherapy

In general, streptococci are very sensitive to penicillin, while enterococci are quite resistant to most antibiotics, except ampicillin or vancomycin. However, pneumococci with partial or complete resistance to penicillin (p. 127), and vancomycin-resistant enterococci, are increasingly common.

Control

A multivalent pneumococcal vaccine is used to protect those particularly at risk, including splenectomised and immunocompromised patients. Locating carriers (nose, throat, skin or perineal carriage) is important in controlling outbreaks, especially in hospitals or closed communities.

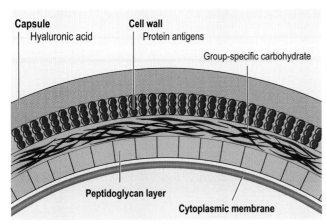

Capsule
  Hyaluronic acid
Cell wall
  Protein antigens
Group-specific carbohydrate
Peptidoglycan layer
Cytoplasmic membrane

Fig. 3 **Structure of *Strep. pyogenes*.**

Streptococci and enterococci

- Streptococci are Gram-positive cocci, usually growing in chains, facultative anaerobes, nutritionally fastidious and catalase negative.
- Enterococci are more resistant than streptococci to bile, salt and antibiotics.
- Identification depends on Gram stain, haemolysis, biochemical tests and Lancefield grouping.
- The complex cell wall and enzymes and toxins have important functions, including adhesion, virulence and spread.
- *Strep. pyogenes* and *Strep. pneumoniae* are aggressive pathogens, invasive and virulent even in normal hosts.
- Other streptococci are opportunistic pathogens, i.e. normal flora that cause disease in abnormal sites or abnormal hosts.
- Disease is caused by invasion and spread, toxin effects and immune mechanisms.

Gram-positive rods: *Corynebacterium, Listeria, Bacillus*

Corynebacteria

Corynebacteria are aerobic (facultatively anaerobic) Gram positive rods. They are non-spore-bearing, non-motile, catalase positive, and ferment various carbohydrates producing lactic acid. The appearance of stained films often resembles Chinese letters (Fig. 1) due to incomplete fission initially during multiplication; *C. diphtheriae* has metachromatic granules, staining a different colour from the rest of the cell.

Only *C. diphtheriae* causes a major disease, diphtheria, now rare where immunisation is effective, as only humans are hosts. Other *corynebacteria* are our normal flora or have animal hosts. *C. minutissimum* causes a superficial skin infection (erythrasma, p. 202) appearing similar to tinea.

Pathogenesis and virulence

Corynebacteria provide a spectrum of pathogenicity from the aggressive primary pathogen *C. diphtheriae* through the normal flora which occasionally become opportunist pathogens (*C. haemolyticum, C. pseudodiphtheriticum, C. xerosis* and *C. jeikeium*) to accidental human infections from animal reservoirs.

Virulence in *C. diphtheriae* is caused by the diphtheria exotoxin, which interferes with protein synthesis; this is only produced when the *tox* gene is transduced into the corynebacterium by a lysogenic bacteriophage *and* when the concentration of iron in the medium is low. All exotoxin is antigenically the same, so one (monovalent) antitoxin is sufficient for treatment.

A second toxin, dermonecrotic toxin, is a sphingomyelinase acting on vascular endothelial cells, increasing vascular permeability.

The role of a third, haemolytic, toxin is uncertain.

Confirmatory tests

Laboratory tests can take a week, so the initial diagnosis of diphtheria must be clinical.

- Gram stain: throat swab often negative
- culture on blood agar is more reliable: three variants occur, *mitis* (small, black, smooth colonies), *intermedius*, and *gravis* (large grey-black, dull colonies), though not correlated with virulence; tellurite is used in selective media
- biochemical tests: *C. diphtheriae* ferments maltose
- toxin production: Elek's immunodiffusion method shows a precipitation line where toxin from a streak of organisms meets antitoxin from a filter paper on an agar plate.

Clinical syndromes and management

C. diphtheriae causes pharyngeal, nasopharyngeal and laryngeal diphtheria (p. 120–121) with a *pseudo-membrane*, or rarely cutaneous diphtheria (Veldt sore, Barcoo rot). The other corynebacteria may cause opportunistic infections (p. 220) or rarely pharyngitis (p. 120).

Diphtheria is completely preventable by immunisation, usually as 'triple antigen'. Antitoxin is essential treatment for clinical diphtheria and must be given as early as possible without waiting for confirmatory tests. Penicillin is used in addition, to kill the bacteria.

Listeria monocytogenes

Listeria monocytogenes is another aerobic (facultatively anaerobic) non-spore-forming Gram-positive rod. Animals are the reservoir. It survives pasteurisation of milk, cheese-making and refrigeration. *L. monocytogenes* causes meningitis, bacteraemia and endocarditis, particularly in pregnancy, babies and the immunosuppressed.

Pathogenesis and virulence

There are no known virulence factors. The important pathogenic feature is its survival protected from host defences as an **intracellular pathogen** in macrophages and monocytes.

Confirmatory tests

- Microscopy: typical rods can be overlooked as commensal corynebacteria; numbers in CSF may be too low for detection in meningitis.
- Culture on blood agar: zone of beta-haemolysis often surrounds colonies (Fig. 2) grown at 25°C.
- Culture in liquid media: unusual tumbling motility is diagnostic.
- Biochemical tests: catalase (+), H_2S production (−).

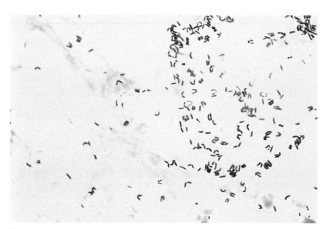

Fig. 1 *C. diphtheriae* with Gram stain showing 'Chinese letter' arrangement.

Fig. 2 *L. monocytogenes* culture on blood agar showing beta-haemolysis.

Clinical syndromes and chemotherapy

Pregnant women may develop bacteraemia, rarely meningitis. Neonates infected in utero develop early-onset **granulomatosis infantiseptica** with disseminated abscesses; if infected after birth, later-onset meningitis develops. Immunosuppressed patients develop **meningitis**, **bacteraemia** or **endocarditis**. Sporadic adult cases of meningitis may be related to cheese or milk products as the organism is common in cattle and goats. The drug of choice is ampicillin, with co-trimoxazole or gentamicin in severe cases.

Bacillus spp.

The genus *Bacillus* consists of aerobic (facultatively anaerobic), Gram-positive rods distinguished by spore formation. The important human pathogens are *B. anthracis* and *B. cereus*. Other *Bacillus* spp. are rare opportunistic pathogens.

B. anthracis

B. anthracis is a large non-motile spore-forming rod. As spores persist in the soil, the usual sources of human infection are animals or their products.

Characteristic **virulence factors** are the capsule, which is anti-phagocytic, and the anthrax toxin. This has three components, the oddly-named protective factor, which with the oedema factor causes severe oedema, and with the lethal factor causes death in the untreated.

Laboratory diagnosis is by finding a large Gram-positive rod, usually single or paired, with a capsule but without spores in clinical specimens, but in long 'bamboo' chains with spores and no capsule in culture. *B. anthracis* differs from other *Bacillus* spp. as the rapidly growing colonies adhere to the media, are non-haemolytic and are 'curly' like a 'medusa head'.

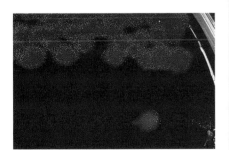

Fig. 3 ***Bacillus cereus* colonies. Culture on horse blood agar.**

The **clinical syndromes** are:

- malignant pustule progressing to massive swelling, systemic symptoms and death (p. 194)
- pulmonary anthrax with rapidly progressive fatal pneumonia (a bio-terrorism threat)
- intestinal anthrax with fatal haemorrhagic diarrhoea from infected meat.

Chemotherapy is by penicillin.

B. cereus

Soil, rice or other foods are the usual source of human infection. Four characteristic **virulence factors** are known: a heat-stable and a heat-labile enterotoxin (necrotic toxin), cerelysin (a haemolysin) and phospholipase C (a lecithinase).

Laboratory diagnosis is by culture (Fig. 3) of incriminated foods in food poisoning, and of the eye, blood or other infected tissues.

Clinical syndromes. These include:

- short-incubation short-duration emetic-type food poisoning from reheated or improperly stored rice (heat-stable toxin, p. 160)
- long-incubation longer-duration diarrhoeal food poisoning (from heat-labile toxin affecting ion transport) from soil-contaminated, undercooked meat or vegetables

- post-traumatic pan-ophthalmitis, usually causing blindness (p. 112)
- rare opportunistic bacteraemia, pneumonia or meningitis.

Chemotherapy is unnecessary for food poisoning, but urgent and difficult because of multi-resistance in the other syndromes: vancomycin or clindamycin, and gentamicin are used empirically until sensitivity results are available.

Erysipelothrix rhusiopathiae

This organism is an aerobic (facultatively anaerobic and micro-aerophilic) non-spore-forming small, slender rod with typical Gram-positive cell structure. It is pleomorphic and often filamentous in culture. Colonies are α-haemolytic, small and grey.

Many animals, especially pigs and fish, are sources of human infection which occurs through a skin abrasion (often in abattoir workers, fishmongers, etc.) producing a distinctive purplish-red spreading skin lesion (erysipeloid, p. 196). Culture of a biopsy specimen is required, as surface swabs are usually negative. Endocarditis is very rare, but case fatality rate is 30%. Chemotherapy is with penicillin or a cephalosporin.

Gram-positive rods

Corynebacteria
- *C. diphtheriae* is an aerobic, non-spore-forming, non-motile, catalase-positive Gram-positive rod.
- There are three colonial types: gravis, intermedius and mitis.
- It causes acute, potentially fatal diphtheria by a potent exotoxin, so urgent treatment is essential with antitoxin and penicillin. Immunisation prevents the disease.
- Rarely, other corynebacteria cause opportunistic disease, e.g. bacteraemia from intravascular devices.

Listeria
- *L. monocytogenes* is an aerobic (facultatively anaerobic) Gram-positive rod. It is non-spore-forming, catalase positive, with characteristic tumbling motility at 25°C. Many animals form the reservoir, and milk or cheese are often sources.
- It is an intracellular organism which particularly infects special groups – pregnant women, newborns, and immunosuppressed patients – though sporadic infections also occur.
- It causes meningitis, multiple abscesses, bacteraemia or endocarditis.
- Ampicillin, with co-trimoxazole or gentamicin, is the treatment of choice.

Bacillus
- These are aerobic (facultatively anaerobic) Gram-positive rods distinguished by spore formation. Soil and animals are the reservoirs.
- *B. anthracis* has an anti-phagocytic capsule and three toxins: protective factor (!), oedema factor and lethal factor. It causes cutaneous, pulmonary or intestinal anthrax with septicaemia, usually fatal.
- *B. cereus* has four toxins and causes two types of food poisoning (emetic and diarrhoeal), serious eye infections and rare opportunistic infections, as may other *Bacillus* spp.

Erysipelothrix rhusiopathiae
- This is an aerobic micro-aerophilic Gram-positive rod found in animals and fish which causes erysipeloid: it is treated with penicillin.

Clostridium

Clostridia are Gram-positive, strictly anaerobic, spore-forming rods, mainly free-living in soil. There are four major human pathogens, but numerous other species occasionally cause infections. The four important pathogens are:

- *C. perfringens*, causing skin, soft tissue, and muscle infections, ranging from simple cellulitis to gas gangrene, and also causing food poisoning and enteritis necroticans ('pig-bel')
- *C. tetani*, the cause of tetanus
- *C. difficile*, implicated in antibiotic-associated colitis
- *C. botulinum*, the cause of botulism.

Features used to distinguish species include colony appearance, the shape and position of spores, motility, biochemical tests and toxin production.

C. perfringens

C. perfringens (formerly *C. welchii*) is a large, spore-forming Gram-positive rod which is an obligate anaerobe, though aerotolerant for up to 72 hours. Unlike most other clostridia it is non-motile, although colonies spread rapidly on agar plates (Fig. 1). It is haemolytic, and metabolically active, doubling in only 8 minutes in ideal conditions! It is found in soil, the gut, the female genital tract and nearby skin.

The occurrence of gas gangrene in war wounds, with extensive tissue damage plus impaired blood supply plus contamination with soil and other foreign matter, led to extensive studies of anaerobic bacterial growth.

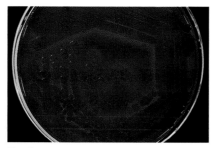

Fig. 1 **C. perfringens culture on blood agar.**

Fig. 2 **Gram stain of clostridia showing short Gram-positive rods.**

Pathogenesis and virulence

C. perfringens produces a huge range of toxins and extracellular enzymes, as might be expected of such a fearsome pathogen. Some of their properties are shown in Table 1 and correlate with five major strain types, A to E: the table is intentionally incomplete, yet still forbidding!

- Alpha toxin is the most important, lysing red and white blood cells, platelets and endothelium, causing severe haemolysis, bleeding and tissue destruction.
- Beta toxin causes vascular leakage and is also important in necrotising enteritis ('pig-bel') (p. 160).
- Delta toxin haemolyses red cells.
- Theta toxin causes haemolysis, pulmonary oedema and cardiac arrhythmias.
- The enzymes help the organism spread rapidly through tissues.
- The enterotoxin is quite different, acting like cholera toxin on the adenylate cyclase system of ion transport to cause fluid loss and diarrhoea (see Fig. 1, p. 50).

Confirmatory tests

Microscopy shows large Gram-positive rods (Fig. 2) usually without spores in swabs, fluid and tissues, but with terminal or sub-terminal spores in media. At times it may stain poorly, even appearing Gram-negative. Appearance is suggestive but not pathognomonic.

Culture should be both anaerobic on blood agar and a cooked meat or thioglycollate broth, and aerobic to detect other pathogens. Rapid, spreading, haemolytic growth is characteristic.

Biochemically, full identification rests on five sugar fermentations and nitrate reduction, but presumptive identification is by two tests: *C. perfringens* causes rapid stormy digestion with acid and gas in litmus milk medium, and the α-toxin (a phospholipase) causes visible opacity on egg yolk medium, inhibited by specific antiserum, the so-called Nagler reaction (Fig. 3).

Clinical syndromes

In skin, soft tissues and muscle there is a spectrum from cellulitis to gas gangrene (Fig. 4) and rapid death (p. 195). In the

Table 1 **Virulence factors produced by clostridia**						
Virulence factor (toxins and enzyme)	Activity	Strain type				
		A	B	C	D	E
Alpha[a]	Phospholipase, haemolytic	++	+	+	+	+
Beta[a]	Capillary leakage, necrosis		++	++		
Delta[a]	Haemolysin		+	+		
Epsilon[a]	Capillary leakage, necrosis		+		++	
Iota[a]	Capillary leakage					+
Theta	Capillary leakage, cardiotoxic	++	+	++	+	
Kappa	Collagenase	++				
Lambda	Protease					
Mu	Hyaluronidase					
Nu	Deoxyribonuclease	+	+	+	+	+
Neuraminidase	Hydrolyses serum protein					
Enterotoxin	Destroys gut ion transport	++				

[a] The first five listed are lethal for experimental animals.

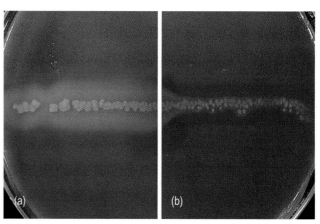

Fig. 3 **Nagler plate. (a)** No antitoxin. **(b)** With antitoxin.

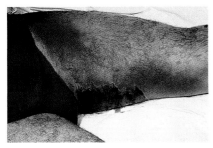

Fig. 4 **Clostridial gas gangrene.**

gut there are two different conditions, infective 'food poisoning', and necrotising enteritis (pig-bel) (p. 160).

Management
Penicillin is given for the tissue infections, but urgent surgery and consultation concerning antitoxin and hyperbaric oxygen are essential. Antibiotics are not needed for food poisoning and are of little help in pig-bel.

C. tetani

C. tetani is a large anaerobic Gram-positive rod; because the spores, when present, are terminal, it resembles a drumstick. It is particularly found in soil.

Tetanus, which is caused by the toxin produced by growing C. tetani, has been known since antiquity, particularly related to war injuries. When a wound is contaminated with tetanus spores, tetanus occurs only if the tissue conditions are suitable for spore germination, i.e. necrosis and anaerobiosis.

Pathogenesis and virulence
Germinating growing organisms produce **tetanospasmin**, one of the two most potent poisons known. It is a heat-labile neurotoxin, of 150 kDa (in a heavy 100 000 kDa chain and a light chain), which is released, binds to peripheral nerve membranes, then moves by retrograde neuronal transport to anterior horn cells where it blocks the release of inhibitory neurotransmitters, thus causing spasms and spastic paralysis.

Confirmatory tests
Diagnosis is clinical, as C. tetani may be isolated from contaminated wounds in which it has not released toxin and, conversely, often cannot be found in the wound (which may be trivial but must be anaerobic) causing tetanus. It may be found in the umbilical cord remnant in neonatal tetanus.

Clinical syndrome and management
The almost unmistakable clinical disease tetanus is described on page 105.

Treatment includes antitoxin, penicillin ± metronidazole, surgical wound care, sedation, and often paralysis and ventilation. Since patients with severe injuries usually receive antitoxin, most cases of tetanus arise from relatively trivial injuries involving contamination with soil or foreign bodies. Active immunisation with tetanus toxoid before injury or after recovery gives excellent immunity.

C. botulinum

C. botulinum is an anaerobic, motile, spore-forming Gram-positive rod with oval, subterminal or central spores. The spores from soil or vegetables are relatively heat resistant.

Pathogenesis and virulence
- *Food-borne* disease is produced (like tetanus) not by infection but by intoxication with an extremely potent heat-labile toxin, usually types A, B or E, in uncooked or improperly cooked foods (the toxin is destroyed by boiling at 100°C for 10 minutes). The heavy chain of the toxin binds to cholinergic nerves, blocking acetylcholine release and hence blocking transmission.
- *Infant botulism* is an actual infection caused as the organisms (often from honey) multiply in the gut and liberate toxin there.
- *Wound botulism* is very rare and is produced by toxin from multiplying organisms in an infected wound.

Confirmatory tests
Diagnosis is primarily clinical but may be confirmed by toxin detection in a mouse assay, or by growth of the organism (made easier by heating the specimen to 80°C for 10 minutes to kill contaminating vegetative organisms).

Clinical syndromes and management
The three forms are food-borne, infant, and wound botulism (p. 158–160, 196). Penicillin treatment is used, but early antitoxin before all the toxin binds to nervous tissue is necessary, and ventilatory support may be needed. Control depends on education in correct cooking and home bottling methods.

C. difficile

C. difficile was only recognised as a pathogen in the early 1970s. It is an obligate anaerobe with typical Gram-positive structure, and resistant spores. It is more antibiotic resistant than other clostridia.

It is part of normal bowel flora in most children and some adults. Its spores persist in hospital and other environments, and some infections are exogenous.

Pathogenesis and virulence
C. difficile produces two toxins, an **enterotoxin** (toxin A) causing secretory, haemorrhagic diarrhoea and a **cytotoxin** (toxin B) causing a destructive cytopathic effect in tissue culture cells. Both cause changes in experimental animals, and each appears important in pathogenesis when the balance of normal flora in the colon is upset by antibiotic therapy.

Confirmatory tests
C. difficile is isolated from stools by anaerobic culture on special selective antibiotic-containing media. Detection (in a tissue culture test) of the cytotoxin is even better evidence of clinical relevance.

Clinical syndrome and management
C. difficile produces antibiotic-associated diarrhoea, varying in severity from several loose stools daily to severe pseudomembranous colitis (p. 159). Withdrawal of the causative antibiotic is sufficient in mild cases, but oral metronidazole, vancomycin or bacitracin is effective in more severe cases, though relapse is common. Control is by judicious selection of antibiotics, and care in hospital practice to avoid cross-infection, e.g. with sigmoidoscopes.

Other clostridia

Other species including C. septicum, C. novyi and C. tertium can cause cellulitis and gangrene similarly to C. perfringens. Apparently spontaneous infection with C. septicum is often a sign of undiagnosed colonic cancer.

Clostridium
- Clostridia are anaerobic spore-forming Gram-positive rods.
- They produce severe disease by numerous very potent toxins.
- C. perfringens causes a range of skin, soft tissue and muscle disease, from simple cellulitis to fatal gas gangrene; it also causes food poisoning.
- C. tetani causes tetanus.
- C. botulinum causes food-borne, infant and wound botulism.
- C. difficile causes antibiotic-associated diarrhoea and pseudomembranous enterocolitis.

Neisseria, Moraxella, Kingella and *Acinetobacter*

These genera contain aerobic Gram-negative cocci including:

- **primary pathogens** like *Neisseria meningitidis*, causing acute and often over-whelming septicaemia and meningitis; *N. gonorrhoeae*, the cause of gonorrhoea; and *Moraxella* (previously *Branhamella*) *catarrhalis*, causing respiratory infections
- **opportunistic pathogens** among our normal flora, rarely causing disease, such as *N. subflava, N. sicca, N. mucosa, K. kingae* and *Actinobacter* spp.

Neisseria

N. gonorrhoeae (gonococcus)

N. gonorrhoeae are Gram-negative cocci which are oval or bean shaped and occur often in pairs with their long sides parallel (Fig. 1). They are fragile and fastidious, dying on drying, and are aerobic and capnophilic (growth enhanced by 5% CO_2). They are oxidase positive. They die rapidly in the environment, and the only known host is mankind.

Pathogenesis and virulence

Figure 2 shows structural features of importance. Protein I has 16 serotypes related to virulence; protein II is found in less virulent strains. Exotoxins are unknown. Gonococci can colonise mucosal surfaces and cause asymptomatic infections, especially in the female genital tract. They can pass through the mucosal cells, invade, and cause inflammation in the underlying tissues. Many strains are killed by serum factors, including IgG, IgM and complement, so disseminated infection to joints, tendons

and skin is unusual. No significant immunity develops, so repeat infections easily occur.

Confirmatory tests

Microscopy is very important. Diagnosis is almost 100% certain if the Gram stain shows intracellular Gram-negative diplococci. False negatives are more common in women and asymptomatic patients.

Culture. Urethral, cervical, rectal and pharyngeal swabs are plated immediately onto warm media. The fragile gonococcus is inhibited by some components of usual media, so isolation is improved by using a selective antibiotic-containing medium (e.g. Thayer-Martin medium) to suppress contaminants, and a rich non-selective medium such as chocolate agar to ensure growth of oxidase positive (Gram-negative) cocci. Joint aspirate may be positive, but skin and blood, even in disseminated disease, are usually negative.

Biochemical tests show acid production from glucose only. Serology is useless. PCR is **P**recise, **C**onclusive, **R**eliable.

Clinical syndromes

The gonococcus is the cause of the venereal disease gonorrhoea (p. 180–186). It infects organs alternately: urethra not vagina, cervix not uterus, fallopian tube not fimbriae (primarily), ovary not posterior abdominal wall. Salpingitis (Fallopian tube infection) leads to tubal block-

age and pelvic inflammatory disease (PID). Urethritis and epididymo-orchitis are the common infections in males. Rectum and pharynx are infected by direct contact with infectious discharge, usually urethral. Disseminated infection is uncommon. Asymptomatic partners are a reservoir of infection, which occurs by direct invasion and local spread.

Chemotherapy

Penicillin G or amoxicillin is still highly effective for sensitive strains, while ceftriaxone or ciprofloxacin is necessary for β-lactamase positive strains (penicillinase-producing *N. gonorrhoeae*, PPNG).

Control

Strain variation and poor antigenicity have precluded an effective vaccine to date, so contact tracing and treatment of all infections, celibacy, monogamy, or safer sex must suffice.

N. meningitidis (meningococcus)

N. meningitidis is a Gram-negative capsulated diplococcus; it is aerobic, capnophilic, fragile and fastidious. It is divided into serogroups by polysaccharide capsular antigens, of which A, B, C, Y and W 135 are most common (these are further divided into serotypes by outer membrane proteins, and immunotypes by lipopolysaccharides). The only known host is humans, and asymptomatic nasopharyngeal carriage occurs.

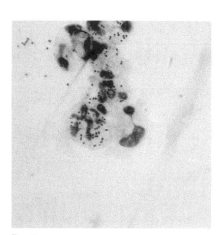

Fig. 1 **N. gonorrhoeae using Gram stain.**
Note the intracellular Gram-negative diplococci, i.e. within neutrophils.

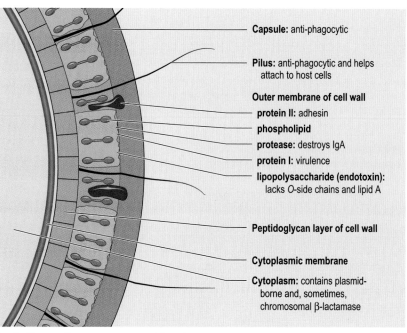

Capsule: anti-phagocytic

Pilus: anti-phagocytic and helps attach to host cells

Outer membrane of cell wall
protein II: adhesin
phospholipid
protease: destroys IgA
protein I: virulence
lipopolysaccharide (endotoxin): lacks O-side chains and lipid A

Peptidoglycan layer of cell wall

Cytoplasmic membrane

Cytoplasm: contains plasmid-borne and, sometimes, chromosomal β-lactamase

Fig. 2 **N. gonorrhoeae: structure and function.**

The meningococcus is very similar structurally to the gonococcus but its more prominent capsule is more protective against antibody-mediated phagocytosis so systemic blood spread is much greater. Continuous production of outer membrane fragments releases great quantities of endotoxin, so shock and haemorrhage are marked (p. 94–95, 142–143).

Infection occurs in three stages, with progression to a further stage often not proceeding:

- growth in the nasopharynx: often asymptomatic
- invasion of blood: petechial rashes, bacteraemia, shock
- invasion of the meninges: meningitis.

Confirmatory tests

Microscopy of CSF samples is often positive for intracellular Gram-negative diplococci in meningococcal meningitis. Culture of blood and CSF is essential but may be negative because of prior antibiotic treatment or inhibitory substances in some media. Colonies are transparent and non-haemolytic; large capsules give mucoid colonies.

Biochemistry is also important. While **g**onococci produce acid from **g**lucose, **m**eningococci also utilise **m**altose (*N. lactamica* also uses **l**actose, and *N. sicca* also uses **s**ucrose, but not lactose).

Serology is useful, as latex agglutination (Fig. 3) detects soluble polysaccharide antigen, especially if empiric antibiotic treatment has made cultures negative. PCR is now widely useful.

Clinical syndromes

Acute meningitis and/or overwhelming septicaemia with haemorrhagic rash and shock are the two major diseases. The Waterhouse-Friderichsen syndrome is meningococcal septicaemia and shock with adrenal haemorrhage and adrenal failure. Rarely, pneumonia, arthritis or subacute low-grade bacteraemia occur.

Chemotherapy

Urgent treatment with penicillin or a third-generation cephalosporin is essential, with appropriate supportive measures.

Control

A polyvalent vaccine is now available but is expensive, and ineffective against the commonest type, B.

Moraxella

Moraxella (subgenus *Branhamella*) are normal flora of the respiratory and genital tracts. The most important member is now called *Moraxella* (subgenus *Branhamella*) *catarrhalis* (for-

merly called *Branhamella catarrhalis*). *Moraxella* are small Gram-negative cocci that tend to grow in pairs end-to-end. Little is known of virulence factors, but about 80% of *M. catarrhalis* produce β-lactamase.

Confirmatory tests

M. catarrhalis is a capsulated Gram-negative coccus, oxidase and catalase positive, which grows on nutrient and blood agar, but does not produce acid from carbohydrates (unlike *Neisseria*).

Clinical syndromes and chemotherapy

M. catarrhalis causes bronchitis, sinusitis, otitis media, sometimes pneumonia and, rarely, osteomyelitis, meningitis or endocarditis. Other *Moraxella* spp. cause eye infections.

Amoxicillin plus clavulanic acid, or erythromycin, tetracycline or co-trimoxazole are each usually effective in treatment.

Kingella

Kingella are found in the human respiratory tract, where asymptomatic carriage occurs. They are small aerobic Gram-negative cocco-bacilli; some are encapsulated. They are oxidase positive but catalase negative, and β-haemolytic on blood agar. Microscopy and culture show these features, and biochemical tests confirm the identity. *K. kingae* is a rare cause of endocarditis and other infections. Penicillin is effective against many strains.

Acinetobacter

The classification of *Acinetobacter* spp. is confused. One acceptable method uses three complexes, *A. calcoaceticus-baumannii* complex (glucose oxidising), *A. lwoffi* (glucose negative) and *A. haemolyticus*. All are small aerobic Gram-negative rods or cocco-bacilli, with some long forms, i.e. they are pleomorphic, ranging from cocco-bacilli to filaments. There are no spores or flagella. They are oxidase negative, unlike all others described here. *Acinetobacter* spp. are normal flora in the respiratory tract, identified by their physical characteristics and by biochemical tests. They sometimes cause hospital-acquired infections, especially ventilator-associated. Community-acquired pneumonia is very rare. *Acinetobacter* spp. are often multi-resistant, though they may respond to sulphonamides, carbapenems or colistin. If sensitive, gentamicin and timentin are used.

> ### Neisseria, Moraxella, Kingella and Acinetobacter
>
> - *Neisseria* are Gram-negative aerobic cocci growing in pairs.
> - *Neisseria* have no exotoxins but numerous virulence factors include capsule, pili, endotoxin and enzymes: gonococci also have proteins I and II.
> - Gonococci are inhibited by serum, so cause local urethral, cervical, tubal, pharyngeal and rectal gonorrhoea, rarely joint or disseminated disease.
> - Meningococci are not inhibited by serum, so spread to cause meningitis and septicaemia with shock and haemorrhage.
> - *Moraxella catarrhalis* is much less virulent and causes broncho-pulmonary infections.
> - The related genera *Kingella* and *Acinetobacter* are of less importance medically.

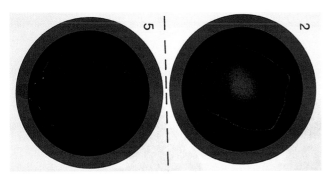

Fig. 3 **N. meningitidis: latex agglutination.**

Haemophilus, Bordetella and Legionella

Haemophilus

H. influenzae

There are many similarities between the three encapsulated organisms *H. influenzae*, *N. meningitidis* and *S. pneumoniae* in virulence factors, pathogenesis and clinical syndromes, though *S. pneumoniae*, being Gram-positive, lacks endotoxin.

H. influenzae is a pleomorphic aerobic Gram-negative coccobacillus which needs accessory growth factors X (haematin) and V (NAD) from blood. It is non-motile and has no spores. Virulent strains have large polysaccharide capsules, with type b the most important of six serotypes, a to f. Humans are the only known host, and non-encapsulated strains are normal respiratory flora in almost all people.

Structural features of importance are:

- the capsule, which is anti-phagocytic
- lipopolysaccharide lipid A of endotoxin, which causes acute inflammation and shock
- a protease that destroys the Fc end of antibody.

Maternal or acquired antibody is strongly protective, so most infections are between age 3 months and 3 years.

Confirmatory tests

Gram stain is characteristic in CSF, pus or sputum (Fig. 1). Culture on chocolate agar (blood agar gently heated to liberate factors X and V and destroy inhibitors), or blood agar with a streak of *Staph. aureus* (to provide X and V) shows small opaque colonies growing best ('satellited') around the streak. Like the gonococcus, it utilises glucose only and is catalase positive.

Serology by latex agglutination confirms the serotype b.

Clinical syndromes

Non-encapsulated strains only cause local disease like bronchitis and otitis media, while capsulated strains, protected from phagocytes, cause meningitis and epiglottitis.

Chemotherapy

At least 20% of strains in most areas now produce β-lactamase, and some also have chromosomally mediated β-lactam resistance, so penicillin and ampicillin are now unreliable; hence a third-generation cephalosporin (or chloramphenicol in poorer communities) is used for serious infections, or ampicillin (if sensitive), co-trimoxazole or cefaclor for milder infections.

Control

Vaccines have been difficult to develop but are now widely available and effective, although antibody response is poorest in the 6–12-month-old child at greatest risk. Rifampicin is used for unvaccinated close contacts of patients with meningitis or epiglottitis.

Other *Haemophilus* spp.

Three other species from the respiratory tract are of some medical importance:

- *H. haemolyticus* because being β-haemolytic it may be mistaken for *S. pyogenes* if the Gram stain is not well decolorised.
- *H. parainfluenzae* (does not require X factor nor CO_2 and ferments sucrose as well as glucose) sometimes causes infective endocarditis and, rarely, other infections similar to those from *H. influenzae*.

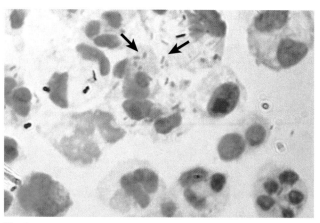

Fig. 1 **H. influenzae: Gram stain of pink cocco-bacilli (few pneumococci also, as purple diplococci).**

- *H. aphrophilus* requires CO_2 but neither X nor V factors, and ferments glucose, sucrose and lactose. Colonies are slow-growing and adherent to chocolate agar, qualities reflected in its rare clinical presentation of subacute endocarditis.

H. ducreyi **is very different**. It does not require V factor or CO_2, is catalase negative and ferments none of the usual three sugars. It causes the sexually transmitted disease chancroid (p. 188). The synonym 'soft sore' is a reminder that the genital lesion is soft, ulcerated and painful, unlike the painless induration of a syphilitic chancre. Gram-stain from the edge of the ulcer or lymph node is more reliable than culture.

Treatment of patient and partner(s) is usually with azithromycin. Ceftriaxone or ciprofloxacin are alternatives.

Bordetella

The genus *Bordetella* comprises tiny Gram-negative, aerobic, nutritionally fastidious rods.

B. pertussis

B. pertussis is non-motile and ferments no sugars. Humans are the only reservoir and source of infection. It causes pertussis, 'whooping cough', a severe but superficial infection of the epithelium of large airways.

Features of importance are:

- fimbriae, which strangely do not assist attachment
- filamentous haemagglutinin, which does assist attachment
- endotoxin, which causes fever and systemic symptoms
- exotoxins (Table 1).

Confirmatory tests

Gram-stain of nasopharyngeal swabs usually shows no organisms, and PCR has replaced direct fluorescent antibody (DFA) staining. Culture needs bedside inoculation of special media, e.g. Bordet-Gengou. Minute colonies grow over 3–4 days. Specific antibody confirms identity.

Clinical syndrome and management

The distinctive disease of pertussis is described on page 123.

Erythromycin and other antibiotics do not alleviate symptoms but diminish infectivity to other humans. Vaccination is

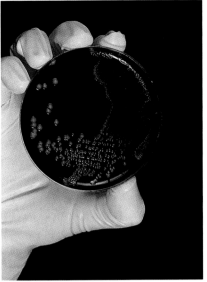
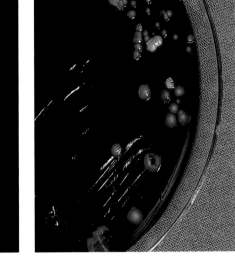

Fig. 2 **L. pneumophila cultured on BCYE agar.**

Table 1 **Virulence factors of B. pertussis**		
Virulence factor	Site of action	Actions
Filamentous haemagglutinin	Host epithelium	Attachment, also RBC agglutination
Endotoxin	Local and systemic	Fever, systemic symptoms
Pertussis toxin (numerous actions, hence many names)	Local and systemic (ADP-ribosylation)	Attachment, blocks cell signals, impairs phagocyte function, lymphocytosis
Tracheal cytotoxin	Ciliated epithelium	Initially ciliastasis, then cell death
Adenylate cyclase toxin	Local conversion of ATP to cAMP	Capillary leak, oedema. Impairs phagocyte function
Dermonecrotic toxin	Local epithelial vasoconstriction	Ischaemia then necrosis

relatively effective, in triple antigen or acellular vaccines, but scare campaigns about side-effects have decreased usage and increased epidemics.

Other *Bordetella* spp.

B. parapertussis causes a minority of cases of pertussis. It is less fastidious than *B. pertussis* and grows on ordinary media, which it may colour brown. It is more active metabolically, being citrate and urease positive.

B. bronchiseptica is an animal pathogen that rarely can cause respiratory infections in humans, including immunocompromised patients. It also grows well on ordinary media, and reduces nitrate as well as being citrate and urease positive.

Legionella

L. pneumophila was eventually isolated from the lungs of delegates to the 1976 American Legion convention in Philadelphia who had developed a new type of pneumonia, which can often be fatal. Other species less commonly cause similar but less severe infections.

Legionellae are small cocco-bacilli, pleomorphic on culture. Virulent strains

are serum resistant, and they survive in macrophages by inhibiting lysosomal fusion. They cause tissue damage, probably by their proteases, lipase, nuclease and phosphatase.

Legionella spp. have a number of unusual features:

- they have a typical Gram-negative cell wall, yet do not stain with Gram's stain (Gimenez and Dieterle silver stain are effective)
- they do not grow on usual media, needing L-cysteine for growth, which

is enhanced by iron and inhibited by sodium and aromatic compounds
- they are widely distributed in water, soil and in the sediment in water systems, and survive 45°C but not 60°C
- they are intracellular parasites, in macrophages.

Confirmatory tests

Antigen detection has largely replaced staining, culture and serology.

- Antigen detection in urine is specific, sensitive and specialised.
- Microscopy. Non-specific stains (Gimenez, Dieterle) are of limited use when other organisms are present in, for example, sputum.
- PCR has replaced the direct fluorescent antibody (DFA) test on clinical specimens.
- Culture. Must be on special media (see above) such as buffered charcoal yeast extract (BCYE) agar, which is buffered to pH 6.9, provides nutrients (L-cysteine and iron), is low in sodium, and absorbs aromatic compounds (Fig. 2). Identification of the species is done in reference laboratories only.
- Serology. This is not reliable diagnostically. Antibodies take 4–8 weeks to appear.

Clinical syndromes and management

Infection may be asymptomatic or result in acute short-lived flu-like 'Pontiac fever', or cause Legionnaires' disease, a severe pneumonia with multi-system (brain, kidney, gut) involvement (p. 127). Azithromycin has replaced erythromycin, plus rifampicin if severe.

Control. Water systems, particularly air-conditioning and evaporative cooling towers and stagnant areas of hot water systems, must be disinfected or flushed regularly to decrease the numbers of *Legionella*, as total sterilisation is usually impossible.

Haemophilus, Bordetella, Legionella

H. influenzae needs X and V factors from blood for growth.

- Virulence factors include an anti-phagocytic capsule and endotoxin.
- It causes meningitis, epiglottitis and other respiratory infections.
- Many strains now produce β-lactamase.

H. ducreyi does not require V factor and causes chancroid.

B. pertussis is a small Gram-negative rod needing special media for growth.

- It has at least four exotoxins as well as endotoxin.
- It causes pertussis (as does *B. parapertussis*, though less often).

L. pneumophila does not stain with usual stains or grow on usual media.

- It lives in the water supplies of buildings, and it does not spread person to person.
- It is an intracellular pathogen causing two different diseases, mild Pontiac fever and severe Legionnaires' disease.
- Treatment is azithromycin ± rifampicin.

Enterobacteriaceae (1)

Aerobic, Gram-negative bacilli can be divided into three broad groups for practical purposes: firstly, the 'coliforms', i.e. intestinal bacteria of the family Enterobacteriaceae (e.g. *Escherichia*, *Shigella*, *Salmonella*, *Citrobacter*, *Klebsiella*, *Enterobacter*, *Serratia*, *Hafnia*, *Proteus*, *Providentia* and *Morganella*); secondly, the parvobacteria (e.g. *Haemophilus*, *Bordetella*, *Brucella*, *Yersinia* and *Pasteurella*) and thirdly, pseudomonads and related bacteria (p. 52–53). The Enterobacteriaceae are all aerobic (facultatively anaerobic) non-spore forming bacilli which live particularly in the intestine and, for convenience, are often called 'coliforms' or 'enteric bacteria'. They cause a range of gastrointestinal, intra-abdominal, urinary, wound and other infections.

Identification of enteric bacteria

Most species are morphologically indistinguishable, being usually straight rods. Otherwise they vary considerably:

- motility: shigellae, yersiniae and klebsiellae are non-motile
- culture: *Proteus* spp. 'swarm' and smell of ammonia; *Klebsiella* spp. produce large mucoid colonies
- biochemical tests: multiple tests distinguish species by differences in metabolism. These tests are usually performed with commercial kits (Fig. 1) or automated machines
- serology: important species are identified by detection of specific antigens by agglutination reactions.

Table 1 shows general features of the main distinguishing biochemical tests; most enteric bacteria are positive for these tests but the exceptions help in identification (Fig. 2). Lack of gas from glucose, non-lactose fermentation (NLF) and positive production of H₂S are all signs of serious pathogens. Other specific tests include ability to grow in KCN, phenylalanine utilisation, ornithine decarboxylation and fermentation of numerous sugars.

Cell structure and function

Figure 3 shows the major structures and their functions in virulence and pathogenesis. All Enterobacteriaceae have H, K and O antigens and endotoxin. Some will produce exotoxins (heat-labile proteins).

Table 1　Biochemical reactions used in identification

Test	Positive result	Exceptions
Acid production from glucose	All	
Gas production from glucose	Most	Shigellae, *Y. pestis*, *S. typhi*
Lactose fermentation	Only *E. coli*, *Klebs*, *Enterobacter*	Salmonellae, shigellae, *Y. pestis*
Catalase positive	All	
Reduce nitrate	All	
Oxidase negative	All	
Production H₂S	Only salmonellae, *Proteus* and *Y. pestis* always +ve	K-E-S-H group always −ve
Urease	*Proteus*, *Morganella*, *Yersinia* spp. strong	K-E-S-H group −ve
Indole production	*E. coli*, *Proteus* spp. strong	*P. mirabilis*, salmonellae, K-E-S-H group
Utilises citrate	Most	*E. coli*, shigellae, morganellae, yersiniae
Gelatin liquefaction	Most	Salmonellae, shigellae
VP	K-E-S-H group	Most negative

K-E-S-H group: *Klebsiella*, *Enterobacter*, *Serratia*, *Hafnia* spp. −ve, negative; +ve, positive.

Table 2　Sensitivity of Enterobacteriaceae (no urines), and increasing resistance in 7 years

Organism	No. of patients	Sensitivity (%)							
		AMOX	CEF 1	SuTM	TIM	CEF 3	CIP	GENT	MERO
E. coli	154	47	**63**	82	85	94	93	97	98
Klebsiella	78	0	82	99	96	94	100	99	99
Enterobacter	79	0	0	**70**	**03**	53	89	**78**	97
Serratia	79	0	0	**82**	**76**	65	65	77	77
Citrobacter	17	0	65	88	**65**	82	94	100	100
Proteus	21	76	95	86	100	100	100	98	100
Providentia	6	0	0	67	NT	NT	83	100	NT
Morganella	27	0	0	100	**71**	**71**	100	100	100
Shigella	5	0	**20**	40	**20**	100	100	100	100
Salmonella	16	94	94	100	100	100	94	100	100
Total	482								
Pseudomonas, NOT CF	325	0	0	0	71	83	76	85	86
Pseudomonas, CF	402	0	0	0	84	81	40	26	81

AMOX, amoxicillin; CEF1, cephalothin; SuTM, co-trimoxazole; TIM, timentin; CEF 3, ceftriaxone (ceftazidime for *Pseudomonas*); CIP, ciprofloxacin; GENT, gentamicin; MERO, meropenem; NT, not tested. ESCPPM see p. 218. CF = Cystic Fibrosis; NOT CF = Not Cystic Fibrosis. **Bold** = 15% more resistant than 1998. Tested in 8 months at The Alfred Hospital, (Monash University), Melbourne, Australia, 2006.

Antibiotic sensitivity

Resistance to antibiotics is becoming an increasing problem in dealing with infections particularly when hospital cross-infection or community spread is rapid. Table 2 gives figures for a complex tertiary hospital. General features of Enterobacteriaceae isolates are:

- *E. coli*, *Klebsiella*, *Enterobacter* and now *Serratia* spp. are the most common in hospitals
- *E. coli*, *Klebsiella* and *Proteus* spp. are in general more sensitive; *Enterobacter*, *Serratia* and *Citrobacter* spp. are in general more resistant to antibiotics
- order of likely efficacy is meropenem, gentamicin/ciprofloxacin, third-generation cephalosporin, then co-trimoxazole or timentin
- amoxicillin, cephalothin and ticarcillin should not be used alone without sensitivity results.

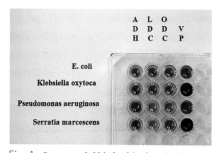

Fig. 1　**Commercial kit for biochemical reactions.**

Escherichia coli

E. coli is a common component of the aerobic bowel flora and causes urinary, wound, lung, meningeal and septicaemic infections. Some strains are important causes of travellers' diarrhoea and the haemolytic-uraemic syndrome.

Identification of *E. coli* and its variants is important because:

- it is normal commensal flora that must be distinguished from intestinal pathogens
- its presence in water supplies is evidence of faecal contamination
- it can be a pathogen.

Pathogenesis and virulence
Entero-pathogenic *E. coli* strains (EPEC) are classified by their O antigens (and subdivided by H and K antigens). Important strains are:

- enteroadhesive (EAEC)
- enteroinvasive (EIEC)
- enterotoxigenic (ETEC): exotoxins
- enterohaemorrhagic (EHEC): cytotoxic verotoxin.

Confirmatory tests
Microscopy and staining shows a motile Gram-negative rod. Culture shows dry flat lactose-fermenting colonies on Mac-Conkey agar (Fig. 2a), and often haemolytic colonies on blood agar. Biochemical tests used include those in Table 1. Note that *E. coli* is citrate-H_2S-urea-VP negative, indole positive and ferments both glucose and lactose with gas. It is motile, unlike *Shigella* spp.

Clinical syndromes
There are four entirely different groups of clinical disease caused by *E. coli*:

- neonatal meningitis from maternal bowel flora and cross-infection (p. 94)
- organ system infections, from the patient's own normal flora or from cross infection, causing UTI, wound, intraperitoneal, bloodstream or lung infections (p. 142, 164 and 174)
- gastroenteritis or dysentery from the EPEC strains noted above (EAEC, EHEC, EIEC, ETEC) (p. 160)
- haemolytic uraemic syndrome (p. 160).

Chemotherapy
Ampicillin and co-trimoxazole resistance are now common. Gentamicin remains reliable. Newer penicillins and cephalosporins may be used.

Control
This depends on hygiene, hospital infection control and the availability of pure food and water.

Shigella
There are four species, *S. flexneri*, *S. sonnei*, *S. boydii* and the most virulent, *S. dysenteriae*. They are non-motile, aerobic Gram-negative rods that are citrate, H_2S, urea, VP and often indole negative and do not produce gas from glucose, nor ferment lactose. As few as 200 organisms can cause bacillary dysentery. Spread is primarily direct faecal–oral (i.e. person to person), rarely via food or water.

Shigellae produce an enterotoxin (shiga toxin) which gives diarrhoea, and are invasive into colonic mucosa. *S. dysenteriae* has a neurotoxin, so headache, meningismus (meningeal symptoms without meningitis) and even fits occur.

Confirmatory tests
Microscopy of stool samples shows many white blood cells but few if any organisms. Culture and biochemistry show no motility, no gas from glucose and no lactose fermentation (Fig. 2b). Serology distinguishes serotypes of all except *S. sonnei*.

Clinical syndromes
Shigella spp. all cause bacillary dysentery, ranging from mild to fatal (p. 161).

Chemotherapy
Only *S. dysenteriae* infections usually need antibiotics to control infection, though antibiotics decrease infectivity in all. Resistance to ampicillin, co-trimoxazole, tetracycline and even chloramphenicol is now widespread, so quinolones, later cephalosporins or gentamicin are used.

Control
Good hygiene, especially hand-washing, is essential.

Citrobacter
The most common *Citrobacter* sp. *C. freundii*, is similar to salmonellae in being H_2S positive, and indole and VP negative, but it is a late lactose fermenter. It is commonly present as normal bowel flora and has low virulence. Clinical syndromes are uncommon, but *Citrobacter* can cause hospital-acquired infections, especially in immunocompromised patients. Gentamicin, ciprofloxacin or a third-generation cephalosporin are usually prescribed.

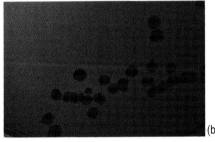
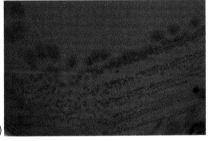

(a)   (b)

Fig. 2 **Lactose fermentation to distinguish species: (a) *E. coli* positive (pink), (b) *Shigella flexneri* negative (colourless).**

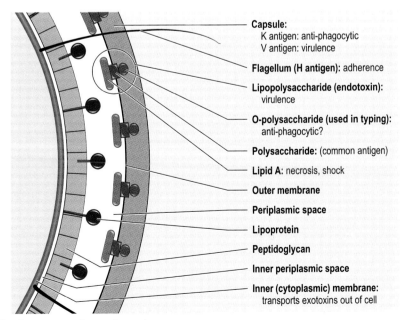

Capsule:
  K antigen: anti-phagocytic
  V antigen: virulence

Flagellum (H antigen): adherence

Lipopolysaccharide (endotoxin): virulence

O-polysaccharide (used in typing): anti-phagocytic?

Polysaccharide: (common antigen)

Lipid A: necrosis, shock

Outer membrane

Periplasmic space

Lipoprotein

Peptidoglycan

Inner periplasmic space

Inner (cytoplasmic) membrane: transports exotoxins out of cell

Fig. 3 **Structure of Enterobacteriaceae.**

Enterobacteriaceae (2)

Salmonella

Salmonella spp. are motile aerobic Gram-negative rods that infect humans, animals and birds. Classification is difficult, as the 2000+ serotypes based on O, H and K antigens (previously separate species) are very useful epidemiologically in tracing outbreaks and yet are not species by the usual rules. One classification has only three species: *S. cholerae-suis* (the type species, basic for nomenclature), *S. typhi* (the cause of typhoid fever, very different from all the others), and *S. enteritidis* ('of enteritis', all the others, causing gastroenteritis). This last group contains a number of serotypes called *Arizona*, formerly a separate related genus, then a sub-genus.

Salmonellae can be divided into two groups, epidemiologically and clinically:

- *S. typhi* and *S. paratyphi* serotypes: these infect humans only, producing severe illness with septicaemic as well as intestinal symptoms (enteric fever)
- all others: primarily animal pathogens, widespread in food animals, eggs and animal feed; these cause local gastroenteritis (salmonella food poisoning).

Structural features of importance are like *E. coli* except the K antigen of *S. typhi* is called Vi (for virulence, though other virulence factors are also important).

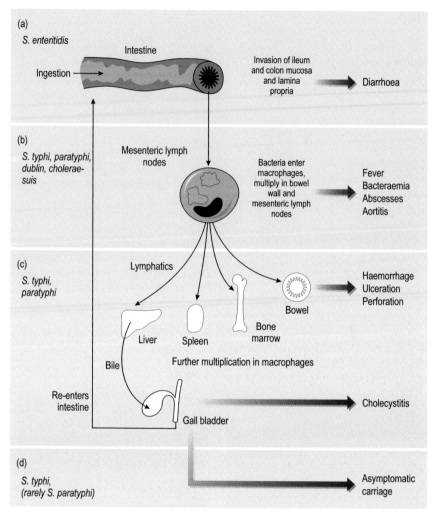

Fig. 1 **Pathogenesis of salmonella infections.**

Confirmatory tests

Salmonellae are citrate positive, produce H_2S gas from glucose (except *S. typhi*) and are non-lactose fermenters. Stool cultures are diagnostic in gastroenteritis, while typhoid fever often needs stool, urine and blood cultures ± the Widal agglutination test with specific antisera.

Clinical syndromes

Pathogenesis follows very different patterns (Fig. 1).

a. **Localised gastroenteritis** (p. 160) without systemic spread (caused by *S. enteritidis* serotypes) results from local invasion (by the bacteria) of the epithelial cells of the gut, then migration to the lamina propria layer where they multiply and stimulate active fluid secretion into the gut lumen.
b. **Bacteraemia** (p. 142) particularly from *S. typhi, S. paratyphi, S. cholerae-suis* and *S. dublin.* Focal abscesses are common.

c. **Systemic 'enteric fever' (typhoid)** (p. 155) where organisms invade the gut mucosa, multiply in macrophages, are carried by them to liver, spleen and bone marrow, where further multiplication causes systemic illness. Liver infection spreads in the bile to the gallbladder, and thence again to the bowel. Colonic mucosal infection progresses to haemorrhage, ulceration and sometimes perforation. This sequence explains the 10-day incubation period and the prolonged illness (Fig. 1). Typhoid fever is due to *S. typhi,* with milder paratyphoid fever from paratyphoid A, B and C serotypes.
d. **Asymptomatic carriage** (p. 155), especially in the gallbladder, with *S. typhi.*

Chemotherapy

Usually no chemotherapy is used for gastroenteritis. Owing to increasing antibiotic resistance, ciprofloxacin is replacing chloramphenicol, co-trimoxazole and ampicillin in treating typhoid. Ciprofloxacin or norfloxacin is used for carriers.

Control

Hygiene in food preparation and storage is essential, and vaccination is available in endemic areas or for travellers.

Klebsiella

Klebsiella spp. are non-motile, capsulated aerobic Gram-negative rods which are citrate and VP positive but indole, H_2S and urea negative, and produce gas by fermenting many sugars including glucose and lactose. Their classification has had many changes: *K. pneumoniae* (including the former *K. aerogenes*) is the commonest clinical isolate and *K. oxytoca* the next commonest. They are normal flora in the gut, and are found in soil, grain and water. *K. ozaenae*, *K. rhinoscleromatis* and *K. granulomatis* are clearly different biochemically and clinically.

A prominent anti-phagocytic capsule causing large mucoid colonies is usual. The cell wall is typical of Gram-negative bacteria, and there are K, O and H antigens and endotoxin as in *E. coli* (Fig. 3, p. 47).

Laboratory identification depends on Gram stain, culture and biochemical tests. Serotyping is rarely used.

Clinical syndromes

- *K. pneumoniae* causes a primary, cavitating, serious pneumonia (Fig. 1, p. 128).
- *K. pneumoniae* and *K. oxytoca* are important in hospital-acquired infections (p. 218) of urine, wounds and respiratory tract from the hospital environment, gut colonisation and other infected patients.
- *K. rhinoscleromatis* causes rhinoscleroma, an unusual chronic infection of the nose and adjacent tissues (p. 122)
- *K. ozaenae* is associated with ozaena, a foul-smelling purulent atrophic rhinitis
- *K. (formerly Calymmatobacterium) granulomatis* causes granuloma inguinale (p. 188–189).

Chemotherapy

Most strains produce penicillinases, so gentamicin, quinolones, third-generation cephalosporins or timentin are used.

Control

Cross-infection measures are necessary, and eradication of hospital reservoirs is desirable.

Enterobacter, Serratia and Hafnia

Enterobacter are very similar to *Klebsiella* except that they are motile, and ornithine positive. They are divided into several species by their biochemistry, especially by arginine and lysine decarboxylase (e.g. *E. cloacae*, *E. aerogenes*, *E. sakazakii*). They are found as faecal flora and in soil, sewage and water. *Serratia* have the same major reactions but usually are pigmented bright pink or red (Fig. 2). They, with *Hafnia*, are distinguished from *Enterobacter* by sorbitol fermentation and DNase production. They are found in faeces, soil, sewage and water.

Their structure and function are unexceptional, and their virulence is relatively low. Laboratory identification is by Gram stain, culture, and biochemical characteristics.

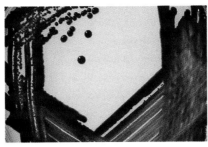

Fig. 2 *Serratia marcescens* **with bright red pigment.**

Clinical syndromes

They are seldom primary pathogens but as opportunists can cause hospital-acquired wound, blood, lung and urinary tract (UTI) infections, especially in immunocompromised patients (p. 218–221).

Chemotherapy

For infections, gentamicin or quinolones are used; third-generation cephalosporins are becoming unreliable owing to the organisms' extended spectrum beta-lactamases (ESBLs).

Control

This depends on hygiene, hand-washing and elimination of sources.

Proteus, Providentia and Morganella

All are aerobic, motile, non-spore-forming Gram-negative rods (Fig. 3) and, alone among Enterobacteriaceae, all are phenylalanine deaminase positive. A commonly accepted division is into *P. mirabilis* (the commonest) and *P. vulgaris* (next commonest) as urease positive, H_2S and indole positive and VP negative with marked swarming over agar without discrete colony formation. *P. mirabilis* is indole negative. *Providentia* are similar in major reactions except that they are urease negative and do not swarm. *M. morganii* is like *P. vulgaris* in

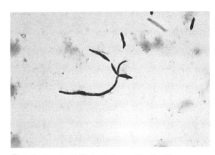

Fig. 3 *P. mirabilis* **in urine: affected by antibiotic.**

major reactions except that it is citrate negative. They are all found in human faeces and in soil.

Features of importance are:

- urease which splits urea in urine, raises urine pH and encourages renal stone formation
- pili may assist both attachment and phagocytosis
- flagellar action may assist spread.

Laboratory identification depends on Gram stain, culture and biochemical tests as above.

Clinical syndromes

Of this group, *P. mirabilis* is the commonest in community acquired UTI; the others are more important in hospital-acquired infections (UTI, wound, blood, and lung). The source is infected patients, not the environment or gut colonisation (contrast with *Klebsiella*) (p. 218–221).

Chemotherapy

P. mirabilis has been more sensitive to antibiotics, but resistance is increasing even to third-generation cephalosporins and often gentamicin, a quinolone or sometimes meropenem is needed for any of these genera.

Control

This is particularly by hygiene and hand-washing.

Enterobacteriaceae

- They are all aerobic, non-spore-forming Gram-negative rods usually found in the gut.
- They are distinguished by biochemical tests, especially citrate, H_2S, indole, VP, urea, sugar fermentation, and by serology.
- Virulence factors include capsular K, flagellar H and somatic O antigens, endotoxin, and some have exotoxins.
- A few are aggressive primary pathogens causing bacillary dysentery and typhoid fever, gastroenteritis, meningitis, pneumonia and urinary infections, but more are opportunist pathogens infecting hospitalised and immunocompromised patients.
- Gentamicin, quinolones and later cephalosporins are often necessary because of antibiotic resistance.
- Control is rarely by vaccine, usually by hygiene and hand-washing.

Vibrio, Campylobacter, Helicobacter, Aeromonas, Plesiomonas

These organisms form, with *Neisseria* and *Pseudomonas*, one of only three groups of **oxidase positive** Gram-negative pathogens.

Vibrio

Vibrios are short, curved, asporogenous, aerobic (facultatively anaerobic), Gram-negative rods. Special features are their comma shape, motility by a polar flagellum, oxidase positivity and salt-tolerance. Major pathogenic species are *Vibrio cholerae*, *V. parahaemolyticus*, *V. vulnificus* and *V. alginolyticus*. They live in fresh, brackish or salt water and infect humans directly or via shell-fish or raw fish.

They have typical Gram-negative cell structure. The somatic O antigens of *V. cholerae* give six serogroups. Most pathogenic strains are O1, further divided into two biotypes, 'cholerae' and 'El Tor', and three serologic subgroups, useful epidemiologically. All antigens are poorly immunogenic, so repeat infections occur, and vaccines are relatively ineffective.

Pathogenesis and virulence

Virulence of *V. cholerae* results from the potent cholera toxin which produces massive secretory diarrhoea (Fig. 1). In addition, cyclic AMP inhibits chemotaxis and phagocytosis. *V. cholerae* is thus an exceptional (and exceptionally effective) pathogen able, like *C. tetani*, to kill by up-regulating a normal biochemical host pathway without cell damage or invasion.

Other vibrios are pathogenic by tissue invasion, though *V. parahaemolyticus* has a mild enterotoxin.

Confirmatory tests

Gram stain is characteristic. Culture of fresh specimens is best on special media such as thiosulphate-citrate-bile-sucrose (TCBS) agar, giving sucrose-positive (Fig. 2) yellow colonies for *V. cholerae* and *V. alginolyticus*, sucrose-negative blue-green colonies for *V. parahaemolyticus* and *V. vulnificus*. Further biochemistry and serology are confirmatory.

Clinical syndromes and management

Syndromes depend on the species:

- *V. cholerae* causes cholera (p. 161) (by toxin)

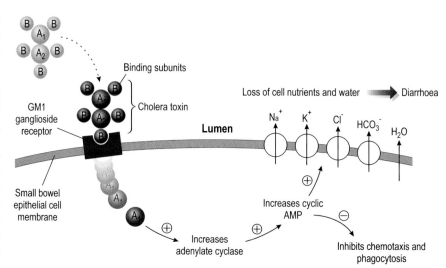

Fig. 1 **The action of cholera toxin.** A_1, active toxin subunit; A_2 binds A_1 to B; B binding subunit to GM1.

- *V. parahaemolyticus* causes gastroenteritis (p. 161) (by toxin and invasion)
- *V. vulnificus* causes severe spreading cellulitis, or septicaemia with unusual skin lesions (by local invasion and distant spread)
- *V. alginolyticus* causes superficial wound, eye and ear infections (by local invasion).

Fluid and electrolyte replacement is the more important treatment for cholera but tetracycline shortens the course. Ampicillin or co-trimoxazole is also effective.

Cholera *epidemics* can only occur with poor hygiene. Vaccines give limited short-term protection. Control involves avoiding exposure, and the provision of pure drinking water.

Campylobacter

Campylobacters were long considered to be mainly animal pathogens, but with microaerophilic faecal cultures at 42°C, *C. jejuni* was recognised as the commonest cause of bacterial gastroenteritis.

Campylobacters are curved, asporogenous, microaerophilic or anaerobic Gram-negative rods. Special features are their curved shape, motility by a polar flagellum, oxidase positivity and need for only 3–15% oxygen. They are unusual metabolically as they use energy from TCA intermediates or amino acids and they neither ferment nor oxidise carbohydrates. Hence they are inactive in many routine biochemical tests. Major

pathogenic species are *C. jejuni*, *C. coli*, *C. lari* (formerly *laridis*), and *C. foetus* (with two subspecies). The pathogenicity of other species is being established. As with salmonellae there are large animal reservoirs of campylobacters; infections result from consumption of contaminated food including meat, and milk from bottles with tops pecked by birds. Rarely, homosexual men have acquired infection sexually.

Like salmonellae, they are not resistant to gastric HCl, so the infective dose is relatively high, usually 10 000 organisms or more. They infect the jejunum, ileum and colon. Probably both tissue invasion and a cytolytic endotoxin are important in pathogenesis. IgG, IgM and IgA antibodies develop and may be protective. *C. foetus* resists complement and antibody-mediated killing in serum much more than *C. jejuni*, so systemic spread occurs.

Confirmatory tests

Gram stain is characteristic ('campyle' means curved), but phase-contrast microscopy may be necessary to detect darting motility. Culture needs the special microaerophilic atmosphere, a temperature of 42°C, and selective media. Identification of species is by biochemical tests including nitrate, H_2S and hippurate hydrolysis, and by antibiotic sensitivity.

Clinical syndromes and management

C. jejuni and, rarely, other species cause enterocolitis (p. 160).

Septicaemia, organ damage (pneumonia, meningitis) and vascular endothelial infections occur with *C. foetus*.

Fluid and electrolyte replacement are important but erythromycin is helpful if given early in enterocolitis. Gentamicin is used for serious infections.

Control
This depends on good food-handling practices and hand-washing.

Helicobacter pylori

Helicobacter pylori is the major causative factor in chronic gastritis, gastric ulcer and duodenal ulcer.

Initially classified as a campylobacter, it is a curved, motile, microaerophilic Gram-negative rod (Fig. 3a), unable to grow at 42°C, strongly urease positive (Fig. 3b) and nitrate negative.

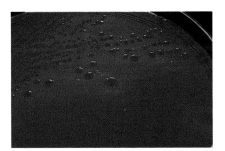

Fig. 2 *Vibrio cholerae* **culture on TCBS medium, yellow colonies.**

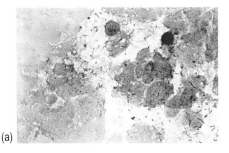

(a)

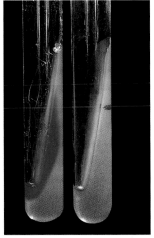

(b)

Fig. 3 *Helicobacter pylori:* **(a) Gram stain and (b) urease reaction.**

Motility assists the organism to move to the chemotactic factors haemin and urea in gastric pits. Urease generates NH_4^+ from urea, neutralising gastric acid. Haemin stimulates further growth of *H. pylori*, then enzyme and mediator release cause chronic inflammation. Little immunity develops, and relapse is frequent.

Confirmatory tests
Non-invasive tests for diagnosis, and for successful treatment, are the C14-urea breath test, and immunoassay detection of *H. pylori* antigen in stool. Invasive tests after endoscopy are the modified Giemsa stain on gastric histology specimens, and strong, rapid urea production (Fig. 3b), which are uniquely diagnostic. Culture (on selective media at 37°C, in a microaerophilic atmosphere) and antibiotic sensitivity tests are not done routinely. Serology by ELISA is only helpful with individual patients if negative, as 30–80% of people are positive without active disease.

Clinical syndromes
These include chronic gastritis, gastric ulcers, dysplasia and cancer, and duodenal ulcers.

Chemotherapy
Various combination regimens are effective. Triple therapy with amoxicillin, clarithromycin and a proton pump inhibitor (omeprazole) probably gives most cures and fewest relapses. Bismuth is unpleasant, and resistance to metronidazole common.

Control
Until the reservoir and route of transmission are known, no logical control measures are possible.

Aeromonas

Aeromonas spp. are short, asporogenous, aerobic (facultatively anaerobic), Gram-negative rods. Special features are their motility by a polar flagellum, oxidase positivity and production of gas by sugar fermentation. Major pathogenic species are *A. hydrophila* and *A. liquefaciens*. Their habitat is water. Virulence is relatively low, and pathogenesis usually by an enterotoxin.

Laboratory identification is by culture on blood agar and MacConkey's medium, Gram stain, oxidase reaction, and biochemical tests including fermentation of sucrose, mannitol and inositol, and ornithine-lysine-arginine tests to differentiate them from pseudomonads, *Plesiomonas*, vibrios and other enteric pathogens.

Aeromonas spp. cause gastroenteritis in normal hosts, and systemic opportunistic infections in compromised hosts (p. 195, 220). Chemotherapy, if necessary, is usually by gentamicin, co-trimoxazole, tetracycline or chloramphenicol. Control depends on avoidance of infected water.

Plesiomonas

P. shigelloides is the only species in the genus; it is a short, asporogenous, aerobic (facultatively anaerobic), Gram-negative rod. Special features are its motility using several polar flagella, oxidase positivity, and no production of gas by sugar fermentation. Its habitat is brackish water, hence shellfish.

An O antigen is related to some *Shigella sonnei*. Virulence is relatively low, and pathogenesis is probably by localised invasion.

Laboratory identification depends on the tests listed above under *Aeromonas*. It causes gastroenteritis, or rarely cellulitis or systemic infection.

Chemotherapy, if necessary, is usually by co-trimoxazole, gentamicin, tetracycline or chloramphenicol. Control is by avoidance of infected shellfish.

Vibrio, Campylobacter, Helicobacter, Aeromonas and Plesiomonas

- All are motile, oxidase-positive, aerobic or microaerophilic Gram-negative rods, often associated with water.

Except for *Helicobacter pylori*, acting locally in gastric and duodenal ulceration:

- They cause disease by enterotoxins or by local invasion, rarely by distant spread and invasion.
- The laboratory should be notified if they are suspected, to use special media or techniques, and oxidase and other biochemical tests.
- Gastrointestinal infection is most common, but systemic infection can occur, especially in compromised hosts.
- Chemotherapy is usually tetracycline, gentamicin or co-trimoxazole.

Pseudomonads and rare Gram-negative rods

'Pseudomonads' is an umbrella term for *Pseudomonas* species plus new genera (previously *Pseudomonas*) including *Burkholderia* and *Stenotrophomonas*. All are an entirely different family from the Enterobacteriaceae ('coliforms').

Table 1 Pathogenesis

| Primary pathogens | Opportunist pathogens | | Accidental infection from animal flora |
	Environmental	Normal flora	
B. pseudomallei	P. aeruginosa	H. actinomycetemcomitans	S. minor
B. mallei	Other pseudomonads	C. hominis	S. moniliformis
K. granulomatis	S. maltophilia	E. corrodens	
	Chryseobacterium spp.		
	C. violaceum		

Pseudomonas and *Burkholderia*

These are Gram-negative rods but, unlike 'coliforms', are:

- strict aerobes (a few can grow anaerobically using nitrate)
- non-lactose fermenting and motile
- oxidase positive, with oxidative metabolism, never fermentative
- able to survive with few nutrients, e.g. acetate, glucose
- widely distributed, therefore in nature, in fluids, in hospitals
- normal bowel flora in few healthy people
- opportunist pathogens infecting those with impaired defences (except for the primary pathogens *Burkholderia pseudomallei* and *B. mallei*) (Table 1).

Their structure is typical of Gram-negative bacteria. From a fluid reservoir by various routes they need a portal of entry such as burnt skin, intravenous drug abuse or medical use, instrumentation or disease. Then their numerous virulence factors (Table 2) overcome weakened host defences, including neutropenia or immune defects.

Confirmatory tests

Gram stain shows slender Gram-negative rods (Fig. 1). Culture is easy on blood or MacConkey agar. *P. aeruginosa* has flat, spreading matt or mucoid colonies, green pigmentation, and a typical grape-like sweetish smell.

Biochemical tests including gelatin, arginine, poly-β-hydroxybutyrate and use of various carbon sources determine the species. Pyocin typing, serotyping and PFGE are research tools.

Clinical syndromes

- *P. aeruginosa* causes lung infections (especially in cystic fibrosis, p. 125), septicaemia (p. 142), wound and burn (p. 196–197), ear (p. 106) and other organ infections.

Table 2 Virulence factors of pseudomonads

Virulence factor	Actions
Common to many Gram-negative bacteria	
Capsule, polysaccharide	Attachment, anti-phagocytic
Fimbriae	Attachment (respiratory tract)
Endotoxin	Fever, shock, DIC
Proteases	Tissue damage, antibody and neutrophil inhibition
Specific to pseudomonads	
Elastase	Vascular endothelial damage, neutrophil inhibition
Exotoxin A, and exoenzyme S (stable)	Protein synthesis inhibition, cell damage, dermonecrosis
Leucocidin	Phagocyte inhibition
Phospholipase C	Haemolysis, tissue damage

- Other *Pseudomonas* spp. mainly cause opportunistic infections, with wound infections, bacteraemia or organ infections, e.g. pneumonia.
- *B. cepacia* (and *Ralstonia* and *Pandoraea* spp.) cause severe pulmonary infections in cystic fibrosis.
- *B. pseudomallei* causes melioidosis, a serious systemic infection (p. 134).
- *B. mallei* is a zoonosis causing glanders in horses; rarely it causes suppurative lesions, pneumonia, or fatal septicaemia in humans.

Chemotherapy

Usually two antibiotics are used, as pseudomonads are intrinsically quite resistant, and host defences are often impaired. Gentamicin (or tobramycin) with either an anti-pseudomonal penicillin like ticarcillin or a third-generation cephalosporin, especially ceftazidime, are usual.

Stenotrophomonas and *Comamonas*

Like *Pseudomonas*, these are strictly aerobic, asporogenous, motile, Gram-negative rods but are oxidase negative (or weakly positive) and have more complex minimal growth requirements. The most important is *Stenotrophomonas maltophilia* (formerly *Xanthomonas maltophilia*), which produces acid with malt-

Fig. 1 ***Pseudomonas aeruginosa*: Gram stain.**

ose, not glucose. It is also found in fluids – water, milk and frozen foods. Characteristic virulence factors and pathogenesis are little studied.

Confirmation is by culture and biochemical tests as for *Pseudomonas* spp.

Clinical presentation is as opportunistic infections from fluids and the environment, including bacteraemia, wound, lung, urinary and other organ system infections, often hospital acquired (p. 218).

Chemotherapy is often difficult, as resistance to aminoglycosides, imipenem and aztreonam is characteristic, and sensitivity to cephalosporins unpredictable. Surprisingly, most are sensitive to co-trimoxazole.

Rare Gram-negative rods

The following organisms are unrelated to the pseudomonads and, mostly, to each other. They are listed here for

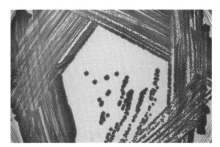

Fig. 2 *Chryseobacterium* showing pigmented colonies.

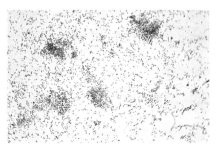

Fig. 3 *Haemophilus actinomycetemcomitans.*

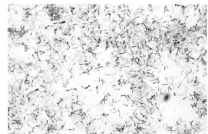

Fig. 4 *Cardiobacterium hominis.*

convenience, being uncommon Gram-negative organisms which at times cause important diseases. Table 1 shows the different patterns.

Chryseobacterium (formerly Flavobacterium) spp.

These are non-motile, aerobic, oxidase-positive, weakly fermentative Gram-negative rods which are widespread in water in the environment and, hence, can contaminate hospital fluids, causing hospital-acquired opportunist infections of bloodstream, lungs and meninges. *C. meningosepticum* is the commonest. They grow easily on routine media and are identified by usual biochemical tests, including citrate, indole, urea, MR/VP, gelatin and sugars, and distinctive yellow ('flavo') pigment (Fig. 2).

Treatment is often difficult because of resistance to penicillins, cephalosporins and aminoglycosides. They may be sensitive to rifampicin, co-trimoxazole and (unusually for Gram-negative bacteria) erythromycin and vancomycin. Control is by using sterile, uncontaminated fluids.

Chromobacterium spp.

These bacteria are pigmented ('chromo' means colour), and similar to pseudomonads and *Chryseobacterium* spp; they are differentiated biochemically.

They also are found widely in environmental water so cause similar opportunistic infections. In addition, *C. violaceum* in warm climates causes infection in swimmers, probably through skin wounds, resulting in systemic sepsis and liver abscesses, often fatal. Treatment may be with gentamicin, chloramphenicol or (surprisingly) vancomycin.

Haemophilus (formerly Actinobacillus) actinomycetemcomitans

The extraordinary former name means the 'ray-shaped bacillus accompanying actinomycetes', as it was first found with actinomycosis. It is a small, capnophilic Gram-negative cocco-bacillus often taking 7 days to grow, even on special media (Fig. 3). It is normal oral flora, and causes local rapidly destructive juvenile periodontitis. Bacteraemia can lead to endocarditis (HACEK group, p. 140–141), endarteritis, organ infections or abscesses.

Abscesses may respond to tetracycline or chloramphenicol, while endocarditis needs bactericidal drugs in combination, usually a penicillin and an aminoglycoside.

Cardiobacterium hominis

This also is a small, capnophilic, slow-growing (1–2 weeks) Gram-negative bacillus (Fig. 4), part of normal oral flora, causing subacute endocarditis from dental disease or procedures.

It grows on blood or chocolate agar, not on MacConkey agar. It is identified biochemically.

Treatment with penicillin for 4–6 weeks is usually successful.

Eikenella corrodens

This is another small, capnophilic, relatively slow growing (2–3 days) Gram-negative rod; 45% of isolates pit ('corrode') the agar surface. It is oxidase and nitrate positive. Being normal mouth and respiratory flora, it (1) infects human bites; (2) causes endocarditis or disseminated polymicrobial infection after dental procedures, and (3) can cause opportunistic infections in patients with oral disease or immune deficiency. It also has unusual sensitivities for a Gram-negative aerobe: it is sensitive to penicillins and resistant to aminoglycosides. It is also resistant to clindamycin and metronidazole, often inappropriately used together in treating bite infections.

Klebsiella (formerly Calymmatobacterium) granulomatis

This unusual capsulated Gram-negative bacterium is difficult to grow and hence poorly characterised. It is diagnosed from tissue smears or sections, usually within macrophages in groups of 15–30 organisms called Donovan bodies.

It causes granuloma inguinale (p. 188–189) by sexual transmission or, occasionally, by trauma. Treatment now is weekly azithromycin for 4–6 weeks.

Spirillum minor and Streptobacillus moniliformis

S. minor is a non-culturable spiral Gram-negative rod with characteristic darting motility from its polar flagella; *S. moniliformis* is a non-motile, pleomorphic, capnophilic Gram-negative cocco-bacillus in chains or filaments, growing best with 20% serum. They are normal oral flora in the rat and either one causes rat bite fever (p. 197), which is treated with penicillin for 10–14 days.

Pseudomonads and rare Gram-negative rods

- **Pseudomonads** are strict aerobes widely distributed in nature.
- They are mainly opportunist pathogens infecting those with impaired defences.
- Virulence factors enable spread of infection from the site of entry, including septicaemia.
- **Some rare Gram-negative rods** are environmental organisms causing hospital-acquired infections from contaminated fluids or equipment.
- **Other rare Gram-negative rods** are normal or animal flora causing opportunistic infections including dental infections, endocarditis, systemic infections or infected bites

Bacteroides, Fusobacterium and other anaerobes

The family Bacteroidaceae are obligate anaerobic, non-sporing Gram-negative bacteria, of variable morphology. A major part of normal oropharyngeal, bowel and genital tract flora, they cause infections if introduced to sterile tissues.

Bacteroides and related genera

The obligate anaerobes of the family Bacteroidaceae are classified into over a dozen genera of which *Bacteroides, Fusobacterium, Prevotella* (Fig. 1) and *Porphyromonas* (Fig. 2) are clinically important. There have been many changes in classification from the original genera (Table 1). All are non-sporing, and growth requires reduced oxygen tension.

Bacteroides produce mixtures of acetic, formic, lactic and other acids from peptones or glucose; fusobacteria produce butyric acid as a major product. Further biochemical tests determine the species and other genera. Their predominant locations as normal flora in mouth, bowel and vagina are also shown in Table 1.

Bacteroides have a typical Gram-negative cell structure except that the **lipopolys**accharide (LPS) of *Bacteroides* does not have endotoxin activity because it lacks two unique carbohydrates. *B. fragilis*, although a minor member of normal flora, becomes the major pathogen because of its numerous virulence factors including a prominent capsule, relative aerotolerance and many enzymes (Table 2).

The pathogenesis of infection is multifactorial: usually the introduction of a mixture of aerobes and anaerobes into sterile tissues produces damage and anaerobic conditions, multiplication of anaerobes, and abscess formation by enzymic action.

Confirmatory tests

Gram stain on pus showing thin pleomorphic pale-staining Gram-negative rods is highly suggestive (Fig. 3). Culture is in specific media, e.g. cooked meat broth, and on agar plates in an anaerobic jar or chamber (Fig. 4).

Biochemical tests provide definitive identification. Gas liquid chromatography (GLC) detects the acetic, butyric, propionic and other acids formed by metabolism; it is a specialised rapid test for the presence of many anaerobes. It helps to diagnose a particular species only in pure culture, not in clinical polymicrobic specimens.

Clinical syndromes

The hallmarks of anaerobic infection are abscess formation and foul pus from polymicrobial, endogenous infection. These include inhalation pneumonia, lung abscess (p. 130), intra-abdominal and pelvic abscesses (p. 164–165), all from adjacent normal flora.

Chemotherapy

Metronidazole is effective against almost all clinically significant anaerobes. Resistance to the previously effective clindamycin and tetracyclines is now common in *B. fragilis*. Some cephalosporins (cefoxitin, cefotetan) are reasonably effective, but various β-lactamases are now widespread.

Table 1 Name changes of anaerobic bacteria, and usual habitat as normal flora

Current name	Previous name(s)	Normal flora in			
		Mouth	Small bowel	Large bowel	Vagina
Fusobacterium nucleatum subspecies *nucleatum*	*Fusobacterium nucleatum*	+	+	+	+
Peptostreptococcus spp.	Most peptococci	+	+	+	+
Porphyromonas asaccharolytica	*Bacteroides asaccharolyticus*	+	–	–	–
Porphyromonas gingivalis	*Bacteroides gingivalis*	+	–	–	–
Prevotella intermedia	*Bacteroides intermedius*	+	–	–	–
Prevotella melaninogenica	*Bacteroides melaninogenicus*	+	+	–	–
Bacteroides fragilis group*	Subspp were spp.	–	–	+	–
Prevotella bivia	*Bacteroides bivius*	–	–	–	+
Prevotella disiens	*Bacteroides disiens*	–	–	–	+

*B. fragilis group includes five subspecies, *B. fragilis* subsp. *fragilis, B. fragilis* subsp. *distasonis, B. fragilis* subsp. *ovalis, B fragilis* subsp. *thetaiotamicron,* and *B. fragilis* subsp. *vulgatus.*

Table 2 Virulence factors and pathogenesis

Virulence factor	Action	*B. fragilis* group	*P. melaninogenica*	*Fusobacterium* spp.
Structural factors				
Capsule (polysaccharide)	Anti-phagocytic, adherence	+++	±	–
Fimbriae	Adherence	–	+	+
Lipopolysaccharide	Endotoxin	NO!	–	+
	WBC migration	+	+	+
	WBC chemotaxis	+	+	+
Enzymes				
Catalase, superoxide dismutase	Aerotolerance	+	+	+
β-Lactamases	Anti-antibiotic	+++	++	+
Collagenase	Lyses collagen	+	+	–
DNAase	Liquefies pus	+	+	+
Fibrinolysin	Lyses fibrin	+	+	–
Neuraminidase	Hydrolyses protein	+	+	–
Ig proteases	Inactivate antibody	–	+	–
Chondroitin sulphatase, heparinase and hyaluronidase	Reduce cell adhesion	+	–	–

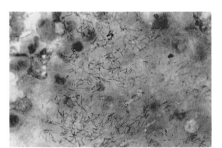

Fig. 1 *Prevotella disiens* **Gram stain.**

Control

Chemoprophylaxis including anti-anaerobic drugs before colonic and other high-risk surgery is essential and now routine.

Peptococcus and *Peptostreptococcus*

These Gram-*positive* cocci are obligate anaerobes which can use peptones or amino acids as their sole energy source.

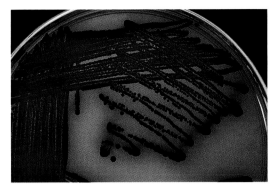

Fig. 2 *Porphyromonas asaccharolytica* **culture.**

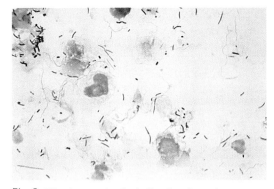

Fig. 3 **Mixed anaerobes including *Fusobacterium* sp. (Gram stain).**

Reclassification in 1983 left only one species in *Peptococcus* (*P. niger*, named from its black colonies), with all others transferred to join the peptostreptococci, of which *P. anaerobius* is commonest. All clinically important species are, like Bacteroidaceae, normal flora in the mouth and upper respiratory tract, the bowel and the vagina.

Peptococcus and *Peptostreptococcus* differ from *Bacteroides* in at least four important ways:

- they are Gram-positive
- they are less virulent, and usually only found in mixed infections with other bacteria, including *Bacteroides*
- they actually outnumber the anaerobic Gram-*negative* bacilli in the vagina, hence are prominent in pelvic infections
- they are normal skin flora, hence found in surgical and wound infections.

Laboratory identification is by Gram stain, anaerobic culture, biochemical tests and sometimes GLC.

Clinical syndromes

As with the Bacteroidaceae, the hallmarks of anaerobic infection are abscess formation and foul pus from polymicrobial, endogenous infection. Anaerobic cocci form about 25% of the isolates in such infections. These include inhalation pneumonia, lung abscess, intra-abdominal and pelvic abscesses (see above), plus surgical and wound infections, all from adjacent normal flora.

Chemotherapy and control

Therapy is usually with penicillins, cephalosporins or clindamycin. Metronidazole is less effective.

Control is by perioperative chemoprophylaxis, as for Bacteroidaceae.

Veillonella

Veillonella parvula is an anaerobic Gram-*negative* coccus, but otherwise has many similarities with the peptostreptococci:

- normal flora in mouth, colon and vagina
- low virulence

- polymicrobial infections (but only 1% of anaerobic isolates)
- clinical laboratory methods similar
- clinical infections in normally sterile lungs, abdomen and pelvis by spread from adjacent normal flora
- chemotherapy by penicillins, cephalosporins or clindamycin (metronidazole is usually effective)
- control by chemoprophylaxis.

Aerococcus

Aerococcus viridans is *microaerophilic* and Gram-positive but is listed here for convenience. It is slow growing, α-haemolytic, weakly catalase positive, and identification is by biochemical tests. Unlike the other bacteria described here, it is not part of our normal flora, but an environmental organism, found in the air, dust and surfaces. Therefore it is occasionally an opportunist pathogen in wounds but is usually only a contaminant; treatment with penicillin, erythromycin or a cephalosporin is therefore seldom necessary.

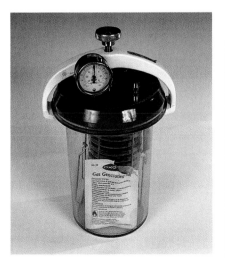

Fig. 4 **Anaerobic jar used for culture.**

Bacteroides, Fusobacterium and other anaerobes

- ***Bacteroides*** and ***Fusobacterium*** spp. are obligate anaerobic non-sporing Gram-negative bacilli.
- They are normal flora in oropharynx, bowel and vagina and cause polymicrobic infections (with foul pus in abscesses) by numerous virulence factors when they are spread to adjacent tissues.
- Chemotherapy or prophylaxis is usually metronidazole or selected cephalosporins.
- **Peptococci** and **peptostreptococci** are obligate anaerobic non-sporing Gram-positive cocci.
- They are normal flora in oropharynx, bowel and especially vagina and skin, and are part of polymicrobic infections when spread to adjacent tissues.
- Chemotherapy or prophylaxis is usually penicillins or cephalosporins.
- **Veillonellae** are obligate anaerobic non-sporing Gram-negative cocci, similar to the above but less virulent and, hence, less important.
- **Aerococci** are microaerophilic Gram-positive cocci quite different from all the above, being environmental airborne organisms, usually found only as contaminants.

Zoonotic bacteria

Zoonoses are human diseases caused by a pathogen with an animal reservoir. This excludes diseases like malaria where humans are essential in the pathogen's life cycle. Table 1 lists some important zoonoses caused by bacteria. See later pages for zoonoses caused by fungi, viruses, helminths and protozoa.

Brucella

Brucellae are small, non-spore-forming, non-motile, non-capsulated strictly aerobic Gram-negative cocco-bacilli, needing several vitamins yet still slow to grow. *B. abortus* needs added CO_2. They are catalase, oxidase, nitrate and urea positive; citrate, indole and VP negative. There are four medically important species, differentiated biochemically and by growth or inhibition by two dyes, basic fuchsin and thionin.

Brucellae are animal pathogens which infect humans by direct contact (farmers, vets, abattoir workers), or through unpasteurised milk or cheese, or through inhalation (laboratory workers).

Virulence and pathogenesis
The marked difference in virulence of different species is not well understood:

- 'smooth' organisms are more virulent than 'rough' but have no detectable capsule
- they are intracellular pathogens, protected from many host defences
- they cause degeneration and lysis of neutrophils and macrophages by unknown mechanisms, blocked by antibody from previous infection.

The pathogenesis is better understood, for brucellae are phagocytosed into macrophages and carried to the reticuloendothelial system (liver, spleen and lymph nodes), where they multiply, form granulomata and spread by bacteraemia to cause destructive lesions in bones, joints and other tissues (p. 209).

Confirmatory tests
Staining is of little use because of their small size. Culture is more useful, but the laboratory must be notified to use rich blood media and prolonged incubation (and CO_2 for *B. abortus*, described by Bang). Staff take great care to avoid laboratory infections!

Serology is helpful. The standard (tube) agglutination test (SAT or STA) mainly measures IgM (not to *B. canis*) and so is positive in acute disease; false positives from cross-reactivity occur from cholera vaccination, cholera and tularaemia. The complement fixation test (CFT) mainly measures IgG so is positive in subacute and chronic disease, when SAT can have become negative.

Clinical syndromes (p. 212)
The course of infection may be subclinical, acute, subacute, relapsing or chronic. The intensity may be mild (*B. abortus*, *B. canis*), or severe (*B. melitensis*, *B. suis*).

The manifestations are extremely variable but combine:

- undulant fever (one name of the disease, p. 212)
- systemic symptoms such as weakness and weight loss
- widespread or focal organ involvement.

'If your joints give you a pang,
And your gum falls away
from your fang,
If you shiver and shake,
And your testicles ache,
You've *Brucella abortus* (Bang).'

Chemotherapy
Doxycycline plus either rifampicin or gentamicin is now standard.

Control
Eradication campaigns particularly in cattle have been very successful in numerous countries.

Yersinia spp.

Y. enterocolitica
Y. enterocolitica is a non-lactose fermenting, aerobic, Gram-negative rod in the family Enterobacteriaceae. It is motile at 22°C but not at 37°C. It is found in numerous domestic animals, in water, milk and other foods. It is identified biochemically and serologically. Characteristics of virulence and pathogenesis are not well understood but include V and W antigens, endotoxin and an enterotoxin, serum resistance and penetration of epithelium. After ingestion, it causes enterocolitis and mesenteric lymphadenitis.

Laboratory isolation is unlikely from faeces without cold 'enrichment' at 4°C for several weeks. Culture from tissues is easier but slow. Serology is only useful retrospectively.

Clinical syndromes include enterocolitis (p. 161) or Reiter's syndrome (p. 180–181). Septicaemia even in immunocompromised patients is rare.

Chemotherapy is of doubtful value in the self-limited enterocolitis. In septicaemia (mortality 50%), gentamicin, a third-generation cephalosporin or chloramphenicol is given. Control is by hygiene to prevent water- and food-borne infections.

Y. pseudotuberculosis
Y. pseudotuberculosis was first isolated from humans in 1953. It is similar to *Y. enterocolitica* but can be distinguished biochemically and serologically. It is

Table 1 Sources, spread and syndromes

Organism	Epidemiological source	Transmission from source	Pathogenic mechanism	Clinical syndrome
Brucella spp.	Cattle, goats, sheep, dogs, pigs	Direct contact, ingestion (inhalation)	Distant spread	Brucellosis
Yersinia enterocolitica	Animals, meat, milk	Ingestion	Local invasion	Enterocolitis
Y. pestis	Rat, flea (humans)	Flea bite, inhalation (1–10 bacteria!)	Local spread Distant spread Aspiration	Bubonic plague Septicaemic plague Pneumonic plague
Pasteurella multocida	Cats, dogs	Animal bite, inhalation	Local spread Aspiration Distant spread	Cellulitis Pneumonia Opportunist
Francisella tularensis	Rabbits, ticks, rodents, water	Bites, ingestion, contact	Local spread Distant spread	Ulceroglandular, oculoglandular Typhoidal tularaemia
Bacillus anthracis (p. 39)	Cattle, goats, horses, sheep, pigs	Contact, inhalation, ingestion	Local spread Distant spread	Anthrax, septicaemia (p. 194)
Salmonella spp. (p. 48)	Many animals	Ingestion	Local invasion Distant spread	Gastroenteritis (p. 160) Typhoid fever (p. 155)
Leptospira interrogans (p. 59)	Mammals	Infected animal urine	Distant spread	Leptospirosis (p. 212)
Borrelia burgdorferi (p. 58)	Wild mammals	Tick bite	Local and distant spread	Lyme disease (p. 154)

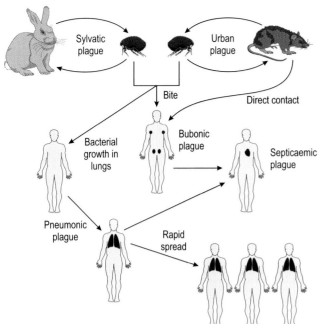

Fig. 1 **Spread of plague.**

found in many wild and domestic animals and birds, water and milk. It causes pseudotuberculosis. Its virulence and pathogenesis result from an endotoxin and its ability to invade and to survive intracellularly.

Y. pseudotuberculosis causes mesenteric adenitis, mimicking acute appendicitis. Rarely, erythema nodosum or septicaemia occur. Chemotherapy when needed is ciprofloxacin, or ampicillin plus gentamicin, and control is by avoiding animal faeces or infected milk.

Y. pestis

Plague is known from the 6th century pandemic. The organism was discovered in Hong Kong in the third pandemic, 1894.

Y. pestis (formerly *Pasteurella pestis*) is also an aerobic Gram-negative rod, but it is non-motile, and has bipolar staining. It has two epidemiologic cycles, sylvatic (forest) plague in wild mammals and their fleas, and urban plague in rats and their fleas. Humans are infected from the animals (now more usual), from fleas (classically) or from humans with pneumonic plague (rare but terrible) (Fig. 1 and p. 212–213).

Laboratory identification is by Gram-stain of lymph node aspirate (positive in 85% of cases), and blood culture.

The organism is readily phagocytosed, but survives and multiplies within the cells (causing enlarged painful lymph nodes), is released and is then resistant to host defences. Endotoxaemia, shock, haemorrhage and 'Black Death' follow. Clinical presentation is as:

- bubonic plague: swollen nodes then systemic symptoms
- septicaemic plague: fever, prostration and death in 2 days
- pneumonic plague: fever, x-ray changes, pneumonia, death.

Chemotherapy is with streptomycin ± tetracycline, and control is best achieved by avoidance of infection, and selective prophylaxis with tetracycline for close contacts.

Pasteurella

P. multocida is the major human pathogen in this genus, which is part of the same family as *Haemophilus*. Pasteurellae are aerobic, non-motile Gram-negative rods that are catalase and oxidase positive, ferment sugars with acid, not gas production. *P. multocida* are carried in the respiratory tract of and are pathogenic to many animals ('multocida = killing many').

Laboratory identification is by Gram stain, culture on blood or chocolate agar, and routine biochemical tests.

Clinical syndromes are:

- cellulitis (rarely osteomyelitis, p. 207) from an animal bite (p. 197)
- opportunist infections in immunocompromised patients
- respiratory infection from inhalation (rare).

Chemotherapy is with penicillin or a cephalosporin, and control is by animal avoidance!

Francisella tularensis

F. tularensis is a tiny fastidious aerobic Gram-negative pleomorphic cocco-bacillus occurring with several **biovars** (**bio**chemical **var**ieties). It causes tularaemia in rabbits, rodents and ticks, and in humans by four routes:

- animal or tick bites
- animal contact
- infected meat or water (10 million organisms needed)
- inhalation (only 10–50 organisms needed).

Virulence depends on an antiphagocytic capsule, on endotoxin and on protection from antibody while intracellular. Bacteraemia follows entry, then transport and multiplication in phagocytes is followed by focal necrosis and granulomata in infected organs.

For laboratory identification, Gram stain is usually unsuccessful, and culture is difficult, delayed and dangerous. Serology is, therefore, the usual method of diagnosis but does not distinguish recent from previous infection.

Clinical syndromes (p. 213) depend mainly on the route of infection:

- ulceroglandular or glandular from bite or skin contact
- oculoglandular or oropharyngeal from local infection
- intestinal from ingestion, or pulmonary from inhalation
- typhoidal (febrile, systemic) from any route.

Chemotherapy is by streptomycin or gentamicin, and control is by avoiding the reservoirs and vectors, or experimental vaccine.

Brucella
- Infection is by direct contact, usually occupational, or by ingestion.
- Diagnosis is by culture (dangerous) and serology.
- Brucellosis is often a long-continued systemic infection with organisms multiplying inside the cells of the reticuloendothelial system producing a granulomatous reaction, then spreading to many systems.
- Chemotherapy is with tetracycline and streptomycin, but is often ineffective with relapses occurring.

Yersinia
- Infect humans from animals and their products.
- *Y. enterocolitica* principally causes enterocolitis, *Y. pseudotuberculosis* causes pseudotuberculosis, principally mesenteric adenitis.
- *Y. pestis* causes bubonic, septicaemic and pneumonic plague.
- Chemotherapy is tetracycline, streptomycin or gentamicin.
- Control is avoidance of the animal reservoir, or vector.

Pasteurella
- *P. multocida* is pathogenic to many animals, usually infects humans by an animal bite, and is treated usually by a penicillin.

Francisella
- *F. tularensis* is dangerous to culture and causes tularaemia in humans when caught from animals, e.g. from rabbits or ticks.
- Disease is ulcerative, glandular, local or systemic ('typhoidal') and is treated with streptomycin or gentamicin.

Spirochaetes: treponemes, borreliae, leptospires

The family Spirochaetaceae include three medically important genera: *Treponema*, *Borrelia* and *Leptospira*. These bacteria differ considerably from all those already considered:

- spiral shape: long, thin and poorly staining
- cell wall Gram-negative-like but has no lipopolysaccharide (LPS)
- culture difficult or impossible in the laboratory
- virulence and pathogenesis thus little understood
- diagnosis by special microscopy and serology, not by Gram stain and culture.

Treponema pallidum

Syphilis was probably brought to Europe by Columbus' sailors 500 years ago. The long, thin spiral is about 0.15μm wide and 12μm long, with internal axial fibrils inserted at each end (Fig. 1) resulting in rapid corkscrew movements and periodic angular bending of the cell body. It is actually classified as *T. pallidum* subspecies *pallidum* but is usually called simply *T. pallidum*. It is very fragile, does not live in culture and dies quickly with drying or heat. It infects only humans and rabbits.

Virulence and pathogenesis

Study of virulence and pathogenesis is limited by failure of laboratory culture (except in rabbit testes). Treponemes enter through intact or abraded skin or mucous membrane, then multiply locally causing tissue destruction, i.e. an ulcer called the **primary chancre**. This heals while the organism spreads systemically, giving the **secondary stage** of fever, 'flu', rash (Fig. 2) and lymphadenopathy 2–6 weeks later. In 70% of patients this passes to **asymptomatic latent syphilis** for 3–30 years, then **tertiary syphilis** develops. This is vasculitis and chronic inflammation, by both direct spirochaetal action (gumma formation) and by cell-mediated hypersensitivity to spirochaetal antigens without live spirochaetes. Antibody is not protective, though useful in diagnosis.

Confirmatory tests

Diagnosis is usually by serology, though immediate dark-ground microscopy (DGM) of exudate from skin ulcers or genital mucous membrane is reliable if positive. (DGM is not suitable for mouth swabs, as non-*pallidum* spirochaetes are normal flora.)

Serology diagnoses spirochaetal disease, not syphilis uniquely. The tests are (1) *non-specific*, such as the VDRL and RPR (rapid plasma reagin) for IgG and IgM 'reagin' antibodies to lipids from damaged host cells (Fig. 3); (2) *specific*, using antitreponemal antibody in the TPHA or TPPA (*T. pallidum* Haem- or Particle-Agglutination), EIA (Enzyme Immuno-Assay) or FTA-ABS (fluorescent treponemal antibody absorption) tests.

All tests may be negative in primary syphilis, become positive during the secondary stage, and, by definition, one at least must be positive in latent syphilis. The FTA becomes negative in 5% and the VDRL in up to 50% of patients with tertiary syphilis. *The non-specific, but not the specific, tests become negative with treatment.* The specific tests are, therefore, used to diagnose if a patient ever had syphilis, while the non-specific are used to assess treatment success.

Clinical syndrome

Syphilis is described on pages 98–99, 112, 189 and 203. Endemic syphilis spread non-venereally by direct contact is called Bejel (p. 203).

Chemotherapy

Fortunately penicillin remains very effective in primary, secondary, untreated latent, and tertiary syphilis with live spirochaetes and gumma formation. Tertiary syphilis with few or no live spirochaetes, such as tabes dorsalis or meningovascular syphilis (p. 98–99), of course, does not respond as well.

Control

Congenital syphilis is controlled by routine antenatal testing and treatment of infected mothers. Venereal syphilis is partly controlled by treatment of infectious patients and their partners, by less promiscuity and by condom use. There is no vaccine.

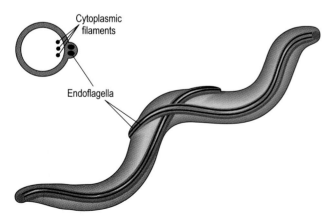

Fig. 1 **T. pallidum structure.** Organisms are long and helical shaped with their flagella between the cell wall and the outer membrane. The flagella originate at each end of the cell and wrap around it in a spiral to overlap at the middle of the cell. From the flagellar basal bodies, cytoplasmic filaments originate.

Cytoplasmic filaments

Endoflagella

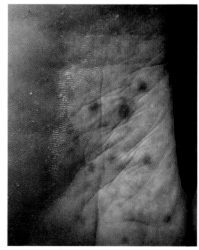

Fig. 2 **Rash of secondary syphilis (sole of foot).**

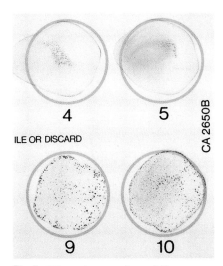

Fig. 3 **RPR serology test for syphilis.**

Other treponemes

T. pertenue

T. pertenue is almost indistinguishable from *T. pallidum* and is correctly named *T. pallidum* subsp. *pertenue*. Why it causes **yaws** rather than syphilis is a mystery. Laboratory identification is by DGM and serology. Clinical presentation is yaws, occurring in three stages, with widespread skin nodules at early stages, and bony and other lesions late if untreated (p. 203).

Chemotherapy is by penicillin, with remarkable response. Control is by mass penicillin campaigns in endemic areas.

T. carateum

T. carateum is similar to *T. pallidum* structurally and in methods of identification. Its virulence factors are unknown. It causes **pinta**, a depigmenting skin disease in South and Central America (p. 203). Chemotherapy is by penicillin, and control is by treating infected patients and contacts.

Borrelia spp.

The borreliae of the relapsing fevers were gradually recognised over the last century. In 1975 two alert mothers in Lyme and Old Lyme, USA, recognised a new arthritis, now called Lyme disease. Borreliae are microaerophilic, fastidious, slow-growing, weakly Gram-negative spiral bacilli, rather bigger than treponemes, with multiple internal periplasmic flagella. The *B. burgdorferi* group infects hard *Ixodes* ticks, *B. recurrentis* infects the human body louse (*Pediculus humanus*) while the others infect soft *Ornithodorus* ticks.

Being difficult to culture, little is known of virulence. No toxins are known. Antigenic variation in waves of borreliae emerging from tissues protects them from host antibody, hence the recurrent fevers. The late organ damage in Lyme disease may be due to direct borrelial action or to immunologic cross-reactivity to host antigens shared with *B. burgdorferi*.

Confirmatory tests

Relapsing fever is diagnosed by seeing borreliae in Giemsa stained blood films taken during fever. Culture is slow, specialised and seldom useful. Serology by ELISA, IFA or PCR for Lyme disease is used.

Clinical syndromes

Clinical syndromes (p. 154) vary with infecting species:

- *B. burgdorferi* group (*B. burgdorferi* itself, *B. afzelii*, and *B. garinii*): Lyme disease
- *B. recurrentis*: epidemic louse-borne relapsing fever
- other *Borrelia* spp. (about 15): tick-borne relapsing fever.

Chemotherapy

Tetracycline is the usual therapy, though chloramphenicol can be used in relapsing fever, and penicillin in Lyme disease.

Control

Vaccines are being developed, but control now is by avoiding tick and louse bites, and by rodent and lice control.

Leptospira interrogans

The genus *Leptospira* now has only two species, the pathogenic *L. interrogans* ('shaped like a question mark') with over 170 serovars causing leptospirosis and the saprophytic *L. biflexa*.

Leptospires are helical, motile, obligate anaerobic organisms, staining poorly with Gram stain. Virulence is not well understood. The kidneys of many animals including rats, cattle and dogs are infected, often lifelong and asymptomatically, and human infection occurs from their urine. After entry through intact or abraded skin or mucosa, leptospires spread via the blood to many tissues, damaging the vascular endothelium, causing fever, haemorrhage and reddened conjunctivae (see Fig. 2, p. 213). Phagocytosis occurs, then antibodies clear leptospires from the blood. Then immune damage causes organ damage.

Laboratory identification is sometimes by dark ground microscopy (DGM), rarely by culture and usually by serology. However agglutinating antibodies only appear 1–2 weeks after infection.

Infection may be asymptomatic, or a flu-like illness, or biphasic with progress to meningitis, haemorrhages, hepatic or renal failure (p. 212). Chemotherapy with penicillin is only helpful early, when diagnosis is hardest. Control is by rat control and avoidance of water contaminated with animal urine, especially by farmers, vets, adventurers and abattoir workers.

Treponemes

- *T. pallidum* is a non-cultivable spirochaete which causes syphilis.
- It can be diagnosed by dark ground microscopy, or more usually by serology, which can also be used to monitor disease progress and treatment.
- Untreated syphilis progresses in stages: primary chancre; secondary fever and rash; an asymptomatic latent stage (3–30 years); and a tertiary stage with vasculitis and chronic inflammation damaging brain, heart and other organs in four distinct clinical patterns.
- Syphilis is treated with penicillin.
- *T. pertenue* causes yaws with skin nodules progressing to bony lesions if untreated.
- *T. carateum* causes pinta, with skin depigmentation.

Borreliae

- These spiral organisms are very difficult to culture, thus diagnosed by microscopy or serology.
- They cause Lyme disease (*B. burgdorferi*), epidemic louse-borne relapsing fever (*B. recurrentis*) and endemic tick-borne relapsing fever (other *Borrelia* spp.).

Leptospirae

- *L. interrogans* are long, thin, spiral bacteria, difficult to culture, hence diagnosed by serology and microscopy. There are over 170 serovars.
- They cause leptospirosis by contact with infected animals or their urine.
- Human infection is often asymptomatic, may be flu-like with myalgia, or may be serious with haemorrhage and organ failure.
- Early penicillin treatment may help.

Mycobacteria

Mycobacteria are non-motile, non-sporing, strictly aerobic rods. The cell wall differs from other bacterial genera in having an outer lipid layer (25% by weight) which makes it resistant to acid decolorisation (i.e. *acid-fast*) (Fig. 1).

This cell wall gives mycobacteria great resistance to:

- environmental stresses like heat, cold, and drying, resulting in infectivity over months or years
- disinfectants, hence dangerous in hospitals
- usual stains and acid, hence identification requires special acid-fast stains
- nutrient uptake, hence slow growth and special culture media
- host defences, hence high infectivity, intracellular bacteria, chronic inflammation, delayed hypersensitivity, initial inapparent disease, late reactivation, chronic host damage and disease
- antibiotics, hence special anti*myco*bacterials.

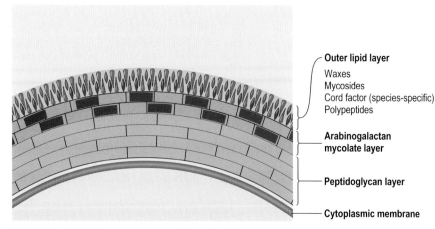

Fig. 1 **The distinctive components of the cell wall.**

Outer lipid layer
Waxes
Mycosides
Cord factor (species-specific)
Polypeptides

Arabinogalactan
mycolate layer

Peptidoglycan layer

Cytoplasmic membrane

M. tuberculosis (MTB)

Tuberculosis (TB) is found in the bones of Egyptian mummies 4000 years old. Growth on special media takes 2–6 weeks. Biochemical tests are used to classify the species. Only humans are naturally infected, by person-to-person spread, usually through aerosols. The closely-related *M. bovis* from cattle infects through unpasteurised milk.

Virulence and pathogenesis

No toxins are known, and virulence depends on its cell wall, its intracellular nature and resistance to host defences; pathogenesis is the same in all tissues, though, of course, the clinical disease varies with the organs infected. Once inhaled, ingested or implanted, the tubercle bacillus ('MTB'), enters macrophages, multiplies and is disseminated to regional lymph nodes; tissue damage is by **tubercles** which are small granulomata of epithelioid cells and macrophages as multinucleated giant (Langhans) cells (Fig. 2). Central cheesy necrosis is called **caseation**; macroscopically this causes **cavitation**. Damage may be local, or MTB may be disseminated by the bloodstream to organs including kidneys, meninges, bones and joints, where the

multiplication and damage continues. Cell-mediated immunity is important, while antibodies are not protective.

Confirmatory tests

The diagnosis of TB is suggested by clinical signs, and supported by chest x-ray changes and a positive reaction in the Mantoux or Quantiferon tests. These tests are confirmed by microscopy using acid-fast techniques such as Ziehl–Neelsen (Fig. 3) on sputum and tissues (less reliable on urine). Culture is slow (2–6 weeks) and requires special media. Further biochemical tests define the species, PCR is specific, and antibiotic sensitivity tests assist treatment.

Clinical syndromes

Pulmonary TB (p. 132) is the commonest form of infection; extra-pulmonary TB occurs mainly in lymph nodes (25%) (p. 137), pleura (20%), genitourinary tract (15%), bone and joint (10%), miliary (10%), meningeal (5%), and elsewhere.

Chemotherapy

This is with three or four special drugs initially, reduced in number after 1 or 2 months or when sensitivity results are available. 'Short' courses of 6 or 9 months are now more usual (p. 232). Multi-drug resistant TB is an increasing problem.

Control

This is by treatment of infectious patients, examination of contacts, isoniazid chemoprophylaxis for recent Man-

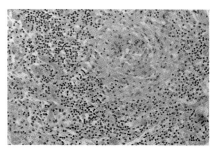

Fig. 2 **Miliary tuberculosis showing rounded granulomata in lung with peripheral epithelioid cells and two central giant cells.**

toux converters, and socioeconomic and health services improvements. In some countries, mass radiography and mass BCG immunisation are used.

M. leprae

The leprosy bacillus was the first ever recognised as a cause of human disease, seen in tissues by Hansen in 1874. *M. leprae* is an obligate intracellular pathogen of humans. The strongly acid-fast parallel-sided rods 0.4µm × 1–8µm do not grow in artificial media, only in mouse foot-pads and the armadillo, i.e. at temperatures lower than 37°C.

Little is known of virulence factors. Pathogenesis is likewise difficult to study but is much influenced by the host response, with active delayed-type hypersensitivity (DTH) in tuberculoid leprosy, but anergy (loss of immune function) in lepromatous leprosy (p. 104, 202).

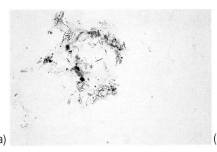
(a)

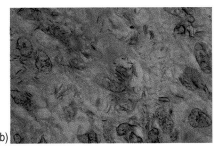
(b)

Fig. 3 **Acid-fast stain: (a) *M. tuberculosis*, (b) *M. leprae*.**

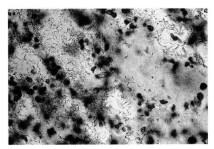

Fig. 4 ***M. ulcerans*: acid-fast stain.**

Confirmatory tests

Nasal mucosal smears, skin snips from eyebrows and other sites (and nerve or other deep biopsies from lepromatous leprosy only) are stained with acid-fast stains (Fig. 3b).

Culture and serology are useless, but histology is used for non-lepromatous leprosy.

Clinical syndromes

There is a spectrum of disease (p. 104) from *lepromatous* leprosy (LL) with chronic inflammation particularly of the skin and mucous membranes, through *borderline* disease to *tuberculoid* disease (TT) with infiltration of peripheral nerves leading to anaesthesia and secondary trophic changes (Fig. 2, p. 104).

Chemotherapy and control

Chemotherapy is usually with rifampicin, dapsone and clofazimine. Control depends more on chemotherapy than isolation, as leprosy is not highly infectious except for the nasal discharge in LL patients.

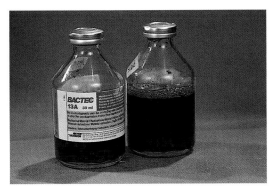

Fig. 5 **Mycobacterial blood cultures.**

Atypical mycobacteria

The atypical mycobacteria are acid-fast rods, distinguished into species by special biochemical tests. The Runyon classification divided them into four groups depending on pigmentation and rate of growth (Table 1). They are environmental organisms of variable pathogenicity, usually by local invasion, followed by dissemination in immunocompromised patients. Their lower virulence compared with *M. tuberculosis* and *M. leprae* is largely unexplained.

Confirmatory tests

Microscopy and acid-fast stains are important for rapid diagnosis (Fig. 4); culture is slow but shortened to 8–14 days by the 'Bactec' system (Fig. 5). Biochemical tests speciate. Specific nuclear probes for MAC and others are available.

Clinical syndromes

More immunocompromised patients means more atypical mycobacterial infections. They cause pulmonary infection (*M. kansasii*), skin and soft tissue ulcers (*M. ulcerans, marinum*), and systemic infections [*M. avium-intracellulare* complex (MAC)] in AIDS (p. 149–151).

Chemotherapy and control

Chemotherapy is difficult, as many strains are multiresistant. Control is also difficult, as mycobacteria are widespread in the environment and particularly infect the immunocompromised.

Table 1 **Runyon classification of some atypical mycobacteria**

Group and examples	Pigmentation	Growth rate[a]	Optimal temperature for growth (°C)
Group I			
M. kansasii	Photochromogens[b]	Slow	37
M. marinum	Photochromogens[b]	Moderate	32
Group II			
M. scrofulaceum	Scotochromogens[c]	Slow	37
Group III			
M. avium-intracellulare	None	Slow	37
M. ulcerans	None	Slow	32
Group IV			
M. chelonae	None	Rapid	37
M. fortuitum	None	Rapid	37

[a] Rapid growth is about 2 weeks by conventional methods; slow growth is 4–6 weeks.
[b] Photochromogens produce vivid yellow carotenoids only with light;
[c] Scotochromogens produce pigment in the dark as well.

Mycobacteria

- Mycobacteria have a special cell wall rich in lipids, making them very resistant to environmental stresses, host defences, disinfectants, stains and antibiotics.

- They are slow-growing and need special laboratory techniques including 'acid-fast' stains and specific media.

- They are intracellular bacteria, particularly in macrophages, where they multiply, disseminate and cause tissue damage as granulomata, with central caseation in tuberculosis.

- *M. tuberculosis* causes the various forms of tuberculosis.

- *M. leprae* causes the various forms of leprosy.

- The atypical mycobacteria are environmental species that can contaminate, or colonise, or cause pulmonary or systemic infections or skin and soft tissue ulcers. They are prominent in infections of the immunocompromised.

Actinomyces, *Nocardia* and rare Gram-positive bacilli

Actinomyces

Actinomyces are Gram-positive anaerobic bacteria, which require rich media, are capnophilic, grow slowly and need temperatures around 37°C for growth. These features correlate with their habitat, the human oral cavity, and contrast with *Nocardia*.

Actinomyces means 'ray fungus' referring to their apparently fungal form with branching filaments in tissues (Fig. 1). However, these break into bacilli and coccoid forms, and their cell structure is clearly procaryotic, with no nuclear membrane and a Gram-positive cell wall. Disease begins when these normal flora enter adjacent sterile tissues by implantation or inhalation.

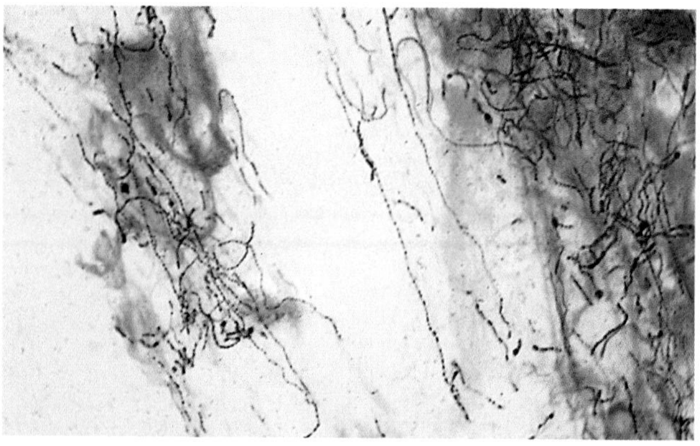

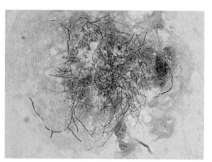

Fig. 1 *Actinomyces israelii*: Gram stain.

Confirmatory tests

This depends on Gram stain of granules in the pus (for organisms are elsewhere scanty), on anaerobic culture with 10% CO_2 for at least 2 weeks, and biochemical differentiation of species. Histopathology or culture from tissues is advisable because isolates from surfaces may be only other normal flora.

Clinical syndromes

Actinomycosis occurs worldwide in five major forms:

- cervico-facial (by local invasion, p. 122)
- abdominal (by local invasion)
- mycetoma (by implantation, p. 202)
- thoracic (by inhalation, p. 134)
- disseminated disease (including brain, p. 102).

The pathological features are **s**welling, **s**low progression, **s**inus formation, **s**clerosis, **s**carring and **s**ulphur yellow granules in the pus.

Chemotherapy and control

Treatment is prolonged penicillin or co-amoxiclav. Control is by dental care and appropriate chemoprophylaxis.

Tropheryma whippelii

Currently uncultivable, this Gram-positive rod seen in gut tissue sections is probably an actinomycete causing the multisystem Whipple's disease of fever, malabsorption and arthralgia. Improvement

follows penicillin ± gentamicin then oral doxycycline treatment, but relapses occur.

Nocardia

Nocardia are Gram-positive and weakly acid-fast aerobic soil bacteria (Fig. 2), which grow on simple media over a wide temperature range. Filaments are better seen in liquid media. Infection is by inhalation or soil implantation.

Confirmatory tests

Identification depends on Gram stain, acid-fast stains (using weak acid only), and prolonged aerobic culture. Biochemical tests speciate.

Clinical syndromes

Pulmonary pseudotuberculosis and brain abscesses occur especially in the immunocompromised, while mycetoma follows skin implantation (p. 75, 202). Unlike actinomycosis, sinuses are not a feature and sulphur granules do not occur. Suppuration and scarring with granulation tissue occur, but granulomata as in tuberculosis do not.

Chemotherapy and control

Chemotherapy is usually with sulphonamides, and control involves care of soil-contaminated wounds and of immunocompromised patients.

Rare Gram-positive bacilli

Lactobacillus, *Propionibacterium*, *Eubacterium* and *Bifidobacterium* spp. are Gram-positive bacilli, at times bifid or branching; most are obligate anaerobes, being normal flora of the skin (propionibacteria), bowel and vagina. Virulence is minimal.

Pathogenesis is only understood for *P. acnes* in acne, where propionic acid production in the follicle causes irritation and comedone formation.

Confirmatory tests

These are usually Gram stain (Fig. 3), anaerobic culture and biochemical testing.

Clinical syndromes

These bacteria are:

- common skin contaminants in blood cultures or swabs
- opportunist pathogens (rarely) in endocarditis or device-related infections
- found with other pathogens in mixed infections
- a major factor in acne (*P. acnes*).

Chemotherapy

This is usually unnecessary, but penicillins, clindamycin and vancomycin are usually active.

Actinomyces
- Anaerobic, Gram-positive, branching, pleomorphic bacteria, slow growing and fastidious.
- Part of normal oral flora, they cause cervico-facial infections, mycetoma if implanted, thoracic infections if inhaled, or disseminated infection.
- Treatment is prolonged penicillin or co-amoxiclav.

Nocardia
- Aerobic, Gram-positive, weakly acid-fast, soil bacteria.
- Slow growing, they cause mycetoma if implanted, pulmonary cavitation if inhaled, and abscesses if disseminated.
- Sulphonamides are drugs of choice.

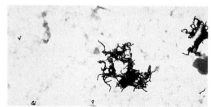

Fig. 2 *Nocardia asteroides*: acid-fast stain.

Fig. 3 Gram stain of propionibacteria.

Mycoplasma and Ureaplasma

Mycoplasmataceae is a family of small bacteria with three genera, *Mycoplasma*, *Ureaplasma*, and *Acholeplasma* (unimportant) They have at least four unique properties:

- the smallest free-living organisms (diameter only 0.2–0.7µm)
- no cell wall, so do not stain with Gram stain and are resistant to cell-wall-active antibiotics like penicillin
- cell membrane is unusual, containing sterols which must be provided for growth in media
- generation time about 6 hours.

They were originally thought to be viruses, but are definitely bacteria with prokaryotic cell structure and division by binary fission.

Mycoplasmata are ubiquitous, frequently contaminating tissue cultures. *M. pneumoniae* in humans is probably found only in those infected, but about one in six sexually active adults is colonised with *M. hominis*, and between 50% and 75% with *U. urealyticum*. Many other human mycoplasmata have been found, but their role in disease is questionable. Virulence varies between species: *M. pneumoniae* has a special terminal protein called P1 which adheres (Fig. 1) to a specific glycoprotein receptor in respiratory epithelium near the base of the cilia and microvilli. Cilial movement then stops, and mucosal (not alveolar) damage occurs by ill-understood tissue toxins including H_2O_2. Inflammatory infiltrate is lymphocytic, not neutrophilic, and the mycoplasmata remain extracellular. The pathogenesis is thus very different from pneumococcal or other pyogenic pneumonias.

Confirmatory tests

Staining is too poor and culture too slow – over 1 week; colonies on specific soft agar have a 'fried egg' appearance (Fig. 2).

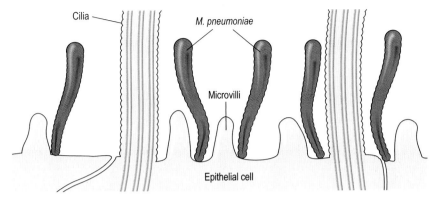

Fig. 1 **M. pneumoniae attachment to respiratory epithelium.**

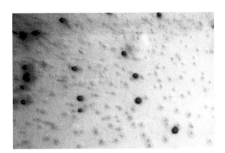

Fig. 2 **Mixed Mycoplasma and Ureaplasma spp. on culture.**

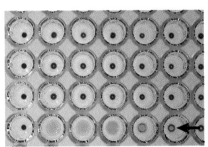

Fig. 3 **M. pneumoniae antibody detection by particle agglutination.**

M. pneumoniae PCR is now routine. Serology (Fig. 3) is the other diagnostic test, either for non-specific cold agglutinins (an early IgM antibody which agglutinates red cells at 4°C) or for specific complement-fixing IgG, which peaks at 4–8 weeks, has numerous false negatives (positive only in two-thirds of patients) and has false positives in, e.g., influenza.

Clinical syndromes

- *M. pneumoniae* is an important cause of atypical pneumonia in young people (p. 126–127); it is considered atypical compared with classical pneumococcal pneumonia because it is slower to develop, less serious, not lobar, not responsive to penicillin and slower to recover. Erythema multiforme rash (Fig. 4) may occur.
- *M. hominis* causes urinary infections, pelvic inflammatory disease and puerperal infections (p. 184).
- *U. urealyticum* probably causes half of non-chlamydial non-gonococcal urethritis (p. 180).

Chemotherapy

This is usually with erythromycin, though tetracycline is useful in adults. Prevention of infection is by avoiding close contact with respiratory infections, and by condom use or sexual continence.

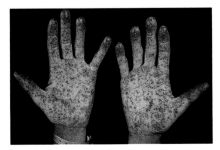

Fig. 4 **M. pneumoniae erythema multiforme skin rash.**

Mycoplasma and Ureaplasma

- *Mycoplasma* and *Ureaplasma* are unique, very small bacteria with no cell wall, a sterol-containing cell membrane and very slow growth.

- They are therefore difficult to stain and culture, and are resistant to cell-wall-active antibiotics like penicillin. Diagnosis is by PCR and serology.

- *M. pneumoniae* causes atypical pneumonia, while *M. hominis* causes genitourinary infections, and *U. urealyticum* causes urethritis: all mucosal surface infections.

- Treatment is by erythromycin or tetracycline.

Chlamydia and *Chlamydophila*

These are small, obligate intracellular bacteria which <u>like</u> most bacteria:

- have a cell wall with inner and outer membranes
- have procaryotic ribosomes, RNA and DNA
- synthesise their own macromolecules
- are susceptible to antibacterials.

<u>Unlike</u> other bacteria, they:

- have no peptidoglycan in their cell wall
- are unable to synthesise ATP
- lack oxidative enzymes such as flavoproteins and cytochromes so are 'energy parasites' and cannot replicate extracellularly.

They therefore have a dimorphic life cycle. The first form is the **elementary body** (EB), which is small (0.3–0.4µm), spherical and stable to environmental stresses. It exists extracellularly as the infective form, rather like clostridial spores or amoebic cysts. The second form is the **reticulate body** (RB), which is the fragile intracellular replicating form with an internal net-like structure.

Chlamydia trachomatis causes four groups of infections (Table 1).

Three species form a new genus *Chlamydophila*:

- *C. pneumoniae* causes respiratory infections
- *C. psittaci* causes psittacosis, a pneumonia from birds
- *C. abortus* from domestic animals causes human abortion, stillbirth, or maternal sepsis.

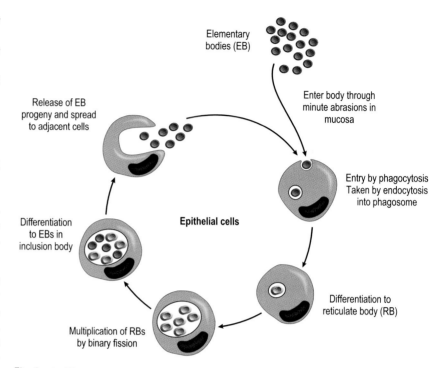

Fig. 1 **The life cycle of *Chlamydia* and *Chlamydophila*.**

Table 1 **Chlamydial infections**

Organism source	Epidemiological source	Pathogenic mechanism	Clinical syndrome
C. trachomatis			
Serovars A-C	Infected eyes	Local invasion	Trachoma
B, D-K	Urogenital infection	Local invasion	Urethritis
		Local invasion	Genital infections
	Genital	Mother to child	Perinatal infections
L_1, L_2, L_3	Genital infection	Lymphatic spread	Lymphogranuloma venereum (LGV)
C. pneumoniae	Respiratory infections	Local invasion	Respiratory tract infections, pneumonia
C. psittaci	Birds	Local invasion, distant spread	Psittacosis with pneumonia
C. abortus	Sheep and goats	Local invasion, transplacental spread	Abortion, stillbirth, severe maternal sepsis

Chlamydia trachomatis

Trachoma was known over 2000 years ago. *C. trachomatis* has at least 15 antigenically different serotypes (serovars):

- 12+ of the trachoma biovar, including A, B, Ba and C causing trachoma itself, and B plus D to K causing genital and neonatal disease
- three (L_1, L_2, L_3) of the LGV biovar (Table 1).

All are human pathogens, spreading by direct contact, with no animal host, though insects can be a vector for trachoma.

Pathogenesis

The life cycle of chlamydiae is shown in Figure 1. Unless antibody-coated, the surface components of the EB prevent the usual fusion of the phagosome with lysosomes, so they are not destroyed. In lymphogranuloma venereum (LGV), the same cycle occurs, but in <u>macrophages</u> that are carried to regional lymph nodes, which become enlarged and tender.

Confirmatory tests

Microscopy on urethral, cervical and eye swabs (Fig. 2) is more effective using direct immunofluorescence (DIF, Fig. 3) than Gram or Giemsa stains. In LGV, lymph node aspirate is used. Culture shows a glycogen-positive inclusion body, but is outmoded.

PCR on urine is replacing antigen detection by ELISA, only reliable in specimens from symptomatic women. Antibody detection is useless, as only genus-specific antigen is usually available which does not distinguish present from past disease.

Clinical syndromes

C. trachomatis causes four groups of infections:

- trachoma (p. 111)
- numerous 'non-specific' genital tract infections (p. 180–186)
- infections from the genital tract during childbirth (p. 215)
- a specific STD, lymphogranuloma venereum (p. 189).

Chemotherapy

Chemotherapy is azithromycin for genital infection, otherwise tetracycline or

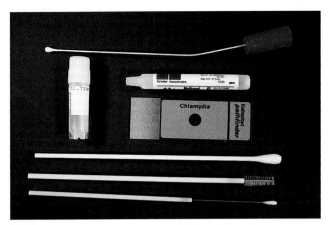
Fig. 2 **Kit for bedside collection of swabs for *Chlamydia*.**

Fig. 3 **Direct immunofluorescent microscopy of chlamydiae.**

erythromycin, which are effective but slow. Control depends on the treatment of infections, safer sex practices and improved socioeconomic conditions.

Chlamydophila pneumoniae

C. pneumoniae was first described in 1986 as the TWAR agent in Taiwan.

C. pneumoniae is by DNA homology a separate genus from Chlamydia, but shares the same unique biological qualities. It is a worldwide human pathogen. No animal host is known.

Pathogenesis is similar to C. trachomatis, but affecting respiratory rather than genital mucosa or conjunctiva.

Confirmatory tests
Microscopy by direct immunofluorescence is available in some centres and is quick and specific. Culture is replaced by PCR. Serology by microimmunofluorescence is specific.

Clinical syndromes
C. pneumoniae is a common cause of 'atypical' pneumonia, clinically very like mycoplasmal pneumonia. It also causes bronchitis and upper respiratory infections.

Chemotherapy
Chemotherapy with tetracycline or a macrolide is effective. There are no specific control measures.

Chlamydophila psittaci

C. psittaci has entirely different epidemiology from other chlamydiae, as it infects many wild and pet birds, which may be ill or asymptomatic. The organism is on their feathers and in dried bird faeces. The infective dose to humans by inhalation is small, as infection has occurred after short exposure in an area previously occupied by an infected bird. Humans kissing love-birds can also become infected!

Virulence and pathogenesis
While structure and function are typical of the two genera, the pathogenesis of psittacosis is different, for this virulent pathogen causes a *systemic* disease, not simply a mucosal or epithelial one. Infection occurs by inhalation, but organisms are carried from the lungs to the reticuloendothelial cells in liver and spleen. Replication occurs there with focal necrosis, then

blood-borne spread occurs back to lungs and to other organs including meninges and brain, heart, gut and adrenals. Inflammation is lymphocytic with macrophages containing glycogen-negative cytoplasmic inclusions, surrounded by oedema, haemorrhage and necrosis.

Confirmatory tests
Microscopy is unhelpful and culture is dangerous. PCR is usually helpful. Serology gives the diagnosis after 2 or 3 weeks, by a rise in titre in paired acute and convalescent sera.

Clinical syndrome
The pathogenesis explains the long incubation period and systemic symptoms of malaise and myalgia, marked headache and mentation changes, macular rash and multiple organomegaly (especially splenomegaly), mucoid sputum and marked pneumonia.

Chemotherapy
Tetracycline is the usual treatment, but macrolides are also effective.

Control
Psittacosis is only a risk disease for those in contact with birds, particularly pet psittacines (birds with hooked beaks, e.g. parrots).

Chlamydia and Chlamydophila
- These are unique obligate intracellular bacteria, unable to synthesise ATP and hence dependent on host cells.
- They exist in two forms: a robust extracellular infective elementary body (EB) and a fragile intracellular replicating reticular body (RB).
- C. trachomatis causes trachoma, non-gonococcal urethritis, cervicitis and other genital infections, neonatal infections from an infected mother, and lymphogranuloma venereum.
- C. pneumoniae causes respiratory infections including 'atypical' pneumonia.
- C. psittaci causes psittacosis, a systemic disease with pneumonia, from infected birds.
- C. abortus causes abortion, stillbirth or severe maternal sepsis.
- Chlamydial infections are treated with azithromycin, tetracycline or a macrolide.

Rickettsiae and bartonellae

In the family Rickettsiaceae there are four medically important genera: *Rickettsia, Orientia, Coxiella* and *Ehrlichia*, which cause a number of diseases including the typhus group and Rocky Mountain spotted fever (RMSF). *Bartonella* (formerly *Rochalimaea*) differ by growing in cell-free cultures. Rickettsiae are small aerobic bacteria which <u>like</u> other bacteria:

- have a cell wall with inner and outer membranes
- have procaryotic ribosomes
- have RNA and DNA
- synthesise their own macromolecules
- have peptidoglycan in the cell wall.

<u>Unlike</u> most bacteria, they lack enzymes for energy metabolism, hence are obligate intracellular parasites, and cannot replicate extracellularly. They require ATP, coenzyme A and NAD from the host cell, and exchange some of their ADP for host ATP. Their *dimorphic life cycle* involves an animal or human reservoir plus an arthropod vector (Fig. 1), so rickettsial diseases each have a special geographic distribution.

Virulence and pathogenesis
Virulence varies between species, possible factors being:

- lipopolysaccharide, like other typical Gram-negative rods
- toxin, ill-defined, of dubious importance
- phospholipase A to dissolve the phagosomal membrane (Fig. 1)
- intracellular replication causing cell destruction and death.

Pathogenesis is similar in all but *Coxiella* infections (Fig. 1). Doubling time is slow, about 8 hours, but in 40–48 hours the host cell dies, ruptures and liberates large numbers of rickettsiae to infect further cells. <u>Vasculitis</u> (damage to small blood vessels) is the most striking feature (Fig. 2b). Antibody, either natural or vaccine-induced, prevents escape from the phagosome so the rickettsiae are destroyed by lysosomal enzymes.

Confirmatory tests
Microscopy is generally not useful except for *R. rickettsii* where direct immunofluorescent (DIF) microscopy of skin biopsies is quick and specific.

Culture is difficult and dangerous, hence rare. Serology is the main identifying method. The Weil-Felix agglutination test uses patterns of cross-reactivity of anti-rickettsial antibodies with antigens in *Proteus vulgaris* strains. Complement fixation tests (CFT) will also differentiate some species. IF, Latex and EIA are now available commercially.

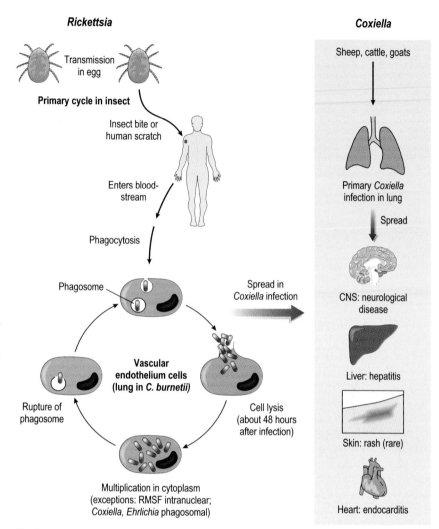

Fig. 1 **Typical events in *Rickettsia* and *Coxiella* infection.**

Table 1 **Rickettsiae: diseases, causative organisms, hosts, vectors, regions**				
Disease	**Organism**	**Host**	**Vector**	**Regions**
Typhus group				
Epidemic typhus	*R. prowazeckii*	Humans	Body louse	Africa, Americas
Murine typhus	*R. typhi*	Rats, mammals	Rat flea	Tropics/subtropics
Scrub typhus group				
Scrub typhus	*O. tsutsugamushi*	Rats	Mites	Asia, Pacific
Spotted fever group (SF) (partial list)				
RMSF	*R. rickettsii*	Rodents, dogs	*Dermacentor*	Americas
Queensland Tick Typhus	*R. australis*	Unknown	*Ixodes* ticks	N. Australia
Boutonneuse fever	*R. conorii*	Rats, mammals	Ticks	Mediterranean
Flinders Island SF	*R. honei*	Reptiles?	Reptile tick	S-E Australia
Rickettsial pox	*R. akari*	House mice	Mouse mite	Urban (USA, etc)
Ehrlichiosis				
Sennetsu fever	*E. sennetsu*	Fish?	Fish?	Japan
Granulocytic and monocytic cell ehrlichiosis	*E. chaffeensis* and *E. phagocytophila*	Humans, mice, deer and dogs	Ticks	USA, Europe

R. prowazeckii

R. prowazeckii causes epidemic louse-borne typhus. Unlike other rickettsioses, humans are the principal host because the vector is the human louse, *Pediculus*

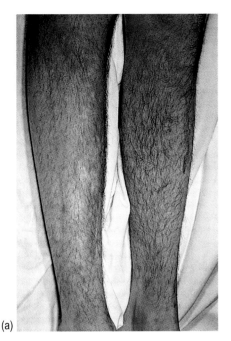

(a)

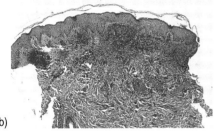

(b)

Fig. 2 **Rocky Mountain spotted fever.**
(a) Rash on legs. **(b)** Vasculitis in skin biopsy.

humanus var *corporis*. All major epidemics of typhus have occurred with wars or famine, predisposing to louse infestation.

Diagnosis is primarily clinical, but serology can confirm.

Clinically, epidemic typhus has mortality in the malnourished of over 60%, and is characterised by fever, headache, prostration and a rash beginning on the trunk and spreading to the extremities (the pattern in all rickettsial rashes except RMSF).

Brill-Zinsser disease is a mild recrudescence 20–40 years later.

Chemotherapy is tetracycline or chloramphenicol.

Control of lice with DDT, permethrin or malathion is essential. A vaccine is available for special risk groups.

R. typhi

R. typhi causes endemic murine typhus. The natural reservoir is the rat. Transmission is by the rat flea, *Xenopsylla cheopis*, which defaecates on feeding, then rickettsiae in the faeces enter humans through the bite wound or scratches. Rat and flea survive!

Diagnosis is usually clinical. Weil-Felix serology distinguishes murine typhus from RMSF, but not from epidemic typhus, which needs specific specialised indirect immunofluorescence.

Clinically, murine typhus is similar to epidemic typhus, but milder. It is distinguished from RMSF by (1) being an urban disease of late summer and autumn with no tick exposure, while RMSF occurs in spring-summer after tick exposure; (2) a rash which spreads from trunk to extremities, whereas RMSF does the reverse; and (3) a positive CFT, which usually differentiates.

Chemotherapy is tetracycline or chloramphenicol.

Control involves rat and flea control.

R. rickettsii

R. rickettsii, the cause of Rocky Mountain spotted fever (RMSF), is present in many animals, including mammals, birds and dogs in endemic areas in the USA. It is transmitted by ticks, especially *Dermacentor andersoni* and *D. variabilis*, the dog tick.

Diagnosis initially must be clinical. DIF microscopy of skin biopsy and serology follow.

Clinically, rash begins on the extremities (Fig. 2) and spreads centrally; headache, fever, myalgia, and prostration occur acutely, while mental clouding, splenomegaly, pulmonary oedema, disseminated intravascular coagulation (DIC), shock and death follow in patients diagnosed or treated late.

Chemotherapy is tetracycline or chloramphenicol, with supportive care.

Control depends on tick avoidance or their early removal.

Coxiella burnetii

Q fever (for query, as the cause was unknown) was first described in Queensland, Australia. The cause, *C. burnetii*, was discovered later.

C. burnetii is in a separate genus because spore-like structures unique among the Rickettsiaceae make it very robust, surviving in the environment for many months, hence infecting humans directly by inhalation, without an arthropod vector. A further difference is its existence in two phases: (I) when isolated from animals and in Q fever endocarditis, and (II) when grown in eggs.

Virulence is high, with a low infective dose.

Pathogenesis (Fig. 1) is different from all other Rickettsiaceae. It is inhaled, and replicates in the lungs causing, in 20 days, an 'atypical' interstitial pneumonia. It also disseminates by the bloodstream and causes granulomata, in the liver particularly. Thirdly, it infects abnormal 'native' and prosthetic heart valves and perivalvular tissues.

Diagnosis is serological. Phase II antibodies develop first: IgM in 2–3 weeks, then IgG after 12 weeks, persisting often for 12 months. Titres of phase I antibody higher than phase II are found in chronic disease, particularly endocarditis.

Clinically, infection is usually occupational, particularly abattoir workers. The commonest syndrome is atypical pneumonia with systemic disease including hepatitis. Endocarditis is fortunately rare.

Chemotherapy for the acute illness is tetracycline (or chloramphenicol or erythromycin). Endocarditis is extremely difficult to treat even with combined surgery and antibiotics: tetracycline with a second drug such as rifampicin or ciprofloxacin for 2–5 years may be needed.

Control is by an Australian vaccine.

Bartonellae

Bartonellae are very small Gram-negative bacilli related to rickettsiae. Three species are:

- *B. bacilliformis*. Causes oroya fever, a serious infection of erythrocytes, hence anaemia and death. Survivors may have verruga peruana, with ulcerating haemorrhagic skin nodules. Sand-flies spread it from infected humans in S. America.
- *B.* (formerly *Rochalimaea*) *henselae*. Causes cat scratch fever (p. 197) (as rarely does the related *Afipia felis*), also bacillary angiomatosis and bacillary peliosis in AIDS (p. 149–151).
- *B.* (formerly *Rochalimaea*) *quintana*. Causes trench fever, infamous in World War I. The body louse spreads it in deprived populations still.

Rickettsiaceae

- Rickettsiae are small obligate intracellular bacteria.
- Most have an animal host and an arthropod vector, hence a specific geographical distribution.
- Pathogenesis is similar with vasculitis, except in Q fever with pneumonia and hepatitis (*Coxiella burnetii*).
- Diagnosis is clinical, then usually serological.
- Tetracycline is the usual treatment.

Aspergillus and *Candida*

Aspergillus and *Candida*, two common fungal genera, are similar in two respects:

- they cause opportunistic infections in immunocompromised hosts
- they do not cause invasive infections in normal hosts.

However, they also differ in two important respects:

- *Aspergillus* spp. are filamentous fungi, while *Candida* spp. are yeasts.
- *Aspergillus* spp. are environmental fungi, while *Candida* spp. are normal flora.

Aspergillus

Although *Aspergillus* infection has been known for a century, opportunistic invasive disease is now more common because of the greater number of patients immunocompromised by **d**isease, **d**rugs or **d**efects in the skin–mucous membrane barrier.

Aspergillus spp. are branching, septate, filamentous fungi, 7–10µm in diameter, and several hundred micrometres long. They are classified by their sexual structures, but distinguished in clinical medicine by their asexual structures including the shape of the conidiophore, the supporting vesicle and phialides (sterigmata), and the conidiospores (Fig. 1). The most important species causing human disease are *A. fumigatus* (Latin for 'smoky', referring to the smoky blue-grey mycelium, Fig. 2), and *A. flavus*, meaning yellow (colonies). They tolerate temperatures up to 50°C, and so grow widely in soil and warm decaying vegetation including compost heaps and haystacks, resulting in easy dispersal into the air.

They have typical fungal eucaryotic cell structure with a nucleus and varied cytoplasmic structures (p. 6). Different species differ in virulence and produce disease by all three fungal pathogenic mechanisms: mycotoxins, hypersensitivity and invasion, particularly of blood vessel walls (p. 8–9).

Confirmatory tests

Both false-positive and false-negative results are frequent because:

- *Aspergillus* species are common in the environment and so are common contaminants of clinical specimens in the absence of disease
- serious infections are usually enclosed in deep tissues
- they grow poorly in blood cultures and some other media.

Definitive diagnosis therefore depends on histopathology showing septate hyphae with dichotomous branching (bifurcating into two at acute angles), plus Gram stain and repeated cultural isolation.

Clinical syndromes

The three pathogenic mechanisms lead to:

- mycotoxicosis from coumarin-like aflatoxins, causing bleeding
- hypersensitivity causing allergic rhinitis, asthma or hypersensitivity pneumonia by inhalation
- local infection such as bronchopulmonary aspergillosis
- invasive opportunistic infection in the immunocompromised host, with a fungus ball in a pulmonary cavity, severe pneumonia, vascular infection or disseminated abscesses in organs such as brain, kidneys, liver, skin or bone (Table 1 and p. 157, Fig. 1).

Pseudallescheria boydii and *Scedosporium* spp. cause similar local and invasive infections.

Chemotherapy

Voriconazole is now preferred to amphotericin B initially. Itraconazole orally is used to complete therapy in selected patients.

Control

Usually impossible, except by removal from the cause in allergic disease, or filtered air and exclusion of plants and soil for highly immunosuppressed patients.

Candida

Superficial candidal infections are less troublesome now because of better control of predisposing factors, better diagnosis and better treatment, but systemic invasive candidiasis is more common, for the reasons given for invasive aspergillosis.

Candida are small round yeasts which multiply by budding (blastoconidia formation), forming pseudohyphae ('germ tubes', Fig. 3). They are classified into species by carbohydrate assimilation and fermentations. *C. albicans* is the commonest and with *C. tropicalis*, *C. (Torulopsis) glabrata* and *C. parapsilosis* is part of the normal oropharyngeal, gut and vaginal flora, but *Candida* are uncommon on the skin unless it is macerated or damaged.

Table 1 **Sources, spread and syndrome**			
Organism	**Epidemiological source**	**Pathological mechanism**	**Clinical syndrome**
A. fumigatus and *Aspergillus* spp.	Air, soil, mouldy vegetation	Toxin production	Bleeding
		Hypersensitivity	Asthma, pneumonia
		Opportunistic direct invasion	Pneumonia, fungus ball
		Systemic spread	Organ abscesses
C. albicans and other spp.	Own normal flora	Opportunistic local infection	Skin, mucosal infection
		Systemic spread	Organ infections

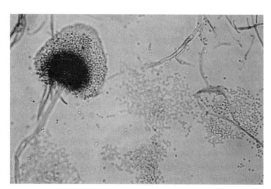

Fig. 1 **Aspergillus.** Hyphae and conidiophore.

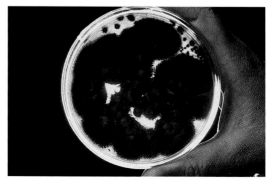

Fig. 2 **A. fumigatus.** Culture.

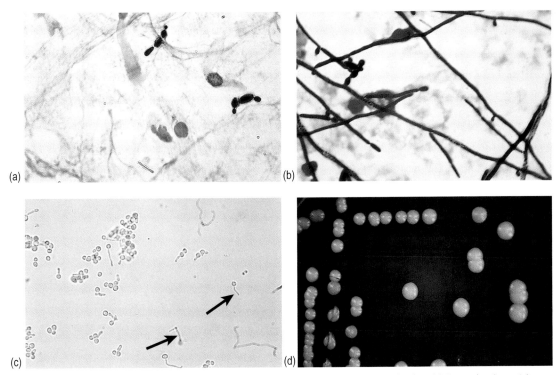

Fig. 3 **C. albicans. (a)** Gram stain of sputum. **(b)** Blood culture showing enormous pseudo-hyphae. **(c)** Germ tubes (no stain). **(d)** Colonies cultured on Sabouraud's medium.

Virulence and pathogenesis

Candida spp. have typical fungal cell structure (p. 6). They have minimal virulence for normal hosts, and pathogenesis depends on one or more defects in host defence, including:

- impaired skin–mucous membrane defences caused by mechanical breaches including catheters, by changes in normal flora owing to disease or drugs, or by maceration, trauma or disease
- impaired neutrophil or eosinophil function
- impaired monocyte or macrophage function
- impaired lymphocyte function
- impaired alternative complement pathway.

Antibody is usually produced but is probably not protective. The known adherence of *Candida* spp. to many cells may be important.

Confirmatory tests (Fig. 3)

Typical Gram stain, culture on usual laboratory media such as blood agar, and germ tube formation in serum in 2–3 hours are the usual tests for *C. albicans*, with carbohydrate assimilation and fermentation tests for other species. Although *C. albicans* can grow in vented blood culture bottles, disseminated candidiasis often has negative blood cultures initially. CT scan of liver and spleen often shows characteristic small, regular

lesions (p. 157, Fig. 2), so histopathology of biopsies is needed less often.

Clinical syndromes

These include (Table 1):

- local skin or nail disease including napkin rash, intertrigo or paronychia (p. 159, Fig. 6), occurring in hosts with only locally impaired defences
- local mucous membrane disease such as oral thrush or vaginitis (p. 187, Fig. 2) with locally impaired defences
- local but severe chronic mucocutaneous candidiasis (CMC) in children with specific T-cell defects
- organ system infection, including CNS, pulmonary, cardiovascular, uri-

nary, eye, bone, joint or disseminated infection, in the immunocompromised patient (p. 220–221).

Chemotherapy

Local imidazoles or nystatin are used for local infections, ketoconazole for CMC. Deep, systemic or disseminated infections need specialised treatment with amphotericin B, fluconazole or caspofungin.

Control

This depends on treating or removing the predisposing defects in host defences. Chemoprophylaxis is used in vulnerable patients.

Aspergillus

- Heat-tolerant, environmental, septate filamentous fungi.
- *A. fumigatus* is the commonest pathogen.
- *Aspergillus* spp. cause disease by mycotoxins, by hypersensitivity and by opportunistic invasion of the immunocompromised patient.
- Voriconazole is preferred to amphotericin B as standard treatment. Oral itraconazole may follow. Systemic infection is often fatal.

Candida

- Round yeasts which multiply by budding.
- *C. albicans* is the commonest yeast in the normal flora of the oropharynx, gut and vagina but is not found on normal skin.
- Local infection of skin, nails or mucous membrane occurs when local, first-line defences are impaired.
- Systemic opportunistic infection occurs in the immunocompromised patient.
- Imidazoles or nystatin are used for local infections and for prophylaxis. Systemic infections need amphotericin B, fluconazole or caspofungin.

Cryptococcus and *Histoplasma*

In contrast to *Aspergillus* and *Candida*, both *Cryptococcus neoformans* and *Histoplasma capsulatum* cause disease (systemic mycoses) in normal hosts, as well as severe or fatal disease in immunocompromised patients.

Cryptococcus neoformans

C. neoformans has two varieties, var *neoformans* and var *gattii*, which differ genetically, biochemically and ecologically. Both however are monomorphic, being yeasts in both culture and tissues (unlike the other four fungi causing systemic mycoses, see below and p. 72–73). The sexual forms are varieties of *Filobasidiella neoformans*. *Cryptococcus* is found worldwide in pigeon excreta and nests (the organism's urease allows the use of nitrogen sources) and in Eucalyptus trees. It infects humans (but not the pigeons!) by inhalation (Fig. 1).

Cryptococci have a typical round yeast structure, with a large characteristic mucopolysaccharide capsule, important in pathogenicity and helpful in diagnosis (Fig. 2). Infections with var. *gattii* are endemic or occupational in normal hosts, while var. *neoformans* patients have immune defects, usually of T-cell and macrophage function, less often of neutrophil, B cell or complement. CNS infections are prominent because soluble serum anti-cryptococcal factors are absent in CSF, CSF is a good growth medium, and CNS inflammation is minimal, partly because the CSF contains no complement.

Confirmatory tests

Microscopy of the CSF is often positive when Indian ink is used as a negative stain to show the clear capsulated cryptococci against a black background (Fig. 3). Gram stain and microscopy of sputum are less reliable. Culture should always be done, whatever the microscopy.

Biochemical tests including urease confirm the identification. Antigen detection by latex agglutination is sensitive and 90% reliable on serum and CSF.

CT scan is often diagnostic, especially in immunocompromised patients (e.g. in AIDS) with cerebral lesions (p. 98, Fig. 1c). Histopathology may be needed for unusual lesions.

Clinical syndromes

Inhalation may lead to an asymptomatic pulmonary lesion, rarely to a primary

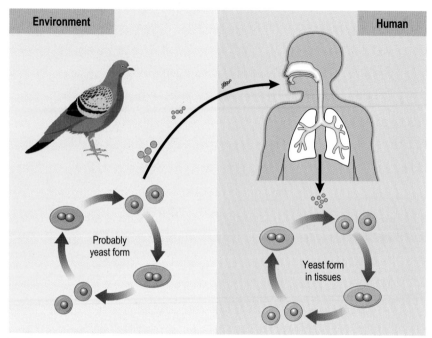

Fig. 1 *C. neoformans* **infection.**

pneumonia, or, most frequently, to meningitis or cerebral infection with single or multiple scattered lesions (p. 98–99, Figs 1 & 2). Skin (Fig. 4, p. 221), bone or visceral lesions also occur.

Chemotherapy

Treatment is often amphotericin B plus flucytosine, but fluconazole is useful, especially for maintenance. Unusual lesions may need excision for diagnosis.

Control

Fluconazole is used for long-term prophylaxis in the immunocompromised patient, particularly in AIDS.

Histoplasma capsulatum

'Tutankhamen's curse', the disease affecting those who opened his tomb, was probably histoplasmosis from spores still viable after 3245 years!

H. capsulatum is a dimorphic fungus, with a filamentous spore-forming mould form in the environment and in culture at 25°C, and the pathogenic yeast form in tissues and macrophages (Fig. 4). The sexual stage is an ascomycete, *Ajellomyces capsulatum*. *H. capsulatum* var. *capsulatum* is found in most countries, but highly endemic areas include the Ohio-Mississippi valleys in the USA. *H. capsulatum* var. *duboisii* is found in Africa. The mould grows in soil, nitrogen-enriched from bird or bat droppings, and humans

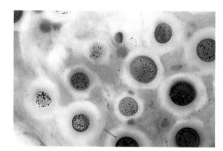

Fig. 2 **Encapsulated *C. neoformans*.**

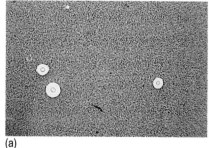

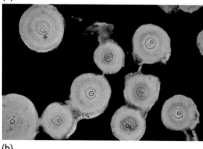

(a)

(b)

Fig. 3 *C. neoformans:* **Indian ink stain.** **(a)** Low power. **(b)** High power.

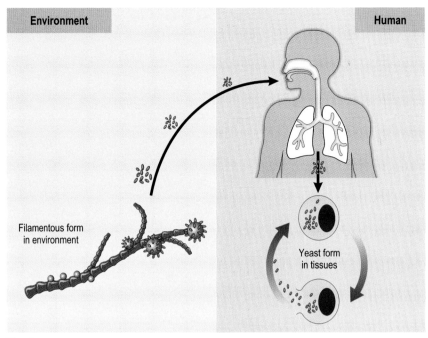

Fig. 4 *H. capsulatum* **infection.**

Table 1 **The interaction between organism and host in *H. capsulatum* infection**				
Organism	**Infecting dose**	**Host tissue**	**Host defence**	**Clinical result**
var. *capsulatum*: usual organism, lesser virulence	Usual	Normal (lung)	Immune	Asymptomatic infection, 90%
			Non-immune	Flu-like illness
	High	Normal	Non-immune	Latent infection
	Usual or high	Normal	Excessive response	Acute pulmonary histoplasmosis
	Usual	Normal	Impaired response	Peri-pulmonary fibrosis
	Usual	Normal	First normal, then impaired response	Disseminated histoplasmosis Re-activation and dissemination
	Usual	Chronic lung disease	Local defect	Chronic pulmonary histoplasmosis
var. *duboisii*: unusual organism, greater virulence	Usual	Normal	Normal	Bone and subcutaneous histoplasmosis

heal, giving rise to diagnostic calcification. Immunity is cell-mediated and wanes with time, though repeated attacks are less severe.

Confirmatory tests

The diagnosis is initially clinical in those exposed, especially in an endemic area, and chest x-ray showing small scattered infiltrates plus hilar lymphadenopathy is characteristic. Calcification is common on healing (Fig. 5).

Microscopy of sputum is not useful, and culture is slow, dangerous, and only useful in chronic disease.

Histopathology with silver stains is usually diagnostic but seldom necessary.

Serology is useful; the complement fixation test is standard on paired sera. Immunodiffusion in agar gel is more specific but less sensitive. Dissemination is detected by rapid antigen tests.

Clinical syndromes

These provide a wonderful illustration of the interaction between the organism's forces (infective dose, varying virulence and tissue trophism) and the host first-line defences (healthy or diseased tissues) and subsequent immune response (normal, or impaired, or initially normal then impaired, or excessive) (Table 1).

Chemotherapy

Treatment for severe or prolonged disease is parenteral amphotericin B or voriconazole. Oral voriconazole or itraconazole can follow.

Control

This depends on avoiding exposure, or using itraconazole as long-term suppression in chronic disease.

are infected by spore inhalation, especially when first exposed during work or leisure.

The filaments are thin, branching and septate, the spore being either tuberculate macroconidia or round microconidia. The yeast form is ovoid, about 2μm × 3μm. No toxins are known. Inhaled spores germinate to the yeast form, which is ingested by macrophages and transported to mediastinal lymph nodes, spleen and liver. Granulomata form and

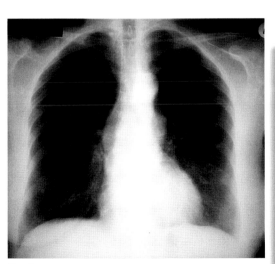

Fig. 5 **Histoplasmosis healed in lung showing scattered small calcified spots.**

Cryptococcus

- *C. neoformans* is a monomorphic yeast with a characteristic capsule, found particularly in pigeon droppings.

- var. *gattii* infects humans with a normal immune system by inhalation, while var. *neoformans* mainly infects the immunocompromised.

- Infection causes pulmonary masses (often asymptomatic), chronic meningitis, cerebral masses or systemic spread.

- Classical treatment is amphotericin B plus flucytosine, though fluconazole is now more used.

Histoplasma

- *H. capsulatum* is a dimorphic fungus: the filamentous mould form is found in soil with bird or bat droppings, and highly endemic areas are notorious.

- Humans are infected by inhalation of spores; these germinate to the yeast form, which is ingested by macrophages.

- The clinical disease depends on the dose inhaled, the immune state and local lung disease.

- Amphotericin B or voriconazole is the usual treatment.

Blastomyces, Coccidioides, Paracoccidioides

Blastomyces dermatitidis

B. dermatitidis (like *H. capsulatum*) is a dimorphic fungus with a filamentous spore-bearing mould form in the environment and on culture at 25°C, and a pathogenic yeast form in tissues (Fig. 1). The sexual form is an ascomycete called *Ajellomyces dermatitidis*. The organism, and hence blastomycosis, is endemic only in parts of North America and Africa. The mould is difficult to find in soil, and infects humans, dogs and horses by inhalation (Table 1).

The pyriform or pear-shaped macroconidia are 2–4μm in diameter; the yeast is bigger (8–15μm) and divides by *single* broadly based buds. No toxins are known and the pathogenesis is initially like histoplasmosis, with yeasts inhaled and spread by macrophages, followed by granuloma formation. However, calcification does not follow, and chronic suppuration is common.

Confirmatory tests

Microscopy of abscess pus shows broad-based budding yeasts, and culture is relatively easy. Serology is unhelpful (unlike histoplasmosis), but histopathology if necessary is usually diagnostic.

Clinical syndromes and management

Asymptomatic pulmonary infection is probably common. Treatment is essential if skin or bone infection, or the less common symptomatic pulmonary or visceral disease, develop.

Chemotherapy

Itraconazole is used for most infections, but amphotericin is necessary for severe disease.

Coccidioides immitis

C. immitis is a dimorphic fungus, with a filamentous spore-forming mould form in the environment and on culture at 25°C, and a pathogenic yeast form in tissues (Fig. 2). The sexual form is unknown. The scattered endemic foci are in southwest USA, Central and S. America. It is a soil organism, infecting by inhalation (Table 1).

Alternate cells in the filaments develop into barrel-shaped arthrospores (arthroconidia), while the second characteristic structure is the large (20–70μm) spherule in the infected tissues (Fig. 3). The spherule is filled with endospores which develop into further spherules, so the budding typical of the other systemic mycoses is absent. Granuloma formation resembling tuberculosis is usual.

Table 1 The systemic mycoses

Organism	Epidemiological source, route, area	Pathogenic mechanism	Clinical syndrome
Blastomyces dermatitidis	Soil and old buildings By inhalation N. America, Africa, Middle East	Local (inapparent) Distant spread	(Pulmonary) Bone and skin
Coccidioides immitis	Soil, dust storms By inhalation USA, Central and S. America	Local infection Distant spread	Pulmonary or none CNS, bone, skin
Paracoccidioides brasiliensis	Soil (probably) By inhalation, (?implantation) S. and Central America	Local (inapparent) Distant spread	(Pulmonary) Nose and mouth
Cryptococcus neoformans	Pigeon droppings By inhalation Worldwide	Local invasion Distant spread	Pulmonary CNS infection (Bone, skin)
Histoplasma capsulatum	Soil from birds and bats By inhalation Worldwide, mainly Americas and Africa	Local invasion Distant spread	Pulmonary Disseminated disease Bone, subcutaneous tissue in Africa

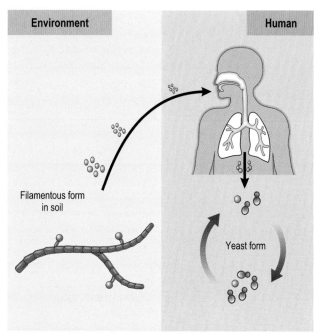

Fig. 1 **Environmental filamentous and pathogenic yeast forms of *B. dermatitidis*.**

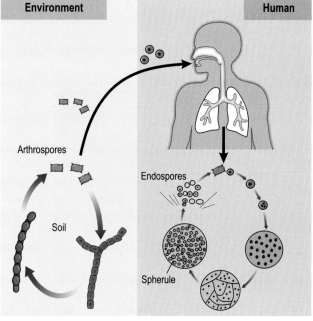

Fig. 2 **Environmental filamentous and pathogenic yeast forms of *C. immitis*.**

Confirmatory tests

Microscopy of sputum may show spherules with endospores. Culture is only done with special facilities because of the risk of laboratory-acquired infections.

Serology by latex agglutination or agar immunodiffusion is useful, and CFT may be used to follow progress. Histopathology is diagnostic if necessary (Fig. 3).

Clinical syndromes

Probably 60% of infections are asymptomatic, while the remainder result in an acute pulmonary infection at times with erythema nodosum or arthralgia. Most heal, but about 1% progress to chronic pulmonary disease or disseminated CNS, bone or skin disease.

Chemotherapy

Initial treatment is usually amphotericin B, then itraconazole long-term, or fluconazole for meningitis.

Paracoccidioides brasiliensis

P. brasiliensis (like *H. capsulatum*) is a dimorphic fungus with a filamentous spore-bearing mould form on culture at 25°C, and a pathogenic yeast form in tissues (Fig. 4). The sexual form is unknown. The organism, and hence paracoccidioidomycosis (South American blastomycosis), is endemic only in parts of Central and South America, especially Brazil. The mould is extremely difficult to find in soil, and probably infects humans by inhalation, though local implantation is possible.

The mycelium and sporulation have no special characteristics. The yeast size varies from 4µm to 40µm, and budding is multiple and circumferential, giving a 'pilot's wheel' formation, in contrast to histoplasmosis.

The mycelium-yeast transformation is inhibited by 17β-oestradiol, probably why adult females are rarely infected. No toxins are known, and infection leads to granuloma formation, chronic suppuration and hyperplasia. Cellular immunity is depressed by infection, and improves with recovery.

Confirmatory tests

Microscopy of abscess pus shows 'pilot's wheel' yeasts and culture is on Sabouraud-dextrose agar at 25°C.

Serology is by immunodiffusion or CFT. Histopathology, if necessary, is usually diagnostic. Skin testing is often negative on diagnosis.

Clinical syndromes and management

This is a progressive chronic disease, mainly in adult males. Primary pulmonary disease is often asymptomatic, and years later chronic 'mulberry' mucous membrane or warty skin ulcers develop. Lymph nodes, adrenals and other viscera can be infected.

Chemotherapy

Itraconazole is replacing ketoconazole. Amphotericin plus sulphonamides are reserved for intolerance, failure or cost reasons.

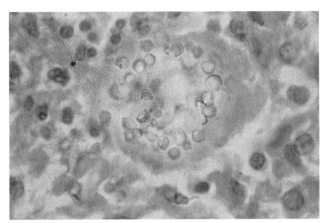

Fig. 3 **Tissue section showing *C. immitis* spherules.**

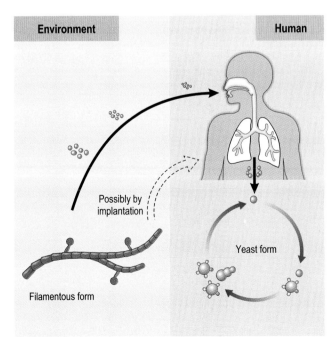

Fig. 4 **Environmental filamentous and pathogenic yeast forms of *P. brasiliensis.***

Blastomyces dermatitidis
- A dimorphic fungus endemic in parts of N. America and Africa.
- A soil organism causing blastomycosis by inhalation.
- Symptomatic pulmonary infection is rare, and chronic bone and skin disease is usual, with broad-based single-budding yeasts and granuloma formation.
- Itraconazole is used for most infections, amphotericin for severe disease.

Coccidioides immitis
- A dimorphic fungus endemic in areas of the Americas.
- A soil organism causing coccidioidomycosis by inhalation.
- Asymptomatic pulmonary infection is commonest, followed by symptomatic pulmonary disease; progressive or systemic disease is rare.
- Arthroconidia and tissue spherules are characteristic, with granulomata.
- Amphotericin is needed for systemic or severe disease, then itraconazole.

Paracoccidioides brasiliensis
- A dimorphic fungus endemic in S. America.
- A soil organism, it probably infects by inhalation, or possibly implantation.
- Chronic progressive skin and mucous membrane ulcers are usual; pulmonary and systemic disease occur rarely.
- *Multiple* budding gives a 'pilot's wheel' appearance microscopically, and granulomata occur.
- Itraconazole is replacing ketoconazole, or amphotericin plus sulphonamides in treatment.

Fungi infecting skin and adjacent tissues

Superficial mycoses

The superficial mycoses are fungal infections of the outermost layers of skin, and of hair.

Tinea versicolor (pityriasis versicolor)

This results from skin infection by *Malassezia furfur* (*Pityrosporum orbiculare*), a lipophilic yeast. Budding yeasts up to 8µm across and short mycelial fragments ('spaghetti and meat balls') are seen in KOH-treated skin scrapings from the scaly hypopigmented infection. Culture requires a medium rich in fatty acids and is not undertaken routinely.

Tinea versicolor (p. 198) should be differentiated from erythrasma, caused by *Corynebacterium minutissimum* (p. 202), which fluoresces pink under UV light.

Tinea nigra of the skin

Exophiala (previously *Cladosporium*) *werneckii*, a dimorphic fungus containing melanin, causes green-black colonies and brown-black skin lesions. Initially double-celled oval yeasts grow (seen in KOH mounts), then hyphae and conidia as the culture ages. The black skin lesions are described on page 198.

Black piedra of the hair

Piedraia hortae, an ascomycete, has its sexual stage on the hair, showing 2–8 slender ascospores in each ascus. Culture gives green-black or red-black colonies with chlamydospores. The hard black hair nodules and treatment by clipping are described on page 198.

White piedra of the hair

White piedra is caused by *Trichosporon beigelii*, a dimorphic fungus. The creamy-white mycelial collar on the hair shaft is of septate hyphae, which break to form arthroconidia. Culture (on media without inhibitory cycloheximide) gives soft white colonies, becoming wrinkled yellow-grey with age. The arthroconidia become rounded blastoconidia, showing the dimorphic nature of the fungus. Full identification is by biochemical tests. Clinical features are on page 198.

Cutaneous mycoses

Fungi known (wrongly) as dermatophytes ('skin plants') infect the kera-

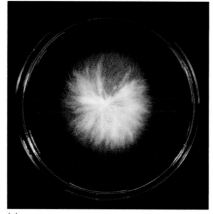

(a)

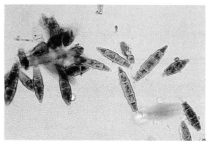

Fig. 2 **Macroconidia of *M. gypseum*.**

tinised surface of the body producing 'tinea' or 'ringworm'. The infections are named after the body area affected:

- tinea capitis: scalp
- tinea barbae: beard
- tinea corporis: body
- tinea cruris: groin
- tinea pedis: feet (athlete's foot)
- tinea unguium (nails).

About 40 species from three genera – *Trichophyton*, *Microsporum* and *Epidermophyton* – are involved (Table 1); many contain keratinases and infect only keratin-containing tissue. The sexual stage of *Microsporum* and *Trichophyton* are ascomycetes, genus *Arthroderma*.

Certain generalisations may be made about Table 1:
- Each species of *Trichophyton* and *Microsporum* can cause infection of skin, hair or nails.
- *T. rubrum*, *T. mentagrophytes* and *M. canis* are most common, but frequency varies widely between tropical and temperate areas.
- *T. schoenleinii* uniquely causes **favus** at the hair follicle.
- *Epidermophyton* does not cause tinea capitis or barbae and very rarely causes tinea unguium.

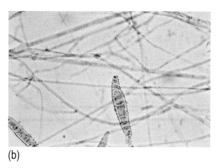

(b)

Fig. 1 ***Microsporum canis*. (a)** Surface view of colony. **(b)** Macroconidia.

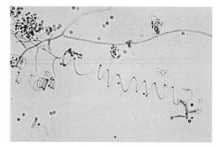

Fig. 3 **Microconidia of *T. mentagrophytes*.**

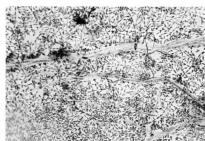

Fig. 4 ***Paecilomyces lilacinus*: a rare cause of hyalohyphomycosis.**

- Some zoophilic species may be recognised by their names; these particularly infect the skin and hair of children, and the beard areas of rural men, owing to greater contact. They usually provoke greater host inflammatory response in humans.
- Geophilic species particularly infect the head of children, again related to their greater contact with soil.

Confirmatory tests

Scrapings from the lesions are treated with KOH to dissolve the keratin and expose the fungal bodies on direct microscopy (Figs 1–3):

- *Trichophyton*: abundant microconidia; rare, smooth, thin-walled macroconidia
- *Microsporum*: many, rough thick-walled macroconidia; rarely any microconidia
- *Epidermophyton*: many smooth-walled macroconidia; no microconidia.

Identification to species level requires culture on selective media, e.g. Sabouraud-cycloheximide agar.

Clinical syndromes

Tinea of the skin, hair and nails is described on page 198. Chemotherapy is by topical antifungals including imidazoles such as clotrimazole. Oral terbinafine, itraconazole or griseofulvin is used for hair, nail and severe skin disease.

Subcutaneous mycoses and mycetoma

These uncommon diseases unfortunately have numerous causative fungi (Table 2), many of which have several synonyms. These mycoses are due to the implantation of soil fungi into the subcutaneous tissues by penetrating trauma, particularly in the tropics. They usually remain localised, except for hyalohyphomycosis, sporotrichosis, and mycetoma.

They are classified into:
- chromoblastomycosis
- phaeohyphomycosis
- hyalohyphomycosis
- lobomycosis
- rhinosporidiosis
- subcutaneous zygomycosis
- sporotrichosis (lymphocutaneous)
- eumycotic mycetoma.

The common causes and diagnostic mycology are summarised in Table 2.

Confirmatory tests

Culture of grains or pus from sinuses, or of excised tissue, and histopathology are specialised but usually diagnostic. The clinical syndrome and geographic area are also helpful.

Clinical syndromes

All cause subcutaneous lesions which often progress to involve the overlying skin. Sporotrichosis and mycetoma spread locally. Hyalohyphomycosis can disseminate (p. 202, 204).

Chemotherapy

Excision is often needed for localised subcutaneous mycoses, though flucyto-sine is sometimes useful in chromoblastomycosis. Disseminated hyalohyphomycosis needs amphotericin B and voriconazole. Mycetoma needs precise microbiologic diagnosis, and specialised medical and surgical treatment. Subcutaneous sporotrichosis is treated with potassium iodide, and extracutaneous sporotrichosis with itraconazole or amphotericin B.

Table 1 **Cutaneous mycoses**

Fungus	Ecology	Clinical disease
Trichophyton		
T. concentricum	A	Tinea corporis
T. equinum, T. mentagrophytes var mentagrophytes, T. verrucosum	Z	Barbae-capitis
T. mentagrophytes var interdigitale, T. rubrum	A	Pedis-manuum, corporis-cruris
T. schoenleinii, T. tonsurans	A	Favus, Tinea capitis
T. violaceum	A	Barbae-capitis
Microsporum		
M. audouinii	A	Tinea capitis
M. canis	Z	Barbae-capitis, corporis
M. equinum, M. gallinae	Z	Tinea capitis
M. ferrugineum	A	Tinea capitis
M. fulvum, M. gypseum, M. nanum	G	Tinea capitis
Epidermophyton		
E. floccosum	A	Pedis-manuum, corporis-cruris

A, anthropophilic (human source); G, geophilic (soil source); Z, zoophilic (animal source).

Table 2 **Subcutaneous mycoses and mycetoma**

Disease	Dominant causative fungi	Diagnostic mycology
Chromoblastomycosis (Chromomycosis)	Cladosporium carrionii, Fonsecaea pedrosoi, F. compacta, Phialophora verrucosa, Wangiella dermatitidis	Dematiaceous (melanin-pigmented) fungi: identified by type of sporulation; Histopathology shows pseudo-epitheliomatous hyperplasia, and golden-brown spherical 'sclerotic' bodies
Phaeohyphomycosis (phaeomycotic cyst)	Alternaria alternata, Curvularia geniculata, Wangiella dermatitidis and others	Dematiaceous fungi; short hyphal fragments, without hyperplasia on histology (Fig. 4)
Hyalohyphomycosis	Fusarium solani / Penicillium marneffii	Hyaline septate mould. Culture / Hyaline septate mould. Culture
Lobomycosis	Loboa loboi	Lemon-shaped yeasts in pairs or short chains; never cultured
(Rhinosporidiosis)	Rhinosporidium seeberi (Now not a fungus!)	(Thick-walled cysts (10–200µm) called spherules, filled with 'spores'; never cultured)
Subcutaneous zygomycosis	Conidiobolus coronatus, Basidiobolus ranarum	Culture after excision shows typical conidia
Sporotrichosis (lymphocutaneous, spreads along lymphatics)	Sporothrix schenckii	Dimorphic: mould at 25°C, and yeast at 37°C and in tissues; conidia form typical rosettes
Eumycotic mycetoma: penetrates deeply to muscle, tendon and even bone	Madurella grisea, M. mycetomatis, Pseudallescheria boydii	Culture and structure of fungi grown from grains from sinuses; distinguish from bacterial mycetoma (p. 62, 202)

Superficial fungal infections
- Superficial mycoses are caused by four specific fungi and result in hypopigmentation or black skin, or black or white hairs.
- Diagnosis is clinical and by microscopy.
- Infected skin is treated topically, and infected hair clipped or shaved.

Cutaneous fungal infections ('Tinea')
- Cutaneous mycoses result from infection by *Microsporum, Trichophyton* or *Epidermophyton* spp.
- Sources are humans, animals or the soil.
- Diagnosis is by microscopy and culture.
- Treatment is topical for mild skin disease, or oral terbinafine, itraconazole or griseofulvin for hair, nail or severe skin disease.

Subcutaneous fungal infections and mycetoma
- Subcutaneous mycoses and mycetoma are caused by many fungi after penetrating trauma.
- Mostly localised, but hyalohyphomycosis, sporotrichosis and mycetoma can spread.
- Chemotherapy and often excision is required.

Fungi causing invasive zygomycosis (mucormycosis)

Zygomycosis is infection with fungi of the class Zygomycetes, which includes the orders Mucorales and Entomophthorales. Mucormycosis is invasive infection with fungi of the order Mucorales, including the genera *Mucor, Rhizopus, Rhizomucor* and *Absidia*. Entomophthoromycosis is infection with fungi of the other order, including *Basidiobolus* and *Conidiobolus* (Subcutaneous zygomycosis, p. 75).

Life cycle and pathogenesis

The Mucorales, like *Aspergillus*, are monomorphic fungi, with only the mycelial form in all environments. The hyphae (Fig. 1) are non-septate, very big (10–15μm across) and branch at right angles (unlike *Aspergillus*, which are septate, smaller and branch at acute angles).

Mucorales are soil organisms which grow easily on bread and fruit, and infection occurs usually by inhalation, rarely by implantation in wounds or burns.

Human infections are usually with *Rhizopus arrhizus* (*R. oryzae*) or *Absidia corymbifera*. These invade tissues, particularly blood vessels, causing infarction and necrosis.

Virulence is increased by acidosis and corticosteroids, so diabetics and immunosuppressed patients are most at risk.

Confirmatory tests

As they are common surface contaminants, diagnosis of infection needs *repeated culture* from non-sterile sites like deep tissues, or *histopathology* (Fig. 2). These fungi cannot be distinguished from each other without culture. Rhizoids (roots) form from stolons (runners). The sporangiophores carry sporangia, containing spores (sporangiospores) (Fig. 1).

- *Rhizopus*: stalks of sporangiophores are opposite the rhizoids
- *Absidia*: stalks of sporangiophores are not opposite the rhizoids
- *Mucor*: no rhizoids.

Clinical syndromes

Recently there has been an increase in generalised infections caused by fungi. Mucormycosis affects brain and lung most often. **Rhinocerebral zygomycosis** or mucormycosis is the commonest and most feared form of this rare

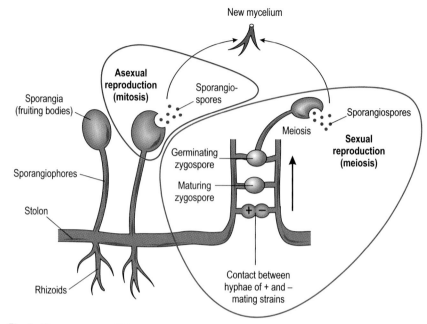

Fig. 1 **The structure and life cycle of a zygomycete.**

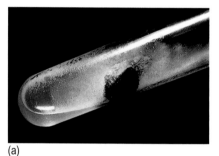
(a)

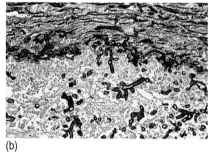
(b)

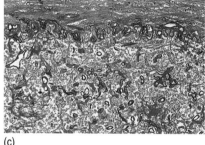
(c)

Fig. 2 **Mucormycosis. (a)** Skin biopsy. **(b)** Histology, staining with H & E. **(c)** Histology, staining with silver iodide.

infection (p. 103). Other rare syndromes are pulmonary (rather like aspergillosis), disseminated, gastrointestinal, wound, skin or visceral. Infected patients are usually diabetic, on steroids, or immunosuppressed by disease or drugs.

Chemotherapy and control

Amphotericin B is essential. Control of the predisposing factors helps to prevent infection; early excisional surgery is usually required.

> ### Fungi causing zygomycosis
>
> - Zygomycosis is infection with fungi of the class Zygomycetes, including mucormycosis from *Rhizopus, Mucor, Absidia* and *Rhizomucor* of the Order Mucorales.
> - Infection from these environmental organisms is by inhalation usually, implantation rarely. Acidosis and corticosteroids enhance their growth.
> - Invasion is characteristic, often vascular.
> - Rhinocerebral mucormycosis is the commonest, often fatal, form, but pulmonary, systemic and local infections can occur.
> - Treatment is by amphotericin B, excision, and correction of predisposing factors, including diabetes and immunosuppression.

Arthropods

The arthropods are invertebrates not microorganisms but they play an important role in human infections in several ways.

- **mechanical vectors** are involved in disease transmission but are not essential for the survival of the pathogen, e.g. house flies with bacterial enteric pathogens
- **biological vectors** are host for an essential part of the life cycle of the pathogen they transmit, e.g. the mosquito host for *Plasmodium* spp., which cause malaria
- **reservoirs**: some arthropods act as reservoirs for maintaining microorganisms between hosts, e.g. lice and *R. prowazekii*, causing typhus.
- **true infections** of the skin, e.g. lice.

Table 1 lists some infections, covered elsewhere in this book, where an arthropod vector is involved.

Arthropod infections

Pediculus humanus and *Phthirus pubis*
Lice are blood-sucking insects that live on human skin: three main types are *Pediculus humanus* var *corporis*, the human body louse; *Pediculus humanus* var *capitis*, the human head louse; and *Phthirus pubis*, the human pubic louse.

The lice are about 3mm long and have a 3-week reproductive cycle: 1 week for eggs to hatch and 2 weeks to maturity.

Three major diseases carried are (p. 66, 67, 154):

- **epidemic typhus fever** (*Rickettsia prowazeckii*): body louse vector
- **trench fever** (*Bartonella quintana*): body louse host
- **epidemic relapsing fever** (*Borrelia recurrentis*): body louse vector.

Table 1 **Some diseases transmitted by arthropod vectors**		
Disease	**Pathogen**	**Vector**
Tularaemia (p.213)	*Francisella tularensis*	Ticks, deer flies
Plague (p. 212)	*Yersinia pestis*	Flea
Lyme disease (p. 154)	*Borrelia burgdorferi*	Tick
Epidemic typhus (p. 66)	*Rickettsia prowazekii*	Body louse
Rocky Mountain spotted fever (p. 67)	*R. rickettsii*	Tick
Malaria (p. 152)	*Plasmodium* spp.	Mosquito (Anopheles)
Sleeping sickness (p. 153)	*Trypanosoma brucei/gambiense*	Tsetse fly
Chagas' disease (p. 138)	*T. cruzi*	Reduviid bug
Filariasis (p. 205)	*Wuchereria bancrofti*	Mosquito
Loiasis (p. 111)	*Loa loa*	Mango fly
Dengue, YF, encephalitis (p. 100, 146)	Arboviruses (400+)	Mosquito

Three predisposing factors are poor hygiene, close contact and shared possessions or partners. Head lice pass rapidly among children in schools and nurseries.

Three indicators of lice infestation are bites, nits (the whitish eggs on hairs, Fig. 1) or lice (especially the pubic type). Three common clinical clues are:

- pruritus: intense, prolonged and widespread
- haemorrhagic bites: especially near folds of clothes
- secondary bacterial infection.

Three rarer clinical clues are:

- blepharitis, from pubic (!) lice and bacterial infection
- maculae caerulae (literally, sky-blue spots) on the abdomen and thighs from pubic lice, possibly by a haemolysin
- vagabond's disease, marked by chronicity, hyperpigmentation and lichenification of the skin.

Three control measures are prevention of overcrowding, improved hygiene (washing clothing and bedding) and insecticides: malathion, permethrin, or DDT in past epidemic situations, plus removing the nits by special fine-toothed combs.

Sarcoptes scabiei
The mite *S. scabiei* causes **scabies**, a parasitic skin infection. The mite lives in the epidermis of human skin and the females lay eggs in the stratum corneum. After a few days the eggs hatch and the larvae mature to spread across the skin. The preferred areas are the wrists and between the fingers, and infection causes severe itching, particularly at night. Secondary bacterial infections can occur where the skin is broken by scratching. The mites themselves do not cause itch directly; hypersensitivity reactions to the mites and their faeces are the powerful mechanism (Fig. 2).

Norwegian scabies appears very different clinically, with grossly thickened skin and thin scales in the immunosuppressed. Thick nails, pyoderma and pigmentation follow.

Scabies is transferred person to person by close contact, and from fomites such as clothes and bedding. Permethrin kills the mites, and hygiene and improved living conditions reduce spread.

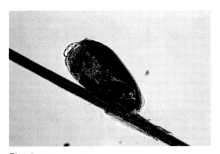

Fig. 1 **Nit on hair.**

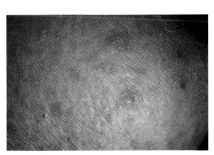

Fig. 2 **Scabies.**

Arthropods
- Can be mechanical vectors, biological vectors, reservoirs or cause infections themselves.
- Lice cause infections, and can carry epidemic typhus, trench fever and relapsing fever.
- *Sarcoptes scabiei* cause scabies, with severe nocturnal itch.

Sporozoa: *Plasmodium, Toxoplasma, Cryptosporidium*

Protozoa contain four major groups: sporozoa (including coccidia, p. 78–79), amoebae (p. 80), ciliates (p. 81) and flagellates (p. 81–83).

Plasmodia

Plasmodia are sporozoan parasites of humans and animals, and cause malaria in humans. Four species infect humans:

- *P. falciparum*: causes malignant tertian malaria, the most severe type and the predominant type in the tropics
- *P. vivax*: causes benign tertian malaria, the most widely distributed form and the predominant type in temperate areas
- *P. malariae*: causes quartan malaria (72-hour cycle)
- *P. ovale*: is a cause of tertian malaria in West Africa and is relatively uncommon (tertian malaria has 48-hour cycles of fever).

Life cycle and pathogenesis

Female *Anopheles* mosquitoes transmit the infection. The life cycle of plasmodia is complex, with a sexual cycle occurring in the mosquito, and two asexual (schizogony) phases in the human (Fig. 1), initially in the liver and then in the blood.

The liver cycle in the human produces merozoites that can either enter new liver cells to repeat the cycle of production, or can enter red blood cells (RBC). The liver phase may persist for long periods in *P. vivax* and *P. ovale*, so relapses from these forms may occur although the parasite has been eliminated from peripheral blood.

The asexual stage in red blood cells consists of numerous forms diagnostic in blood films (RBC cycle, Fig. 1). Episodes of fever occur when further merozoites are released from RBC. The intervals between the bouts of fever depend on the time taken to complete the asexual cycle in the blood.

Some merozoites in RBC develop into male and female gametocytes which are ingested by mosquitoes to complete the life cycle.

Partial immunity from previous infections, and the sickle cell trait, decrease the severity of infection.

Confirmatory tests

Thick and thin blood films stained by Leishman or Giemsa show the malarial parasites (MP) in sequential development:

1. ring forms (trophozoites), usually as small round structures with a clear centre and a chromatin dot at one side
2. rosettes, which are schizonts containing daughter merozoites
3. gametocytes, rarely seen.

Each species has specific morphology, e.g. the gametocytes of *P. falciparum* are crescentic while the trophozoites of *P. vivax* (meaning 'living') are amoeboid.

Rapid Antigen Detection, and PCR are promising second line tests.

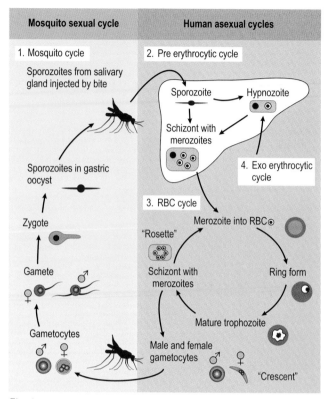

Fig. 1   *Plasmodium* **life cycle.**

Clinical syndromes

Acute malaria is a medical emergency (p. 104, 152).

Chemotherapy

This is complex (p. 152). Recent WHO or Health Department recommendations must be followed. Primaquin is used to kill liver 'hypnozoites'.

Control

This depends on mosquito control, protection from bites, and chemoprophylaxis in the non-immune during and after visits to endemic areas.

Toxoplasma gondii

T. gondii is a coccidian parasite of cats. The sexual cycle is in the cat (Fig. 2a), producing **oocytes** in the faeces that infect intermediate hosts – humans, many mammals and some reptiles. Islands without cats have no human toxoplasmosis, which appears if cats are introduced.

In the human or animal host, the asexual cycle produces slender **tachyzoites**, which infect cells (often macrophages and endothelial cells), or shorter broader dormant **bradyzoites**, which form large tissue cysts (Fig. 2b) with hundreds of organisms in tissues. These account for latency, and are infectious to other animals if the tissue is eaten.

The asexual cycle also occurs in cats, perpetuating infection.

Humans are infected by ingesting **oocysts** in food soiled with cat faeces, by eating raw or undercooked meat (e.g. lamb, mutton) containing **tissue cysts**, or by **transplacental** infection (congenital infection, p. 214–215).

All strains appear of equal virulence. They survive initially in macrophages by preventing phagosome-lysosome activity and fusion, but are killed by activated macrophages.

Confirmatory tests

Serology for IgM and IgG was the major diagnostic method, now being replaced by PCR.

CT brain scans in AIDS and other immunosuppressed patients are often characteristic. Histopathology and/or PCR on biopsies are diagnostic, if necessary.

Clinical syndromes (p. 213)

- Most infections are asymptomatic: about 40% of adults have positive serology but recall no infection.
- A mononucleosis-like syndrome can occur with acute infection.
- Local tissue cysts form.
- Recrudescence of latent infection occurs with immunosuppression, e.g. in transplant or AIDS patients.

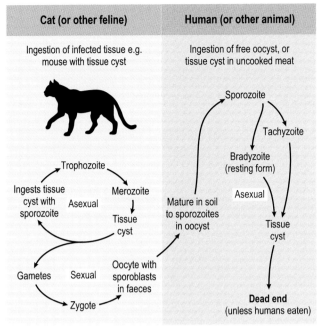

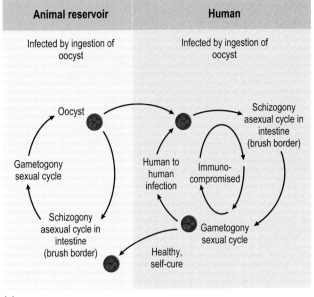

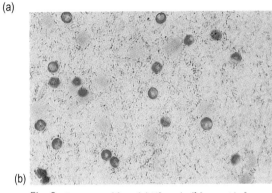

Fig. 3 ***Cryptosporidum.* (a)** Life cycle; **(b)** oocyst in faeces stained by acid-fast stain (*Cryptosporidum parvum*).

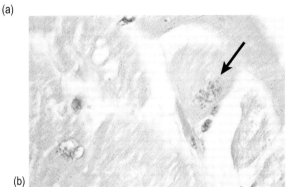

Fig. 2 ***Toxoplasma.* (a)** Life cycle; **(b)** tissue cyst.

- Congenital infection acquired in utero from an infected mother causes chorioretinitis, convulsions, cerebral atrophy and calcification (Figs 2, 3, and 4, p. 215).

Chemotherapy

A combination of pyrimethamine and sulphadiazine is the usual treatment, while clindamycin, clarithromycin or spiramycin are alternatives. Treatment is only suppressive as tissue cysts are resistant.

Control

Meat should be properly cooked, and hands washed after handling cats or their litter, after preparing raw meat, and before eating. It is believed that humans are usually infected by eating food contaminated with oocysts. Cats are a health hazard particularly to women of childbearing age.

Cryptosporidium spp.

Cryptosporidium spp. are coccidia, found worldwide. They are animal parasites which infect humans, from contaminated water, calves, and by contact.

Virulence and pathogenesis

Cryptosporidia have a simple life cycle (Fig. 3a). Only one or two cycles occur in normal hosts, but many cycles in the immunocompromised patient.

The fertilised oocyst in faeces is diagnostic; it stains, unexpectedly, with acid-fast stains (Fig. 3b).

Clinical syndromes

Patients usually present with diarrhoea that lasts 1–2 weeks; in immunocompromised patients prolonged severe diarrhoea is caused by the multiple replication cycles.

Chemotherapy and control

Nitazoxanide is the first effective treatment, replacing paromomycin. Handwashing and safer sexual practices offer some protection.

Cyclospora cayetanensis and *Isospora belli*

These coccidia are rare causes of prolonged diarrhoea in the immunocompromised, including AIDS patients. They are diagnosed by stool staining and microscopy, and treated with nitazoxanide or co-trimoxazole.

Sporozoan parasites

- Sporozoan parasites have life cycles with distinct sexual and asexual phases; the sexual phase occurs in the primary host (often non-human) and the asexual proliferation phase gives rise to the clinical symptoms.
- Chemotherapy is not always effective. Control is by avoiding infection, reducing mosquito bites (malaria), and careful handling of food and water.
- Malaria is caused by *Plasmodium* spp. which infect humans via the bite of the female *Anopheles* mosquito.

- Treatment for malaria includes drug regimens that must vary with parasite drug resistance. Chemoprophylaxis is used for travellers.
- *T. gondii* is a cat parasite that causes toxoplasmosis in humans. Infection of the fetus or in the immunocompromised has severe consequences.
- *Cryptosporidium, Cyclospora* or *Isospora* spp. cause diarrhoea that is usually severe in the immunocompromised.

Amoebae: *Entamoeba, Naegleria, Acanthamoeba*

Entamoeba histolytica

E. histolytica is the pathogenic amoeba causing **amoebic dysentery**, occurring mainly in developing countries. Initial attacks are virulent: local colonic invasion causes acute dysentery (diarrhoea with blood plus mucus). Some immunity develops, so in endemic countries, mild chronic or intermittent diarrhoea or asymptomatic cyst passing are more common.

E. histolytica lives in the mucosa of the large intestine producing local necrosis and ulcers. Local and distant spread can occur, with tissue lysis ('histolytica') causing distant abscesses. Transmission is usually faecal–oral, sometimes ano–oral, rarely ano–penile in homosexuals.

The fragile, motile erythrocytophagic ('able to eat red blood cells') **trophozoite** comes from resistant non-motile **cysts** which survive outside the body for years. *E. dispar* is microscopically identical.

Confirmatory tests

Careful and expert microscopy on three or more fresh stool specimens may be needed to find trophozoites or cysts (Fig. 1), and distinguish pathogenic *E. histolytica* from non-pathogens like *Entamoeba coli* (Table 1). Cysts (Fig. 1) do not prove active disease.

Serology is most useful in non-endemic countries and for extraintestinal amoebiasis, using IgM detection for acute disease. Stool antigen tests are improving, but PCR is still impractical.

CT scans of liver and brain, and chest x-rays define spread.

Clinical syndromes

Amoebic infection ranges from asymptomatic cyst passage to acute dysentery to chronic intermittent dysentery, and to extraintestinal liver, lung and brain abscesses, or cutaneous infections (p. 103, 162, 168, 204).

Chemotherapy

Metronidazole is standard, but adding intestinal antiseptics such as diloxanide furoate improves cure rates. Abscesses seldom need drainage now.

Control

Hygiene includes hand-washing after defaecation, and careful preparation of food. Safer sex practices are also partly protective.

Other intestinal amoeba

Entamoeba coli, Entamoeba hartmanni, Endolimax nana, Iodamoeba butschlii are all considered non-pathogenic but microscopically must be differentiated carefully from *E. histolytica. Entamoeba polecki* from pigs may cause brief, mild diarrhoea. *Dientamoeba fragilis* is now classified as a flagellate (p. 81).

Naegleria fowleri

N. fowleri is a free-living amoeba widely distributed in fresh water, especially where bacterial contamination occurs. The trophozoite is slow moving, but a mobile flagellate form occurs in culture, and a cyst form in unfavourable conditions.

N. fowleri is highly virulent and causes **amoebic meningoencephalitis** (Fig. 2) by inhalation and penetration through the nasal mucosa and the cribriform plate.

Confirmatory tests

Microscopy of CSF shows the causative amoebae with many polymorphs. Trophozoites are 10–20μm across, move slowly and have a large central karyosome in a round nucleus – features distinguishing them from monocytes. Protein is elevated, glucose low.

Clinical syndrome

Acute amoebic meningoencephalitis is rapidly progressive and fatal in 3–4 days unless treated early and vigorously.

Chemotherapy

Intravenous high-dose amphotericin B is essential and may be supplemented intrathecally, plus oral rifampicin and an imidazole.

Acanthamoeba spp.

These are also free-living amoebae, rather smaller than *Naegleria* and with foamy cytoplasm. They are found in contaminated water, soil and the human oral cavity. They cause either a more chronic **granulomatous meningoencephalitis** in immunocompromised patients, or **corneal infection** after trauma, surgery, or contact lens contamination.

Amphotericin B is surprisingly ineffective; flucytosine and imidazoles are used.

Balamuthia mandrillaris

This free-living amoeba is a rare cause of **granulomatous meningoencephalitis** in people with normal or impaired immunity. Treatment is as for *Acanthamoeba* infection.

Table 1	**Distinguishing *Entamoeba* spp.**		
	E. histolytica / E. dispar	**E. coli**	**E. nana**
Trophozoite size (μm)	15–50	10–30	6–12
Nuclear karyosome	Central	Eccentric	Massive
Nuclear chromatin	Peripheral, fine	Clumped, coarse	Indistinct
Ingested RBC	Yes	No	No
Cyst size (μm)	8–20	10–30	8–10
Cyst nuclei	1–4	1–8	1–4
Chromatoidal bars	Rounded	Split-enz	None

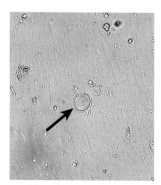

Fig. 1 *Entamoeba histolytica* cyst in stool.

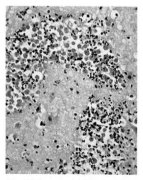

Fig. 2 **Amoebic encephalitis.**

Amoebae

- Pathogenic amoebae occur as amoeboid trophozoites or as resistant long-living cysts.

- Humans carry many non-pathogenic intestinal amoebae; *E. histolytica* causes amoebic dysentery and can spread to distant organs causing abscesses.

- Free-living amoebae *N. fowleri* and *Acanthamoeba* spp. are found in fresh water and cause severe meningoencephalitis.

- *Acanthamoeba* spp. also cause keratitis after trauma, surgery, or contact lens contamination.

Intestinal and vaginal flagellates and ciliates

Giardia lamblia

This flagellate protozoan (= *G. intestinalis*, *G. duodenalis*) is distinctive both in morphology and in infecting the duodenum and small intestine. Like amoebae, it has a fragile **trophozoite** (Fig. 1), a tougher infective **cyst** (Fig. 2) and divides by binary fission. Ingested cysts liberate trophozoites that adhere to the intestinal mucosa by a ventral sucking disc causing local damage and malabsorption in heavy infection.

The reservoirs of infection are water, humans and animals including beavers. Infection is by water or food, or by faecal–oral or ano–oral spread. Large outbreaks of giardiasis have occurred. It varies from asymptomatic infection to acute watery diarrhoea to chronic intermittent diarrhoea with malabsorption.

Diagnosis is by stool microscopy, which shows the distinctive cysts more often than trophozoites. The distinctive 'face with moustache' trophozoite is distinctive (Fig. 1). Repeated specimens are often necessary because of intermittent excretion. Rarely a duodenal aspirate or biopsy with smear is needed.

Giardiasis is treated with metronidazole or quinacrine, albendazole or nitazoxanide; repeat courses may be needed. Control depends on good hygiene including hand-washing. Cysts resist usual water chlorination levels.

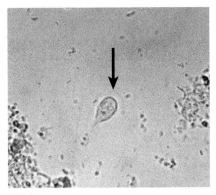

Fig. 1 *G. lamblia* trophozoite.

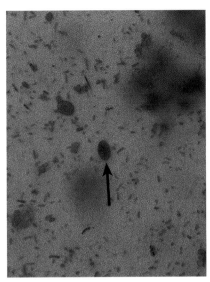

Fig. 2 *G. lamblia* cyst.

Dientamoeba fragilis

This flagellate has several unusual characteristics:

- it is a highly motile trichomonad, not an amoeba, despite its name
- no cyst form is known
- the delicate trophozoite is probably transmitted person-to-person protected inside eggs of the pinworm, *Enterobius vermicularis*!
- it is bi-nucleate, with 4–6 chromatin granules in each.

D. fragilis causes mild local damage to the proximal colon and rarely causes abdominal and diarrhoeal symptoms. Diagnosis is by stool microscopy, and treatment is metronidazole, doxycycline or iodoquin. Control is by hygienic measures and pinworm treatment.

Balantidium coli

B. coli is the largest protozoan infecting mammals; the trophozoite is 50–200µm in diameter, structurally complex, and forms a resistant cyst that transmits disease. It is a parasite of pigs, infecting humans by the faecal–oral route, then from person to person. It invades the colonic mucosa, causing dysentery with blood and mucus in the stools.

Diagnosis is by stool microscopy, treatment is by tetracycline, metronidazole, or iodoquin, and control is by hygiene including hand-washing.

Trichomonas vaginalis

T. vaginalis is a urogenital flagellate. It is very common in the vagina of sexually active women, and transmission is usually sexual, occasionally by fomites.

The trophozoite reproduces by binary fission, and no cyst form is known. Some strains have greater virulence, and pathogenesis involves epithelial adhesion, damage and microulceration. Asymptomatic infection is common in both women (vaginal) and men (urethral). Vaginitis with frothy watery yellow discharge is the most common symptomatic disease, while symptomatic urethritis, prostatitis or epididymitis are rare.

Direct microscopy of vaginal or urethral discharge by the wet mount technique shows the distinctive motile trophozoite.

Metronidazole is given to the patient and all sexual partners. During pregnancy, clotrimazole may be safer but is less effective.

Safer sexual practices and care with shared personal articles help control transmission.

Intestinal and vaginal flagellates and ciliates

- *G. lamblia* occurs in trophozoite and cyst form; it is found in water and it spreads rapidly person to person causing large outbreaks of giardiasis.
- Giardiasis usually causes diarrhoea and may result in malabsorption; several courses of metronidazole, albendazole, nitazoxanide or quinacrine may be needed.
- *D. fragilis* rarely causes diarrhoea but *B. coli* causes dysentery.
- *T. vaginalis* is a sexually transmitted urogenital flagellate causing vaginitis and sometimes urethritis; treatment should include sexual partners.

Blood and tissue flagellates

Haemoflagellates are protozoa with flagella which infect blood and tissues; they are transmitted by biting flies or bugs, usually from animal reservoirs (see p. 24, 77).

Leishmania

The genus *Leishmania* includes variants not considered here, hence the term 'complex' in *Leishmania donovani* complex, *L. tropica* complex, *L. brasiliensis* complex and *L. mexicana* complex. All are intracellular parasites of humans, **transmitted by sandfly bites**.

Life cycle and pathogenesis

Leishmaniae have a simple life cycle (Fig. 1) with only two forms:

- a rounded (2–3μm), replicating **amastigote** with nucleus, parabasal body and kinetoplast, but no flagellum, in the mammalian host cells; replication is by binary fission
- an elongated (2 × 20μm) flagellated **promastigote** in the insect (sandfly) host.

All are virulent, causing severe disease in normal hosts. Pathogenesis begins with local destruction and invasion of macrophages; dissemination to spleen, liver and other lymphoid tissues occurs in the visceral form, and to mucosa and skin in the mucocutaneous and cutaneous types. Activation of T-cells and cell-mediated immunity are important in host resistance.

Confirmatory tests

While clinical diagnosis is often possible in endemic areas, definite diagnosis depends on microscopy and specific staining (Giemsa, Wright) for amastigotes:

- in bone marrow, called Leishman-Donovan (LD) bodies (Fig. 2), or other aspirate in kala-azar
- in ulcer scrapings, aspirates or biopsies in 'Old World' cutaneous disease (Fig. 3)
- in punch biopsies (smear plus histopathology) in 'New World' cutaneous and mucocutaneous disease.

Clinical syndromes

Four types of leishmaniasis occur (p. 152, 205):

- *L. donovani* complex causes kala-azar (visceral) and post-kala-azar dermal leishmaniasis

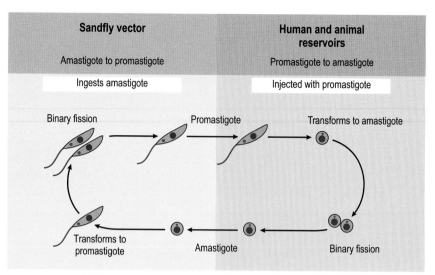

Sandfly vector — Amastigote to promastigote — Ingests amastigote

Human and animal reservoirs — Promastigote to amastigote — Injected with promastigote

Binary fission → Promastigote → Transforms to amastigote

Transforms to promastigote ← Amastigote ← Binary fission

Fig. 1 **Leishmania life cycle.**

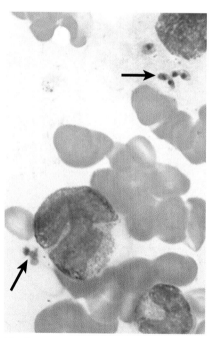

Fig. 2 **LD bodies in bone marrow.**

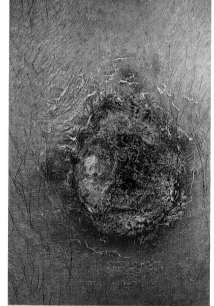

Fig. 3 **Cutaneous leishmaniasis sore.**

- *L. tropica* complex causes oriental sore (cutaneous leishmaniasis)
- *L. mexicana* complex causes American (New World) cutaneous leishmaniasis
- *L. brasiliensis* complex causes mucocutaneous leishmaniasis.

Visceral disease is characterised by fever and anaemia, with high mortality. The cutaneous forms involve granulomatous and ulcerative sores.

Chemotherapy

Stibogluconate (used in the Old World) or the equivalent meglumine antimoniate (used in the New World) are used for all except Ethiopian disease. Alternatives

are pentamidine or oral miltefosine in visceral disease, local heat in Oriental disease, and amphotericin B in American and Ethiopian disease.

Control

This depends on sandfly control, particularly around houses, and protection from biting.

Trypanosoma

Human trypanosomes include two variants of *Trypanosoma brucei*, *T. brucei gambiense* and *T. brucei rhodesiense*, plus *T. cruzi*.

T. brucei causes the cattle disease, nagana, and <u>human sleeping sickness</u>. *T. brucei* live and multiply in the human bloodstream and invade the CNS to cause sleeping sickness. *T. cruzi* is an intracellular parasite of humans, causing acute and chronic <u>Chagas' disease</u>, with cardiac and gut involvement. Both are spread by insect vectors, the tsetse fly for *T. brucei* and the reduviid ('kissing') bugs for *T. cruzi*. The reservoir hosts are wild animals and cattle in some areas; in other areas the animal host is unknown.

Life cycle and pathogenesis

T. brucei have a simple life cycle (Fig. 4), with only two stages:

- the **trypomastigote** in human blood. Usually as a long slender (3 × 30μm)

form with nucleus, parabasal body and kinetoplast, flagellum and full-length undulating flagellar membrane. It is somewhat polymorphic, so short broad forms without a flagellum, and intermediate forms occur. Replication is by binary fission.
- the **epimastigote** in the tsetse fly with only a partial undulating membrane.

In *T. cruzi* (Fig. 5) there is a third stage, the **amastigote**, which is the invasive, dividing, destructive tissue stage in humans.

The pathogenic trypanosomes are virulent, causing severe disease in normal hosts. Pathogenesis begins with variable local destruction (the trypanoma) and invasion of the bloodstream, followed by invasion and destruction of cerebral tissue (*T. brucei*) or cardiac, oesophageal or colonic tissue (*T. cruzi*). *T. brucei* largely avoids host response by changing its surface antigens (glycoproteins) during bouts of parasitaemia.

Confirmatory tests

While clinical diagnosis is often possible in endemic areas, definite diagnosis depends on microscopy and specific staining (Giemsa) for amastigotes in anticoagulated blood, blood films or lymph node aspirates. Culture is often necessary in Chagas' disease where parasitaemia is less or absent. Serology is of some use.

Clinical syndromes

Details of the trypanoma, acute disease and progressive encephalitis of sleeping sickness from *T. brucei*, and of Chagas' disease from *T. cruzi* are covered on pages 105, 138, 153.

Chemotherapy

Suramin is the drug of choice for early *T. brucei* infections, the alternative being pentamidine. Toxic organic arsenicals such as melarsoprol are needed for CNS infection. Benznidazole is the drug of choice in *T. cruzi* infections.

Control

This depends on tsetse fly and reduviid bug control, particularly around houses, protection from biting, and treatment of infected humans.

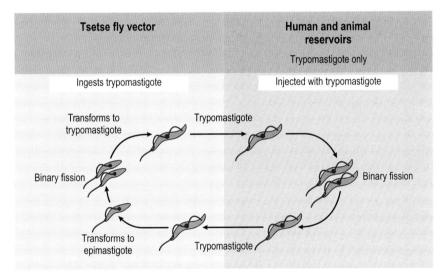

Fig. 4 *Trypanosoma brucei* **life cycle.**

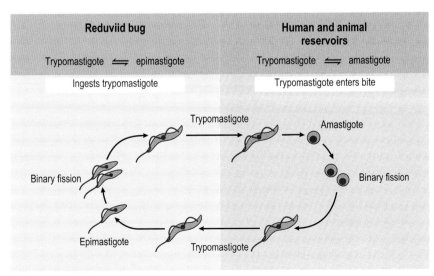

Fig. 5 *Trypanosoma cruzi* **life cycle.**

> ## Blood and tissue flagellates
>
> - Leishmaniasis can be visceral (kala-azar), cutaneous (oriental sore) or mucocutaneous depending on the *Leishmania* spp. involved. All are transmitted by sandfly bites, and infections are diagnosed by microscopy of bone marrow, splenic, skin or mucosal ulcer specimens.
>
> - *T. brucei* variants cause sleeping sickness in humans, spread by tsetse flies. Initial local trypanoma is followed by encephalitis. Parasites are detected in blood films.
>
> - *T. cruzi* causes Chagas' disease in Latin America and is spread by reduviid ('kissing') bugs. Diagnosis is by microscopy of blood in early disease, or by culture in chronic disease with cardiac involvement, mega-oesophagus or mega-colon.

Intestinal nematodes (worms)

Helminths contain three groups: nematodes (p. 84–87), cestodes (p. 88–89) and trematodes (p. 90–91). Some of the intestinal nematodes have an obligatory soil phase, others can have direct person-to-person spread or autoinfection. Infection is either by ingestion or skin penetration.

Enterobius vermicularis (pinworm or threadworm)

The pinworm, a very common intestinal helminth, is small (male 2.5mm, female 10mm) like a piece of cotton thread. Unlike most other worms, it is more common in temperate climates because it spreads person-to-person by direct contact or fomites, and occasionally by inhalation of egg-contaminated dust.

Life cycle and pathogenesis. Unusually, pinworms have no obligatory soil cycle, nor do they multiply *in* the body! The gravid female lays 10000 to 15000 bean-shaped eggs (50 × 25µm) in a few minutes on the peri-anal skin then dies. So eggs are found on underclothes, on bedding, or under scratching finger-nails, or ingested or, occasionally, inhaled (Fig. 1a). The eggs can also carry *Dientamoeba fragilis* (p. 81).

Clinical syndrome. Light infections are asymptomatic; peri-anal female worms cause itching (pruritus ani, p. 163) or vaginal irritation.

Confirmatory tests. Microscopy of adhesive tape previously pressed to the anus shows the typical egg (Fig. 2a). The adult worms may be seen macroscopically.

Chemotherapy. Treatment with pyrantel pamoate or mebendazole is given to the whole family.

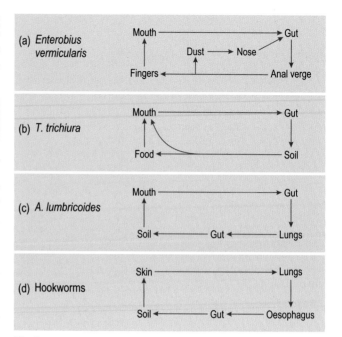

Fig. 1 **Life cycle of five helminths (including two hookworms).**

Control involves family treatment, hand and nail hygiene, washing of bedding and night attire, and vacuuming to remove any eggs in dust.

Trichuris trichiura (whipworm)

Shaped like a whip (the tail) with a handle (the body), this worm is 3–5cm long. Found worldwide, it is most common where human faeces enrich soil directly, so spread is indirectly faecal–oral, with no animal reservoir.

Life cycle and pathogenesis. The life-cycle is simple (Fig. 1b): ingested eggs hatch in the small bowel, the larvae migrate to the caecum, the adult fertilised female lays 5000 to 10000 eggs daily and lives up to 7 years! Eggs passed in faeces must develop in the soil for 3 weeks to be infectious when ingested. Secondary bacterial infection can occur where the adult worm head penetrates caecal mucosa.

Clinical syndromes. Symptoms range from none to mild abdominal discomfort to bloody diarrhoea to rectal prolapse (p. 163). Luminal worms in appendicitis may not be causal.

Confirmatory test. Microscopy of stool shows the typical 'tea-tray'-shaped eggs, elongated ovals with bi-terminal plugs (Fig. 2b).

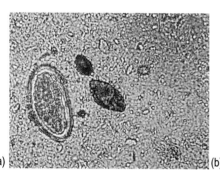
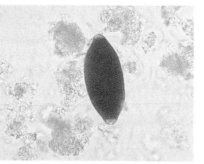
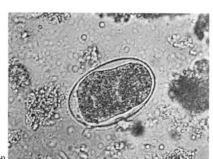

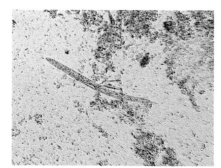

Fig. 2 **Helminth eggs in faeces, wet preparations. (a)** *E. vermicularis.* **(b)** *T. trichiura.*
(c) *A. lumbricoides.* **(d)** Hookworm.

Fig. 3 **Strongyloides larva.**

Chemotherapy. This is by mebendazole or albendazole.

Control. This is by better sanitation and personal hygiene.

Ascaris lumbricoides (roundworm)

Shaped like a big earthworm 25–30cm long, the roundworm is most common where human faeces enrich soil directly. Maturation of the egg in soil is essential, so spread is indirectly faecal–oral. There is no animal reservoir.

Life cycle and pathogenesis. The life-cycle involves an additional stage: pulmonary migration (Fig. 1c). The adult fertilised female lays up to 200 000 eggs daily for up to 1 year! Pathogenesis can include partial or complete mechanical obstruction to bowel, bile ducts or appendix, pneumonitis during pulmonary migration, or secondary bacterial infection when the adult worm head penetrates the small bowel (p. 162–163).

Clinical syndromes. Symptoms range from none to abdominal discomfort to bowel obstruction, obstructive jaundice, appendicitis or peritonitis.

Confirmatory tests. Microscopy of stool shows the typical brownish oval eggs, about 45 × 70µm, either fertilised or unfertilised, with or without (decorticated) their rough outer shell (Fig. 2c).

Chemotherapy. Pyrantel pamoate, mebendazole or albendazole are used.

Control involves education, and better sanitation and personal hygiene, especially in food handlers.

Ancylostoma duodenale and Necator americanus (hookworms)

A. duodenale, the Old World hookworm, is a little larger (1.2 × 0.6mm) than *N. americanus*, the New World hookworm, (1 × 0.4mm) and has a different mouth. Both are most common where human faeces enrich soil directly. Maturation of the egg in soil is essential, so spread is indirectly faecal–skin. There is no animal reservoir.

Life cycle and pathogenesis. The life-cycle includes both skin penetration and pulmonary migration (Fig. 1d). The adult worms are about 1cm long and live attached to intestinal mucous membranes by four hooked teeth. The adult fertilised female lays about 10 000 (*Necator*) to 30 000 (*Ancylostoma*) eggs daily for about 5 years. Pathogenesis is by the ingestion of blood from the human bowel mucosa, from 0.03 ml (*Necator*) to 0.3ml (*Ancylostoma*) per worm per day: over 100ml daily for a worm burden of 500 adults!

Clinical syndromes. Symptoms are itch at skin entry sites, allergic pneumonitis and, particularly, those of iron-deficiency anaemia (p. 163).

Confirmatory tests. Microscopy of stool shows the typical unstained oval eggs, about 40 × 70µm, containing a developing larva (Fig. 2d).

Chemotherapy and control. Pyrantel pamoate, mebendazole or albendazole, plus iron, are used in chemotherapy. Education, better sanitation, personal hygiene and the wearing of shoes should improve control.

Strongyloides stercoralis

This little skin-penetrating nematode (female 2.5mm long, male only 0.7mm) can cause severe disease. It is most common where human faeces enrich soil directly, for infective larvae pass in the faeces (Fig. 3). Maturation of the larvae in soil is *not* essential, so spread can be directly faecal to skin or mouth, or by direct anal contact (including sexual contact), or by autoinfection (see below). There is no animal reservoir.

Life cycle and pathogenesis. The life cycle (Fig. 4) adds three further features to the cycle seen in the hookworm:

■ The female may dispense with the male, and lay fertile eggs parthenogenetically in the small bowel

■ The rhabditiform larvae hatch in the human bowel and are passed in the faeces to become infective filariform larvae or free-living adults in the soil

■ Rhabditiform larvae may become filariform larvae while still in the bowel and cause **autoinfection** through the small bowel mucosa or peri-anal skin.

Pathogenesis is by allergy in skin and lungs, by local bowel damage and invasion, and by disseminated infection in the immunocompromised patient (p. 220–221). At times, this is complicated by septicaemia from accompanying intestinal bacterial pathogens.

Clinical syndromes. Symptoms are itch at skin entry sites, allergic pneumonitis, abdominal symptoms, and disseminated infection in immunocompromised patients.

Confirmatory tests. Microscopy of repeated stool specimens or duodenal aspirate shows the filariform larvae, about 200–300µm long (Fig. 3), with a longer oesophagus than hookworm larvae.

Chemotherapy. Ivermectin is now the drug of choice; albendazole is the alternative.

Control is enhanced by education, better sanitation, personal hygiene and the wearing of shoes. In endemic areas, patients for immunosuppressive therapy should be screened by at least three stool microscopies.

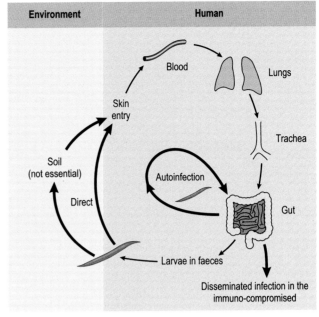

Fig. 4 **Life cycle of S. stercoralis.**

Intestinal nematodes

■ Worm infections are common worldwide, with differing geographic distribution depending on the life cycle.

■ Four have obligatory soil cycles, while pinworm and *S. stercoralis* do not, so spread directly person-to-person.

■ They cause disease variously by allergy, mechanical obstruction, local bowel damage, blood loss, secondary bacterial infection and dissemination.

■ Diagnosis is by stool microscopy, or anal adhesive tape microscopy for pinworm.

■ Anthelminthics include pyrantel pamoate, mebendazole, albendazole and ivermectin.

■ Control is by education, better sanitation, personal hygiene, therapy of infected people, and wearing shoes.

Tissue nematodes (worms)

The nematodes (p. 12) infecting the bloodstream, lymphatics and tissues are considered in four groups:

- filarial worms
- Guinea worm
- worms causing larva migrans
- *Trichinella spiralis*.

Filarial worms

Wuchereria bancrofti and *Brugia malayi*

These are sheathed filariae having many similarities, so are considered together. They occur in tropical Africa and Asia, the Pacific and South America, are transmitted by mosquito bites, and cause classical Bancroftian filariasis. They are coiled thread-like worms, 4–10cm long. The life cycle is shown in Figure 1.

Infection is shown by detecting microfilariae in blood films obtained at night, except for the diurnal Pacific infection.

Clinically (p. 205), hypersensitivity reactions cause lymphangitis and fever, and lymphatic obstruction may cause elephantiasis (Fig. 2). Diethylcarbamazine (DEC) can be used cautiously but there is no cure. Control is by decreasing mosquito bites, and mass chemotherapy with DEC or ivermectin.

Loa loa (African eye worm)

Loa loa is found in West and Central Africa. It is spread from infected humans by the bite of *Chrysops* spp. mango flies. The life cycle is similar to that of *W. bancrofti* (Fig. 1) but with several differences:

- insect host bites in daytime
- larvae burrow through skin when deposited on it, rather than being directly injected by the insect
- microfilariae (*Microfilaria diurna*) appear late (3–4 years) and are diurnal (during daytime)
- adult worms move in subcutaneous tissues near tendons (and across the front of the eye) for up to 20 years after infection (p. 111)
- allergic reactions to filarial toxins cause 'Calabar swellings' lasting 3 days on the hands, forearms or elsewhere.

Blood films show diurnal microfilaria, in adults more than children. Eosinophilia is usual, and serology usually positive. Chemotherapy is diethylcarbamazine or ivermectin, with or without surgery, and control is by education, avoiding fly bites, and mass treatment.

Onchocerca volvulus (river blindness worm)

Onchocerciasis, leading to 'river blindness', affects about 25 million people in areas in West and Central Africa, and Central and South America. The disease is transmitted by the bite of blood-sucking black flies, especially *Simulium damnosum*.

The life cycle, with stages in fly larvae and human, follows the familiar pattern. The adults live mainly in subcutaneous nodules, and the microfilariae migrate to various parts of the body. They rarely enter the blood. In heavy infections, eye invasion causes blindness. The diagnosis is made by finding microfilariae in skin snips or in the eye, or adult worms in biopsies. Eosinophilia is common.

The classical clinical triad is dermatitis, nodules and keratitis (p. 111). Yearly ivermectin kills microfilariae, not adult worms. Control is by fly control programmes and ivermectin mass treatment.

Dracunculus medinensis (guinea worm)

The guinea worm is found in Africa, the Middle East and South Asia, and infection is by drinking water containing infected crustacea. It invades soft tissues, usually in the leg. The female

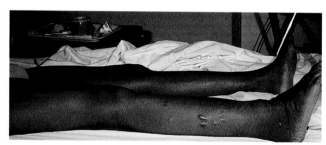

Fig. 2 **Filarial elephantiasis.**

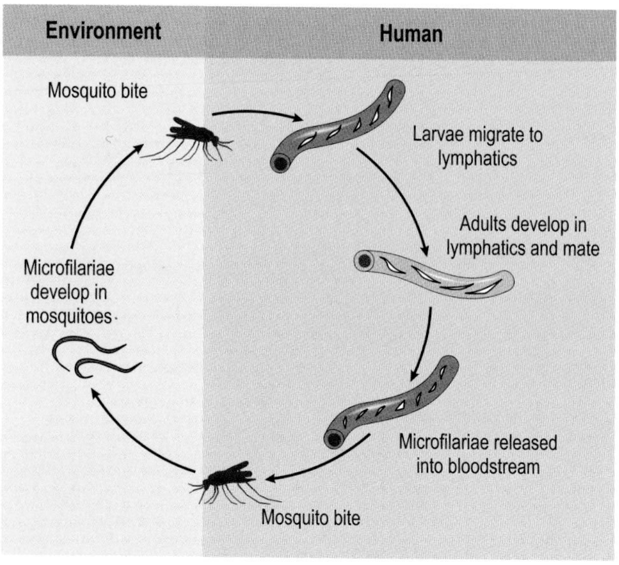

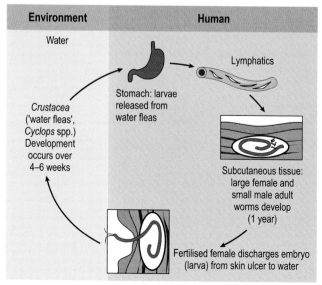

Fig. 1 **Life cycle of the filarial worms.**

Fig. 3 **Life cycle of *Dracunculus medinensis* (guinea worm).**

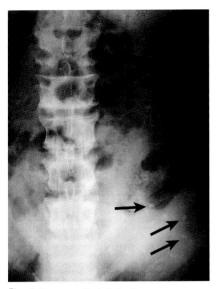

Fig. 4 **Dracunculiasis infection (calcification).**

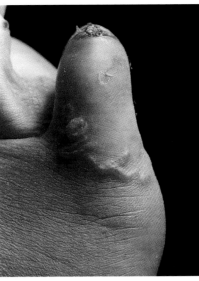

Fig. 5 **Cutaneous larva migrans.**

migrating larvae (Fig. 5). *Dirofilaria immitis*, the mosquito-borne dog heart worm, is one example; others are *Angiostrongylus, Gnathostoma* or *Anisakis* spp.

Four others follow:

Ancylostoma caninum and *A. braziliense* (dog/cat hookworms)

These hookworms (and other animal hookworms) sometimes infect humans, particularly children. Hookworm eggs hatch in soil or sand, and the filariform larvae can penetrate skin, then migrate subcutaneously for weeks or months, causing cutaneous larva migrans (p. 204), with pruritus on infection ('ground itch'), then erythema and vesicles moving 1–2 cm daily ('creeping eruption'). Diagnosis is usually clinical, rarely by biopsy, and treatment is thiabendazole.

is 60–90 cm long (rarely 120 cm), only 2–3 mm thick and is mainly a huge uterus packed with up to 3 million embryos!

The life cycle is shown in Figure 3. Diagnosis is made by detecting embryos in washings of the ulcer, and x-rays (Fig. 4) with or without radio-opaque injection can show the adult. Eosinophilia is frequent. A skin ulcer with a worm visible at the base is very distinctive (p. 204–205).

Chemotherapy by niridazole reduces inflammation and assists surgical removal. Classically the ulcer is wetted daily and the worm extracted by winding it gradually round a stick. However, septic complications are common. Control depends on education and clean water.

Larva migrans (cutaneous or visceral)

Some nematodes, primarily of animals, can infect humans 'accidentally'; because the human is an abnormal host, the normal life cycle cannot be completed and disease is caused by the

Toxocara canis and *T. cati* (dog and cat ascaris)

Infection is by ingestion of ascarid eggs from faecally-contaminated soil, especially by children. The eggs hatch in the human gut producing larvae that penetrate the gut wall, reach the bloodstream and migrate into various tissues to produce visceral larva migrans (p. 155). Pathology includes haemorrhage, necrosis and granulomata, especially in lungs, liver and eyes, producing pneumonitis, hepatitis and retinitis.

Diagnosis is clinical, confirmed serologically. Infected pets are found by stool tests. Treatment is by albendazole. Control is by treatment of pets and disposal of animal faeces.

Trichinella spiralis (pig threadworm)

This infects humans when they eat incompletely cooked pork or bear meat containing encysted larvae (Fig. 6). Again, the life cycle is incomplete in the human 'dead-end' host.

Diagnosis is initially clinical but may be confirmed by finding encysted larvae in muscle biopsies or infected pork. Antibody rises after 3–4 weeks are detected by serology in some countries.

Clinical syndromes include abdominal symptoms, fever, periorbital oedema, splinter haemorrhages, myalgia and life-threatening cerebral or cardiac involvement (p. 213).

Chemotherapy is with albendazole with or without steroids. Control prevents pig infections from infected food, and cooking pork kills the encysted larvae.

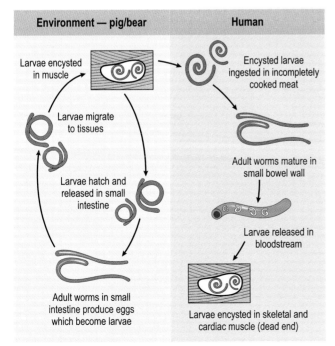

Fig. 6 **Life cycle of *Trichinella spiralis* (pig threadworm).**

> ## Tissue nematodes
>
> - Filarial infections are diagnosed by detecting microfilariae in blood films (taken at the right time of day or night), or larvae, or adult worms in ulcers or tissue biopsies.
> - Symptoms arise from hypersensitivity reactions, secondary blockage of lymphatics, or tissue damage.
> - Treatment is often unsatisfactory, whether by surgery or chemotherapy.
> - As filarial infections are spread via intermediate hosts (often biting insects) control can be attempted at this step.
> - Dead-end infections result from accidental infection of humans with larvae or eggs from soil or larvae encysted in meat. Clinical symptoms result from cutaneous or visceral larva migrans or encysting larvae in skeletal or cardiac muscle.

Cestodes (tapeworms)

Cestodes are flat segmented worms (tapeworms), and humans can be infected in two modes:

- As **definitive** hosts of the adult worm in the gut after ingesting encysted larvae in incompletely cooked meat; this produces mild or moderate intestinal disease in all but *Echinococcus*.
- As **intermediate** hosts of larvae in tissues after ingesting eggs in faecally contaminated food; this produces tissue disease from encysted larvae (e.g. cysticercosis) with space-occupying lesions (SOL).

Taenia saginata (beef tapeworm)

T. saginata is a common intestinal tapeworm found wherever human faeces contaminate pastures, and raw or undercooked larvae-infected beef is eaten, so it does not occur in Hindus or vegetarians.

The life cycle is illustrated in Figure 1. The egg, indistinguishable from *T. solium* eggs, is round, 40μm across and has three pairs of internal hooklets (Fig. 2). The worm can exceed 10 metres in length, and the segments (proglottids) each contain nervous, muscular, excretory and male and female genital systems, the uterus having 15–30 lateral branches (*T. solium* has 7–12).

Clinical syndromes. Distress is either abdominal from the worm, or mental from seeing the proglottids in faeces or the bed!

Confirmatory tests. Stool microscopy for the egg confirms a tapeworm infection. The tiny scolex (head) or the 1 × 1.5 cm proglottid confirms the species.

Chemotherapy. Praziquantel or niclosamide are effective orally. After treatment to expel the worm the faeces should be examined to ensure that the head is expelled, otherwise the worm will regenerate.

Control is by education, sanitation, meat inspection and proper cooking of beef (or not eating beef).

Taenia solium (pork tapeworm)

Taenia solium is a large intestinal tapeworm, common wherever human faeces contaminate pastures, and raw or undercooked larvae-infected pork is eaten, so it does not occur in Muslims or vegetarians.

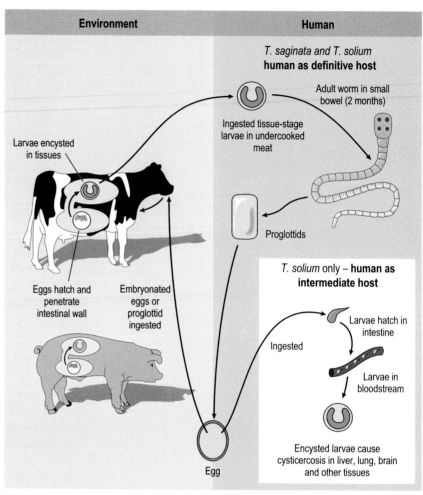

Fig. 1 **Life-cycles of *Taenia saginata* and *T. solium*.**

The egg is indistinguishable from *T. saginata* eggs (Fig. 2). The worm can exceed 6 metres in length, and the segments (proglottids) are similar to *T. saginata* except that the uterus has 7–12 lateral branches.

Life cycle and pathogenesis. The normal life cycle in which humans are the definitive host occurs exactly as with *T. saginata*. However, the larval stage, which would normally occur in the pig, can develop in humans if the eggs are ingested in faecally-contaminated water or plants. Larvae from the egg go through the bowel wall to the bloodstream, thence to brain, muscle, eye or other tissues. This results in serious disease from the encysted larval tissue stage (**cysticercosis**) in brain (p. 103), liver or other tissues. Eventual degeneration of the cyst causes an inflammatory reaction with worsening of symptoms in the human dead-end host.

Clinical syndromes. Abdominal symptoms are non-specific. CNS symptoms

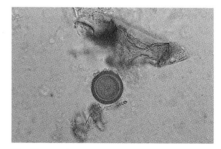

Fig. 2 ***Taenia* spp. egg from faeces.**

from encysted larvae include fits, strokes, and cranial nerve or visual impairment.

Confirmatory tests. Intestinal worms are diagnosed as for *T. saginata*. Cysticercosis is diagnosed by x-ray, CT or brain scans, MRI or by surgery.

Chemotherapy. Albendazole is the first choice for cysticercosis, niclosamide for intestinal disease, or praziquantel for either. Steroids reduce inflammation.

Control is by education, sanitation, meat inspection and proper cooking of pork (or not eating pork).

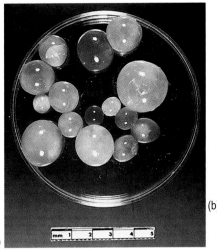

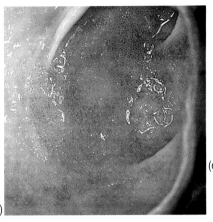

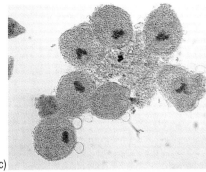

(c)

Fig. 3 *Echinococcus granulosus.* **(a)** Hydatid brood capsules removed from the cyst. **(b)** 'Hydatid sand' within the cyst. **(c)** Seven hydatid scolices within the laminated membrane (latter not visible).

Echinococcus spp. (hydatid worms)

Humans are not definitive hosts of the hydatid worm. Humans become (dead-end) intermediate hosts for the encysted larvae after being infected by eggs in canine faeces. Canines are the definitive reservoir host, and herbivores such as sheep and cattle are the usual intermediate hosts. So human disease is commonest in sheep-rearing countries.

Two species infect humans: the more usual *E. granulosus* (Fig. 3), forming hydatid cysts, and the invasive *E. multilocularis*, spreading like a malignancy.

The egg is very similar to *Taenia* eggs. The adult worm is small, only 3–9 mm long, with only four proglottids.

Life cycle and pathogenesis. The life cycle is like that of *T. solium* but only the intermediate stage occurs in humans. Larvae hatch from eggs in the human gut and travel in the portal vein to the liver. Those not lodging there travel to the lungs, and, if still not filtered out, to the brain and other tissues. The larvae of *E. granulosus* develop to hydatid cysts with a host-derived laminated membrane and *inner* germinal layer, giving rise to brood capsules containing daughter cysts each containing an embryo larva as a scolex with hooklets (Fig. 3). In *E. multilocularis*, the germinal mem-

brane is *outermost* so no cyst is formed, and the disease spreads like a malignancy.

Confirmatory tests. Serology particularly for Arc 5 in a gel immunodiffusion test is highly specific; latex agglutination and other serology are used for screening or supplementary testing. CT and liver and brain scans are used for localisation. Old liver cysts calcify.

Clinical syndromes. Symptoms are usually caused by a SOL in liver (p. 169), brain (p. 103), lung (p. 134) or other tissues.

Chemotherapy. Albendazole is useful, but surgery or cyst aspiration is still often necessary, being very careful not to spill infective cyst contents.

Control. Treating adult worms in farm herbivores, preventing dogs from eating raw infected animal (e.g. sheep) viscera, and hand-washing after dog or soil contact, are important means of control.

Hymenolepis nana (dwarf tapeworm)

Dwarf tapeworm (2–4 cm long) occurs worldwide, especially in children. Unusually, it has *no* intermediate host. Ingested eggs develop to the tissue stage (cysticercoids) in small bowel mucosa, releasing adults into the lumen. Eggs released from proglottids can autoinfect the same host (hence very high worm loads = hyperinfection) or be shed to reinfect by ingestion, *directly*.

Only local gut symptoms occur, and stool microscopy identifies eggs (Fig. 4).

Chemotherapy. Praziquantel is the first choice.

Control depends on education, sanitation, and hand-washing after defaecation.

Diphyllobothrium latum (fish tapeworm)

Fish tapeworm is doubly unusual, in having two intermediate hosts and causing human disease by preventing absorption of vitamins, especially B_{12}. It occurs wherever infected raw (or smoked) fish are eaten.

The adult is huge, 3–10 metres long with 3000–4000 proglottids. The egg is operculated (with a cap over an opening), $40 \times 70\,\mu m$. The eggs release ciliated larvae in water that are eaten by and develop in crustacea ('water fleas', *Cyclops* spp.) The larvae then encyst in the muscles of freshwater fish that eat the water fleas.

Pathogenesis in the human gut is mechanical by the worms' size and also by interfering with vitamin absorption.

Clinical syndromes. Symptoms include abdominal distress, passage of proglottids, and pernicious anaemia from vitamin B_{12} deficiency. Stool microscopy shows the characteristic egg or proglottids.

Chemotherapy. Praziquantel is the drug of choice.

Control depends on sanitation, cooking fish and treating infections.

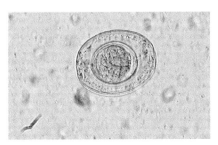

Fig. 4 *Hymenolepis nana* **cyst.**

> ### Cestodes
>
> - Tapeworms infect humans either by ingestion of encysted larvae to produce intestinal worms, or by ingestion of eggs to produce large tissue masses from encysted larvae.
> - Diagnosis is usually by stool microscopy and imaging techniques (CT, scans, etc.), sometimes by serology.
> - Treatment is usually praziquantel, albendazole or niclosamide, with surgery for tissue masses.
> - Control is by sanitation, education and proper cooking.

Trematodes (flukes)

Trematodes (flukes) are flat, leaf-shaped worms. They have an oral muscular sucker and an incomplete digestive system. Schistosomes have separate sexes, but other trematodes are hermaphrodites, i.e. have both male and female sexual organs in one body.

The life cycle of all trematodes occurs in part outside the human body (Fig. 1), and all have reservoir hosts and a first intermediate host in a snail (or other mollusc). Several have a second intermediate host stage in fishes (*Opisthorchis* spp.) or crabs or crayfish (*Paragonimus* spp.). Humans are infected by ingestion of larvae, except schistosomes which infect through the skin. The adults, as their common names indicate, live in bowel, bile duct, liver, lungs or blood vessels. Eosinophilia is common in all fluke infections.

Opisthorchis sinensis (Chinese liver fluke)

O. (previously *Clonorchis*) *sinensis* and related species are found in China, Japan and nearby countries. Humans are infected by eating uncooked fish infected with the larvae (metacercariae). Eggs in human faeces are ingested by the first intermediate host (fresh-water snails) which are eaten by the second intermediate host, fish. Reservoir hosts include dogs, cats and fish-eating animals.

The egg is oval, operculated and small, 15 × 25μm (Fig. 2). The larvae (cercariae) are 500 × 100μm, the adult is about 4 × 25mm.

Clinical syndromes correlate with the life cycle (Fig. 1), and range from no symptoms to abdominal pain, diarrhoea and fever, to obstructive jaundice, cholecystitis, liver abscesses or bile duct carcinoma.

Laboratory identification is by microscopy of stools, showing the distinctive eggs. Praziquantel is the drug of choice in treatment. Control of the parasite depends on education, sanitation and changed cooking or eating habits.

Fasciola hepatica (sheep liver fluke)

F. hepatica and related species are found where sheep and the snail hosts co-exist: Japan, China, Russia, Egypt and South America. Humans are infected by eating water plants, like watercress, contami-

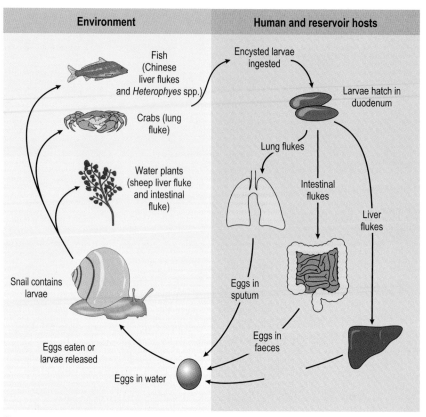

Fig. 1 **Life cycle of flukes.**

nated with the larvae (metacercariae), or raw liver. Reservoir hosts include sheep, cattle and humans.

The egg is oval, operculated and large, 75 × 140μm. The larvae (cercariae) are 0.7mm, the adult is about 2 × 12mm.

Clinical syndromes again correlate with the life cycle:

- Adult flukes from raw sheep liver cause pharyngitis ('halzoun').
- early tender hepatomegaly from larval migration
- adults in the bile ducts cause cholangitis and obstruction
- adults in the liver cause necrosis ('liver rot'), bacterial infection and cirrhosis.

Stool microscopy shows the eggs, indistinguishable from *F. buski*.

Praziquantel is the drug of choice; bithionol is an alternative. Control depends on education, sanitation, and avoiding uncooked water plants or raw sheep liver!

Fasciolopsis buski (giant intestinal fluke)

F. buski and related species (e.g. *Heterophyes*, *Metagonimus* spp.) are found where

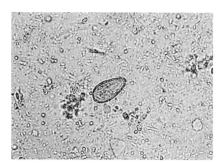

Fig. 2 *Opisthorchis sinensis* **ovum.**

the snail hosts exist: China, South East Asia and India. Humans are infected by eating raw fish or plants like water chestnuts contaminated with the larvae (metacercariae). Reservoir hosts include pigs, dogs and humans.

The egg is oval, operculated and large, 75 × 140μm. The larvae (cercariae) are 0.7mm, the giant adult is about 3 × 12cm.

The intestinal fluke produces abdominal pain, diarrhoea, malabsorption and even obstruction.

Stool microscopy shows the eggs, indistinguishable from *F. hepatica*.

Praziquantel is the treatment of choice; niclosamide is the alternative. Control depends on education, sanitation and avoiding uncooked water plants or raw fish. The snails and definitive hosts are difficult to control.

Paragonimus westermani (lung fluke)

P. westermani and related species are found where the snail hosts exist and the crab or crayfish hosts are eaten uncooked: Asia, India, Africa and Latin America. Humans are infected by eating uncooked crabs, crayfish or reservoir hosts infected with the larvae (metacercariae). Reservoir hosts include pigs, boars and monkeys.

The egg is oval, operculated and quite large, 60 × 100μm. The larvae (cercariae) are 70 × 200μm; the adult is about 7 × 18mm.

Migration of the larvae (adolescercariae) through the diaphragm, pleura and lung to the bronchioles forms cystic cavities where the adult flukes develop. This results in pulmonary cavitation and bronchiectasis, bronchitis, and pleural effusions (p. 135). Spread to the spinal cord, brain and other tissues can occur, causing fits or paralysis.

Sputum microscopy shows the eggs. Chest x-rays are abnormal.

Chemotherapy uses praziquantel as first choice; bithionol is the alternative. Control depends on education, sanitation, and avoiding uncooked crabs and crayfish. The snails and definitive hosts are difficult to control.

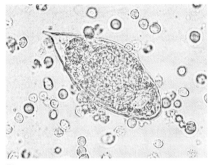

Fig. 3 *Schistosoma haematobium* ovum seen in faeces.

Schistosoma spp. (schistosomes)

The three major pathogenic species of blood flukes are S. *haematobium*, causing vesicular (bladder, Fig. 3, p. 13) schistosomiasis with haematuria, and S. *mansoni* and S. *japonicum*, causing intestinal schistosomiasis with hepatosplenomegaly. They are found where humans and the snail hosts co-exist (Table 1). Humans are infected by larvae (cercariae) penetrating the skin. Reservoir hosts include primates, rodents, domestic animals and humans.

The diagnostic differences between the eggs (Fig. 3) of the three species are listed in Table 1. Unlike other trematodes, all have no operculum. The larvae (cercariae) are 0.8mm, the adult is about 1 × 15mm.

The life cycle has one intermediate host, freshwater snails (Fig. 4).

Disease again correlates with the life cycle. Initially there is skin itch and allergy on skin penetration, then hepatitis, followed by either bladder symptoms including haematuria from S. *haematobium*, or abdominal disease including dysentery, portal hypertension and gross hepatosplenomegaly with the two other, mesenteric vein species (p. 153).

Eggs may spread to cause pulmonary, cerebral and spinal cord granulomata. Carcinoma of the bladder is common with chronic S. *haematobium* infection.

Stool or urine microscopy shows the distinctive eggs (Fig. 3).

Praziquantel is the drug of choice; oxamniquin is an alternative in S. *mansoni* infections. Control is difficult and depends on education, sanitation, mass treatment or molluscicides against the snails in some circumstances. Vaccine development continues.

Table 1 Different characteristics of three major schistosomes			
Characteristic	S. haematobium	S. mansoni	S. japonicum
Distribution	Africa, India, Middle East	Africa, Arabia, S. America, West Indies	Japan, China, SE Asia
Reservoir hosts	Monkeys	Primates/rodents	Many animals
Egg size (μm)	80–180 × 60	110–170 × 60	70–100 × 55
Egg spine	Terminal	Lateral	Tiny lateral
Veins infected	Urogenital	Inferior mesenteric	Both mesenteric
Egg excretion	Urine	Faeces	Faeces
Chronic disease	Urinary (late cancer)	Hepatosplenic (spinal, lung)	Hepatosplenic (cerebral)

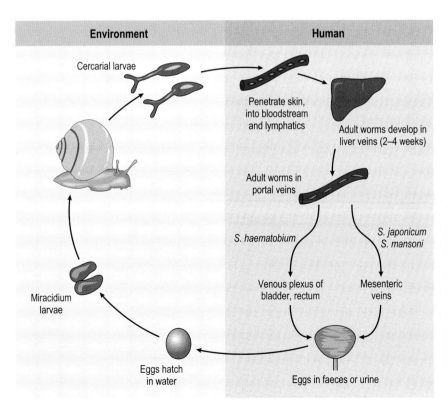

Fig. 4 **Life cycle of schistosomes.**

Environment — Human

Cercarial larvae

Penetrate skin, into bloodstream and lymphatics

Adult worms develop in liver veins (2–4 weeks)

Adult worms in portal veins

S. haematobium

S. japonicum
S. mansoni

Venous plexus of bladder, rectum

Mesenteric veins

Eggs in faeces or urine

Miracidium larvae

Eggs hatch in water

Trematodes

- Flukes infect humans either by ingestion of encysted larvae to produce intestinal, bile duct or lung flukes (adult worms) or by skin penetration to produce intravascular and tissue schistosomiasis.

- Diagnosis is usually by stool, urine or sputum microscopy, sometimes assisted by imaging techniques (x-ray, CT, etc.), serology or biopsy.

- Treatment is by praziquantel or specialised alternatives.

- Control is by sanitation, education and proper food preparation or cooking, and minimising water and snail contact.

Viruses

Classification

There are two useful major, separate classifications: structural and biological.

Structural classification is primarily by:

- the <u>nucleic acid</u> – whether it is DNA or RNA, single- or double-stranded, linear or circular, or in one piece, diploid or segmented
- the <u>nucleo-capsid shape</u>, and
- the absence or presence of an <u>envelope</u>.

A summary of these features and resultant clinical syndromes is in Tables 1 and 2.

Details of virus composition and structure, the effects on the human host cell, virus replication and genetics, and the stages of virus infection are described on pages 14–19.

Details of the resultant clinical syndromes are in the pages listed in Tables 1 and 2.

Biological classification uses several criteria (transmission, target organ, chronicity of disease, malignant potential), so is untidy with overlap. It is particularly into:

- <u>Enteric</u> viruses (ingested and multiply in gut, though may then infect elsewhere: e.g. caliciviruses, rotaviruses, most enteroviruses, some adenoviruses, qv)
- <u>Respiratory viruses</u> (inhaled, multiply in respiratory tract, and usually infect there: orthomyxoviruses, paramyxoviruses, coronaviruses, rhinoviruses, most adenoviruses, and some enteroviruses, qv)
- <u>Contact viruses</u> (implanted, e.g. Herpes simplex, papillomaviruses, most poxviruses, HIV)

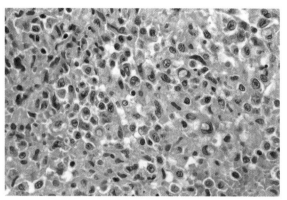

Fig. 1 **Cerebral lymphoma from EBV in AIDS – histology shows huge numbers of lymphoma cells.**

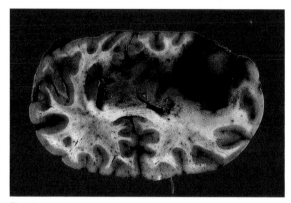

Fig. 2 **Cerebral lymphoma from EBV in AIDS at necropsy showing several tumours.**

Table 1 **Classification, characteristics and clinical syndromes of DNA viruses**					
A. DNA Viruses	**Size (nm)**	**Virion shape**	**Genome shape**	**Appearance (stylised)**	**Page**
a. Non-enveloped, single-stranded					

1. Parvovirus
    Parvovirus B19 infections include Erythema
    infectiosum, anaemia, arthritis, foetal hydrops
	22	Icosahedral	Linear		145

b. Non-enveloped, double-stranded					

2. Papovaviruses
    Papillomaviruses: Warts; Cervical cancer
    Polyomaviruses:
      BK virus
      JC virus: Progressive Multifocal
      Leuco-encephalopathy (PML)
	50	Icosahedral	Circular		182,188
					
					101

3. Adenoviruses Respiratory infections, gut infections, conjunctivitis	80	Icosahedral	Linear		108,116 161
c. Enveloped, double-stranded					
4. Hepadnaviruses: Hepatitis B	42	Spheric or filamentous	Circular		170 171

5. Herpesviruses
    H. simplex; H. zoster and varicella; EBV; CMV;
    Roseola infantum; Kaposi's sarcoma; (herpes B).
	100–200	Icosahedral	Linear		200
					144

6. Poxviruses
    Smallpox
    Molluscum contagiosum, monkeypox, vaccinia
    Parapoxvirus infections (orf and milker's nodes).
	250 × 350
	(Brick)
		Complex	Linear		148
					201

- Arboviruses (arthropod-borne, see particularly p. 96–97, 146–148)
- Non-arbovirus zoonoses (e.g. Rabies, other lyssa viruses)
- Hepatitis viruses (see p. 170–172)
- Slow viruses (see p. 100–101)
- Tumour viruses which include:
  – Papillomaviruses (see Cervical infections, p. 182–183)
- Hepatitis B virus (see Hepatocellular carcinoma, p. 171)
- Hepatitis C virus (see Hepatocellular carcinoma, p. 172)
- Epstein–Barr virus (Figs 1 and 2, and see Burkitt's lymphoma and other tumours, p. 145, 150)
- Herpes virus 8 (see Kaposi's sarcoma, p. 150)
- HTLV I and HTLV II (p. 149).

Table 2 **Classification, characteristics and clinical syndromes of RNA viruses and prions**

B. RNA Viruses	Size (nm)	Virion shape	Genome shape	Appearance (stylised)	Page
a. Non-enveloped, single-stranded					
1. **Picornaviruses**					
i. **Rhinoviruses** Common cold	25–30	Icosahedral	Linear, +		116
ii. **Enteroviruses**	25–30	Icosahedral	Linear, +		
Poliovirus Poliomyelitis					97
Hepatitis A virus Hepatitis A					170
Coxsackie- and ECHO viruses Herpangina, Hand, Foot and Mouth Disease, Intercostal myositis, Meningitis/paralysis, Myo/pericarditis, Neonatal infection, Rash, Respiratory infection					200 144
2. **Astrovirus and caliciviruses** including **Norwalk virus** Gastroenteritis, Hepatitis E	28–38	Icosahedral	Linear, +		161 172
b. Non-enveloped, double-stranded					
3. **Reoviruses** including **Rotavirus,** Diarrhoeal disease, Colorado tick fever (arbovirus)	60–80	Icosahedral	Linear, 10 segments		161 146
c. Enveloped, single-stranded					
4. **Retroviruses: HIV, HTLV 1 and 2** HIV/AIDS, Lymphoma, leukaemia	80–110	Icosahedral (Spheric)	Linear, + 2 segments		149, 151 101
5. i. **Toga (Alphavirus)** E & W Equine Encepahalitis Rubella (Non-Arbo Togavirus)	40–70	Icosahedral	Linear, +		100, 146 148
ii. **Flaviviruses,** Yellow fever, dengue, West Nile Hepatitis C (Non-Arbo Flavirus)	40–50	Icosahedral	Linear, +	If arthropod borne, are called **Arbo**viruses	117 147 171 146
iii. **Bunyaviruses** Californian encephalitis, Hanta V.	90–110	Helical (Spherical)	Circular, Negative 3 segments		
iv. **Rhabdoviruses** Rabies and other Lyssaviruses (Non-Arboviruses).	75 × 180	Helical (Bullet)	Linear, Negative		96
6. i. **Orthomyoviruses: Influenza viruses** Influenza	80–120	Helical (Spherical)	Linear, Negative 8 segments		116
ii. **Paramyxoviruses** include **Parainfluenza Respiratory Synctial Virus (RSV), Metapneumovirus** Croup, bronchitis, bronchiolitis **Measles, mumps viruses:** Measles, mumps **Hendra, Nipah viruses:** pneumonia, encephalitis	150–300	Helical	Linear, Negative		116 145, 101 96
iii. **Coronaviruses** Respiratory infections especially colds. SARS	60–220	Helical (Spherical)	Linear, Positive		116-117
7. **Delta virus** Hepatitis D	37	Spherical	Circular, Negative		172
8. i. **Arenaviruses:** Lassa fever, LCM	80–130	Helical (Spherical)	Circular, Negative		147
ii. **Filoviruses:** Ebola and Marburg fevers	80 × 180	Helical (Filament)	Linear, Negative		147
C. Prions					
1. **Transmissible spongiform encephalopathies** Creutzfeldt-Jacob disease, kuru, (scrapie)	<30	Filaments	Not viral		101

Note: Both icosahedral and helical viruses can appear spherical when enveloped.

Acute meningitis

Acute meningitis is acute inflammation, developing over a few hours or days, of the meninges (Fig. 1), particularly the arachnoid mater overlying the cerebrum, the adjacent area of which may also be inflamed (cerebritis). Meningitis is usually spontaneous in normal hosts but can occur after trauma, surgery, or delivery, or in the immunocompromised. Organisms enter the CNS by three routes:

■ via the bloodstream after inhalation, through bites (*Rickettsiae*) or through the placenta (congenital infections)
■ via the olfactory bulb (amoebic infections, p. 80)
■ via direct inoculation (surgery or trauma).

Causative organisms

The important causative agents are shown in Table 1; the first three account for three-quarters of bacterial meningitis and common virulence factors include a polysaccharide capsule.

Meningitis usually occurs in single episodes but epidemics occur in crowded conditions or where asymptomatic carriers are responsible.

Clinical features

Headache, fever, and neck stiffness occur in all types of acute meningitis. Clouding

of consciousness and vomiting are common as intracranial pressure increases, which can cause VI nerve pareses (Fig. 2) as a false localising sign.

1. Clinical clues suggest the causative organism:

■ petechial rash (Fig. 3) and shock with the meningococcus, rarely with the pneumococcus or S. *aureus*
■ otitis media with S. *pyogenes*, S. *pneumoniae* or H. *influenzae*
■ rash with viral or rickettsial infections (Rocky Mountain spotted fever, RMSF)
■ myalgia and occupational exposure with leptospirosis
■ special rash of erythema chronicum migrans (ECM) in Lyme disease.

2. Special situations suggest causative organisms.

■ CSF leak from ear or nose after closed cranial trauma: this is pneumococcal in about 75% of cases and is usually prevented by chemoprophylaxis

■ CSF shunt for hydrocephalus: usually coagulase-negative staphylococci (55%) or S. *aureus* (25%) implanted with the shunt
■ immunocompromised patient: *Listeria*, *Pseudomonas* or other Gram-negative rods, fungi such as *Cryptococcus*, or parasites like *Toxoplasma*
■ neonatal: *E. coli* and group B streptococci cause about 75%.
■ postoperative: *Pseudomonas* or other Gram-negative rods can be more common than staphylococci
■ recurrent meningitis:
 – underlying anatomic abnormality
 – parameningeal focus
 – immunocompromised patient
 – unrelated viral meningitis attacks (rare)
 – Mollaret's meningitis: benign, unknown cause, ?HSV.

3. Differential diagnoses needing different treatment include:

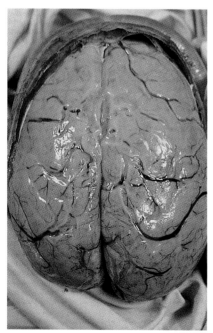

Fig. 1 **Pneumococcal meningitis.** Thick pus is seen over the vertex of this brain at autopsy.

Table 1 **Pyogenic and 'aseptic' meningitis**			
Causative organism	**Clinical clues**	**Chemotherapy**	**Control and prophylaxis**
PYOGENIC MENINGITIS			
Most common			
Haemophilus influenzae	Children, severe	Ceftriaxone	Rifampicin, vaccine
Neisseria meningitidis	Rash and shock	Penicillin	Rifampicin
Streptococcus pneumoniae	Severe	Penicillin or ceftriaxone	Vaccine
Common bacteria			
Gp A streptococci	Otitis media	Penicillin	Penicillin
Gp B streptococci	Neonatal	Ceftriaxone	Obstetric care
Gram-negative rods	Neonatal, immunocompromised	Ceftriaxone ± aminoglycoside	Obstetric care
Staphylococci	Trauma, surgery	Flucloxacillin	Operative
ASEPTIC MENINGITIS			
Unusual bacteria			
Actinomyces or *Nocardia* spp.	Brain abscess	Penicillin or sulphonamide	Dental
Anaerobes	Abscess or focus	Metronidazole	Surgery
Brucella spp.	Encephalitis also	Doxycycline and rifampicin	Animal vaccination
Listeria monocytogenes	Immunocompromised	Ampicillin	Avoid dairy foods
M. tuberculosis	Rarely acute	Triple	BCG
Mycoplasma pneumoniae	Respiratory also	Tetracycline	
Rickettsiae (RMSF)	Rash and shock	Tetracycline	Avoid vector
Spirochaetes			
Borrelia burgdorferi	Very variable	Tetracycline	Avoid vector
Treponema pallidum	Rarely acute	Penicillin	Safer sex
Leptospires	Systemic, myalgic	Penicillin	Animal control
Viral (see below)	Usually mild	None	(Vaccines)
Fungal			
Cryptococcus neoformans	Immunocompromised	Amphotericin B and fluconazole	Fluconazole
Parasitic			
Toxoplasma gondii	Immunocompromised	Pyrimethamine and co-trimoxazole	Pyrimethamine and sulphonamide
Amoebic			
Naegleria fowleri	Swimming	Amphotericin B	Chlorination
Acanthamoeba spp.	Immunocompromised	Sulphonamide and flucytosine	Chlorination?
Viruses include Enteroviruses (ECHO, Coxsackie), Herpes viruses (HSV, VZV, CMV, EBV), HIV, Mumps, Adenovirus			

- cerebral abscess
- parameningeal focus: in middle ear, mastoid or sinuses, or subdural, extradural or paraspinal abscess, sometimes with adjacent osteomyelitis
- suppurative thrombophlebitis.

Confirmatory tests

The pathogen is suggested by the **clinical features** above, and confirmed by **urgent lumbar puncture** for cell count, Gram stain and culture, antigen and PCR tests, and CSF glucose and protein levels, even if empiric antibiotics have been given. Important findings include:

- Cell count above 1500 with > 60% neutrophils favours bacterial meningitis, and one below 1000 with < 10% neutrophils favours viral or partially treated bacterial meningitis. There is overlap, especially in early disease.
- Gram stain of centrifuged CSF shows organisms in about 80% of patients with untreated bacterial meningitis, and antigen detection or PCR are specific when positive.
- Culture, including chocolate agar for *Haemophilus*, is for sensitivity tests, and additionally useful if Gram stain is unhelpful.
- Protein is highest and glucose lowest in bacterial meningitis.

Blood cultures and other cultures depending on **Clinical Clues** and **Special Situations** (see above) are essential. Imaging by CT scan or MRI is necessary if focal neurologic signs are present, suggesting an abscess or other focal lesion (p. 102–103). Special stains and serology are needed for specific pathogens.

A repeat LP is necessary in 6–12 hours if the first was non-specific, antibiotics were withheld and the patient worsens.

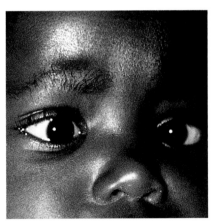

Fig. 2 **Sixth nerve pareses from raised intracranial pressure caused by *Haemophilus* meningitis.**

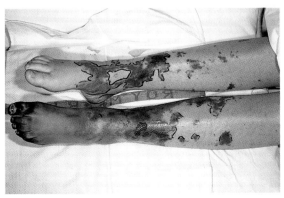

Fig. 3 **Petechial rash in meningococcal meningitis.**

Aseptic meningitis

Aseptic meningitis is meningitis with increased cells, particularly lymphocytes, but no growth in usual CSF cultures, and is caused by:

- non-viable partially treated pyogenic bacteria
- non-pyogenic unusual bacteria (Table 1)
- non-bacterial infections: viral, fungal, amoebic or parasitic
- non-meningeal infection: encephalitis, cerebral or para-meningeal abscess
- non-infective causes: e.g. **c**arcinomatous, **c**hemical (including drugs), '**c**ollagen' disease, **c**hronic subdural haematoma or **c**ysts.

Treatment

If microbial diagnosis is known, the drugs of choice are listed in Table 1.

If microbial diagnosis unknown, chemotherapy is chosen by the clinically suspected cause (Table 1); usually a third-generation cephalosporin is given if the pathogen is unknown, except for:

- CSF shunt-related infection: vancomycin is used initially
- immunocompromised patients need specific rapid investigations (e.g. cryptococcal antigen), specialist advice and initial broad therapy, which may include amphotericin and fluconazole, and/or sulphas and pyrimethamine.
- neonatal treatment usually involves giving gentamicin and/or ampicillin until the microbial diagnosis is known
- postoperative infection: flucloxacillin or vancomycin is added to ceftriaxone for better anti-staphylococcal cover.

Other management

This often includes dexamethasone and monitoring of intracranial pressure, or removal of infected shunts. An implanted reservoir to give intraventricular aminoglycoside, vancomycin or amphotericin is rarely needed.

Control and prevention

Rifampicin is given to the close contacts and the patient with *Haemophilus* (for 4 days) or meningococcal meningitis (2 days) to prevent secondary cases. Routine childhood vaccination is available in developed countries against *H. influenzae* type b, and meningococcal vaccine is available for high-risk situations.

Acute meningitis

- The commonest bacterial causes are *Neisseria meningitidis*, *Streptococcus pneumoniae* and *Haemophilus influenzae*, but other causes are other bacteria, fungi, parasites and viruses.
- The pathogen is suggested by certain Clinical Clues and Special Situations, and confirmed by lumbar puncture.
- Headache, fever, and neck stiffness occur in all types of acute meningitis.
- Clinical Clues include rash, myalgia, shock, or a source such as otitis media or respiratory infection.
- Special Situations include CSF leak, CSF shunt, immunosuppression, neonatally, or postoperatively.
- Urgent lumbar puncture is essential, and guides treatment.
- Directed chemotherapy depends on the organism, while empiric chemotherapy for an unknown organism depends on the Clinical Clues and Special Situation.

Acute encephalitis and poliomyelitis

Classification: Encephalitis may be chronic (p. 100–101) or acute, which may be infective or immune; the immune types are called acute disseminated encephalomyelitis, see below.

Acute encephalitis

Causative organisms

- Herpes simplex virus is the commonest cause in developed countries (Type 2 in neonates, Type 1 in adults).
- Arboviruses are important in different geographic areas, e.g. West Nile in Africa, Middle East and North America; Japanese B encephalitis in SE Asia, PNG and now Australia; and Murray Valley and Kunjin encephalitis in Australia.
- Other causative herpes viruses include CMV, EBV, VZV and Herpes B.
- HIV, as part of the acute sero-conversion illness, rarely causes encephalitis.
- Other viruses of lesser or regional importance include entero- and adenoviruses, influenza, rabies and other lyssa viruses, and Hendra, Nipah, and Cache Valley viruses.
- Trypanosomes cause 'sleeping sickness' in Africa (p. 82–83, 104–105).
- Bacteria rarely cause encephalitis (in contrast to meningitis), but the intracellular organisms causing listeriosis, melioidosis, mycoplasma infections, nocardiosis, rickettsioses, spirochaetal infections, toxoplasmosis and tuberculosis are rare causes.

Clinical features are a prodrome of fever, malaise and headache, then cerebral dysfunction, localised especially to the temporal lobe with Herpes simplex, but usually global: so there are disturbances of consciousness (drowsiness, stupor, coma), mentation (confusion, delirium), movement (fits, focal motor signs, aphasia) and behaviour. Sensory changes and meningeal irritation are uncommon. Rabies may have a 'dumb' phase, or a 'furious' phase, and hydrophobia or aerophobia (Fig. 1) are characteristic.

Confirmatory tests are lumbar puncture (often showing 'aseptic' meningitis, see Table 1 on p. 94), CSF PCR for relevant viruses (HSV, enteroviruses, arboviruses, VZV) and imaging by CT or MRI. EEG is little used now. Store serum and CSF, or do specific serology or PCR if special or rare pathogens are suspected. Rabies is diagnosed by fluorescent antibody tests on neck skin biopsy, Negri bodies in corneal scrapings (or the brain at PM), or antibody detection in serum or CSF.

Chemotherapy is urgent and important for Herpes simplex encephalitis, as prognosis is directly related to early treatment with i.v. aciclovir, followed by oral valaciclovir or famciclovir. Ganciclovir is used in CMV CNS infections (Fig. 2) with less effect.

There is no effective therapy for arbovirus, Hendra or Nipah virus infections, nor for established rabies or lyssa virus infections.

Control and prevention. Rabies or Lyssa virus infections are prevented by rabies vaccine given post-exposure but before symptoms develop, or pre-exposure in high-risk people.

Acute disseminated encephalomyelitis (ADEM)

Classification. This may be either **post-infectious** or **post-vaccine encephalomyelitis**. They are believed to be immune-mediated, with white matter demyelination (Fig. 3) and perivascular inflammation.

Causative organisms include measles, rubella or varicella, influenza or rarely other viral respiratory or gut infections. It has occurred after vaccinia or rabies immunisation.

Clinical features are like acute viral encephalitis (above), but occur *7–21 days after* the viral infection or vaccine. Recovery is usual without sequelae. Note that encephalitis from measles is of three types:

- During acute measles from actual viral infection of the brain, often with sequelae
- Post-infectious, 7–21 days later, immune mediated, usually no sequelae
- Subacute Sclerosing Pan-Encephalitis, (SSPE), occurring years later as a rare but severe, progressive, and fatal disease (p. 100).

Confirmatory tests are often unnecessary if the time relationship to the precipitating infection or vaccination is clear. If not, investigate as for acute encephalitis above.

Chemotherapy is ineffective, but steroids are used to help cerebral oedema.

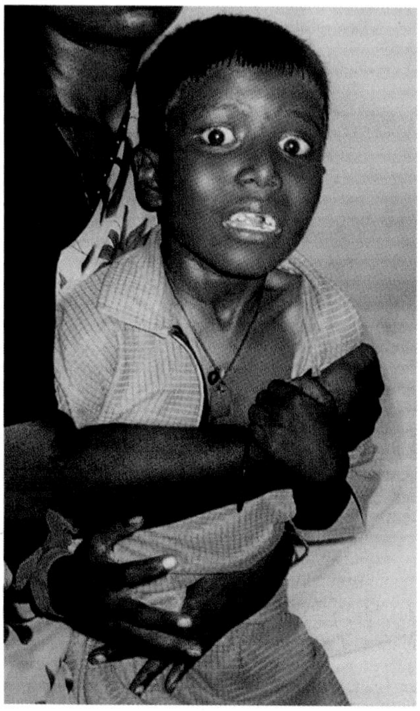

Fig. 1 **Aerophobia (fear when fan turned on) in rabies.**

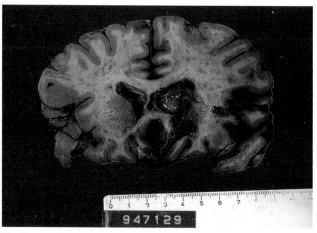

Fig. 2 **Cytomegalovirus ventriculitis on right side.**

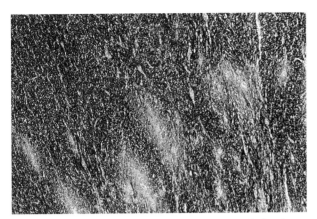

Fig. 3 **Acute disseminated encephalomyelitis (ADEM), showing peri-vascular demyelination (the numerous cleared white areas).**

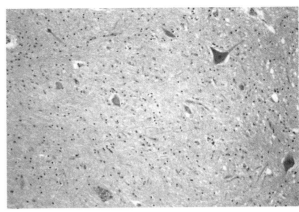

Fig. 4 **Polio, showing almost total loss of large triangular anterior horn cells.**

Control and prevention. These conditions are seldom seen now because:

- Measles-mumps-rubella (MMR) vaccine has greatly decreased these three diseases
- Varicella vaccine is becoming more widely used
- Improved rabies vaccine has a much lower ADEM rate than earlier vaccines
- Smallpox eradication has made vaccinia ('smallpox') vaccination rare.

Acute poliomyelitis

Classification. Polio is classified into four grades of increasing severity:

- Inapparent infection, with no symptoms or signs – commonest in non-immunised young children in endemic areas of the developing world
- Abortive infection, when only a mild febrile illness occurs, with sore throat, headache, nausea or vomiting, but no neurological disease, with full recovery
- Non-paralytic polio, with fever, headache and neck stiffness, i.e. aseptic meningitis but no paralysis; spontaneous resolution is usual
- Paralytic polio, with aseptic meningitis and infection of the anterior horn cells (AHC) of the spinal cord giving flaccid paralysis, often with brain-stem infection ('bulbar polio') causing life-threatening respiratory paralysis. There is little or no recovery from full paralysis with destroyed AHC, but not all AHC of individual muscles may be affected, so some muscles are weak rather than paralysed.

Causative organisms. The poliovirus is an enterovirus, i.e. a non-enveloped single-stranded RNA picornavirus with an icosahedral nucleocapsid (see Table 2, p. 93). There are only three serotypes, so vaccines are effective. Immunity is type-specific, lifelong after natural infection, and long-lasting after immunisation.

Humans are the only host, with infection by the faecal–oral route. The virus spreads from the gut via the bloodstream to the motor neurons in the anterior horns of the spinal cord (Fig. 4) and to the brain stem. Retrograde spread up axons also occurs. Paralysis is due to neuronal death, not muscle infection. The virus may be excreted for some months, but permanent carriage is unknown.

Clinical features. These are described above. In addition, a post-polio syndrome occurs many years after acute polio, with severe worsening of the residual weakness in the affected muscles. The mechanism is unknown.

Confirmatory tests. These are usually unnecessary for paralytic polio, but the virus can be found in the throat, stool or CSF by culture showing a typical cytopathogenic effect (CPE), while serology shows an antibody rise.

Chemotherapy. No antiviral drugs are effective. Symptomatic therapy may be needed for headache and nausea. Physiotherapy is very important to maximise muscle power, and respiratory support is needed for bulbar polio.

Control. Two types of excellent vaccine are available:

- The oral live attenuated Sabin vaccine has two advantages – it is easy to give, and stops faecal–oral transmission by causing protective secretory IgA in the gut, so is favoured for eradication campaigns. However it has four disadvantages – refrigerated storage because it is live; rarely, reversion to a virulent 'wild' strain causes polio; other gut viruses can reduce its replication and hence reduce protection; and immunodeficient people may develop polio.
- The injectable inactivated 'killed' Salk vaccine has none of these disadvantages, while an enhanced version now induces some gut IgA.

Acute encephalitis
- Acute encephalitis is usually viral, particularly herpes simplex or an arbovirus depending on the geographic area. Rarer viral causes are other herpes viruses, rabies, HIV, enteroviruses, and influenza. It is rarely due to bacteria (intracellular). Trypanosomes in Africa cause acute encephalitis, called sleeping sickness.
- Clinically there is a prodrome, then cerebral dysfunction with disturbed mentation, consciousness, movement and behaviour.
- Confirmation is by LP, imaging, PCR and serology.
- Chemotherapy is aciclovir for HSV, ganciclovir for CMV.
- Control is by avoidance of insect and animal bites, and rabies vaccine pre- or post-exposure.

Acute disseminated encephalomyelitis (ADEM)
- This is a rare immune reaction occurring 7–21 days after viral infection or vaccine
- Causes are usually measles, rubella, varicella, or vaccinia or rabies vaccine.
- Clinically it is like acute encephalitis except for the 7–21 day interval.
- Confirmation is often unnecessary, and treatment is supportive only.

Acute poliomyelitis
- Clinically this may be inapparent, abortive, non-paralytic, or paralytic.
- Classically, paralytic is lower motor neuron flaccid paralysis, and bulbar polio causes respiratory paralysis.
- Cause is the polio virus, a non-enveloped SS RNA enterovirus.
- Confirmatory tests are usually unnecessary, and no chemotherapy helps.
- Control is by oral or injected polio vaccine.

Chronic diffuse non-viral CNS infections

Chronic infections of the CNS are characterised by development over weeks or months. They are classified into diffuse infections (meningitis and meningoencephalitis) and focal infections (p. 102–103).

Diffuse infections are usually bacterial or viral (p. 100–101), rarely fungal or parasitic; there are three main non-viral causes:

■ *Cryptococcus neoformans*: cryptococcosis
■ *Treponema pallidum*: syphilis
■ *Mycobacterium tuberculosis*: tuberculosis.

Other less common pathogens are *Borrelia burgdorferi*, *Trypanosoma* spp. (p. 82–83, 153) and, rarely, *Angiostrongylus cantonensis* or *Brucella* spp.

Clinical features

In chronic meningitis, as with acute meningitis, headache, fever, clouding of consciousness and neck stiffness are usual. In meningoencephalitis, cerebral disturbances occur. Intractable vomiting and visual changes signal raised intracranial pressure.

Differential diagnosis
This includes cerebral tumour, subdural or subarachnoid haemorrhage, multiple sclerosis, metabolic encephalopathies or autoimmune diseases.

Confirmatory tests
Lumbar puncture (LP) is the key to diagnosis, but should not be done if a *focal* infection is indicated by CT or MRI. The fluid is tested for cell counts, staining, culture, PCR, serology, plus CSF and serum glucose and protein. Mantoux, chest x-ray or CT scans may be helpful.

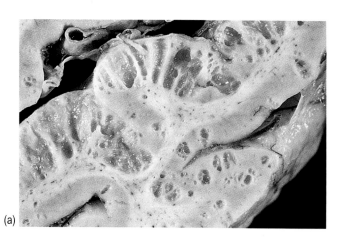

(a)

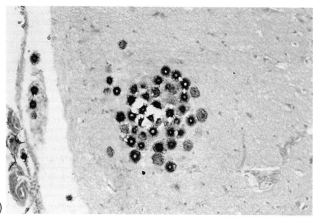

(b)

Specific diseases

Cryptococcosis
The fungus *Cryptococcus neoformans* (p. 70) causes both meningitis and multiple abscesses in the CNS (Fig. 1). It also causes pulmonary, bone and skin lesions, and more acute systemic disease (cryptococcaemia) in the immunocompromised, e.g. in AIDS.

Clinically, in CNS infection, fever and headache are not marked, while changes in mentation, behaviour and memory are prominent. Cranial nerve involvement can cause visual impairment or facial weakness; other focal lesions are rare. As with any cause of raised intracranial pressure, VI nerve paresis may be a false localising sign (Fig. 2).

Confirmation is by LP, which shows the characteristic capsulated fungi (see Fig. 2, p. 70). Latex agglutination detects antigen in CSF or blood.

Chemotherapy is usually by amphotericin B ± flucytosine, then fluconazole. Continuing secondary prophylaxis by lower-dose fluconazole is needed in the immunocompromised.

Syphilis
Syphilis is a systemic spirochaetal disease caused by *Treponema pallidum* (p. 58).

In **primary syphilis**, asymptomatic invasion of the CNS may occur and current treatment aims to treat this. In **secondary syphilis**, acute 'aseptic' meningitis may occur. In **latent syphilis**, by definition there are no symptoms and CSF syphilis serology is negative, though serum is positive.

In **tertiary neurosyphilis** there are five categories:

1. Asymptomatic with positive CSF serology.
2. Meningo-vascular with chronic meningitis or meningoencephalitis from endarteritis obliterans of meninges, brain or spinal cord.

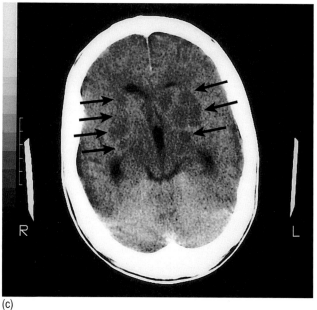

(c)

Fig. 1 **C. neoformans: cerebral infection. (a)** Multiple gelatinous masses. **(b)** Organisms stained blue in brain tissue. **(c)** CT scan.

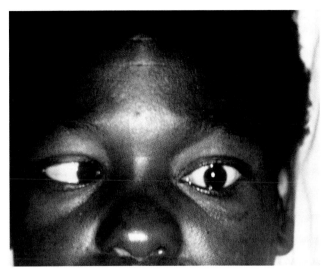

Fig. 2 *C. neoformans*: sixth nerve paresis.

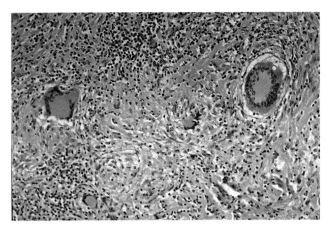

Fig. 3 *M. tuberculosis*: tubercles with giant cells.

3. General paresis of the insane (GPI) with cerebral cortical destruction causing changes in **p**ersonality, **a**ffect, **r**eflexes (hyperactive), **e**ye (Argyll Robertson pupils, reacting to accommodation, not light), **s**ensorium (delusions, hallucinations), **i**ntellect and **s**peech.
4. Tabes dorsalis with spinal posterior column and dorsal root destruction causing bladder dysfunction, Romberg's sign, ataxia, impotence, and neuropathy (both cranial and peripheral) with loss of vibration and position sense.
5. Gumma, a localised necrosis, with symptoms and signs dependent on its position.

Diagnosis is clinical and serological, LP being essential. Treatment is by at least 3 weeks i.v. penicillin. Ceftriaxone or tetracycline are unproven alternatives in penicillin allergy. Prevention is by treatment of primary or secondary disease.

Tuberculosis
Tuberculosis is a chronic bacterial disease (Fig. 3) caused by *Mycobacterium tuberculosis* (p. 60). It causes a chronic meningitis with the usual symptoms or, rarely, localised masses called tuberculomata. Rarely, the meningitis is acute. Spread can cause cerebral, cerebellar or spinal symptoms and signs.

Diagnosis depends on LP; the usual findings are 100–1500 cells, mainly lymphocytes, elevated protein and low sugar; bacteria are only visible on AF stain in about one-third of the first LPs, which must be repeated if doubt remains.

Treatment is by intensive triple or quadruple therapy including isoniazid and rifampicin.

Eosinophilic meningitis
Eosinophilic meningitis is an unusual disease found in south-east Asia and the Pacific, caused by the parasite *Angiostrongylus cantonensis*, the rat lungworm, which has an unusual life cycle, from rats to slugs and snails to rats. Humans are accidentally infected by ingesting raw snails or contaminated raw vegetables. Human infection is often asymptomatic, or the ingested larvae migrate to the CNS, causing severe headache, vomiting, neck stiffness and often cranial nerve lesions. Unusually for meningitis, fever is minimal or absent.

LP is unusual because the pleocytosis (500 or more) is eosinophilic (10–50%) and lymphocytic. Larvae or young adult worms are seldom found in the CSF, and serology may not distinguish it from other parasitic infections of the CNS (p. 102–105). There is no specific therapy, and most patients recover in 3–8 weeks.

Lyme disease
Lyme disease is a systemic spirochaetal disease caused by *Borrelia* spp., usually *B. burgdorferi* (p. 58–59). Infected tick bites cause a specific rash then CNS involvement, with initial acute meningismus (headache, neck pain and stiffness without meningitis on LP). Fluctuating chronic meningitis or meningoencephalitis follows, often with cranial or peripheral nerve lesions, rarely myelitis (spinal cord).

LP shows mild (100–300) lymphocytosis. Diagnosis is clinical and serological. Treatment is by i.v. penicillin or ceftriaxone. Control is by avoidance of tick bite in endemic areas.

Brucellosis
Brucellosis is a chronic or relapsing systemic bacterial infection caused by one of the *Brucella* spp. (p. 56). It can cause a chronic meningitis, which gives the usual symptoms, or more commonly meningoencephalitis, where headache and lassitude, cranial nerve lesions and neuropsychiatric symptoms (particularly depression) are common. LP has an unusual picture, with mainly monocytes in the pleocytosis (elevated cell count) of some hundreds, and prolonged culture in CO_2 is positive in about 50%. Serology is helpful but not always diagnostic. Treatment is doxycycline with streptomycin (best proof of efficacy), gentamicin (safer, easier) or rifampicin (safest, easiest). Control is aimed at infected animals and animal products including cheese.

> ### *Chronic diffuse non-viral CNS infections*
> - Chronic meningitis and meningoencephalitis are infections developing over weeks or months.
> - Main non-viral causes are cryptococcosis, syphilis and tuberculosis.
> - Chronic meningitis causes headache and vomiting, changes in conscious state and neck stiffness, while meningoencephalitis causes changes in mentation.
> - Diagnosis is principally by lumbar puncture showing increased cells (often not neutrophils), with special stains and cultures. Serology and imaging help with specific diagnoses.

Chronic diffuse viral and prion CNS diseases

Chronic encephalitis

Classification. This uncommon syndrome is characterised by insidious onset and progressive cerebral disease. A non-infectious encephalopathy (carcinoma, vasculitis, drugs) must be separated from true infective encephalitis due to bacteria, fungi or parasites (p. 98–99) or a virus or prion where either the agent or the host is abnormal, i.e.:

- a common virus such as an enterovirus or adenovirus (p. 96–97), in an uncommon patient with abnormal immunity
- a virus causing immune deficiency – see HIV (p. 149–151)
- an unusual 'slow virus' (defective measles virus, JC virus, HTLV 1) causing a specific disease (SSPE, PML, TSP, see below), or
- a very unusual agent called a prion, see below.

Subacute sclerosing panencephalitis (SSPE)

Causative organism is a defective (mutant) measles virus unable to complete replication. Abnormal host immunity is also probably important.

Clinical features are chronic personality changes progressing to dementia and death 2–20 years after measles. The rare occurrence after measles vaccine was probably due to prior, unrecognised subclinical measles.

Confirmatory tests are very high measles antibody in serum and CSF, and MRI or brain biopsy showing widespread inflammatory lesions.

Chemotherapy is ineffective.

Control and prevention is by widespread measles vaccination, which has almost abolished SSPE.

Progressive multifocal leucoencephalopathy (PML)

Causative organism is the JC papovavirus. About 50% of normal people have latent infection, and disease results when re-activation occurs in the immunocompromised, especially in AIDS. Oligodendrocytes are killed, and astrocytes form syncytia.

Clinical features are pareses, visual impairment and mental state changes

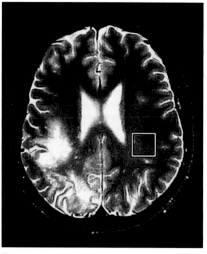

Fig. 1 **Progressive multi-focal leucoencephalopathy (PML) on MRI, showing coalescing lesions in white matter.**

progressing to blindness, dementia and death within 6 months.

Confirmatory tests are characteristic disseminated white matter demyelination on CT or MRI (Fig. 1) or necropsy (Fig. 2), while PCR on CSF, urine or brain is definitive.

Chemotherapy is usually ineffective, though cidofovir may be useful.

Control and prevention is by Highly Active Anti Retroviral Treatment (HAART) of AIDS, and minimising or avoiding immunosuppression in other diseases.

Tropical spastic paraparesis (TSP)

Also called HTLV-associated myelopathy (HAM).

Causative organism is the Human T-cell Lymphotropic Virus-1 (HTLV-1), and possibly HTLV-2. These are enveloped retroviruses with reverse transcriptase and two copies of single-stranded positive-polarity RNA, like HIV (p. 149).

Clinical features are chronic lower limb weakness, disturbed gait, low back pain and often impaired bladder and bowel control progressing over some years.

Confirmatory tests are HTLV-1 antibody in serum and CSF, while PCR detects infected cells. MRI shows non-specific demyelination.

Chemotherapy is ineffective.

Control and prevention is by screening blood for transfusion, by condom use, and by discouraging breast-feeding by infected women.

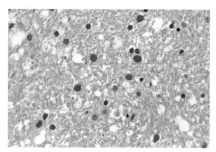

Fig. 2 **Progressive multi-focal leucoencephalopathy (PML) histopathology showing swollen basophilic nuclear inclusions.**

Transmissible spongiform encephalopathies (TSE)

Classification. These 'slow', i.e. chronic, diseases are caused not by viruses but by *prions*, which are infectious particles composed entirely of protein, with no detectable RNA or DNA. The most important human TSE is **Creutzfeldt–Jakob Disease (CJD)** and its **Variant CJD (vCJD)**, discussed below. Others, all very rare, are **Kuru, Gerstmann–Straussler–Scheinker (GSS) Syndrome** and **Fatal Familial Insomnia** (Table 1). Three 'slow' transmissible diseases in animals are **Scrapie** and **Visna** in sheep, and **Bovine Spongiform Encephalopathy** (BSE, 'Mad Cow Disease') in cattle.

Causative organism and mechanism. Normal brain contains normal prion protein, called PrP^c for Prion Protein Cellular. It is probably involved in signal transduction in neurons, is coded by a normal cellular gene, and has an alpha-helical conformation. Enhanced by a specific cellular RNA, this alpha-helical conformation changes to an abnormal beta-pleated sheet which is the Prion Protein Scrapie, PrP^{sc}. This forms filaments causing neuronal dysfunction and death. This abnormal prion protein further recruits alpha-helical forms and 'reproduces' by changing their conformation to more beta-pleated forms, causing more neuronal damage and death.

Creutzfeldt–Jakob Disease (CJD)
CJD arises in three different ways:

- **Infective**, transmitted from infected tissue by human growth hormone made from human pituitary glands,

Table 1 **Human prion diseases (TSEs)**

Disease	Pathogenesis	Cause	Clinical disease
Creutzfeldt–Jakob disease (CJD)	1. Infectious/transmissible	Iatrogenic (instruments, grafts, growth hormone)	Myoclonic jerks, ataxia, speech and visual loss, pareses & dementia
	2. Sporadic	Commonest. Cause unknown – ?mutation	
	3. Genetic	Germ cell mutation	
Variant CJD (vCJD)	Infectious/transmissible	Eating brain-contaminated beef from cattle with 'mad cow disease'	Younger, longer course, psychiatric and sensory disturbances prominent
Kuru	Infectious/transmissible	Eating or handling brain from infected people	Ataxia, tremors, but not dementia
Gerstmann–Straussler–Scheinker (GSS) syndrome	Genetic	Germ cell mutations in prion protein gene	Spastic paraparesis and cerebellar ataxia
Fatal familial insomnia (FFI)	Genetic	Germ cell mutation in prion protein gene	Insomnia, autonomic dysfunction, dementia

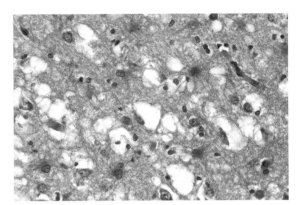

Fig. 3 **Creutzfeldt–Jakob disease brain showing spongiform changes from neuronal vacuolation and loss, with no inflammation.**

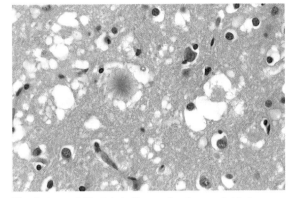

Fig. 4 **Creutzfeldt–Jakob disease showing amyloid plaques.**

by corneal and dura mater grafts, by brain electrodes or contaminated neurosurgical instruments
- **Hereditary**, by genetic mutation in germ cells (about 10% of cases)
- **Sporadic**, by spontaneous mutation in about 1 per million people.

Clinical features are summarised in Table 1.

- **Classic Creutzfeldt–Jakob Disease (CJD)** usually presents between 50–70 years of age with progressive dementia (confusion, memory loss, behavioural changes), often with myoclonic jerks, pareses, ataxia, and visual or speech loss. The patient becomes mute, motionless and incontinent before welcome death in 6–12 months.
- **Variant Creutzfeldt–Jakob Disease (vCJD)** usually affects younger people, and psychiatric and sensory changes are prominent, unlike classic CJD. Progression is somewhat slower, with death in 12–18 months.

Confirmatory tests. Prions cause no inflammatory or immune response, being chemically normal body protein, though conformationally abnormal. Brain biopsies thus show spongiform changes from neuronal vacuolation and loss, with no inflammation (Fig. 3), and amyloid plaques occur (Fig. 4). Tonsillar biopsy is often positive in vCJD, saving brain biopsy. There are no serologic tests, because there is no immune response, therefore no human antibody. Immunohistochemical tests use antibody made in animals in which human prions are immunogenic. There are no culture tests. CSF often contains a normal brain protein called 14-3-3, but no inflammatory cells.

Chemotherapy is currently useless, though acridines such as quinacrine that are active in cell culture are being investigated.

Control and prevention. The infectious forms are prevented by blocking transmission.

Prions are resistant to formaldehyde, boiling, usual autoclaving and ultraviolet light, but inactivated by protein-destroying disinfectants including hypochlorite, phenols, NaOH and ether, and by repeated long-cycle maximum temperature-pressure autoclaving.

Transmission of classical CJD is blocked by excluding those possibly infected from blood or tissue donation, by using disposable instruments when possible for any procedures, and by special autoclaving or strong hypochlorite if instruments cannot be discarded.

Transmission of variant CJD is blocked by excluding possibly infected sheep organs from bovine food, slaughtering or excluding infected animals from human food, and eating Australian beef.

Hereditary forms of CJD, GSS and FFI may be prevented by carrier detection (when possible) and genetic counselling.

Kuru has been almost eradicated by changed cultural practices in the Fore people of Papua New Guinea.

Chronic encephalitis and prion diseases

- Chronic encephalitis may be caused by a 'usual' virus in an unusual, i.e. immunocompromised, patient.
- Subacute sclerosing panencephalitis is a fatal dementia from a variant measles virus.
- Progressive multifocal leucoencephalopathy is a fatal dementia due to JC virus in an abnormal immunocompromised patient, e.g. with AIDS.
- Tropical spastic paraparesis is a rare paralysing infection by HTLV 1, a retrovirus.
- Transmissible spongiform encephalopathies include the dementing Creutzfeldt–Jakob Disease (CJD), its variant vCJD, and several other rare diseases. They are due to unique agents called prions, which are protein, contain no DNA or RNA, but 'reproduce' by conformational change.

CNS abscesses and other focal infections

Focal infective lesions of the CNS are characterised by a mass lesion, also called a space-occupying lesion (SOL). The distinction from meningitis and diffuse infective cerebral lesions (preceding topics) is doubly important, firstly because lumbar puncture is contraindicated with a mass lesion, and secondly because surgery is often needed.

Focal lesions may be classified into **abscesses** (with pus), usually bacterial or fungal and often needing surgery, **cysts**, usually parasitic and seldom needing surgery, or **necrosis**, usually viral (p. 96–97), in which global dysfunction usually overshadows focal features except with HSV (p. 96, 200). Table 1 lists causative organisms.

Clinical features

Focal lesions present rather like meningitis or diffuse lesions with headache, fever and altered conscious state, but with three important distinctions:

- neck stiffness is absent or slight
- focal signs are present
- evidence of raised intracranial pressure (severe vomiting, papilloedema) is much more prominent.

Differential diagnosis is from noninfective focal lesions, including tumour, infarcts or haemorrhage.

Confirmatory tests

Lumbar puncture is contraindicated for three reasons: it is potentially dangerous because intracranial pressure (ICP) is usually raised even if papilloedema is not visible, it is seldom helpful, and it may be misleading.

Imaging by CT or MRI is the basis of diagnosis (Fig. 1). If not available, a brain scan (or skull x-ray if a calcified pineal gland is displaced) can confirm a mass lesion but give minimal detail.

The causative organism is obtained by aspiration or surgery, or deduced from serology. Aspirate or surgically removed tissue is tested by staining, culture and biochemical tests for the suspected pathogen.

ABSCESSES

These usually have one of three sources as predisposing factors:

- **parameningeal infection** (40–50%): paranasal sinuses, ear, mastoid or dental infections, with sub- or extradural abscess and/or osteomyelitis; less com-

monly, face or scalp infections (including head tongs or ICP or fetal monitors) or meningitis
- **distant infection with septicaemic spread** (25%): especially from lungs or with cardiac right–left shunts
- **head surgery or trauma.**

Parasitic cysts and viral necrosis occur from haematogenous spread. Peripheral nerves bring some viruses – polio, rabies, VZV.

Brain abscesses

Anaerobes

Anaerobes, such as peptostreptococci and *Bacteroides* spp. (p. 54, 55), often mixed with aerobes such as streptococci and Gram-negative enteric bacilli, are by far the commonest organisms. Confirmatory laboratory tests depend on rapid transport of adequate anaerobic and aerobic samples followed by specific anaerobic and aerobic culture. Chemotherapy pending culture results is usually penicillin plus metronidazole; if Gram-negative aerobes are likely, e.g. secondary to ear or sinus infections, a third-generation cephalosporin such as ceftriaxone is added. Early surgical consultation concerning aspiration or incision and drainage is essential. The source, particularly parameningeal foci and septicaemic spread from distant foci, must be sought and treated.

Table 1 Major causes of focal CNS infections

Category and causative organism	Clinical features and incidence	Chemotherapy (usually with surgery)
Bacteria		
Actinomyces or *Nocardia*	Immunocompromised	Penicillin or sulphonamide
Anaerobes	Common, 50–75%	Penicillin or metronidazole
especially *Bacteroides*	Common, 20–30%	Metronidazole
Staphylococci	Postoperative	Flucloxacillin
Streptococci (especially micro-aerophilic)	Frequent 20%	Penicillin
Gram-negative rods	Ear, sinus or abdominal focus	Ceftriaxone
Mixed	Common, 40–50%	Ceftriaxone + metronidazole
M. tuberculosis	Tuberculoma rare	Triple therapy
T. pallidum	Gumma very rare	Penicillin
Fungi		
Aspergillosis	Immunocompromised	Amphotericin + voriconazole
Candidiasis	Immunocompromised	Amphotericin + fluconazole
Cryptococcosis	Immunocompromised	Amphotericin + 5-flucytosine or fluconazole
Systemic mycoses	Geographic area	Amphotericin + itraconazole
Invasive zygomycosis	Diabetes, leukaemia	Amphotericin + azole
Parasites		
Cysticercosis	Cyst, endemic area	Praziquantel
E. histolytica	Abscess, endemic area	Metronidazole
Hydatid disease	Cysts, endemic area	Albendazole
Toxoplasmosis	Immunocompromised	Pyrimethamine + sulphas
Viruses		
HSV, CMV, arboviruses, PML	Encephalitis, HIV	Aciclovir, ganciclovir, none

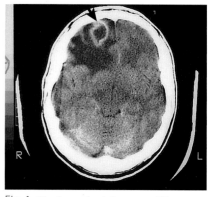

Fig. 1 **Single cerebral abscess on CT.**

Staphylococci

Staphylococci (p. 34) are particularly important in brain abscesses after trauma or neurosurgery, are diagnosed by routine techniques, and are treated by flucloxacillin unless meticillin-resistant, when vancomycin is used.

Actinomyces and *Nocardia* spp.

Actinomyces and *Nocardia* (p. 62) are rare causes of brain abscess. Both are chronic bacterial infections, though more acute in the immunocompromised. Cervicofacial infection and sinus formation are characteristic of actinomycosis, while pulmonary disease resembling tuberculosis plus multiple, multiloculated abscesses are more typical of nocardiosis. Prolonged anaerobic culture (for *Actinomyces*) and aerobic culture (for *Nocardia*)

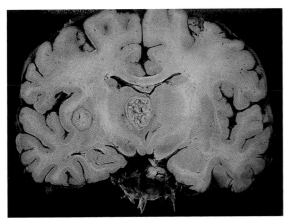

Fig. 2 **Cerebral tuberculomata.**

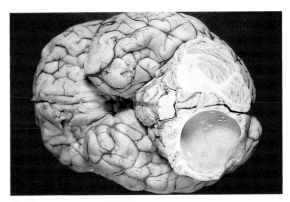

Fig. 4 **Hydatid cyst of brain.**

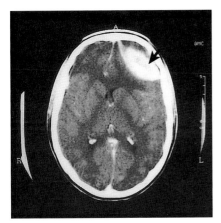

Fig. 3 **Extradural abscess.**

are needed to grow the branching Gram-positive, weakly acid-fast filaments. Chemotherapy is long-term penicillin for actinomycosis, and sulphonamide for nocardiosis. Thick-walled abscesses often require surgery.

Syphilis

Syphilis (*Treponema pallidum,* p. 58) is a very rare cause of a focal lesion (a gumma, p. 99) and is diagnosed by imaging and syphilis serology. Chemotherapy is high-dose i.v. penicillin for 14 days.

Tuberculosis

Tuberculosis (p. 60, 132) also rarely produces one or more focal lesions (plural: tuberculomata, Fig. 2), diagnosed by imaging, a positive Mantoux, evidence of tuberculosis elsewhere, and AFB stain and culture if surgery is needed. Treatment is by triple therapy.

Fungal abscesses

Fungal abscesses (Table 1) are uncommon, and in aspergillosis, candidiasis or cryptococcosis most often occur in immunocompromised patients with fungaemia. In aspergillosis, blood vessel invasion often causes infarction, and in cryptococcosis meningitis is common

(p. 70, 98). Of the systemic mycoses, blastomycosis, coccidioidomycosis and rarely histoplasmosis (p. 70–73) can cause brain abscesses. Treatment is specific chemotherapy, and surgery as indicated.

Rhinocerebral zygomycosis

This invasive mucormycosis (p. 76) is a rapidly progressive infection mainly in patients with diabetes or haematologic malignancy. Fungus spreads through the nose, sinuses, skull, meninges and brain, causing tissue destruction and necrosis rather than true abscess formation. Unless diagnosed early and the predisposing cause reversed if possible, and the fungus treated vigorously with amphotericin B plus an azole and surgery if possible, it is fatal.

Sub- and extradural abscesses

Abscesses may form just inside the dura mater (subdural abscess: subdural empyaema) or outside it [extradural (Fig. 3): epidural abscess] or both at once. As with brain abscesses, there is usually one of the three predisposing factors (above).

Typically a patient with sinusitis or otitis worsens rapidly, with fever, severe headache, vomiting, altered mental state, and then focal signs plus signs of raised

intracranial pressure. The focal signs may spread to involve a whole cerebral hemisphere. Imaging and surgery are urgent and essential. The usual causative organisms are aerobic and anaerobic streptococci, other anaerobes, and S. *aureus.* If the abscess follows abdominal operation, aerobic Gram-negative rods (GNRs) are common. Chemotherapy is high-dose i.v. flucloxacillin and metronidazole, with gentamicin or ceftriaxone for GNR.

CYSTS

When the haematogenous spread of parasites causes focal lesions in the CNS, these are usually cysts: of tachyzoites in toxoplasmosis (p. 78), of larvae of *Taenia solium* in cysticercosis (p. 88) and of larvae of *Echinococcus granulosus* within brood capsules within a hydatid cyst (Fig. 4) (p. 89). An exception is *Entamoeba histolytica* (p. 80), which does not form tissue cysts but, as its name describes, 'lyses tissue' to form abscesses.

All present as mass lesions with focal signs, and little or no fever or other systemic upset.

Imaging, serology and epidemiology may lead to the diagnosis, or surgery may be needed for both diagnosis and treatment.

CNS abscesses and other focal infections

- Focal infections of the CNS must be distinguished from meningitis and diffuse lesions because lumbar puncture is contraindicated and surgery is often essential.
- Focal lesions may be abscesses (usually bacterial or fungal), cysts (usually parasitic) or necrosis (usually viral).
- Factors predisposing are parameningeal infections, distal infection with haematogenous spread, or local trauma including surgery.
- Bacterial abscesses are usually anaerobic or mixed anaerobic-aerobic.
- Fungal infections are usually candidiasis, cryptococcosis or aspergillosis in immunocompromised patients.
- Parasitic infections include toxoplasmosis, hydatid cysts, cysticercosis and amoebiasis.
- Diagnosis is by imaging (usually CT), microscopy and special cultures of surgical specimens, or serology in special infections.
- Treatment is specific chemotherapy, and usually urgent surgery (not toxoplasmosis).

Nervous system: tropical and rare infections

Neural tissue can be damaged by viruses (p. 96–97, 100–101) and by bacteria, fungi or protozoa (below). Some infect nervous tissues: others produce neurotoxins which impair neuron function.

Botulism

Botulism is a rare but serious disease characterised by flaccid paralysis caused by the neurotoxin of *Clostridium botulinum* (p. 41). This anaerobic Grampositive rod is found almost everywhere in the environment; its heat-resistant spores occur in soil and food, particularly inadequately canned or bottled vegetables, honey and fish. Wound botulism (the rarest form) and infant botulism (from honey) are *infections*, with actual bacterial multiplication in the body before intoxication occurs. Adult food-borne disease, the commonest form, is an *intoxication* from ingested toxin. The toxin enters neurons and prevents the release of acetylcholine.

Clinical features. These include blurred vision with fixed dilated pupils, dry mouth, constipation and abdominal pain, descending flaccid paralysis, respiratory arrest and death in 10–60% of adults, but only 1–5% in infants.

Differential diagnosis. This includes myasthenia gravis, polio and the Guillain–Barré syndrome of ascending polyneuritis.

Confirmatory tests. These are specialised, depending on anaerobic culture or on detection of botulinum toxin in mice.

Chemotherapy. Penicillin is relatively unimportant, treatment depending on antitoxin and respiratory support.

Control and prevention depends on sufficient time at the correct temperatures during food preparation, and not giving honey to infants less than 1 year old.

Leprosy

Leprosy (Hansen's disease) is a chronic infection of the nerves and skin with *Mycobacterium leprae* (p. 60). Disease is classified by the cell-mediated immune (CMI) response (Fig. 1). Infection is by droplet spread from infected nasal secretions, direct skin contact and possibly from breast milk and insect bites.

Clinical features. These vary widely, depending on the classification and extent

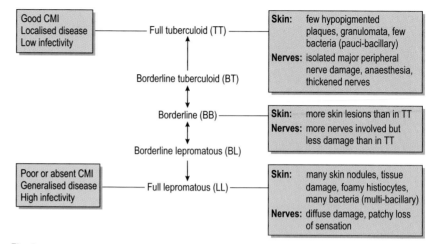

Fig. 1 **Classification of leprosy.**

of disease. Extensive LL causes leonine facies, succulent ear lobes, nasal cartilage destruction, erythema nodosum leprosum (p. 191), polyarthritis and painful peripheral neuritis with, e.g., foot drop, a neuropathic ulcer (Fig. 2) or ulnar nerve involvement causing a 'claw hand' (Fig. 3). Local sensory loss makes the patient susceptible to secondary trauma and bacterial infections.

Confirmatory tests. These depend on seeing acid-fast bacilli in nasal scrapings or skin biopsies, and on histology, as culture is only possible in mouse foot-pads or armadillos (facilitated by the lower body temperature).

Chemotherapy. This is with daily dapsone and monthly rifampicin, plus clofazimine in LL disease. Duration varies from 6–9 months in TT to years or even lifelong in LL. Ofloxacin and clarithromycin are being evaluated. Management of ulcers and disfigurement is important.

Control and prevention. This depends on treatment of infective (LL, BL) patients, and dapsone for their close contacts aged < 16 years.

Malaria

Malaria affects the CNS in two ways:

- cerebral malaria, which is severe and may be fatal (Fig. 4), characterised by widespread changes in cerebral function from capillary plugging caused by *Plasmodium falciparum* (p. 78)
- mild cerebral symptoms from general tissue anoxia occurring in malaria from other species.

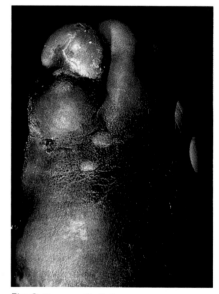

Fig. 2 **Neuropathy in leprosy.**

Clinical features. Cerebral malaria causes severe headache, high fever, rigors, altered behaviour, confusion, hallucinations, disturbed consciousness and at times fits or focal lesions.

Confirmatory tests. These depend on urgent thick and thin stained blood films ± antigen detection.

Chemotherapy. This is by i.v. quinine or artesunate, begun immediately but given slowly. Monitoring of cardiac function and blood glucose is necessary. Follow-up therapy with oral antimalarials is needed, the drug depending on specialist advice.

Control and prevention involves measures against mosquitoes, and chemoprophylaxis with the appropriate antimalarial, varying for different countries.

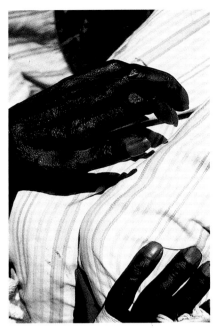

Fig. 3 **Leprosy: claw hand from ulnar nerve lesion.**

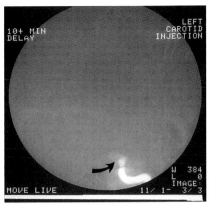

Fig. 4 **Cerebral malaria: angiogram showing no circulation, shortly before death.**

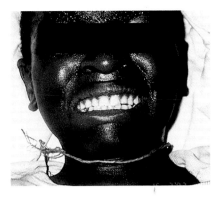

Fig. 5 **Tetanus: risus sardonicus.**

Paragonimiasis

Paragonimiasis is caused by *Paragonimus westermani*, the oriental lung fluke (p. 91). Adult flukes develop in cystic cavities, particularly in the lungs, but also in the brain and other tissues after haematogenous spread. Cerebral paragonimiasis can produce severe disease with visual impairment, fits and motor weakness.

Confirmatory tests. Imaging by brain CT shows the cysts, and sputum microscopy may show the eggs. Eosinophilia is common, as in all fluke infections, and chest x-rays are abnormal.

Chemotherapy. Praziquantel is the drug of choice; bithionol the alternative.

Control depends on education, sanitation and avoiding uncooked crabs and crayfish. The snails and definitive hosts are difficult to control.

Tetanus

Clostridium tetani (p. 41) is a strictly anaerobic Gram-positive rod (with terminal spores) which is not invasive; it multiplies only in the infected wound. It produces a toxin, tetanospasmin, which spreads to the CNS causing severe tetanic (sustained) muscle spasm by blocking inhibitors of neurotransmission. The disease is classified into <u>adult</u> localised or generalised tetanus from soil-contaminated wounds, and <u>neonatal</u> tetanus from soil-contaminated umbilical wounds.

Clinical features. These are almost unmistakable, with progressive muscle stiffness, spasms, then spastic paralysis, giving trismus (lockjaw), sardonic smile (risus sardonicus, Fig. 5), and arching of the back (opisthotonos) in advanced cases. Autonomic involvement gives sweating, salivation, swinging blood pressure and supraventricular or other arrhythmias. Laryngeal or glottal spasm can cause death.

Confirmatory tests. The organism usually cannot be found in the often trivial wound causing this potentially fatal disease.

Management. This is by penicillin, plus antitoxin and supportive measures.

Control and prevention. This is by active immunisation with tetanus toxoid, which gives excellent immunity.

Trypanosomiasis (African)

This is a chronic encephalitis caused by blood and tissue flagellated protozoa (p. 82–83).

Causative organisms. There are two variants of *Trypanosoma brucei*, *T. brucei gambiense* and *T. brucei rhodesiense*, which live and multiply in the human bloodstream and invade the CNS to cause 'sleeping sickness'. Both are spread by tsetse flies, but while the West African (Gambian) form has no known animal reservoir, the East African (Rhodesian) has cattle, sheep and wild animals as reservoir hosts.

Clinical features. These begin with a <u>trypanoma</u> (lump) or ulcer at the site of the tsetse fly bite, followed by acute <u>systemic spread</u> with fever, myalgia, arthralgia and lymphadenopathy. Finally progression to the third, chronic stage of <u>encephalitis</u> occurs with lethargy, tremors, mental impairment, convulsions, paralysis, incontinence and merciful death in 9–18 months.

Confirmatory tests. Microscopy and specific staining (Giemsa) for trypomastigotes in anticoagulated blood, blood films or lymph node aspirates.

Chemotherapy. Suramin is the drug of choice for early *T. brucei* infections, the alternative being pentamidine. Toxic organic arsenicals such as melarsoprol are needed for CNS infection. Eflornithine is a safer but more expensive drug for *T. b. gambiense*.

Control and prevention. This depends on tsetse fly control (particularly around houses), protection from biting, and treatment of infected humans.

Other causes

Numerous **congenital** infections of the unborn fetus can infect the CNS, including the 'Torch' group; **t**oxoplasmosis, **o**thers including HIV and syphilis, **r**ubella, **c**ytomegalovirus and **h**erpes simplex (p. 214–215)

Postinfectious encephalomyelitis is not an infection but an immune response causing demyelination subsequent to a viral or bacterial infection (p. 96–97).

Tropical and rare infections

- Botulism is a flaccid paralysis from a neurotoxin.
- Leprosy causes hypopigmentation, anaesthesia, skin infiltration and nodules.
- Malaria causes fever, headache, confusion, coma and death.
- Paragonimiasis causes multiple cysts, fits and focal signs.
- Tetanus causes spasms, spastic paralysis and death.
- Trypanosomiasis causes 'sleeping sickness' and death.

Otitis, mastoiditis and sinusitis

Otitis externa

Otitis externa (OE) is infection of the external auditory canal. It is **classified** into four types in which the **causative organisms** vary; the commonest are given in parentheses:

- acute localised, often secondary to folliculitis elsewhere (*Staph. aureus*)
- acute diffuse, often secondary to swimming or spa baths (*P. aeruginosa*)
- chronic, usually secondary to chronic otitis media (as chronic OM plus *Candida* spp., rarely TB, syphilis)
- malignant (necrotising) otitis externa, usually secondary to diabetic microangiopathy (*P. aeruginosa*).

Clinical features

- Acute localised OE is usually a painful pustule, often with local lymphadenopathy.
- Acute diffuse OE ('swimmer's ear') is itchy, painful, oedematous and reddened with purulent discharge and sometimes perichondritis.
- Chronic OE is similar with less redness, and if perforated, the ear drum drains. Often there is fungal or other chronic disease elsewhere, particularly in an immunocompromised host.
- Malignant OE is a serious disease. The name easily misleads, for it is not malignant meaning cancerous, but malignant in its progressive, often fatal course. Nor does the condition remain as OE but spreads to surrounding bone, blood vessels, facial nerve and meninges (Fig. 1). Consult with ID physician, ENT surgeon and/or neurosurgeon urgently.

Confirmatory tests

Tests are usually microscopy and culture of the discharge; malignant OE needs full investigation with x-ray, CT scans and MRI, as appropriate, to define the extent and to monitor progress (Fig. 1).

Management

Chemotherapy depends on the diagnosis and organism:

- acute localised: none or flucloxacillin
- acute diffuse: local neomycin or polymyxin
- chronic: local imidazole for fungi; treat OM
- malignant: i.v. tobramycin plus ticarcillin or ceftazidime for weeks or months, often with surgery.

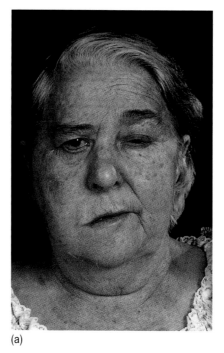

(a)

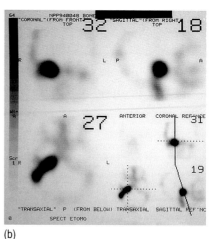

(b)

Fig. 1 **Malignant otitis externa. (a)** Facial (7th) nerve paralysis. **(b)** Bone scan showing 'hot spots' (black) in temporal bone.

Control and prevention

Depends on the predisposing factors: folliculitis, moisture, otitis media, chronic disease elsewhere and diabetes mellitus.

Otitis media

Otitis media (OM) is infection of the middle (media) ear. It is classified into:

- acute suppurative, presenting with pus in the middle ear and often simply called 'otitis media'; it is extremely common in infants and children
- chronic, including both recurrent OM and the very common persisting middle-ear effusion after acute OM, called secretory OM (glue ear) because of the thick consistency of the middle ear fluid.

The two most important **causative organisms** are the usual respiratory pathogens: the pneumococcus S. *pneumoniae* (35%) and *H. influenzae* (20%). *Neisseria* spp., *Moraxella catarrhalis*, *S. aureus*, other streptococci, Gram-negative rods and viruses are less common.

Clinical features

Otitis media not uncommonly follows an upper respiratory infection, presumably spread up the Eustachian tube, and may be accompanied by sinusitis, also by direct spread.

Deep ear pain, headache and fever, then tinnitus and vertigo, are accompanied by a reddened, bulging and immobile ear drum (Fig. 2), hearing loss, then a perforated ear drum and ear discharge if treatment is delayed. Even with apparently adequate treatment, a middle ear effusion often (in 40%) persists for a month or more.

Confirmatory tests

These are unnecessary routinely, but aspiration through the ear drum (tympanocentesis) for microscopy and culture is done if response to treatment is slow.

Management

Chemotherapy is usually either amoxicillin or cefuroxime, with amoxicillin/clavulanate if beta-lactamase-producing *H. influenzae* are common. Tympanostomy tubes (grommets) or adenoidectomy may be needed for 'glue ear' persisting more than 3 months with adequate medical management.

Chemoprophylaxis may be used to prevent recurrent OM in winter and spring, with pneumococcal vaccination.

Mastoiditis

Mastoiditis is infection in the air cells of the mastoid process of the temporal bone. These are connected to the middle ear, so they are extensions of the upper

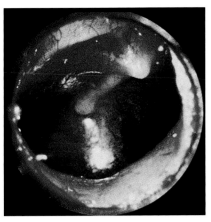

Fig. 2 **Otitis media: red ear drum.**

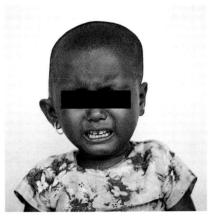

Fig. 3 **Mastoiditis: note displacement of ear.**

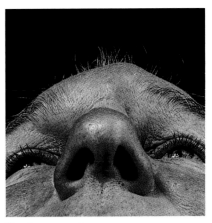

Fig. 4 **Pott's puffy tumour.**

respiratory tract. Therefore mastoiditis is an extension, now rare, of OM. It may be acute or chronic.

Causative organisms
These are as in OM (above).

Clinical features
Clinical features are those of acute OM plus pain, tenderness, redness and then swelling behind the pinna of the ear which is displaced out and down (Fig. 3). Systemic symptoms become more marked. Involvement of nearby vital structures (facial nerve, meninges, venous sinuses) follows if treatment is delayed.

Confirmatory laboratory tests
Tests are x-ray or CT, showing air-cell opacity, then bone destruction.

Chemotherapy
This uses the drugs for OM, or ceftriaxone, given i.v. Drainage by mastoidectomy is needed for unresponsive abscesses.

Control and prevention
This depends on early treatment of OM.

Acute sinusitis

Acute sinusitis is infection in one or more of the paranasal sinuses; maxillary (antral) sinusitis is the most prominent. This, like mastoiditis and OM, is an infection in a bony cavity extending from the upper respiratory tract. The predictable **predisposing factors** are:

- upper respiratory tract infection (URTI), either viral or bacterial
- dental infection, especially upper molar
- nasal deformity, obstruction or infection
- swimming, especially in 'summer sinusitis'
- chronic sinusitis.

The **causative organisms** are similar to those in OM.

Clinical features
Acute sinus pain and tenderness, purulent nasal discharge, nasal obstruction and headache are usual, with fever in 50%. Complete opacity of the sinus on trans-illumination is highly reliable unless chronic sinusitis preceded the acute attack. Acute frontal sinusitis may progress to osteomyelitis and even frontal lobe abscess. Subperiosteal pus causes forehead oedema and swelling called Pott's puffy tumour (Fig. 4) ('tumor' in Latin means swelling, not necessarily malignant).

Confirmatory tests
These include x-rays of the sinuses, with CT if extension to bone, meninges or brain is suspected. Culture of nasal pus may mislead because of normal flora, so antral puncture is needed to isolate the pathogen(s). This is only necessary in severe, unresponsive or recurrent disease.

Management
Chemotherapy is usually either amoxicillin or cefuroxime, with amoxicillin/clavulanate if beta-lactamase-producing *H. influenzae* are common. Nasal decongestants and analgesia alleviate symptoms but not the infection. Frequent recurrent attacks may be prevented by early treatment of URTIs.

Chronic sinusitis

Chronic sinus disease is mainly permanent mucosal damage and poor drainage, with infection a minor component. Causative organisms are similar to those of acute sinusitis except anaerobes are more prominent. Clinical features are minimal; mild pain and chronic nasal discharge are common, with intermittent acute sinusitis. The confirmatory test is an x-ray showing mucosal thickening, and partial or complete sinus opacification. Chemotherapy is given for acute attacks. Surgery may help the chronic state. Control and prevention depends on effective treatment of acute sinusitis.

Otitis, mastoiditis and sinusitis

- Otitis externa can be localised (folliculitis), diffuse (secondary to swimming or other moisture), chronic (fungal, or secondary to chronic otitis media), or so-called malignant (with extension to bone, venous sinuses, facial nerve or meninges). Malignant OE is a severe and often fatal disease requiring urgent treatment.

- Otitis media or acute sinusitis often follow an upper respiratory infection, and the pneumococcus and *H. influenzae* are the commonest causative organisms. Amoxicillin or cefuroxime are, therefore, the usual chemotherapy providing *H. influenzae* is sensitive.

- Persistent effusion (glue ear) may need tympanostomy tubes (grommets) inserted. Chronic sinusitis may need surgery.

- Mastoiditis is a complication of untreated otitis media and can progress to facial nerve paralysis, meningitis and intracranial thrombophlebitis if unrecognised. Treatment is i.v. antibiotics, and drainage if needed.

Superficial ocular infections

Blepharitis

Blepharitis is inflammation of the eyelid and has two forms:

■ *Preseptal (periorbital) cellulitis* is acute, uncommon, and unilateral involving the whole lid anterior to the orbital septum, hence not extending into the orbit. It is usually post-traumatic in adults, or from bacteraemia in children.

Causative organisms. Infection is commonly with *Staph. aureus* or *Strep. pyogenes* in adults, or *H. influenzae* in children under 5 years. Anaerobes infect after human or animal bites.

Clinical features. There is acute purplish swelling, in children after a respiratory infection or in adults after local infection or trauma. Full, painless ocular mobility distinguishes it from *orbital* cellulitis (see below).

Confirmatory tests. Infection is confirmed by local and blood cultures.

Chemotherapy. Children need a third-generation cephalosporin such as ceftriaxone while adults need flucloxacillin.

Control and prevention. This depends on control of local infection or bacteraemia.

■ Chronic, bilateral, marginal blepharitis associated with seborrhoea or rosacea, or ulceration often with coagulase-negative staphylococci. There is chronic itching and scaling. Concomitant skin or scalp seborrhoea is treated with shampoos or ketoconazole cream, while oral doxycycline helps rosacea. Tetracycline or chloramphenicol ointment locally may assist.

Stye and chalazion

A stye (hordeolum) is an acute infection of eyelash follicle glands. A chalazion is an infection of the Meibomian glands deeper in the lid stroma. Causative organisms are *Staph. aureus* and skin flora. Clinical features are pain and swelling, with visible pus in a stye. Confirmatory tests (Gram stain and culture) are seldom necessary. Chemotherapy is initially local, with lash removal for styes, while chalazions may need incisional drainage.

Conjunctivitis

Conjunctivitis is inflammation of the conjunctiva and can be bacterial, viral, or chlamydial in origin, or non-infective.

Causative organisms. *S. aureus*, *S. pneumoniae*, *S. pyogenes*, *Haemophilus* spp., *C. trachomatis* (inclusion conjunctivitis and trachoma, p. 111) and adeno- and enteroviruses are common in adults and children, plus *N. gonorrhoea* in neonates. Ophthalmia neonatorum (p. 215) was once only gonococcal but now is more often chlamydial.

Clinical features. These vary with the cause: discharge is usual, ranging from mild and thin in viral infections, through moderate in most bacterial infections to profuse in gonorrhoeal and chlamydial infections. Pain is not prominent. Follicles are most prominent in trachoma which progress to lid-scarring, plus corneal involvement (p. 111).

Confirmatory tests. Infection is confirmed by Gram stain, chlamydial PCR, and bacterial culture. Viral PCR has replaced culture.

Chemotherapy. This depends on the cause. Trachoma needs oral sulphonamide or tetracycline, gonorrhoea needs i.v. penicillin or ceftriaxone and local saline, while the other bacteria need local bacitracin, neomycin or gentamicin.

Control and prevention. This is only feasible in gonorrhoea and trachoma, depending on treatment of infected mothers, and hygiene.

Keratitis and corneal ulcers

Keratitis is inflammation of the cornea, usually caused by bacterial or viral infection, less commonly by fungal or parasitic infection (Fig. 1). Any can progress to corneal ulceration and so to corneal perforation, aqueous humour loss, and potential permanent blindness.

Causative organisms. Over 60 bacteria, viruses, chlamydia, fungi and parasites have been described as causes of keratitis, but the most important are *S. aureus*, pneumococci and beta-haemolytic streptococci, *Bacillus* spp., and herpes simplex virus. *Pseudomonas* spp., other Gram-negative rods and *Acanthamoeba* spp. are important in infections associated with soft contact lenses. *Staph. aureus* can cause corneal abscesses, e.g. after corneal grafting.

Clinical features. Severe pain, marked conjunctival injection at the limbus, i.e. adjacent to the cornea, grey-white haze or ulceration and blurred vision from central ulcers are characteristic. Pus in the anterior chamber is called hypopyon (Fig. 2). It is important to involve an ophthalmologist.

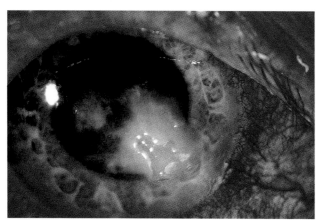

Fig. 1 **Fungal keratitis.**

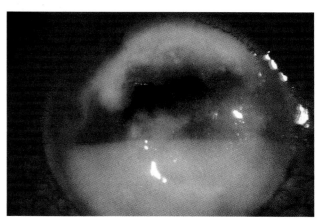

Fig. 2 **Corneal ulcer with hypopyon.**

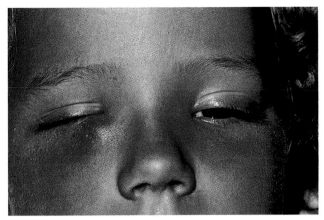

Fig. 3 **Dacryocystitis.**

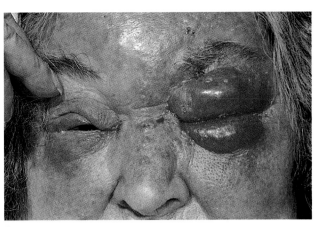

Fig. 4 **Orbital cellulitis with swelling and proptosis.**

Confirmatory tests. Infection is confirmed by microscopy, with special stains if necessary, and culture of corneal swabs or scrapings. Corneal staining with fluorescein can show the distinctive dendritic ulcer of herpes simplex. Corneal biopsy may be necessary for difficult pathogens.

Chemotherapy. This depends on the pathogen. Initially, broad-spectrum local antibiotics such as vancomycin and tobramycin are given for bacterial keratitis, aciclovir for viral, amphotericin B or flucytosine for fungal, and propamidine drops plus oral ketoconazole for amoebic infections.

Control and prevention. Early attention to minor corneal trauma, and scrupulous sterile care with contact lenses and their solutions, are important.

Dacryocystitis, canaliculitis and dacryoadenitis

Dacryocystitis is inflammation of the lacrimal sac (cyst) just below the inner end of the lower eyelid (Fig. 3); canaliculitis is inflammation of the 'little canals' leading from the lacrimal puncta of the inner end of the lids to the lacrimal sac; and dacryoadenitis is inflammation of the main lacrimal gland, anteriorly in the upper-outer part of the orbit.

Causative organisms. Acute dacryocystitis and dacryoadenitis are caused by pneumococci, other streptococci, staphylococci, and *P. aeruginosa*. Long or branching organisms, i.e. *Actinomyces, Aspergillus, Candida* or *Fusobacteria*, cause canaliculitis. Obstruction, whether congenital or from trauma, tumour or dacryoliths (tear stones), predisposes to infection.

Clinical features. Epiphora (overflow of tears) and pain, swelling and redness are characteristic in acute cases.

Confirmatory tests. Gram stain and culture of expressed pus should confirm infection.

Management. Treatment involves local antibiotic eye drops, systemic flucloxacillin in acute cases, local warmth, and consultation with an ophthalmologist concerning probing or incision.

Orbital infections

These are infections in the orbit behind the orbital septum (contrast with *preseptal* cellulitis above). Analogous to brain abscesses, they have one of three sources as predisposing factors:

- adjacent infection, usually ethmoidal (in children) or frontal (in adults) sinusitis in 75%; less commonly from nearby infection such as facial cellulitis, otitis or dental infection
- distant infection with septicaemic spread (rare)
- eye surgery or local penetrating trauma.

Causative organisms. The usual causes have been *S. pneumoniae, S. pyogenes* or *H. influenzae* (now rare). *S. aureus* is common after trauma, anaerobes with necrosis and foul smell are common in chronic infections, while Gram-negative rods and fungi are rare.

Clinical features. These cumulate through five stages:

1. Orbital oedema causes painless swelling of the lids.
2. Orbital cellulitis causes fever, pain, tenderness, redness and painful limited eye movement, with some proptosis (Fig. 4); call an ophthalmologist and infectious diseases physician.
3. Subperiosteal abscess with pus between the periosteum and bone causes displacement of the globe of the eye.

4. Orbital abscess causes ophthalmoplegia (paralysis of ocular movement) and some visual loss.
5. Cavernous sinus thrombosis is potentially fatal and causes severe headache and eye pain, further visual and retinal changes, paresis of 3rd, 4th and 6th cranial nerves, meningitis with neck stiffness, plus high fever, chills and systemic toxicity.

Confirmatory tests. Conjunctival, blood and sinus aspirate stains and cultures are essential. Orbital, sinus and brain CT have replaced x-rays. Meningeal signs make lumbar puncture essential.

Management. This depends on the *source* and the *stage*: initially high-dose i.v. flucloxacillin and ceftriaxone are usual, modified after culture results. Abscesses need drainage, and sinusitis may need specific drainage.

Control and prevention. This depends on early treatment of possible sources.

> ## Superficial ocular infections
>
> - Blepharitis is usually a mild infection needing local treatment only.
> - Styes usually need local ointment and lash removal only, while chalazions often need incision and drainage.
> - Common bacterial conjunctivitis needs only local antibiotics, while trachoma or gonorrhoea need oral or i.v. treatment, respectively.
> - Keratitis, corneal ulcer and corneal abscess are serious, have numerous causes and need specialist advice and treatment.
> - Infections of the lacrimal apparatus need local antibiotics, systemic flucloxacillin, and specialist consultation concerning drainage.
> - Orbital infections are usually **s**econdary to **s**inusitis, are **s**erious and **s**preading, and need **s**pecialist advice and **s**ystemic antibiotics.

Tropical ocular infections

Infections in the tropics affect the eye in one of four ways:

- **Severe prostrating infections**, often accompanied by malnutrition and inadequate medical care, result in exposure keratitis and conjunctivitis, corneal ulcers, iritis and even endophthalmitis, loss of eyesight or the eye. This sequence occurs with infections such as malaria, amoebic or bacillary dysentery, cholera or typhus, and viral infections including measles and smallpox.
- **Wandering worms, larvae or parasites** invade the eye, e.g. *A. cantonensis* (p. 99), dracunculiasis (p. 204–205) or filariasis (p. 205) and many rarer parasites.
- **Systemic diseases infect the eye**, e.g. brucellosis (p. 212), the systemic mycoses (p. 70–73), leishmaniasis (p. 152, 205), plus leprosy, toxocariasis, toxoplasmosis, trypanosomiasis, tularaemia and yaws (see below).
- **Specific infections of the eye**, e.g. loiasis, onchocerciasis and trachoma (see below).

Systemic diseases

Leprosy

Leprosy (p. 60, 104) affects the eye either indirectly through facial nerve paresis causing lagophthalmos (incomplete eyelid closure) or directly by invasion and infection, causing madarosis (loss of eyebrows and eyelashes), superficial punctate keratitis or deeper opaque stromal keratitis, episcleritis with limbal nodules, or iritis with 1 mm 'pearls' (Fig. 1). Posterior chamber involvement is rare unless corneal perforation from keratitis leads to endophthalmitis. Confirmatory tests involve microscopy of skin and nasal tissue. Treatment is local for the specific tissue(s) damaged, plus systemic anti-leprotics (dapsone plus rifampicin). Surgery may be needed.

Toxocariasis

Visceral larva migrans is due to infection with *Toxocara canis* or *T. cati*, the dog and cat round worms (p. 87). Ingestion of ascarid eggs, usually by children, causes pneumonitis, hepatitis and retinitis, rarely irido-cyclitis. Clinical diagnosis is confirmed serologically, and treatment is by mebendazole or diethylcarbamazine. Control depends on keeping children away from infected puppies and kittens, and on treating pets.

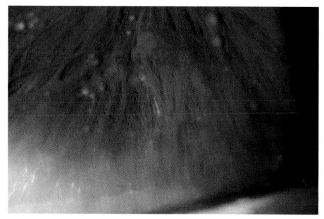

Fig. 1   **Leprosy: iritis pearls.**

Toxoplasmosis

Toxoplasma gondii infection (toxoplasmosis) (p. 78, 213) can affect the eye, causing chorio-retinitis (Fig. 2) or, rarely, irido-cyclitis. Infection can be congenital or acquired (serious in immunosuppression) and is confirmed by serology. Treatment is with sulphadiazine and pyrimethamine. Control depends on good hygiene with cats and meat.

Trypanosomiasis

Unilateral oedema of the eyelids, Romana's sign, is diagnostic in Chagas' disease (p. 138), caused by *T. cruzi*. Eyelid oedema, keratitis and irido-cyclitis occur with the African forms, caused by *T. brucei*, and cranial nerve pareses and papilloedema occur late from the encephalitis (p. 105). Infection is confirmed with serology and treated with benznidazole (*T. cruzi*) or suramin/melarsoprol (*T. brucei*).

Tularaemia

Oculoglandular tularaemia (*Francisella tularensis*, p. 57) is one cause of conjunctivitis, with preauricular and parotid gland swelling (Parinaud's syndrome). Serology confirms the diagnosis, and treatment is with streptomycin or gentamicin.

Yaws

The secondary stage (p. 203) of infection with *Treponema pertenue* (p. 58) may involve the eyebrows and lids. **Gangosa** is

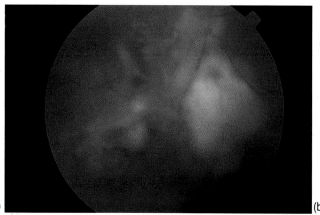
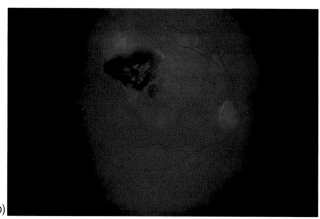

(a)   (b)

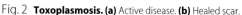

Fig. 2   **Toxoplasmosis. (a)** Active disease. **(b)** Healed scar.

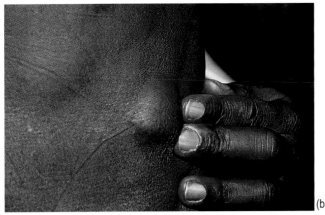

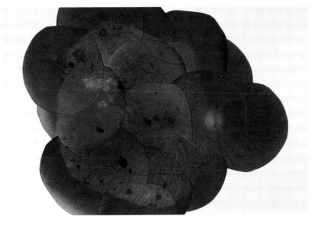

Fig. 3 **Onchocerciasis. (a)** Skin nodule. **(b)** Extensive chorioretinitis.

a dreadful destructive rhino-pharyngitis which can spread to the eyelids and cause exposure keratitis. Treatment is with penicillin.

Specific infections of the eye

Loiasis

Loiasis is a chronic filarial disease in West and Central Africa that particularly affects the eyelids. *Loa loa,* a filarial nematode, is the causative organism (p. 86). Infection is spread between humans by the bite of *Chrysops* spp. flies.

Initially, palpable worms migrate through the subcutaneous tissues including the eyelids and conjunctivae. Subsequently, transient oedematous 'Calabar swellings' appear at various sites, including the eyelids, as a result of allergic reactions to filarial toxins. Confirmatory tests are microfilaria in the blood by day, eosinophilia and serology.

Chemotherapy is ivermectin or diethylcarbamazine. Surgical removal of the worms may be necessary. Control and prevention is by protection from flies, and diethylcarbamazine for 3 days monthly or ivermectin 3-monthly.

Onchocerciasis

Onchocerciasis is a chronic filarial disease in West and Central Africa, and Central and South America which particularly affects the skin and anterior chamber of the eye. The causative organism is *Onchocerca volvulus,* a filarial nematode (p. 86). Infection is spread between humans by the bite of *Simulium* spp. black flies.

Clinical features include skin nodules with depigmentation and atrophy (Fig. 3a), lymphadenopathy and lymphoedema;

eventually, blindness from iritis and secondary glaucoma occur. Conjunctivitis, keratitis and chorioretinitis (Fig. 3b) also occur. Confirmatory laboratory tests are microfilaria in skin or conjunctival snips. Eosinophilia is common.

Chemotherapy is with ivermectin (less often with diethylcarbamazine or suramin). Control and prevention is by fly control, and possibly mass chemoprophylaxis.

Trachoma and other chlamydial infection

Chlamydiae (p. 64) have surface molecules (ligands) that can bind to receptors on conjunctival cells, enabling them to avoid host defences, and resulting in trachoma being the world's most important eye infection. Transmission is eye to eye, directly by droplets or through flies. There are at least 15 different serotypes of chlamydia:

- Serotypes A, B and C cause trachoma, a chronic kerato-conjunctivitis
- D–K cause inclusion conjunctivitis in neonates and adults from genital infections (p. 215)
- L1, L2 and L3 (p. 189) cause ocular lymphogranuloma venereum with keratitis, uveitis and optic neuritis.

Clinical features of trachoma are classified in four stages:

1. TF: trachomatous folliculitis (Fig. 4)
2. TS: trachoma scarring
3. CO: conjunctiva scarred; pannus (blood vessels) over cornea gives corneal opacity
4. TT: trichiasis with ingrowing eyelashes and corneal ulceration.

Confirmatory tests are direct antigen detection, PCR or culture.

Chemotherapy is with azithromycin, alternatively tetracycline, erythromycin or sulphas. Scarring may need surgery. Control and prevention need education and improved living and hygienic standards.

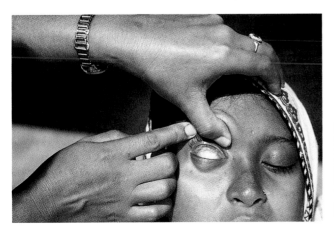

Fig. 4 **Trachoma: everting the upper eyelid to examine the tarsal conjunctiva.**

> *Tropical ocular infections*
>
> - Exposure keratitis can occur in any severe systemic infection, e.g. dysentery, typhoid, typhus.
> - Worm infections can invade the eye accidentally in their migrations, e.g. dracunculiasis and filariasis.
> - Systemic infections, e.g. leprosy and toxocariasis, can cause severe eye disease.
> - Specific infections include loiasis, onchocerciasis and trachoma.
> - All need precise diagnosis and specialist treatment.

Deep eye infections

Deep eye infections are all serious and are caused by a wide range of pathogens so specialist diagnosis and treatment are essential to avoid blindness.

Anterior uveitis (iridocyclitis)

The iris and ciliary body (anterior segment of uveal tract) share the same blood supply, so are commonly inflamed together in a syndrome called iridocyclitis. Many causes are not proven infections (e.g. rheumatoid arthritis).

Causative organisms. These are unusual organisms: *Brucella* spp., chlamydiae and other causes of Reiter's syndrome (p. 180), mycobacteria (*M. leprae*), a Rickettsia (Rocky Mountain spotted fever), spirochaetes (syphilis, Lyme disease and leptospirosis) and viruses (HSV, CMV, VZV).

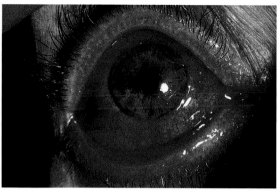

Fig. 1 **Iridocyclitis.**

Clinical features. These are predominantly **p**hotophobia, **p**ain (deep, ocular), **p**upillary constriction, **p**rofuse tears and a **p**lum-red eye with **p**rofound limbal injection (Fig. 1). Call an ophthalmologist.

Confirmatory tests. Slit lamp shows typical keratic precipitates (KPs) and adhesions (synechiae). Serology, special culture and, at times, anterior chamber aspiration for microscopy and special (e.g. viral) tests like PCR are used depending on the suspected pathogen.

Management. This is dictated by the cause of disease. Do not delay.

Chorioretinitis (posterior uveitis)

Inflammation of the choroid usually spreads to the retina, forming chorioretinitis. This is usually chronic and granulomatous, and may be non-infective, e.g. sarcoidosis.

Causative organisms. As with granulomatous disease elsewhere, the usual causes are *Candida* spp., *Cryptococcus neoformans*, *Histoplasma capsulatum*, *M. tuberculosis* or *M. leprae*, *Toxoplasma gondii*, *Toxocara* spp., *T. pallidum*, or viruses (CMV, Fig. 5, p. 151), usually with systemic infection and/or immunoparesis.

Clinical features. Gradual visual loss with lack of pain are the main features. The damaged retina is seen on fundoscopy (Fig. 2).

Confirmatory tests. These depend on the causative systemic disease and are usually serology, antigen detection for cryptococcosis, PCR, special cultures and chest x-ray.

Management. This is dictated by the cause. Do not delay: specialist care is essential.

Endophthalmitis

Endophthalmitis is a feared infection of the intra-ocular contents causing loss of vision or loss of the eye. Unlike the other two deep infections above, it is commonly bacterial, leading to abscess formation after surgery, trauma, corneal ulceration or bacteraemic spread (compare with the sources of cerebral and parameningeal abscesses, p. 102).

Causative organisms. Over 60 causative organisms have been described. Bacteria include staphylococci, streptococci, *Bacillus cereus*, Gram-negative rods and anaerobes. Fungi are involved par-

ticularly in the immunocompromised; genera include *Candida*, *Aspergillus*, *Cryptococcus* and the class *Zygomycetes*. The parasites *O. volvulus*, *T. gondii*, *T. solium* and *Toxocara* spp. can also infect the vitreous body.

Clinical features. Ocular pain and visual loss, with photophobia, headache, fever and systemic illness are characteristic. Signs are swelling of the lids and conjunctivae (chemosis), limited eye movement, pus in the anterior chamber (hypopyon), iritis from local spread, and vitreal opacities (Fig. 3).

Confirmatory tests. These are essential because of the wide range of virulent pathogens. Microscopy and culture of anterior and posterior chamber fluid and any wound is urgent, as is specialist care.

Chemotherapy. Treatment is initially empiric, both intravitreal and systemic, and often subconjunctival or topical also. Initial antibacterial therapy usually includes vancomycin plus gentamicin or ciprofloxacin, while antifungal therapy is usually amphotericin B and flucytosine. Vitrectomy is needed in severe cases, and steroids diminish the destructive immune response when infection is controlled.

Control and prevention. This depends on operative technique, and rapid effective treatment of penetrating wounds, bacteraemia or fungaemia.

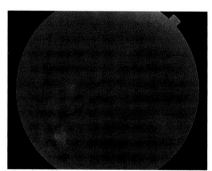

Fig. 2 **Chorioretinitis.**

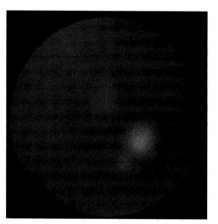

Fig. 3 **Endophthalmitis.**

> ### Deep eye infections
>
> - Deep eye infections are serious, requiring specialist care to save sight.
> - Laboratory identification is important because of the wide range of potential pathogens.
> - Areas infected are the iris and ciliary body, the choroid and retina, and the vitreous body.

Stomatitis

Stomatitis is infection of the oral cavity (mouth), and is usually acute. The normal flora of the mouth can become pathogenic if local or general body defenses are impaired.

- Infections of the teeth are described on page 114.
- Oral manifestations of systemic disease are described in the relevant sections.

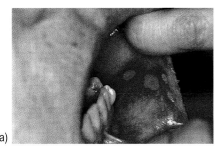

(a)

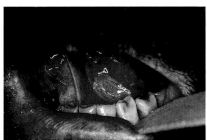

(b)

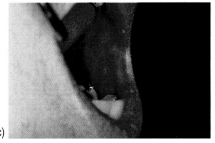

(c)

Fig. 1 **Aphthous ulcers. (a)** Minor. **(b)** Major. **(c)** Herpetiform ulcers.

Aphthous stomatitis

Aphthous stomatitis is characterised by painful recurrent ulcers of the oral mucosa.

Causative organisms. These are not known. Immune mechanisms and local trauma may be involved, as may viruses.

Clinical features. The ulcers are classified in three types (Fig. 1):

- Minor ulcers: small in size (3–5mm), very painful and often anterior and multiple. The ulcers have a yellow-grey base and a bright red edge; they heal in 4–14 days.
- Major ulcers: larger, occur throughout the mouth and are more chronic, taking 4–8 weeks to heal, then relapsing months later.
- Herpetiform ('shaped like a serpent' and *not* caused by Herpesvirus) ulcers: pinhead in size and multiple, appearing in crops.

Confirmatory tests. These are not available, but the clinical appearance is diagnostic (Fig. 1).

Chemotherapy. This is of no use. Local measures and dental attention are indicated. Local steroids are a last resort.

Stomatitis in the immunocompromised

Immunocompromised patients are prone to stomatitis if their oral flora is disturbed (e.g. by broad-spectrum antibiotics), their oral mucosa damaged (e.g. by anti-cancer drugs causing 'mucositis'), or their other lines of defence impaired (e.g. by neutropenia). The stomatitis is classified as fungal, viral or bacterial, though in 'neutropenic stomatitis' only normal flora may be cultured.

Causative organisms. The commonest fungi are *Candida* spp., followed by *Aspergillus* spp. and the feared *Zygomycetes*; the commonest bacteria are anaerobes and mixed Gram-negative rods, while Herpes simplex, CMV and VZV are the commonest viruses.

Clinical features. These are variable and may suggest the causative organism:

- candidiasis ('thrush') shows white patches like a thrush's breast (Fig. 2)
- aspergillosis or zygomycosis cause progressive ulceration and necrosis
- anaerobic infection causes foul odour and tissue destruction.

Confirmatory tests. Microscopy and culture of mouth swabs may confirm infection, but oral flora often make interpretation difficult; biopsy is therefore necessary in progressive infection.

Chemotherapy. This depends on the pathogen and the duration of the predisposing factor(s), e.g. local nystatin or clotrimazole is sufficient for candidiasis if broad-spectrum antibiotics are stopped, while oral fluconazole is needed if neutropenia persists.

Control and prevention. This depends on avoidance or removal of the predisposing factor(s).

Gangrenous stomatitis (noma, cancrum oris)

Gangrenous stomatitis is an uncommon, rapidly destructive infection caused by mixed anaerobes and spirochaetes, and occurs particularly in debilitated children. It begins on the gums and spreads outwards, destroying lips and cheeks, and exposing bone and teeth. Immediate i.v. penicillin is essential. Reparative surgery is usually needed.

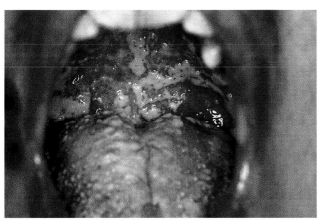

Fig. 2 **Candidal stomatitis.**

Stomatitis

- Aphthous ulcers are painful, recurrent and of uncertain cause.
- Fungal, bacterial and viral infections occur when oral flora is altered, oral mucosa damaged or general defence mechanisms are impaired.
- Gangrenous stomatitis is an uncommon, rapidly destructive disease needing urgent penicillin therapy and specialist care.

Dental and periodontal infections

Tooth and gum structure is shown in Fig. 1. The periodontal structures – ligament and gingiva – support the teeth by attachment to the jaw bones.

Dental, periodontal and related infections (Fig. 1) are classified into:

- **dento-alveolar infections** of the teeth and adjacent alveolar bone
- **periodontal disease**
- **deep fascial space infections**
- **other local spread**
- **metastatic spread by bacteraemia.**

Densely packed bacteria called **bacterial plaque** cause the three major infections of teeth and periodontal tissue: supragingival plaque causes dental caries, and subgingival plaque causes gingivitis and periodontitis. Hyper-responsiveness of some immune mechanisms, and deficiency of others, also contribute to periodontal infections.

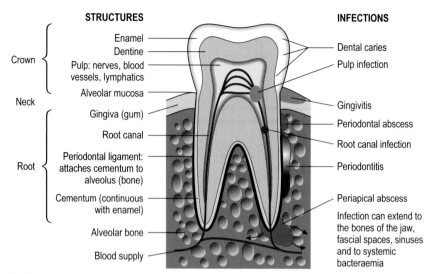

STRUCTURES

INFECTIONS

Crown {
- Enamel
- Dentine
- Pulp: nerves, blood vessels, lymphatics
- Alveolar mucosa

Neck

Root {
- Gingiva (gum)
- Root canal
- Periodontal ligament: attaches cementum to alveolus (bone)
- Cementum (continuous with enamel)
- Alveolar bone
- Blood supply

- Dental caries
- Pulp infection
- Gingivitis
- Periodontal abscess
- Root canal infection
- Periodontitis
- Periapical abscess
- Infection can extend to the bones of the jaw, fascial spaces, sinuses and to systemic bacteraemia

Fig. 1 **Dental and periodontal structures and infections.**

Dento-alveolar infections

Infections of the teeth and adjacent alveolar bone progress from dental caries ('tooth decay'), through pulp infection to periapical abscess and acute alveolar abscess.

Causative organisms
If teeth are not brushed for 1–3 days, many oral bacteria, particularly *Streptococcus mutans*, form dense plaque attached to the thin glycoprotein layer of pellicle on the tooth enamel, especially on the crown and at the gingival margin. Such plaque is removed by brushing, but completely mineralised plaque called dental calculus is not. In unmineralised dental plaque, bacterial metabolism of sucrose, glucose and fructose produces glucans and fructans, which are anaerobically converted to organic acids. The consequent low pH leads to enamel demineralisation and hence to dental caries.

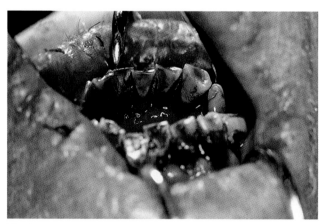

Fig. 2 **Dental caries: extensive decay.**

Clinical features
Caries (Fig. 2) converts hard enamel to soft leathery tissue. Extension to the dentine and pulp causes toothache and temperature sensitivity, while further extension to a periapical abscess (Fig. 3) usually causes severe throbbing pain, often fever, and even swelling and a discharging sinus (Fig. 4). X-rays show the extent of tooth and bone destruction.

Management
Chemotherapy is unhelpful for uncomplicated dental caries, which needs mechanical removal and repair by a dentist; endodontic infection (in the root canal) needs specialised endodontic treatment. Periapical and bone infection need drainage and chemotherapy such as penicillin.

Control and prevention of caries depends on oral or local fluoride, and regular brushing.

Periodontal infections

Infection of the periodontal structures is classified into four types:

Gingivitis. This is a reversible infection of the soft gingival tissues, with no bony infection. All gingivitis is primarily caused by plaque (Fig. 5) but additional secondary factors including anaerobic and spiral bacteria [in 'trench mouth', Vincent's acute necrotising ulcerative gingivitis (ANUG)], hormones, drugs such as phenytoin or ciclosporin, and malnutrition worsen plaque effects.

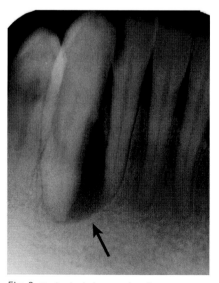

Fig. 3 **Periapical abscess showing rarefaction (dark grey).**

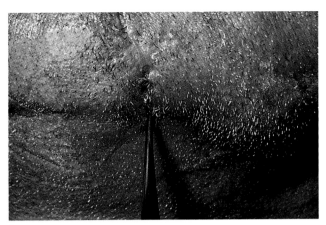

Fig. 4 **Jaw sinus from dental abscess.**

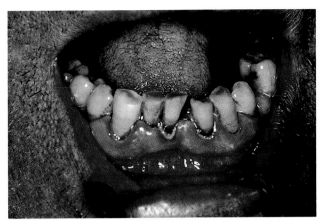

Fig. 5 **Gingivitis with calculus from poor hygiene.**

Periodontitis. This is irreversible infection of hard tissues, i.e. periodontal ligament, cementum and alveolar bone. It is classified into adult (the most common), rapidly progressive, juvenile and prepubertal types.

Periodontal abscess. This complicates periodontitis when infection is trapped between tooth and gum.

Pericoronitis. This is an acute local infection beneath gum flaps covering the crown ('corona') of a partially erupted molar.

Causative organisms

- In gingivitis, as bacterial plaque extends into the pocket between tooth and gingiva, the predominant streptococci and *Actinomyces* spp. are partly replaced by *Bacteroides intermedius* and other anaerobic Gram-negative rods.
- In ANUG there is infection with mixed fusiform anaerobes and spirochaetes (Fig. 6).
- In adult periodontitis, with deeper extension, anaerobes, particularly *B. gingivalis*, predominate.
- In juvenile periodontitis, *B. gingivalis* is replaced by *Haemophilus actinomycetemcomitans* and *Capnocytophaga* spp.
- In periapical and alveolar abscesses, there is usually a mixture of anaerobic oral flora (*Actinomyces, Bacteroides, Fusobacteria* and *Peptostreptococci* spp.) and aerobic streptococci. Enteric Gram-negative rods and staphylococci are uncommon.
- In pericoronitis, there is (again) mixed oral flora.

Clinical features

Gingivitis causes tender, swollen, bleeding, usually painless, gums. In ANUG, there is also foul mouth odour, acute pain and a purulent exudate but no bony resorption. Periodontitis shows progressive gum recession with exposed teeth roots and bony resorption. Abscesses as usual cause throbbing pain, swelling and fever.

X-rays show the extent of bone destruction.

Management

Dental hygiene by regular brushing and flossing minimises plaque formation.

Antibiotics such as penicillin and metronidazole are only useful chemotherapy in gingivitis (particularly ANUG) and abscesses. Local debridement with chlorhexidine gluconate mouthwash, and removal of plaque, calculus and secondary factors such as drugs and malnutrition, are essential.

Other infections

Other infections by spread from tooth, gum or abscess are:

- **Deep fascial space infections.** Direct spread of disease can occur between the deep fascia (p. 119).
- **Other local spread.** Although rare, this can occur to give:
  - sinusitis (p. 107)
  - osteomyelitis (p. 206)
  - cavernous sinus thrombosis (p. 109)
  - suppurative jugular thrombophlebitis (p. 119)
  - carotid artery erosion (p. 119)
  - mediastinitis (p. 119).
- **Metastatic spread by bacteraemia.** Metastatic spread is rare but can cause distant abscesses, infective endocarditis (p. 140) or infected joint prostheses (p. 208).

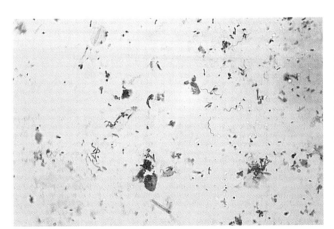

Fig. 6 **Vincent's infection (ANUG): Gram stain of mouth swab.**

> *Dental and periodontal infections*
>
> - Bacterial plaque builds up on teeth that are not cleaned; bacterial action produces acid, which attacks tooth minerals. Calculus is mineralised plaque.
> - Dental caries is caused by supragingival bacterial plaque, while subgingival plaque causes gingivitis and periodontitis.
> - All may be complicated by bacterial abscesses, and by spread to adjacent fascial spaces, to adjacent tissues and, rarely, to distant tissues.
> - Chemotherapy is only useful for specific infections like ANUG, for abscesses, for bacterial infections in adjacent fascial spaces and tissues, and for bacteraemic spread.
> - Control depends on prevention by oral hygiene, including regular brushing and flossing.

Viral respiratory infections

The major respiratory viruses are influenza and parainfluenza, rhino-, RSV, corona- and adenoviruses. They cause two types of respiratory infection – regional infections like pharyngitis, bronchitis or pneumonia (CMV pneumonia, Fig. 1) with bacterial and other causes (p. 118, 123–129), or specific viral infections described in these two pages. The first four specific viral infections are very common, the last three rare at present in humans.

Bronchiolitis

Classification. Bronchiolitis is a lower respiratory tract infection of the bronchioles characterised by wheeze and hyperinflation in children.

Causative organism is the Respiratory Syncytial Virus (RSV) in about 60%, parainfluenzaviruses in over 20%, and adenoviruses (Fig. 2), rhino- or influenzaviruses, or *Mycoplasma pneumoniae* in the remainder. Metapneumovirus is now known to be a common infection, causing bronchiolitis and pneumonia in young children. It is a paramyxovirus like RSV. Though discovered in 2001, serology proves its widespread presence for over 50 years.

Clinical features are acute wheeze, chest wall retraction and hyperinflation in children under 2, usually with fever, rhinorrhoea, cough, tachypnoea and respiratory distress, and some systemic symptoms.

Confirmatory tests. Chest x-ray characteristically shows hyperinflation, at times with pneumonia. PCR and other rapid tests for RSV are replacing culture, which, however, detects other pathogens. Other tests are often unnecessary because of the distinctive clinical picture.

Chemotherapy with ribavirin is seldom given. Oxygen is essential, with ventilation if needed. Steroids and bronchodilators are still unproven, and antibacterials are useless.

Complications are unusual, except for recurrent wheeze or asthma. Bronchiolitis obliterans is rare but devastating, with recurrent bronchiolitis, pneumonia and bronchiectasis.

Control and prevention is not possible. A killed vaccine made disease worse, and no safe vaccine is yet available.

Common cold

Classification. This is not one disease but a syndrome caused by at least five viral families.

Causative organisms are rhinoviruses (40%), coronaviruses (Fig. 3), influenza, parainfluenza viruses and RSV (about 10% each), and other viruses (20%). Incubation period is 1–2 days.

Clinical features are universally known – nasal discharge and obstruction, sneezing, sore throat and cough. Fever is minimal except in children. A red, dripping nose is usual. A 'geographic tongue' (Fig. 4) is relatively common though the mechanism is unexplained.

Confirmatory tests are usually unnecessary unless sinusitis or otitis media develops.

Chemotherapy is useless. First-generation antihistamines plus an NSAID give statistically significant symptom relief.

Control and prevention depends on avoiding sufferers. No vaccine is available.

Croup (laryngo-tracheo-bronchitis, LTB)

Classification. This common illness is laryngo-tracheo-bronchitis in children,

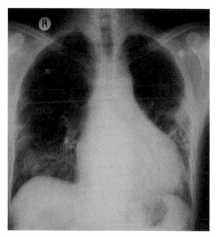

Fig. 1 **CMV pneumonia, with bilateral streaky opacities on chest x-ray.**

usually viral, with sub-glottic infection, dyspnoea and inspiratory stridor.

Causative organisms in children under 5 are parainfluenza viruses (30–40%), influenza viruses, measles, RSV, adeno-, rhino- and enteroviruses (5–10% each), with *Mycoplasma pneumoniae* in older children.

Clinical features. There is often a 2-day prodrome of rhinorrhoea, sore throat and cough. Then "his voice is … harsh and pulling … he awakens with a most unusual cough, rough and stridulous. And now his breathing is laborious, each inspiration being accompanied by a harsh, shrill noise" (Cheyne, 1814). "The sharp stridulous voice (resembling) the crowing of a cock is the true diagnostic sign" (Home, 1765). Tachypnoea is less than with bronchiolitis. Croup fluctuates in severity for 3–4 days. Recurrent attacks called 'spasmodic croup' are not uncommon.

Confirmatory tests are seldom essential unless bacterial epiglottitis is a possible diagnosis. Rapid PCR or immunofluorescence tests are now widely available.

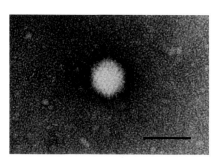

Fig. 2 **An adenovirus, cause of various respiratory infections.** Bar represents 100nm.

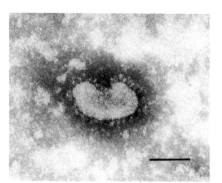

Fig. 3 **A coronavirus, cause of various respiratory infections including SARS.** Bar represents 100nm.

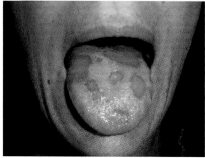

Fig. 4 **Geographic tongue in viral upper respiratory infection.**

Chemotherapy is useless. Oxygenation guided by oximetry is important, and warm humidified air is traditional, though cold night air often gives improvement! Adrenaline is proven to help, as are corticosteroids. Occasionally intubation is needed.

Control and prevention is not feasible, as only measles and influenza vaccines are available.

Influenza (human and avian)

Classification. Influenza is a viral infection of the respiratory tract from the nose to the bronchi, extending to the lungs if complicated by viral or bacterial pneumonia. It occurs in winter epidemics every 1–3 years, and in worldwide pandemics every 20–30 years.

Causative organisms are:

- influenza A (an orthomyxovirus, Fig. 5) in most years, most epidemics and all pandemics
- influenza B in milder epidemics about every 5 years
- influenza C in mild sporadic cases.

Influenza A also infects pigs, birds, horses and even marine mammals.

Clinical features are in three stages:

- Sudden systemic symptoms with abrupt fever, chills, malaise and anorexia. Headache and myalgia are usually severe, with prostration in some
- Respiratory symptoms predominate, with rhinorrhoea, sore throat, a dry cough and often hoarseness
- Convalescence lasts for 10–20 days with cough and lassitude persisting.

Confirmatory tests are unnecessary for most patients, but rapid tests include PCR, DFA, antigen detection with monoclonal antibody, and neuraminidase detection. Cultures detect the virus type and strain. Serology is only useful in retrospect.

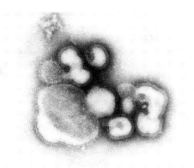

Fig. 5 **An orthomyxovirus, cause of influenza.** Bar represents 100nm.

Chemotherapy. Neuraminidase inhibitors called zanamivir (by inhalation) and oseltamivir (oral) block the release of virus from infected cells if given early (within 48 hours of onset).

Control and prevention. Vaccine protects well if it contains the prevalent strain(s). Domestic animals with 'bird flu' are usually killed.

Hantavirus pulmonary syndrome

Classification. This severe respiratory disease was discovered in 1993 in western USA.

Causative organism. This hantavirus called Sin Nombre ('without a name!') is a bunyavirus with single-stranded RNA in an enveloped helical nucleocapsid. It is transmitted by aerosol spread from the urine and faeces of deer mice, so is a robovirus = *ro*dent *bo*rne.

Clinical features begin like influenza but respiratory failure rapidly follows, with about 40% mortality.

Confirmatory tests are PCR or immunohistochemistry on lung tissue, or serum IgM.

Chemotherapy is not available – ribavirin is ineffective. Treatment is supportive only.

Control and prevention is only by avoiding deer mice, as no vaccine exists.

Hendra virus

Classification. This is a severe human respiratory or cerebral infection transmitted by hand contact or airborne droplets from the intermediate host, infected horses. The fruit bat is the reservoir.

Causative organism is a paramyxovirus originally called equine morbillivirus as it resembles measles virus. The first case occurred in Hendra, Australia. It is a new genus, Henipavirus, which also contains the **Nipah** virus of Malaysia, Singapore and Bangladesh, also a cause of pneumonia or encephalitis (p. 96).

Clinical features are either like influenza, or pneumonia with severe progressive fatal respiratory failure, or aseptic meningitis or fatal encephalitis.

Confirmatory test is usually by ELISA, but electron microscopy and culture have been used.

Chemotherapy. Ribavirin was not used, but improved survival in Nipah virus infection.

Control and prevention depends on gloves and masks when handling sick or dead horses.

Severe acute respiratory syndrome (SARS)

Classification. This is a severe acute respiratory infection which was a global epidemic from March to June 2003, originating in southern China.

Causative organism was a novel coronavirus, SARS-CoV. It was isolated from patients, civet cats and other market animals in S. China. Transmission was by large respiratory droplets through direct and indirect contact. Aerosol transmission was rare.

Clinical features began like influenza with fever, myalgia and headache, but then dry cough, dyspnoea and chest tightness were followed in a week by respiratory deterioration, needing intensive care and ventilator support in some.

Confirmatory tests were principally chest x-ray, normal early, then showing non-specific patchy opacities. PCR was developed, and was positive in most patients tested, particularly later in the infection. Antibody tests as usual gave only retrospective diagnosis.

Chemotherapy with ribavirin was ineffective, while interferon perhaps helped. Steroids were probably of no use.

Control and prevention was by usual infection control measures – surveillance, education, screening of travellers, isolation, direct and indirect contact control, contact tracing and home quarantine.

Viral respiratory infections

- Bronchiolitis is usually due to RSV, with acute wheeze and hyperinflation in children, has no specific treatment but minimal mortality.
- Common cold is a syndrome caused by over 100 viruses: rhino-, corona-, parainfluenza-, RSV and others. Rhinorrhoea, sore throat and cough recover within a week with no specific treatment.
- Croup is usually due to parainfluenza or other viruses, has characteristic difficult breathing and stridor, and recovers with oxygen and supportive therapy.
- Influenza due to the influenza viruses occurs in epidemics and pandemics, has three stages, and now has specific treatment as well as vaccines.
- Rarer infections are the Hantavirus Pulmonary Syndrome, Hendra and Nipah virus Infections and the Severe Acute Respiratory Syndrome (SARS).

Throat infections

Pharyngitis and tonsillitis

Pharyngitis is inflammation of the pharynx, usually caused by infection, and may occur without tonsillitis. Tonsillitis is infection of the tonsils and is often accompanied by pharyngitis, i.e. pharyngotonsillitis. Classification is by the causative organisms.

Causative organisms

The two commonest causes are <u>viruses</u> (rhino-, adeno-, Coxsackie, EBV, HIV, influenza and parainfluenza viruses, about 40%) and <u>streptococci</u> (about 25%), of which about half are the important Group A *S. pyogenes*. Less common (only 1–2%) but therapeutically important are *Corynebacterium diphtheriae* (diphtheria), *Neisseria gonorrhoeae* (gonorrhoea), and *Fusobacteria* spp. with spirochaetes (Vincent's angina). *Mycoplasma* spp. or *Chlamydia pneumoniae* may cause many of the remaining 'culture-negative' 30%.

All are spread person-to-person by direct contact or aerosol, except Vincent's angina which is endogenous.

Clinical features

Streptococcal infection. This varies from mild to severe pharyngitis, characterised by fever, sore throat, enlarged regional lymph glands, a bright red pharynx and uvula (Fig. 1), purulent exudate on the pharyngeal wall, and/or tonsillitis with pus in the follicles (Fig. 2).

Diphtheria. There is a characteristic adherent grey-white membrane and, at times, a musty odour. Untreated, it progresses to systemic toxaemia and respiratory obstruction, especially with laryngeal diphtheria (p. 120–121).

Pharyngeal gonorrhoea. There may be no symptoms (hence the importance of culture) or mildly painful pharyngitis.

Vincent's angina is an infection with mixed anaerobes and spirochaetes, causing foul mouth odour and a purulent exudate. It is often associated with Vincent's gingival infection, called acute necrotising ulcerative gingivitis (ANUG) or 'trench mouth' (p. 114).

Viral pharyngitis is usually mild, with variable associated symptoms and signs depending on the causative virus, e.g. in glandular fever. It is rarely clinically distinguishable from streptococcal infection, except **herpangina** from Coxsackieviruses causes tiny vesicles yet severe symptoms and fever.

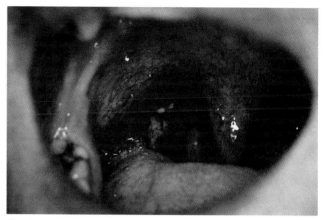
Fig. 1 **Streptococcal pharyngitis.**

Confirmatory tests

Culture and microscopy of throat swabs will identify most bacterial pathogens. Streptococcal and viral causes can be distinguished serologically using rapid specific latex agglutination for the former, and PCR or immunofluorescence for viruses.

Complications

Complications are uncommon if treatment is prompt. They are:

- local spread to give peritonsillitis or peritonsillar abscess (quinsy), and fascial space infections (see below)
- distant spread to give sinusitis, otitis media, mastoiditis (p. 106–107); post-anginal septicaemia (Lemierre's disease); or extension along the carotid sheath to give mediastinal infection (p. 119)
- toxin production: scarlet fever (p. 37, 191)
- immune damage: rheumatic fever (p. 139) and acute glomerulonephritis (p. 178).

Chemotherapy

There is debate whether penicillin should be given before diagnosis of a 'strep throat' is laboratory-proven; on balance, it is better than progressing to rheumatic fever. Penicillin for 10 days is the drug of choice for streptococcal infections, diphtheria and Vincent's angina; ceftriaxone is more effective for gonorrhoeal pharyngitis. Ampicillin should not be given for any pharyngitis or tonsillitis, as it is less effective and provokes a rash in mononucleosis. Antitoxin is essential for diphtheria, with appropriate measures to maintain oxygenation and circulation. Viral infections are treated symptomatically.

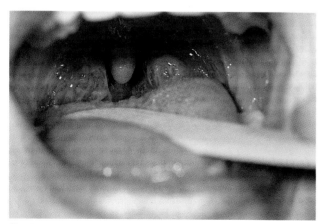
Fig. 2 **Tonsillitis.**

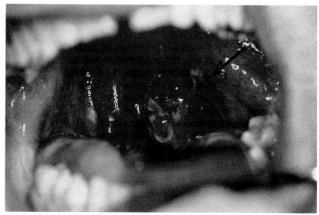
Fig. 3 **Quinsy: puncture mark over swelling from diagnostic aspiration.**

Structures | Groups of fascial spaces

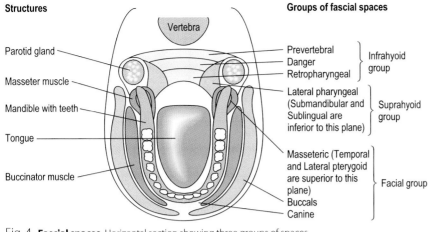

Fig. 4 **Fascial spaces.** Horizontal section showing three groups of spaces.

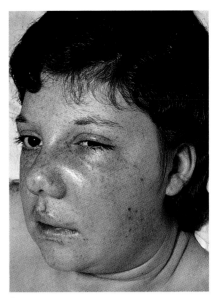

Fig. 5 **Buccal space infection showing facial swelling.**

Control and prevention is only really effective for diphtheria, by immunisation, and for Vincent's infection, by good oral and dental hygiene. All others depend on avoidance of sources of infection.

Peritonsillitis and peritonsillar abscess (quinsy)

Untreated tonsillitis can lead to cellulitis then abscess formation in the peritonsillar tissues by local spread. Rarely there is direct extension along the carotid sheath to the mediastinum. Mixed anaerobes and streptococci are the usual causative organisms.

Clinical features. In addition to tonsillitis, there is more severe pharyngeal pain and fever, with dysphagia (difficult, painful swallowing) and even some respiratory obstruction. There is peritonsillar redness and swelling (Fig. 3), displacing the tonsil medially.

Specialist ENT opinion is necessary, for peritonsillitis needs penicillin and metronidazole, while an abscess must be aspirated or drained surgically.

Fascial space infections

The primary *source* of infections in the fascial spaces is either a dental or periodontal infection (odontogenic infection), or a non-odontogenic infection, such as stomatitis, pharyngotonsillitis, parotitis or sinusitis.

Many of the fascial spaces (Fig. 4) between fascia, muscles, bones and other structures communicate with each other, but the spaces and their infections can be *classified* into three groups (Fig. 4).

Causative organisms

These are usually a mixture of anaerobic oral flora (*Actinomyces*, *Bacteroides*, *Fusobacteria* and *Peptostreptococcus* spp.) and aerobic streptococci. Enteric Gram-negative rods and staphylococci are uncommon.

Clinical features

These obviously differ somewhat with the site, but all show fever and pain, and symptoms from the source (see above). Trismus naturally occurs with masticator space infections. Swelling and brawny induration is early with upper and superficial spaces [temporal, parotid, buccal (Fig. 5), canine, submandibular and sublingual], but late and internal with the other, deeper spaces. These deep and infrahyoid space infections, and Ludwig's angina (p. 121) in the submandibular and sublingual spaces, thus endanger the airway, cause dysphagia and can extend down into the mediastinum. Urgent specialist consultation is essential.

Confirmatory tests

Microscopy and culture of aspirated or operative pus can confirm the causative organisms. Imaging by CT is often necessary.

Chemotherapy

This is important, particularly in the early cellulitic stage, but urgent drainage is necessary if swelling and abscess formation threatens the airway, plus dental treatment for odontogenic infections. Penicillin i.v. is usually sufficient in normal hosts, though metronidazole may be added. Clindamycin can be used in those with hypersensitivity to penicillin. Cefoxitin, timentin or even imipenem may be needed in immunocompromised patients, e.g. with leukaemia.

Control and prevention

This depends on proper oral hygiene and dental treatment.

Post-anginal septicaemia (Lemierre's disease)

Lemierre's disease is a rare but serious complication of Vincent's angina (anaerobic pharyngitis) which occurs when local spread causes septic jugular vein thrombophlebitis, then bacteraemic spread causes lung and other metastatic abscesses. Sometimes there is direct extension along the carotid sheath to the mediastinum. *Fusobacterium necrophorum* is the usual causative organism.

Clinical features

In addition to tonsillitis and/or peritonsillar abscess, there is neck pain, stiffness, tenderness and dysphagia with fever, septicaemia, metastatic infection and death if untreated.

Management

This is usually with penicillin i.v. and metronidazole; appropriate circulatory and respiratory support is needed.

Throat infections

- Pharyngitis and tonsillitis are commonly caused by viruses or streptococci, rarely by gonorrhoea, diphtheria or Vincent's angina.
- The clinical features of streptococcal and viral infections are similar, and a swab for culture and antigen detection is advised.
- Complications of throat infections arise from local spread, distant spread, toxin production and immune mechanisms.
- Antibiotic treatment depends on the pathogen; penicillin is usually given on suspicion of streptococci. Antitoxin is given for diphtheria. Fascial space and other abscesses need drainage plus chemotherapy.

Epiglottitis, diphtheria and Ludwig's angina

Epiglottitis

Epiglottitis is infection of the epiglottis and surrounding tissues, particularly the larynx and subglottic area. It can be very acute and cause respiratory arrest in 4 hours or less.

Causative organisms
The causative organism is nearly always *Haemophilus influenzae* type b (p. 44), rarely other *Haemophilus* spp., pneumococci, streptococci or staphylococci. Epiglottitis develops when virulent *H. influenzae* infects those without specific antibodies, especially unvaccinated children aged 2–4 years who have lost maternal antibodies. Childhood vaccination leaves adults vulnerable.

Clinical features
The distinctive features are **d**ysphagia, **d**rooling, **d**yspnoea, **d**istress (respiratory, circulatory and mental), **d**eveloping obstruction with stridor, and **d**eath if untreated. Sore throat is usual, and patients lean forward and drool because they cannot swallow their secretions. Auscultation early shows inspiratory stridor and tachycardia, then decreased breath sounds and bradycardia as death approaches. The throat should *not* be examined for the classical 'cherry red' epiglottis (Fig. 1), as throat examination may provoke respiratory arrest.

The differential diagnosis includes:

- **croup**, where the child usually has had a preceding URTI, lies supine and has a barking cough (p. 116–117)
- **diphtheria**, with typical adherent grey-white membrane
- **angioneurotic laryngeal oedema** or **foreign body**, where the history should be helpful
- **pharyngeal infections** (p. 118–119), including severe tonsillitis, peritonsillar abscess, or retropharyngeal abscess, revealed if throat examination is safe
- **Ludwig's angina**, which shows submandibular swelling (see below).

Confirmatory tests
There may be no time for investigations before securing the airway. If feasible, a lateral x-ray shows the swollen epiglottis, 'like an adult thumb' (Fig. 2). A high white cell count and positive blood culture may later confirm diagnosis.

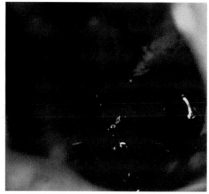

Fig. 1 **Epiglottitis – direct view. NB: this is potentially very dangerous.**

Management
Antibiotics are less urgent than securing the airway, usually by an expert in intubation. Tracheostomy may be necessary if intubation is impossible or unsafe. Ceftriaxone is now the antibiotic of choice, or chloramphenicol if it is unavailable.

Control and prevention.
Rifampicin is given at once to all household contacts and to the patient on recovery to eradicate carriage and prevent secondary cases. Then vaccinate all.

Diphtheria

Diphtheria, caused by toxin-producing strains of *Corynebacterium diphtheriae*, is a rare but important infection of the upper airways that causes respiratory obstruction, and distant effects – particularly on myocardium and nervous tissue. It is classified by the major site of infection (see below). The bacteria multiply locally without spreading. The exotoxin destroys epithelial cells and polymorphs, causing a local ulcer. This toxin enters the bloodstream causing fever, myocarditis (within the first 2 weeks) and polyneuritis (weeks later).

Causative organism
C. diphtheriae (p. 38) is a Gram-positive aerobic rod. It has three colonial variants; small smooth 'mitis' (mild), through 'intermedius', to large rough 'gravis' (grave, severe), that despite their names do not correlate with virulence. It is spread person-to-person by respiratory droplets from patients or asymptomatic carriers.

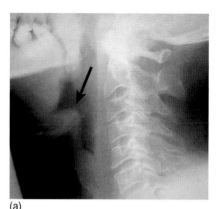
(a)

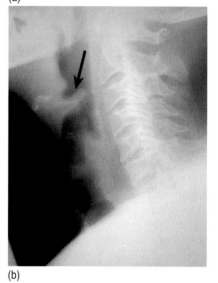
(b)

Fig. 2 **Epiglottitis (lateral x-ray). (a)** Before treatment. **(b)** After treatment.

Clinical features
Nasal diphtheria is usually mild, with purulent nasal discharge and few systemic symptoms. **Pharyngeal diphtheria** is the commonest initial clinical presentation, with sudden onset of fever, malaise and pharyngitis, followed by a prominent *pseudomembrane* of bacteria and necrotic tissue cells on the tonsil and posterior pharynx (Fig. 3). This can spread upwards, with marked systemic symptoms, as **naso-pharyngeal diphtheria**, and/or downwards as **laryngeal** and **bronchial diphtheria**. Respiratory obstruction (Fig. 4) and death may follow rapidly, or, arrhythmias and myocarditis, or neurological complications including peripheral neuritis, follow over 1–6 weeks.

Cutaneous diphtheria (Veldt sore, Barcoo rot) is now very rare. It forms a chronic indolent ulcer, either sponta-

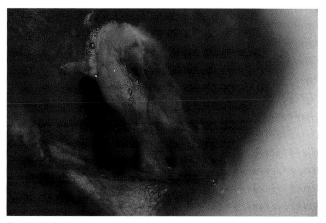

Fig. 3 **Diphtheria: membrane over tonsils.**

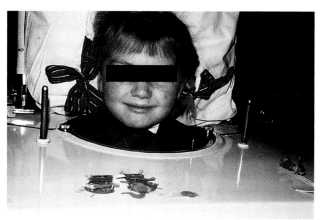

Fig. 5 **Respiratory paralysis in diphtheria treated in tank respirator.**

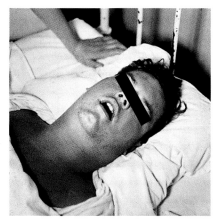

Fig. 4 **Bull neck diphtheria.**

neously or in a wound. Systemic symptoms rarely follow.

Pseudo-diphtheria. Rarely other corynebacteria cause 'pseudo-diphtheria', i.e. pharyngitis with scarlatiniform rash (*C. haemolyticum*, p. 38) or severe diphtheria-like pharyngitis (*C. ulcerans*).

The differential diagnosis of diphtheria includes severe pharyngitis from streptococci, Vincent's angina (anaerobic pharyngitis), Ludwig's angina and infectious mononucleosis (p. 118–119).

Confirmatory tests

Treatment cannot wait on laboratory tests, but throat and nasopharyngeal swabs should be taken for later confirmation. Gram stain is difficult to interpret without great experience, but culture on non-selective and special (tellurite, Loeffler's) media grows the typical colonies for biochemical confirmation. Elek's specific immunodiffusion test shows precipitation where toxin from the patient's organism meets antitoxin from filter paper.

Management

Diphtheria is a life-threatening illness. Immediately the diagnosis is suspected

the patient is isolated to reduce spread, and treatment with antitoxin is started. The airway must be secured. Penicillin i.v. is the drug of choice, while erythromycin is second choice. Cardio-respiratory support may be necessary (Fig. 5).

Control and prevention

Immunisation with killed vaccine, usually as DPT triple antigen with pertussis and tetanus, is highly effective for 10 years. Patient contacts need a booster if immunisation was more than 10 years ago. Erythromycin usually eradicates asymptomatic carriage.

Ludwig's angina

Ludwig's angina is a severe inflammation of both sides of the floor of the mouth in the submandibular and sublingual spaces (p. 121). It results in massive swelling of the neck, and if untreated can lead to airway obstruction and death.

Causative organisms. Anaerobic and aerobic oral flora are thought to be involved.

Clinical features. Submandibular swelling can spread to the neck. Fever is common.

Confirmatory tests. Culture of blood and operative specimens will indicate the particular pathogen(s).

Management. Drainage of the area may be necessary, and tracheostomy if the airway is threatened. Penicillin and metronidazole are antibiotics of choice. Prevention is through oral and dental hygiene.

Epiglottitis
- Epiglottitis affects unvaccinated children and adults; it is usually caused by *Haemophilus influenzae* and is a serious infection with respiratory distress quickly leading to respiratory obstruction.
- The distinctive features are **d**ysphagia, **d**rooling, **d**yspnoea, **d**istress (respiratory, circulatory and mental), **d**eveloping obstruction with stridor, and **d**eath if untreated.
- The throat should not be examined before the airway is secured. Ceftriaxone is now usual treatment.

Diphtheria
- Diphtheria is a serious infection of the upper (and sometimes the lower) airways causing respiratory obstruction and, at times, arrhythmias, myocarditis, peripheral neuritis and death.
- It is caused by *Corynebacterium diphtheriae*, with a potent exotoxin. It is diagnosed clinically and confirmed later by culture, Gram stain, biochemical tests and immunodiffusion for toxin production.
- Treatment is antitoxin and penicillin, with respiratory and cardiac support. Prevention is by immunisation.

Ludwig's angina
- This is infection in the fascial spaces in the floor of the mouth.
- It spreads rapidly, is serious, and speedily causes respiratory obstruction.
- Treatment is penicillin and metronidazole, with tracheostomy if needed.

Tropical and rare oro-facial infections

Cervical lymphadenitis

Enlarged cervical lymph nodes are seen in local infections or in generalised lymphadenopathy.

Mycobacterial infection

This is an important cause of enlargement, often without other signs of disease.

Clinically, the nodes are painless and fluctuant under purplish thin skin (Fig. 1a), and ulcerate if untreated (Fig. 1b).

Confirmatory tests. Staining for acid-fast bacilli, PCR and culture of the pus, and chest x-ray are confirmatory.

Management. Treatment is specific (usually triple) therapy including isoniazid and rifampicin for tuberculosis itself. Atypical mycobacterial infections are more antibiotic resistant and usually need excision. Fluctuant tuberculous nodes should never be incised, or a chronic sinus results, with later scarring.

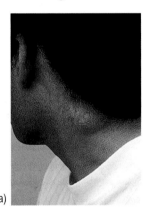

(a)

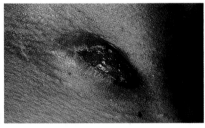

(b)

Fig. 1 **Tuberculous cervical gland (a) enlargement and (b) ulceration.**

Control and prevention is by pasteurisation of milk, immunisation by BCG and prevention of spread from open infections.

Salivary gland infections

Parotitis

Inflammation of the parotid gland can be bacterial or viral (see mumps, p. 144–145).

Acute suppurative parotitis is now uncommon; it follows oral neglect and dehydration from any cause. Local pain, swelling and redness (usually unilateral, Fig. 2a) are accompanied by fever; spread is serious, causing osteomyelitis, airway obstruction and bacteraemia.

Chronic bacterial parotitis is recurrent acute exacerbations of chronic low-grade infection, causing gradual parotid destruction.

Confirmatory tests are microscopy and culture of aspirated or operative pus.

Management involves flucloxacillin and metronidazole for both forms of parotitis. Acute infection needs surgical drainage but advanced chronic destruction or loculated abscesses (Fig. 2b) necessitate parotidectomy.

Salivary gland calculi and sialadenitis

Salivary gland calculi cause duct obstruction and gland infection, with local tenderness and swelling. Penicillin and/or metronidazole are adjuncts to surgery.

Other infections

Actinomycosis

Cervico-facial actinomycosis develops when oral or dental infection, trauma or surgery give a portal of entry for *Actinomyces* spp. from normal oral flora (p. 62) into the tissues.

Clinically a painful lump with purple-red overlying skin necroses to form a sinus. Mild fever and systemic symptoms

occur, and the infection may spread to mandible (Fig. 3), sinuses or orbit, mimicking tuberculosis.

Confirmation is by microscopy and prolonged anaerobic culture of pus, or histopathology.

Chemotherapy is prolonged penicillin, initially intravenous, followed by oral penicillin for 6–12 months.

Control is by dental care and appropriate chemoprophylaxis.

Paracoccidioidomycosis (South American blastomycosis)

This systemic fungal infection is caused by *P. brasiliensis* (p. 73). Chronic 'mulberry' oral or nasal mucous membrane lesions or warty skin ulcers develop years after the primary pulmonary infection. Treatment is with ketoconazole.

Rhinoscleroma

This rare infection is caused by *Klebsiella rhinoscleromatis* (p. 49). Clinically, there is progressive painless nasal deformity and distortion or destruction of respiratory passages. It is treated with streptomycin, oral tetracycline or co-trimoxazole.

Rhinosporidiosis

This was classified as a rare subcutaneous mycosis (p. 75) but the causative organism *Rhinosporidium seeberi* is not actually a fungus. Clinically, there are, on the nasal mucosa, large vascular, friable warts or polyps which are excised.

Gangrenous stomatitis

This rare infection, also called noma or cancrum oris ('cancer of the mouth'), destroys lips and cheeks (p. 113).

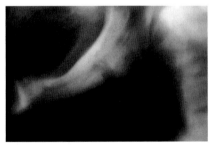

Fig. 3 **Actinomycosis of mandible.**

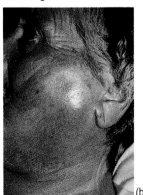

(a)

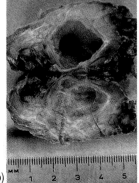

(b)

Fig. 2 **(a) Acute parotitis with swelling. (b) Parotid abscess.**

Tropical and rare oro-facial infections

- Cervico-facial actinomycosis is a chronic bacterial infection from oral or dental disease or trauma.
- Mycobacterial cervical lymphadenitis is either tuberculous or 'atypical' and causes relatively painless fluctuant matted nodes that ulcerate and discharge caseous pus to leave a chronic sinus.
- Parotitis is acute bacterial after oral neglect and dehydration, or chronic with gradual gland destruction, or viral (mumps).
- Paracoccidioidomycosis is a systemic mycosis with oral or nasal warty ulcers.

Laryngitis, tracheitis and pertussis

Laryngitis

Laryngitis is inflammation of the larynx and may occur alone, or with proximal pharyngitis, or distal tracheitis and bronchitis (see p. 116 for croup). It is classified by the causative organisms.

Causative organisms. Laryngitis alone is usually caused by respiratory viruses (influenza, parainfluenza, RSV, rhino-, corona-, and adenoviruses), but bacterial causes include *S. pyogenes*, *H. influenzae*, *Chl. pneumoniae* and *Mycoplasma pneumoniae*. Laryngitis without pharyngitis can occur in diphtheria, tuberculosis and *Moraxella catarrhalis* infections.

Clinical features. Hoarseness is the major symptom, which may progress to aphonia. Fever suggests a bacterial cause. The distinctive membrane of diphtheria (p. 120) is not easily visible in the larynx until almost too late. Infection of the larynx by sputum occurred in 30% of patients with advanced open pulmonary TB and is now sometimes caused by miliary spread. *M. catarrhalis* produces acute hoarseness and mild fever.

Confirmatory tests. Throat swabs and sputum need special microscopy and culture if diphtheria, TB or even rarer causes like syphilis are suspected.

Chemotherapy. Diphtheria needs specific antitoxin and penicillin urgently, and tuberculosis needs specific, usually triple, therapy. *M. catarrhalis* is not uncommonly beta-lactamase producing, and so needs amoxicillin plus clavulanate, or ceftriaxone.

Control and prevention. Diphtheria is preventable by immunisation, and BCG gives some protection from tuberculosis.

Tracheitis

Tracheitis is inflammation of the trachea, which may occur alone or with proximal laryngitis or distal bronchitis.

Causative organisms. Tracheitis alone is usually caused by respiratory viruses (above), but sometimes acute bacterial tracheitis occurs in adults and children, and must be distinguished from epiglottitis or croup. It is usually caused by *S. pyogenes*, *H. influenzae* type b or *S. aureus*.

Clinical features. Substernal pain and cough are the major symptoms. Bacterial tracheitis usually follows tracheal injury or intubation, with acute onset of pain, hoarse cough and fever. Mucosal swell-

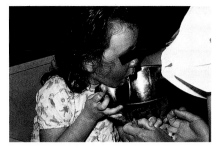
Fig. 1 **Tenacious sputum after cyanotic spasm in pertussis.**

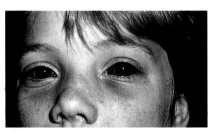
Fig. 3 **Subconjunctival haemorrhages in pertussis.**

ing and copious sputum can cause airway obstruction.

Confirmatory tests. Throat swabs and sputum are used for microscopy and culture.

Chemotherapy. Ceftriaxone is suitable initial treatment for bacterial tracheitis until the specific pathogen is identified.

Control and prevention. This depends on avoiding viral infections, and on tracheal care in hospital.

Pertussis

Pertussis is a severe preventable bacterial infection of the ciliated epithelium of large airways, characterised by spasmodic attacks of coughing.

Causative organism. Most attacks of pertussis are caused by *Bordetella pertussis* with a minority due to *B. parapertussis* (p. 45).

Clinical syndromes. The clinical features occur in three stages:

1. Catarrhal stage: a very infectious stage lasting 1–2 weeks with non-specific symptoms similar to the common cold.
2. Paroxysmal stage: lasts 2–4 weeks with the classic whooping spasms of uncontrollable repetitive cough until breathless or even cyanotic (Fig. 1), then a gasping inspiratory 'whoop' through the narrowed glottis for air, repeated 30–50 times a day. This is

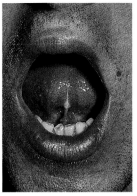
Fig. 2 **Frenal ulcer in pertussis.**

often followed by vomiting and expectoration of tenacious sputum (Fig. 1). Airway obstruction can occur. The forceful cough may produce frenal ulcers (Fig. 2) or subconjunctival (Fig. 3) or other haemorrhages.

3. Convalescent stage: the paroxysms gradually disappear over 3–6 weeks, but pneumonia, fits or encephalopathy may appear.

Confirmatory tests. Confirmatory tests are scarcely necessary in a classic case; the diagnosis may be proved by PCR, rapid direct immunofluorescence, or a per-nasal swab. Blood films show lymphocytosis.

Chemotherapy. Clarithromycin decreases infectivity though it does not shorten the clinical course. It should also be given to susceptible, unvaccinated household contacts.

The vaccine, usually with tetanus and diphtheria in triple antigen, is moderately effective, though unwarranted scare campaigns about its side-effects have diminished acceptability.

Laryngitis, tracheitis and pertussis

- Laryngitis is usually viral, but bacterial causes include common respiratory pathogens, plus diphtheria and tuberculosis.

- Tracheitis is usually viral, but a bacterial cause should be excluded in acute tracheitis after tracheal trauma.

- Pertussis is a severe, preventable bacterial infection characterised by recurrent paroxysms of coughing with 'whooping' inspirations, tenacious sputum and uncommon but serious complications. Clarithromycin decreases infectivity, and vaccination is moderately protective.

Bronchial infections

Bronchial infection may be a primary disease, or secondary to underlying broncho-pulmonary disease.

Acute bronchitis

Bronchitis is inflammation of the bronchi, and may occur alone or with proximal tracheitis or distal pulmonary infection. It is classified by the causative organisms.

Causative organisms
Bronchitis alone is usually caused by respiratory viruses (p. 116), but about 40% is bacterial, usually one of the five common respiratory pathogens – *S. pneumoniae*, *H. influenzae* type b, *Moraxella (Branhamella) catarrhalis*, *Mycoplasma pneumoniae* or *Chlamydophila pneumoniae* – or, rarely, other bacteria.

Clinical features
Cough and purulent sputum are the major symptoms. Fever and noisy respiration are less common. Dyspnoea indicates pre-existing or current lung disease.

Confirmatory tests
Bacterial infections need sputum microscopy and culture. *Mycoplasma*, chlamydial or severe viral infections need PCR.

Chemotherapy and control
A newer macrolide is suitable initial treatment for bacterial bronchitis until laboratory results show the pathogen. Amoxicillin is inactive against *Mycoplasma*, and *C. pneumoniae* needs a tetracycline.

Control and prevention depends on avoiding contact with similar infections. Influenza vaccine is particularly useful in epidemic years.

Acute infections in chronic obstructive pulmonary disease

Chronic obstructive pulmonary disease (COPD) includes emphysema and chronic bronchitis: the latter is defined as the production of sputum on most days for at least 3 months for more than 2 years (if wheeze and bronchospasm accompany the sputum production, it is called asthmatic bronchitis). The role of infection in *chronic bronchitis* is complex: although it is seldom a causative factor, it may be a perpetuating factor and often is an exacerbating factor. As infection is only one factor, along with smoking and occupational dust or fumes, so mucus

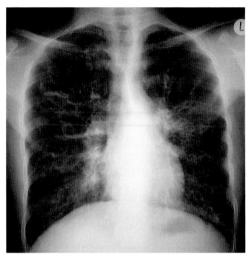
Fig. 1 **Cystic fibrosis: chest radiograph showing bronchiectasis and peripheral air trapping.**

gland hyperplasia with intraluminal mucus and pus are often more prominent than bronchial wall infection, though the usual bacterial respiratory pathogens, particularly pneumococci or *H. influenzae*, are common in intraluminal or expectorated sputum. This chronic multifactorial inflammatory response in the bronchial wall leads to scarring, obstruction and bronchiectasis ('dilated bronchi', see below).

Causative organisms
Acute exacerbations are caused by viruses (including influenza) in about 50%, and by pneumococci or *H. influenzae* in about 40%.

Clinical features
Cough and purulent sputum are the major symptoms. Dyspnoea and wheeze are common because of the pre-existing lung disease. Fever is less common.

Confirmatory tests
Bacterial infections need sputum microscopy and culture. Chest x-ray helps to distinguish bronchial from pneumonic infection.

Chemotherapy and control
Oral amoxicillin, amoxicillin-clavulanate, cephalosporin or doxycycline are reasonable empiric treatment for acute bac-

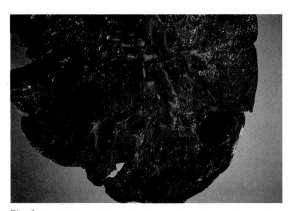
Fig. 2 **Cystic fibrosis lung at autopsy showing cystic spaces and lung destruction.**

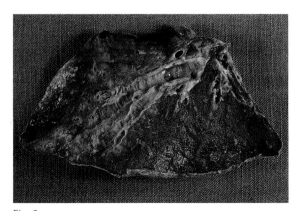
Fig. 3 **Bronchiectasis secondary to tuberculosis at autopsy showing grossly dilated bronchi.**

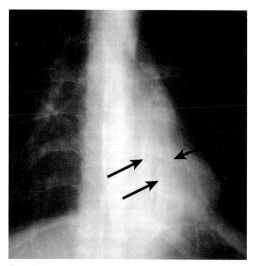

Fig. 4 **Bronchiectasis: chest radiograph showing dilated bronchi behind the cardiac shadow.**

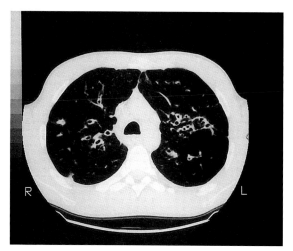

Fig. 5 **Bronchiectasis: CT scan of same patient reveals more extensive disease.**

terial exacerbations. Long-term suppressive antibiotics are not often helpful.

Influenza vaccine is particularly useful in epidemic years.

Acute infections in cystic fibrosis

Cystic fibrosis (mucoviscidosis) is a congenital disease of the pancreas and lungs where abnormally viscid mucus causes bronchial and bronchiolar plugging; this then produces bronchial and pulmonary infection, which causes more mucus plugging, hence more infection, with eventual bronchiectasis (Fig. 1), lung destruction (Fig. 2) and death.

Causative organisms

In childhood *H. influenzae* and *S. aureus* are the prominent pathogens, replaced between age 5 and 18 by *Pseudomonas aeruginosa*, which may be accompanied in late disease by *Burkholderia* (formerly *Pseudomonas*) *cepacia*.

Clinical features

Cough and large amounts of thick purulent sputum are the major symptoms, followed by fever and wheeze. Dyspnoea and cyanosis occur with progression of the lung disease. Systemic symptoms include tiredness, weakness, anorexia and weight loss with bulky malodorous stools.

Confirmatory tests

Acute exacerbations need sputum microscopy, culture and antibiotic sensitivities, for the organisms change with age and antibiotic treatment. Chest x-ray helps to distinguish bronchial from pneumonic infection and shows the development of bronchiectasis and air-trapping from bronchial obstruction (Fig. 1).

Chemotherapy and control

H. influenzae is usually treated with amoxicillin, amoxicillin-clavulanate or cephalosporins, *S. aureus* with amoxicillin-clavulanate or flucloxacillin, and *P. aeruginosa* with gentamicin or tobramycin with ticarcillin or ceftazidime; other, reserve antibiotics such as meropenem or aztreonam are needed as resistance develops.

The use of chronic suppressive antibiotics has considerable disadvantages and some advantages, so active physiotherapy and postural drainage are very important. Lung transplantation is life-prolonging in late disease.

Bronchiectasis

Bronchiectasis means dilated bronchi and is not a disease of itself but the result of bronchial obstruction by secretions or scarring, e.g. after measles, chronic bronchitis, cystic fibrosis or tuberculosis (Fig. 3).

Causative organisms

These are primary from the causative disease, or secondary following the obstruction and dilatation, including particularly the common respiratory pathogens *S. pneumoniae* and *H. influenzae*.

Clinical features

Cough and copious purulent sputum are the major symptoms. Fever and haemoptysis are less common. Dyspnoea results from the underlying lung disease.

Confirmatory tests

Bacterial infections need sputum microscopy, culture and sensitivity tests. Chest x-ray may show the dilated bronchi (Fig. 4), but CT is more sensitive and specific (Fig. 5).

Chemotherapy and control

Oral amoxicillin, amoxicillin-clavulanate, cephalosporin or doxycycline are reasonable empiric treatment for acute exacerbations.

Control and prevention depends on diagnosis and treatment of the predisposing causes.

Bronchial infections

- Bronchial infection may be primary (acute bronchitis), or secondary to underlying broncho-pulmonary disease, such as chronic bronchitis, cystic fibrosis or bronchiectasis.

- Causative organisms include viruses and the five common bacterial pathogens: *S. pneumoniae*, *H. influenzae* type b, *Moraxella catarrhalis*, *Mycoplasma pneumoniae* or *Chlamydophila pneumoniae*. In cystic fibrosis, *S. aureus* and then *P. aeruginosa* are most important.

- Clinical features are cough and sputum, with variable wheeze, fever, haemoptysis and dyspnoea.

- Chest radiographs and CT scan indicate the extent of disease.

- Treatment should be empirical antibiotics initially, with changes when the pathogen has been identified by sputum microscopy, culture and sensitivity tests.

Pneumonia I: in the normal host

Pneumonia means an infection of the lung tissue. There are over 60 different types and causes, which can be **classified** in many ways. For example:

- **Anatomically**: left, right, upper lobe, lower lobe.
- **Bacteriologically** (actually, microbiologically), by the causative organism: pneumococcal, chlamydial, tuberculous, etc.
- **Clinically**, by the age, lung disease, mechanism and immunity:
  1. Neonatal
  2. Previously healthy child or adult
  3. Complicating underlying pulmonary disease
  4. Aspiration – the mechanism, not inhalation as the other five
  5. Hospital-acquired (nosocomial)
  6. Immunocompromised patient.

These four pages (126–129) use the clinical classification.

Pneumonia is commonly **described** as:

- lobar: involves distinct lobe of lung
- broncho-pneumonia: diffuse patchy, spreading throughout lung
- interstitial: invasion of interstitium
- necrotising: cavitation and destruction of parenchyma, forming abscesses.

1. Neonatal pneumonia

Neonatal pneumonia can be of three types:

Congenital pneumonia. Congenital infection is transplacental and can result from syphilis, toxoplasmosis or viruses (including cytomegalovirus, herpes simplex or rubella). Babies are small with specific signs of the causative organism. If possible, treatment is for the pathogen implicated.

Intrapartum pneumonia. This occurs as the result of aspiration of infected amniotic fluid or bacteria from the maternal birth canal. The pathogens are usually group B streptococci (*S. agalactiae*), Gram-negative rods, or *Chlamydia trachomatis*. Intrapartum pneumonia presents with rapid respirations, asphyxia or generalised sepsis; fever is often absent. Immediate high-dose empirical antibiotics are essential: usually an aminoglycoside with either ampicillin or a third-generation cephalosporin. Oxygen and supportive therapy are important.

Postpartum pneumonia. Infection soon after birth is nosocomial from staff or equipment and is usually caused by staphylococci, Gram-negative rods or viruses. The clinical syndrome is one of respiratory distress, including tachypnoea or apnoea, rib retraction and grunting respiration. Treatment is as for intrapartum pneumonia.

Confirmatory tests

These include culture of respiratory secretions and blood, chest x-ray, blood gases and biochemistry. Co-existent meningitis should be considered, with lumbar puncture as necessary. Serology and PCR are done in congenital pneumonia.

Control and prevention

Congenital disease can be prevented or treated more effectively by screening of mothers, especially for syphilis and rubella antibodies. Treatment of maternal infections, and caesarean sections to avoid birth canal pathogens reduce intra- and postpartum risks of infection. Neonatal respiratory suction and prophylactic antibiotics are used in high-risk infants.

2. Pneumonia in the previously healthy

This is conventionally classified into:

- classical or typical pneumococcal pneumonia
- atypical pneumonia.

However, the clinical distinction in real life is not always easy. Classical pneumococcal pneumonia is 'typical' in being of abrupt onset, severe, lobar, and often with pleurisy. It has one microbial cause and has been penicillin responsive. Atypical pneumonia, in contrast, is usually of more gradual onset, less severe, affects one or more segments, seldom gives pleuritic pain, has many microbial causes and is seldom penicillin responsive.

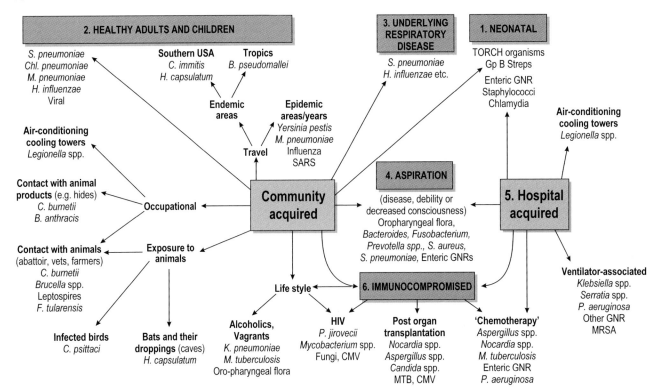

Fig. 1 **Major causes of pneumonia** (see also Fig. 1, p. 128).

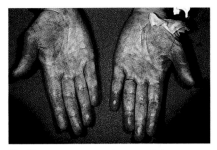
Fig. 2 **Erythema multiforme rash in mycoplasma pneumonia.**

Table 1 **The use of Gram stain to guide initial therapy in pneumonia**		
Major organism in purulent sputum	**Probable pathogen**	**Empiric treatment**
Gram-positive cocci	Diplococci, probably *S. pneumoniae*	Penicillin or ceftriaxone
	Cocci in clusters, probably *S. aureus*	Flucloxacillin
Gram-negative cocco-bacilli	May have capsules, probably *H. influenzae*	Ceftriaxone or cefotaxime (amoxicillin now unreliable)
Gram-negative rods	Resemble 'enterics'	Third-generation cephalosporin ± gentamicin
	Resemble pseudomonads	Ticarcillin + tobramycin

Causative organisms

Classical lobar pneumonia is caused by the pneumococcus (*S. pneumoniae*), while 'atypical' pneumonia has many causes for which the setting in which disease occurs – the epidemiology – may indicate a likely pathogen (Fig. 1).

Clinical syndromes

Classical lobar pneumococcal pneumonia characteristically begins abruptly with a rigor and fever, then dry cough followed by sharp chest pain on inspiration (pleuritic pain, which is shoulder-tip if diaphragmatic pleura is infected). Sputum is initially absent or minimal, streaked with blood ('rusty'). Systemic signs are severe, and the pneumonia is often fatal if untreated.

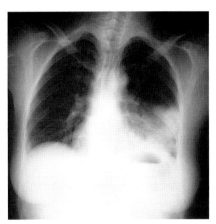
Fig. 3 **Pneumococcal lobar pneumonia.**

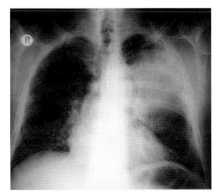
Fig. 4 **Legionella pneumonia in left mid-zone on chest radiograph.**

While 'atypical' pneumonia has many causes and hence variable clinical features, in most temperate areas there are five or six important causes (*Chlamydophila*, *Legionella*, *Mycoplasma*, staphylococcal, TB, viral). These may be severe but are in general of more gradual onset than pneumococcal pneumonia, less severe, affecting one or more segments rather than a whole lobe, seldom giving pleuritic pain and not penicillin responsive.

Similarly, each developing country or tropical area has its particular spectrum of common pneumonias, as do particular occupations or hobbies (Fig. 1).

There are few distinguishing signs, especially in temperate areas, though mycoplasma pneumonia may cause Raynaud's phenomenon, due to cold agglutinins, or erythema multiforme (Fig. 2).

Confirmatory tests

Difficulties arise in deciding what pathogen is involved and, therefore, how best to treat. The choice of test will depend on the epidemiological clues and geographic area but in general will include sputum microscopy by Gram stain (which can guide initial treatment: Table 1) and special stains, sputum and blood cultures. Chest x-ray (Figs 3 and 4), PCR, serology, and sometimes histopathology of tissue are contributory to diagnosis.

Chemotherapy

It is often difficult to choose the initial empiric therapy. Penicillin by injection is the drug of choice for pneumococcal pneumonia unless high-level resistance is known or suspected. Most atypical pneumonias do not respond to penicillin, so alternative treatments are used in particular cases. These are:

- adults: erythromycin plus a third-generation cephalosporin
- children: *H. influenzae* and staphylococci are more likely, so flucloxacillin is substituted for erythromycin
- endemic areas or with epidemiological clues: specific therapy should begin.

In all cases, initial therapy should be reviewed after laboratory results and clinical progress (or deterioration) are assessed.

Control and prevention

Vaccination is available against pneumococci, *H. influenzae*, influenza and TB for the general population, and against plague, Q fever and scrub typhus in specific situations. The animal host can be vaccinated or killed in anthrax, brucellosis, plague and TB.

Pneumonia in the normal host

- Neonatal pneumonia needs urgent investigation and treatment. It can be:
  - congenital, by transplacental infection
  - intrapartum by aspiration of infected amniotic fluid or maternal birth canal organisms
  - postpartum by nosocomial infection from staff or equipment.

- Previously healthy adults and children can be considered to have either typical or 'atypical' pneumonia.

- Classical pneumococcal pneumonia is 'typical' in being of abrupt onset, severe, lobar, often with pleurisy, has one microbial cause and is often penicillin responsive.

- Atypical pneumonia is usually of more gradual onset, less severe, affects one or more segments, seldom gives pleuritic pain, has many microbial causes and is seldom penicillin responsive.

- Atypical pneumonia in most temperate areas has five or six important causes: *Chlamydophila*, *Legionella*, *Mycoplasma*, staphylococcal, TB and viral pneumonia.

- The cause of atypical pneumonia can be suggested by epidemiological clues including occupation, travel or residence, animal exposure and hobbies.

Pneumonia II: in the abnormal host

Pneumonia is often a complication of a pre-existing condition (acute or chronic) which predisposes to the pneumonia (Fig. 1). As a wide range of pathogens can be causative, confirmatory tests are urgent, and initial treatment is empirical.

Confirmatory tests

Sputum microscopy with Gram stain (plus special stains) and sputum culture are essential, as is blood culture if bacteraemia is likely. Chest x-ray indicates areas of consolidation; some particular pathogens show typical features (see below). Blood gases and biochemistry are needed in severe disease, and PCR and serology may be useful. Four major groups of predisposing situations tend to show specific identifying features, as follows:

3. Pneumonia complicating underlying pulmonary disease

Three main types of pulmonary disease can be complicated by pneumonia:

- chronic obstructive pulmonary disease (COPD) (p. 124)
- cystic fibrosis (p. 125)
- viral respiratory infections (p. 116–117).

The presence of COPD in many elderly people makes them vulnerable to pneumonia, the commonest cause of death in the industrialised world. In addition to *S. pneumoniae* and *H. influenzae* (Fig. 1), enteric Gram-negative rods and *S. aureus* infect the elderly, especially in nursing homes.

Clinical syndrome

Abrupt onset and severe disease are usual with pneumococcal pneumonia (p. 126), while other pathogens generally cause more gradual onset of increased cough and sputum, fever and dyspnoea. Haemoptysis and pleuritic pain are less common. Severe pneumonia causes hypoxia and confusion, hypotension and circulatory failure.

Confirmatory tests

Chest x-ray in staphylococcal pneumonia characteristically shows multiple small abscesses which may leave cysts called pneumatocoeles (Fig. 2). Blood gases and biochemistry are needed in severe pneumonia.

Chemotherapy

Initial empiric therapy may be guided by the Gram stain on purulent sputum and is aimed at the likely causes. In COPD,

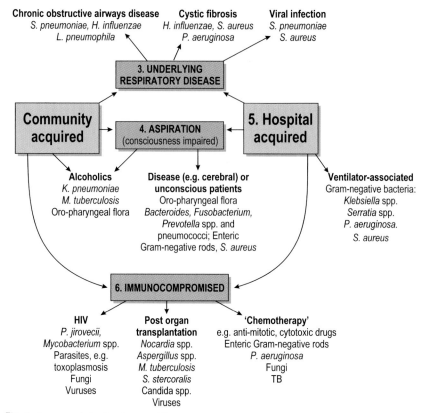

Fig. 1 **Pneumonia in the abnormal host.**

intravenous penicillin or a third-generation cephalosporin is used, in cystic fibrosis ticarcillin and tobramycin, and in post-viral pneumonia penicillin or flucloxacillin. Subsequent specific therapy is guided by the sputum culture results in conjunction with the clinical response, i.e. penicillin or ceftriaxone are the drugs of choice in pneumococcal pneumonia, flucloxacillin in staphylococcal pneumonia, erythromycin +/− rifampicin in legionellosis, etc.

Control and prevention

Pneumococcal and influenza vaccine should be given to patients with COPD, and *Haemophilus* vaccine to children.

4. Aspiration pneumonia

Aspiration of oro-pharyngeal secretions occurs in any disease state where consciousness and hence normal gag and swallowing reflexes are impaired. It may be community acquired, e.g. in alcoholics, or nosocomial, e.g. in cerebral disease. Infection is usually with oro-pharyngeal flora including anaerobes (Fig. 1).

Clinical features

Cough, sputum, fever and tachypnoea develop, with dyspnoea, hypoxia, cyanosis and respiratory and circulatory failure in severe cases.

Confirmatory tests

Sputum examination is less helpful than in other pneumonias, as the principal causative organisms are normal oropharyngeal flora that will be present in expectorated sputum from any cause. Chest x-ray may show unilateral peripheral opacities in all lobes from aspiration while lying on one side (Fig. 3). If aspiration occurs while lying on the back (supine), most secretions enter the right upper lobe bronchus, causing upper lobe pneumonia.

Chemotherapy and control

As sputum examination is unhelpful, chemotherapy is empiric with metronidazole, often with penicillin or timentin, particularly if aspiration occurred in hospital.

Control and prevention depends on adequate care of patients with impaired gag and swallowing reflexes, e.g. the unconscious patient or those with some nervous system conditions such as pseudo-bulbar palsy.

5. Hospital-acquired pneumonia

Pneumonia may occur in any hospitalised patient but is particularly seen in those requiring assisted ventilation. Enteric bac-

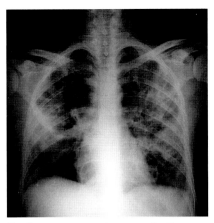

Fig. 2 **Staphylococcal pneumonia.** Chest radiograph showing bilateral abscesses and pneumatocoeles.

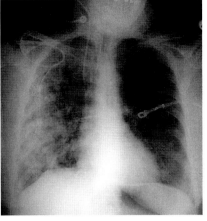

Fig. 3 **Aspiration pneumonia.** Chest radiograph showing right-sided peripheral opacities in all lobes from aspiration while unconscious, lying on the right side.

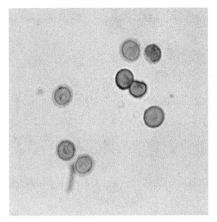

Fig. 4 *Pneumocystis jirovecii* **from 'induced sputum'.**

teria often colonise such patients without causing disease, and their presence in respiratory cultures without chest x-ray changes, neutrophilia or worsening pulmonary function does *not* mean infection. Bacteria are often multi-resistant.

Clinical features
Cough, sputum, dyspnoea and often fever occur in non-intubated patients, while those on ventilators show increased respiratory secretions, increased ventilatory requirements and fever.

Confirmatory tests
Neutrophilia is less common in old, ill patients. Further tests may be needed to exclude pulmonary embolism or other non-infectious lung pathology.

Chemotherapy and control
A third-generation cephalosporin or timentin is often combined with an

aminoglycoside like gentamicin for initial empiric treatment; they are replaced by specific antibiotics when cultures reveal the probable causative organism. Respiratory and cardiac support are often necessary.

Aseptic airway and ventilator care plus physiotherapy help in prevention.

6. Pneumonia in the immunocompromised patient

This is usually a particular subgroup of hospital-acquired pneumonia, though sometimes it is community acquired. It is a special hazard for leukaemic and cancer patients on anti-mitotic chemotherapy, for AIDS and organ transplant patients, as well as for patients on high-dose steroids or cytotoxic drugs. Infection can occur with the full range of organisms from viruses, bacteria and fungi to protozoa and parasites.

Clinical features
The course of the pneumonia is often rapid, with dyspnoea, cough, sputum

and haemoptysis, followed by respiratory failure.

Confirmatory tests
Alveolar sputum induced with nebulised saline is necessary to diagnose *P. jirovecii* (formerly *P. carinii*) pneumonia ('PCP') (Fig. 4). PCP has typically a uniform 'ground glass' appearance in a chest radiograph, while *C. neoformans* may cause a localised 'cryptococcoma' (Fig. 5). Tuberculosis, nocardiosis and staphylococcal pneumonia produce cavities, while aspergillosis often infects pre-existing cavities.

Management
Urgent empiric broad-spectrum antibiotics usually include a beta-lactam such as a third-generation cephalosporin or timentin combined with an aminoglycoside like gentamicin. Specific drugs are used when the pathogen is identified or probable. Respiratory and cardiac support are often necessary.

Chemoprophylaxis is used against TB in Mantoux-positive immunocompromised patients, and against PCP and atypical mycobacteria, while aseptic airway and ventilator care help in prevention.

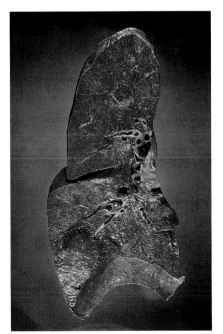

Fig. 5 **Cryptococcoma in lung at post-mortem.**

> *Pneumonia in the abnormal host*
>
> ■ Pneumonia can complicate pre-existing pulmonary diseases:
> – chronic obstructive pulmonary disease: often pneumococcal
> – cystic fibrosis: staphylococci, *H. influenzae* and *P. aeruginosa*
> – viral infection: pneumococcal or staphylococcal.
>
> ■ Aspiration pneumonia is caused by aspirated oro-pharyngeal anaerobes and streptococci in unconscious or incoordinate patients. The position during aspiration determines the lobe(s) infected.
>
> ■ Hospital-acquired pneumonia particularly occurs in ventilated patients, and is usually caused by enteric bacteria, *P. aeruginosa* or *S. aureus*. Chest radiograph changes, neutrophilia or worsening pulmonary function indicate infection rather than simple colonisation.
>
> ■ Pneumonia in the immunocompromised patient is a special hazard for leukaemic, cancer, AIDS and transplant patients as well as patients on high-dose steroids or cytotoxic drugs. There is a wide range of causative organisms.

Lung abscess and empyaema

Lung abscess

Lung abscesses are pus-containing cavities within the lung; they may be single or multiple, uni- or bilateral. *They arise by five routes* (Fig. 1). The commonest is from above, through the bronchi by inhalation (from sinusitis, dental or oral sepsis, bronchitis or bronchiectasis) or by aspiration (lost gag/swallowing reflexes, coma or anaesthesia, oesophageal reflux, foreign body or tumour).

Causative organisms

The likely pathogens (often mixed) depend on the route of infection:

1. From above: usually oro-pharyngeal flora of mixed anaerobes and mixed streptococci, plus Gram-negative rods in hospitalised patients.
2. From below: mixed enteric flora including anaerobes and aerobic Gram-negative rods and cocci; *E. histolytica*. See p. 135 for *P. westermani*, causing paragonimiasis.
3. From within, following pneumonia: *K. pneumoniae*, other Gram-negative rods and *S. aureus* are common; *Legionella* spp., *Actinomyces* and *Nocardia* spp. are rare. See p. 134 for *Pseudomonas pseudomallei*, causing melioidosis.
4. From without: *S. aureus*, skin flora, soil organisms.
5. From remote sources: *S. aureus*, *E. coli*, and anaerobes, especially *Fusobacterium necrophorum* and *B. fragilis*.

Clinical features

Copious foul sputum (indicative of anaerobes) and persistent fever are prominent, with anorexia, malaise and weight loss. Chest pain and dyspnoea are uncommon. Differential diagnosis is from a necrotic cavitating tumour or infarct, infected lung bullae, or rare infections (p. 134) including actinomycosis, aspergillosis, hydatid cyst (Fig. 2) or nocardiosis.

Confirmatory tests

Chest x-ray confirms the diagnosis (Fig. 3). Sputum culture is unhelpful for abscesses from above (aspiration) but may help in other causes. Cultures from blood, wounds or remote sources may help. Direct aspiration under CT control is safe and specific.

Chemotherapy

Metronidazole (because of the usual involvement of anaerobes) plus penicillin is the usual empiric treatment. Clindamycin is active against most anaerobes and staphylococci. Metronidazole plus a third-generation cephalosporin is appropriate if aspiration occurred in hospital. Specific therapy is given if the abscess follows specific pneumonia or septic emboli. Posturing may help drainage, and surgery may hasten cure.

Control and prevention

This depends on preventing infection by the five routes: airway control, treatment of intra-abdominal abscesses, of pneumonia, of chest wounds, and of septicaemia. If treatment is delayed, infection may spread to the pleural cavity, resulting in empyaema.

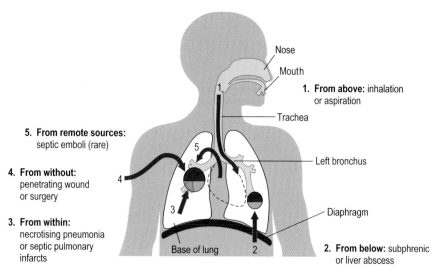

5. **From remote sources:** septic emboli (rare)

4. **From without:** penetrating wound or surgery

3. **From within:** necrotising pneumonia or septic pulmonary infarcts

Nose

Mouth

1. **From above:** inhalation or aspiration

Trachea

Left bronchus

Diaphragm

Base of lung

2. **From below:** subphrenic or liver abscess

Fig. 1 **Pathogenesis of lung abscess: routes of infection.**

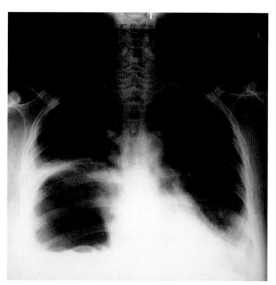

Fig. 2 **Hydatid cyst – note daughter cysts at base.**

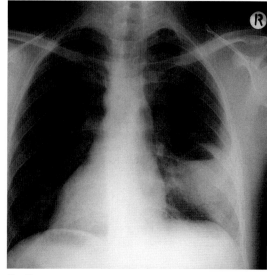

Fig. 3 **Lung abscess on chest radiograph, showing cavity with fluid level in right lower zone.**

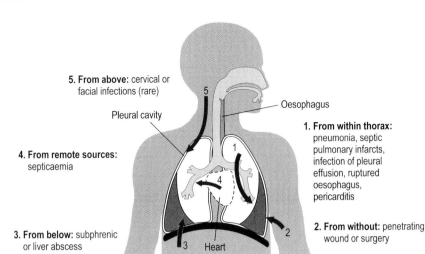

5. **From above:** cervical or facial infections (rare)

Pleural cavity

Oesophagus

1. **From within thorax:** pneumonia, septic pulmonary infarcts, infection of pleural effusion, ruptured oesophagus, pericarditis

4. **From remote sources:** septicaemia

2. **From without:** penetrating wound or surgery

3. **From below:** subphrenic or liver abscess

Heart

Fig. 4 **Pathogenesis of empyaema: routes of infection.**

Empyaema

An empyaema (= pyothorax) is a collection of pus within the pleural cavity, outside the lung. Like a lung abscess, an empyaema *can arise by five routes*, in different order of importance (Fig. 4).

Causative organisms

Again, the common causative organisms depend on the route of infection:

1. From within: anaerobes, particularly *Bacteroides* spp., *F. nucleatum* and peptostreptococci; aerobic streptococci and, after nosocomial pneumonia, enteric Gram-negative rods.
2. From without: *S. aureus* or enteric Gram-negative rods, soil or skin flora.
3. From below: gut anaerobes and enteric GNR.
4. From remote sources: *S. aureus*.
5. From above: respiratory anaerobes and streptococci.

Clinical features

Dyspnoea, chest pain and a dry cough are usual, with sputum production only when the underlying lung is infected. Sometimes there are few systemic symptoms and low-grade fever; usually major systemic symptoms with hectic swinging fevers occur.

Confirmatory tests

Chest x-ray shows the empyaema (Fig. 5), though CT may be needed to differentiate it from a lung abscess. Microscopy of aspirated pus with Gram and special stains, plus aerobic and anaerobic culture reveal the pathogens.

Chemotherapy

Empiric initial treatment is often with metronidazole and a third-generation cephalosporin (or flucloxacillin if staphylococci are probable), then specific antibiotics when the pathogens are known. Adequate medical or surgical drainage is essential, with re-expansion of the lung.

Control and prevention

This depends on preventing infection by the five routes: treatment of pneumonia, of chest wounds, of intra-abdominal abscesses, of septicaemia and of cervical infections.

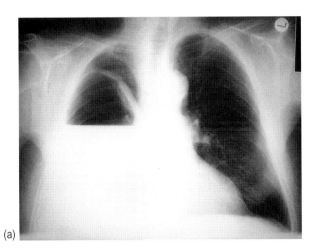

(a)

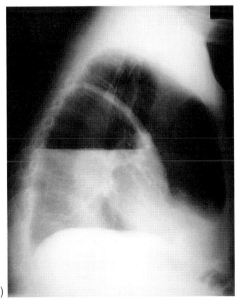

(b)

Fig. 5 **(a) A huge empyaema on chest x-ray. (b) The lateral view shows it is behind the right lung.**

Lung abscess and empyaema

- Lung abscesses arise by one of five routes:
  - most commonly from above, by inhalation or aspiration of oro-pharyngeal flora
  - from below, from intra-abdominal abscesses
  - from within the lung following pneumonia
  - from without the chest, by wounds or surgery
  - from remote sources (rare) through septic emboli.
- An empyaema arises by one of the same five routes as for lung abscess although infection from above is from cervical infections, not by aspiration into the bronchial tree. Infection from within the thorax is the commonest cause.
- Chest x-ray and CT define the abscess(es) or empyaema. The pathogens are identified in aspirate for both diseases.
- Chemotherapy is empirical initially, guided by route of infection.
- Adequate medical or surgical drainage is essential, with re-expansion of the lung.

Tuberculosis and atypical mycobacterial infections

Tuberculosis (TB)

Tuberculosis is a chronic infection of humans and animals. It affects healthy as well as immunocompromised people. It is primarily a lung disease but may begin in or spread to other sites, or form a generalised (miliary tuberculosis) infection. It has three stages:

- primary
- latent
- post-primary (secondary).

1. Primary tuberculosis

Primary tuberculosis usually occurs in childhood by person-to-person aerosol spread of *Mycobacterium tuberculosis* ('MTB', 'tubercle bacilli', p. 60) or, rarely, by *M. bovis*. It is characterised by the **primary complex**, which has two parts, a primary focus of infected tissue plus the associated regional lymphadenopathy. **M**acrophages, **m**ultiplication, **d**issemination and **d**amage are the essential features – the mycobacteria are engulfed by **m**acrophages, in which they can survive and **m**ultiply, and are then **d**isseminated in lymphatics to lymph nodes where a **d**amaging cell-mediated immune response begins. The body reacts to contain the pathogen in infected tissue in **tubercles**, which are small granulomata of epithelioid cells and giant cells: multiplying mycobacteria make macrophages appear as multinucleated giant (Langhans) cells. Central cheesy necrotic damage in tubercles is called **caseation**, and any progression to macroscopic damage causes **cavitation** (p. 60 and Fig. 4a). Unlike most bacterial infections, tubercle bacilli cause little direct damage themselves, and do not produce toxin. Instead, tuberculosis is an example of a disease where the pathology is a consequence of the cell-mediated immune response, attempting to prevent spread of the disease.

Tuberculosis is **acquired** by five mechanisms:

- *Inhalation* is easily commonest, causing the primary focus in the best aerated (middle and lower) zones of the lungs
- *Ingestion* of unpasteurised milk infected with *M. bovis*, causing the primary complex in the small bowel wall and mesenteric lymph nodes
- *Implantation* in the skin, *intercourse* and *intra-uterine transmission* are very rare.

Primary tuberculosis can **evolve** in three ways:

- *Healing* may occur, often with calcification (Fig. 1), without spread elsewhere. The development of cell-mediated immunity (CMI) is shown by a positive Mantoux test, when purified protein derivative (PPD) of *M. tuberculosis* produces a palpable (10mm) lump 72 hours after intradermal injection. A healed calcified pulmonary primary focus is named a Ghon focus.
- *Progressive primary tuberculosis* may develop by local spread through the lung as progressive primary tuberculous pneumonia, or to the pleura as a primary tuberculous effusion (Fig. 2).
- *Miliary spread* (like millet seeds on chest x-ray) occurs through the bloodstream, particularly to lymph nodes, the upper zones of the lungs, to kidneys, bones, central nervous system or genital tract. This may cause severe clinical disease called *miliary tuberculosis* (Fig. 3) or may heal without symptoms, passing to the next, latent, stage.

2. Latent tuberculosis

Latent tuberculosis means there are no symptoms and signs of infection, though the Mantoux test usually remains positive for many years. Latent *infection* may last 10–90 years, being much commoner than clinical *disease*.

3. Post-primary (secondary) tuberculosis

Post-primary, 'adult' (secondary) tuberculosis develops by *reactivation* of dormant infection seeded by miliary spread of primary tuberculosis, in the upper zones of the lungs (Fig. 4), lymph nodes (p. 122), kidneys (p. 179), bones and joints (p. 209, 211), central nervous system (p. 99) or genital tract (p. 186).

Clinical syndromes

- The primary complex is usually asymptomatic, but mild fever and malaise may occur.
- Progressive primary pulmonary tuberculosis causes fever, cough, sputum, haemoptysis and, if extensive, dyspnoea.
- Primary tuberculous effusion causes dyspnoea and fever, with little cough. Any sputum and haemoptysis reflect the underlying lung infection.
- Miliary spread in the primary stage may be asymptomatic, but miliary disease is usually serious, often with pulmonary and meningeal disease together, at times with bone or renal disease also.

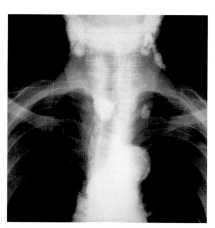

Fig. 1 **Calcified mediastinal and cervical tuberculous lymph nodes.**

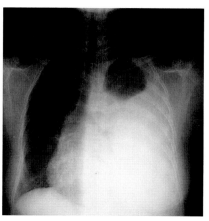

Fig. 2 **Pleural effusion from pulmonary TB, on chest radiograph.**

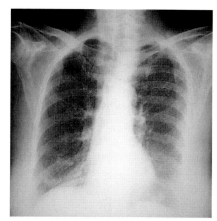

Fig. 3 **Miliary TB on chest radiograph, showing multiple fine opacities 'like millet seeds' in all zones.**

- Latent disease by definition is asymptomatic with a positive Mantoux test. (Note broad similarities but differences of detail with the stages of the other classic chronic infectious disease, syphilis.)
- Post-primary pulmonary TB causes chronic cough, sputum with haemoptysis and fever, and anorexia and progressive wasting, hence the old name, 'consumption'. Dyspnoea and chest pain usually occur late.
- Extrapulmonary TB occurs mainly in lymph nodes (25%) and pleura (20%), genitourinary tract (15%), bone and joint (10%), disseminated (10%) and meninges (5%).

Confirmatory tests

A positive Mantoux or Quantiferon test (quantifying anti-TB gamma interferon) indicates previous exposure to the tubercle bacillus, not necessarily active disease.

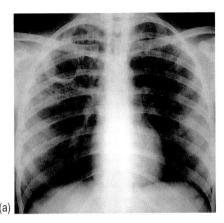

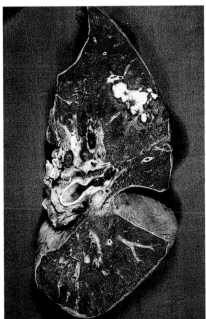

Fig. 4 **Pulmonary fibro-caseous TB.**
(a) Apical fibrosis and cavitation on chest radiograph. **(b)** Autopsy specimen showing fibrosis and cavities.

Conversely, in overwhelming TB, the Mantoux may become negative.

Acid-fast bacilli are presumptive evidence of TB, but as other mycobacteria and *Nocardia* spp. are acid-fast, full identification needs PCR or culture, which is also essential for sensitivity testing.

Chest x-ray (Fig. 4) shows the extent, monitors progress, and detects complications like pleural effusion.

Chemotherapy

This is specialised: triple therapy usually involves rifampicin and isoniazid (INAH) for 6 months, with a third drug, usually pyrazinamide, for the first 2 months. Quadruple therapy with ethambutol, for example, added to the above three can shorten treatment to 6 months in uncomplicated disease caused by sensitive organisms. Directly observed therapy (DOT) twice or thrice weekly in some countries ensures uninterrupted chemotherapy. Incomplete or inadequate treatment leads to drug resistance and even Multi-drug resistant TB in the index patient and those subsequently infected. Adjunctive surgery is still sometimes necessary.

Control and prevention

BCG vaccination is used where TB is prevalent, so vaccinees react quickly to limit infection if it occurs. Chemoprophylaxis with isoniazid for 1 year is given to close contacts of new patients or those recently converting from Mantoux negative to positive, i.e. recent asymptomatic infections.

Atypical mycobacterial infections

About 30 mycobacterial species can cause infections: disease is well known in immunosuppressed patients, particularly in AIDS (p. 149–151). Mycobacteria other than *M. tuberculosis* (MOTT) cause various diseases (Table 1). Species are now differentiated precisely by PCR and biochemical tests rather than the Runyon classification (p. 61).

Management

Chemotherapy depends on the species and sensitivity tests, although the latter are often unreliable. Atypical mycobacteria are often resistant to many antibiotics, so usually combination therapy is required. *M. scrofulaceum* varies in susceptibility, and triple therapy or surgery is usually necessary. *M. chelonei* and *M. fortuitum* are relatively resistant to drugs; amikacin, doxycycline, cefoxitin and clarithromycin may be useful. Surgery to remove all infected tissue is important. Infection from surgery or prostheses is minimised by aseptic techniques.

Table 1 **Some atypical mycobacterial infections**

Species	Disease
M. leprae	Leprosy (p. 60)
M. marinum	Skin infections and deeper infections, 'fish-tank granuloma' (p. 196)
M. kansasii	Lung infections (rare) resembling TB
M. avium-intracellulare	Disseminated infections in AIDS patients (p. 151). Cervical lymphadenitis
M. scrofulaceum	Cervical lymphadenitis (p. 122)
M. ulcerans	Skin infections: Bairnsdale or Buruli ulcers (p. 202)
M. fortuitum and *M. chelonae*	Infections associated with implantation by trauma or surgery

Tuberculosis and atypical mycobacterial infections

- Tuberculosis is a chronic disease caused by *M. tuberculosis* (rarely *M. bovis*). Bacteria multiply in macrophages both at the site of infection (usually in the lung by inhalation) and in the lymph nodes.
- The primary stage involving the primary complex may heal, may spread locally or may spread systemically (miliary).
- After a latent period, post-primary (secondary) disease develops, again most often pulmonary, but at times renal, glandular, skeletal, cerebral or genital.
- Because mycobacteria are often drug resistant, chemotherapy is specialised quadruple or triple therapy for 6–9 months or longer.
- Control is by BCG vaccination, and chemoprophylaxis.
- The atypical mycobacteria can be contaminants or colonising organisms or cause infections: pulmonary (*M. kansasii*), skin and soft tissue ulcers (*M. ulcerans*, *M. marinum*), systemic (*M. avium-intracellulare* in AIDS), or opportunist (*M. chelonae*, *M. fortuitum*).

Tropical or rare respiratory infections

These rare infections are caused by a range of organisms which may cause disease in other organ systems also. The features of lung disease are shown in Table 1.

Actinomycosis

Actinomycosis is a rare, chronic infection by filamentous Gram-positive anaerobic slowly growing *Actinomyces*, usually *A. israelii* (p. 62). Thoracic actinomycosis occurs by inhalation of *Actinomyces* from normal oral flora. The pathological features are **s**low progression, **s**inus formation (late), **s**clerosis, **s**carring and **s**ulphur yellow granules in **s**inus or cavitary pus.

The clinical features are cough, sputum, haemoptysis and chest pain. Fever and systemic symptoms are mild, yet the infection may spread to pleura, mediastinum or chest wall. It may mimic tuberculosis.

Confirmatory tests are Gram's stain of any granules, *prolonged anaerobic* culture of washed sputum or pus, or histopathology on excised tissue.

Chemotherapy and control. Chemotherapy is prolonged intravenous penicillin then oral penicillin for 6–12 months. Control is by dental care and appropriate chemoprophylaxis.

Aspergillosis

Infection of the lung by *Aspergillus* spp. (p. 68) occurs by inhalation; the species most often involved are *A. fumigatus*, *A. niger* and *A. flavus*. Infection is becoming more common because of the increase in immunocompromised patients. Aspergillosis of the lung is classified into three clinical types:

- **Allergic broncho-pulmonary aspergillosis.** This occurs in asthmatics and causes expectorated bronchial plugs (Fig. 1) and some increase in dyspnoea. Episodes may recur for years.
- **Aspergilloma.** This is a fungus ball in a pre-existing cavity or cyst, typically causing haemoptysis, plus the features of the underlying disease.
- **Fulminant pneumonia.** This usually occurs in the immunocompromised host and causes high fever, cough, progressive dyspnoea, respiratory failure and death in 1–3 weeks.

Confirmatory tests. Microscopy will identify hyphae and conidiophores (p. 7).

Table 1 **Features of rare lung infections**				
Disease	**Course in lungs**	**Characteristics**	**Cavitation**	**Complications**
Actinomycosis	Chronic	Lower lobes often	++	Pleura/empyaema
Aspergillosis				
Allergic	Recurrent	Fleeting	–	Bronchiectasis
Aspergilloma	Progressive	Fungus ball	Always	Bleeding, spread
Pneumonia	Fulminant	Expanding, >1 lobe	–	Spread, death
Hydatid disease	Silent	'Cannon ball'	–	Secondary infection
Melioidosis	Fulminant	Like TB, any lobe	+	Sepsis, death
Nocardiosis	Chronic	Like TB, any lobe	+	Pleural spread
Paragonimiasis	Progressive	Mixed, cysts, calcification	+	Fibrosis
Systemic mycoses				
Blastomycosis	Nil or progressive	Dense, segmental	±	Rarely spread
Coccidioidomycosis	Acute or progressive	Variable infiltrate	++	Rarely spread
Cryptococcosis	Nil or cryptococcoma	Globular mass	–	Spread in AIDS
Histoplasmosis	Acute or progressive	Like TB, any lobe	++	Rarely spread, calcification
Paracoccidioidomycosis	Nil or progressive	Fluffy infiltrates		Oro-nasal disease

Culture is needed for identification. Chest x-ray and CT scan define the extent of disease.

Chemotherapy. Amphotericin B and voriconazole are helpful but seldom curative. Aspergillomas are removed surgically.

Control and prevention is seldom feasible except by filtered air for highly immunocompromised patients especially during building works.

Hydatid disease

The causative organism in pulmonary hydatid disease is usually the cestode *Echinococcus granulosus*, rarely *E. multilocularis* (p. 89). Clinically there may be cough or dyspnoea, but often the cyst is asymptomatic, found incidentally on chest x-ray (Fig. 2).

Confirmatory tests are serological, particularly for arc 5 in a gel immunodiffusion test, which is highly specific. X-rays, CT, and liver and brain scans are used for localisation.

Chemotherapy. Chemotherapy with albendazole is useful, but cyst aspiration or surgery is still often necessary, being very careful not to spill the infective cyst contents.

Control and prevention is by treating adult worms in farm herbivores, preventing dogs from eating raw infected animal (e.g. sheep) viscera, and hand-washing after dog or soil contact.

Melioidosis

Melioidosis is caused by *Burkholderia* (formerly *Pseudomonas*) *pseudomallei* from soil (p. 52). It causes cutaneous, pulmo-nary and systemic disease. It is found especially in Southeast Asia, Northern Australia and tropical Africa.

The clinical features are acute or chronic suppurative infection or acute septicaemia. Pulmonary disease occurs most often; this may be inapparent, or an acute fulminant infection with cough, sputum, fever, chest pain, tachypnoea, upper lobe consolidation and cavitation.

Confirmatory tests are microscopy for bipolar staining rods, like 'safety pins', and careful culture.

Chemotherapy. Chemotherapy is with ceftazidime and imi/meropenem for 30 days, followed by co-trimoxazole for 3–6 months.

Control and prevention is by wearing shoes, gloves while gardening, and early energetic wound care.

Nocardiosis

Characteristics of nocardiosis are chronic abscess formation with suppuration and spread, especially in skin and subcutaneous tissues, producing a mycetoma (p. 202), or cavitating pulmonary disease mimicking tuberculosis or actinomycosis. It occurs particularly in immunocompromised patients, e.g. after organ transplantation. Many other organs have been infected by systemic spread.

Causative organism is usually *N. asteroides* (p. 62), rarely other species.

Clinical features of lung disease are chronic cough, thick sputum, chest pain, dyspnoea and fever with moderate systemic symptoms.

Confirmatory tests are Gram stain to show characteristic thin, beaded, branch-

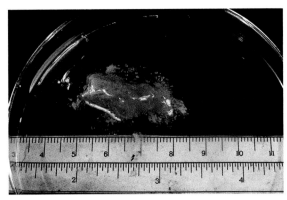

Fig. 1 **Bronchial plug in allergic aspergillosis.**

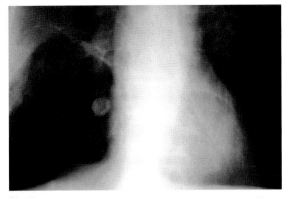

Fig. 2 **Small calcified hydatid cyst in right lung near cardiac border.**

ing Gram-positive filaments, a modified acid-fast stain to show weakly acid fast filaments, and aerobic culture for at least 1 week.

Chemotherapy. Chemotherapy is with long-term sulphonamides, or amikacin plus meropenem.

Control and prevention involves care of soil-contaminated wounds and of immunocompromised patients.

Paragonimiasis

Paragonimiasis is caused by the lung fluke *Paragonimus westermani* (p. 91). Humans are infected by eating encysted larvae in crabs or crayfish. These excyst in the stomach and migrate to cause human pulmonary cavitating infection. Expectorated sputum infects snails, the other intermediate host.

Clinical features are fever, cough, sputum, haemoptysis, dyspnoea and severe chest pain. Fibrosis, bronchiectasis and pleural effusions follow. Worms spread to other organs, especially the nervous system, causing fits, paralyses or blindness.

Confirmatory tests are microscopy of sputum or faeces for the characteristic large operculated eggs, chest x-ray, and CT or other scans of other infected organs.

Chemotherapy. Chemotherapy is with praziquantel, or bithionol as an alternative.

Control and prevention depends on education, sanitation and avoiding uncooked crabs and crayfish. The snails and definitive hosts are difficult to control.

Systemic mycoses

Five major fungi cause systemic mycoses (p. 70–73). Respiratory disease is acute at the time of infection in coccidioidomycosis and histoplasmosis; progressive pulmonary disease is rare.

Blastomycosis

Blastomyces dermatitidis is a dimorphic soil fungus endemic in parts of N. America and Africa. It infects by inhalation. Asymptomatic lung infection is common, but symptomatic lung disease is rare. Chronic bone and skin disease is usual, with broad-based budding yeasts and granuloma formation. Itraconazole is used for most infections, amphotericin for severe infections.

Coccidioidomycosis

Coccidioides immitis is a dimorphic soil fungus endemic in areas of the Americas and infects by inhalation. Asymptomatic pulmonary infection is most common, followed by symptomatic pulmonary disease; progressive or systemic disease is rare. Arthroconidia and tissue spherules filled with spores are characteristic; granulomata resembling tuberculosis occur. Amphotericin is usual initial therapy, then itraconazole.

Cryptococcosis

Cryptococcus neoformans is a monomorphic yeast with a characteristic capsule, found particularly in pigeon droppings. It infects humans by inhalation. It can infect humans with a normal immune system, though 50% of those infected have a detectable immune deficiency.

Infection causes pulmonary masses (often asymptomatic), chronic meningitis or organ masses. Classical treatment is amphotericin plus flucytosine, though fluconazole is used both acutely and for long-term suppression in the immunocompromised patient.

Histoplasmosis

Histoplasma capsulatum is a dimorphic fungus; the filamentous mould form is found in soil with bird or bat droppings, and certain endemic areas are notorious for histoplasmosis. Spores are inhaled and germinate to the yeast, which is ingested by macrophages. The clinical disease depends on the dose inhaled, the immune state and local lung disease (p. 71). Treatment is voriconazole or amphotericin B, or oral itraconazole.

Paracoccidioidomycosis

Paracoccidioides brasiliensis is a dimorphic fungus endemic in S. America. It is probably a soil organism and may infect by inhalation or possibly by implantation. Chronic progressive skin and mucous membrane ulcers are usual; pulmonary or systemic disease is rare. Multiple budding gives a 'pilot's wheel' appearance microscopically, with granulomata. Itraconazole is replacing amphotericin plus sulphonamides in treatment.

Tropical or rare respiratory infections

- Actinomycosis is a rare chronic cavitating pneumonia.
- Aspergillosis can involve:
  – allergic broncho-pulmonary aspergillosis in asthmatics
  – aspergilloma (fungus ball) in a pre-existing cavity or cyst
  – fulminant pneumonia, usually in the immunocompromised host.
- Hydatid disease has rounded 'cannon ball' lung cysts.
- Melioidosis is a fulminant fatal cavitating pneumonia.
- Nocardiosis is a chronic cavitating pneumonia similar to tuberculosis.
- Paragonimiasis causes progressive cavitating lung damage.
- Of the systemic mycoses, only coccidioidomycosis and histoplasmosis are characterised by acute pulmonary disease at the time of infection; progressive pulmonary disease is rare in all systemic mycoses.

Suppurative thrombophlebitis / lymphangitis / lymphadenitis

Suppurative thrombophlebitis

Suppurative or septic thrombophlebitis is venous infection with thrombosis ('thrombophlebitis' without an adjective is venous thrombosis with inflammation rather than infection). It is classified into:

- superficial
- pelvic
- portal (called 'pylephlebitis')
- intracranial.

It arises from intravenous catheters and other intravascular devices, from intravenous drug use (IVDU), or from local skin or tissue infections. It gives rise to local spread, or distant spread by bacteraemia or septic emboli (Table 1).

Causative organisms

- In superficial infection, *S. aureus* and coagulase negative staphylococci are now less common than enteric Gram-negative rods (GNRs), especially *Klebsiella* or *Enterobacter* spp. *Candida albicans* occurs particularly with parenteral nutrition or IVDU.
- In pelvic infection, streptococci and anaerobes predominate.
- In pylephlebitis, enteric GNRs, enterococci and anaerobes are dominant.
- In intracranial infection, *S. aureus* and/or respiratory flora are usual.

Clinical features

Superficial septic thrombophlebitis when acute (Fig. 1) causes local redness, swelling, tenderness and pain, with pus from any puncture or sinus. Subacute infection, especially in burns patients, may have mainly systemic manifestations with fever and shock, and few local signs. Both lead to bacteraemia, septic emboli and distant abscesses, especially pulmonary.

Pelvic thrombophlebitis follows childbirth, abortion or pelvic surgery, and again causes mainly systemic signs with high fever, chills, and vomiting, few abdominal signs, then septic pulmonary emboli and lung abscesses.

Portal thrombophlebitis follows appendicitis or other intra-abdominal infection, causes high fever and signs of sepsis, and leads to septic emboli and liver abscesses.

Intracranial thrombophlebitis can be in the cortical veins or the cavernous, lateral, sagittal or petrosal venous sinuses. It follows local facial, oral, ear or paranasal sinus infection, and causes (depending on the venous sinus involved), peri-orbital swelling (Fig. 2), various cranial nerve lesions, limb weakness, sensory impairment, fits and coma. Urgent neurological and surgical consultation is essential. Uncontrolled infection is fatal.

Confirmatory tests

Microscopy and culture of pus if present, and several blood cultures are essential. Chest x-ray may show lung abscesses and pleural fluid. In pelvic, portal or intracranial thrombosis, CT scanning or other special imaging is usually needed.

Chemotherapy

- Superficial suppurative thrombophlebitis needs surgical excision as well as appropriate antibiotics for cure.
- Pelvic thrombophlebitis responds slowly to antibiotics such as penicillin and metronidazole, while abscesses need drainage, and the infected veins may need ligation.

- Pylephlebitis needs appropriate antibiotics against gut flora, such as ampicillin, gentamicin and metronidazole, plus removal of the cause, and drainage of abscesses.
- Intracranial suppurative thrombophlebitis needs flucloxacillin plus metronidazole, surgery for the source and any abscesses, and control of intra-cranial pressure and of fits.

Control and prevention

This depends on early recognition and treatment of the cause.

Lymphangitis

This is characterised by inflammation of the lymphatics, usually subcutaneous. It is classified into **acute**, which is usually bacterial, or **chronic**, usually fungal, mycobacterial or filarial.

Causative organisms

Acute lymphangitis (Fig. 3) is usually due to *S. pyogenes* or rarely to *S. aureus* after injury, *Pasteurella multocida* after animal bites, or *Wuchereria bancrofti* after mosquito bites.

Chronic lymphangitis is often due to *Sporothrix schenckii*, also to *M. marinum*, *Nocardia* spp. (Fig. 4), or *W. bancrofti* (p. 86).

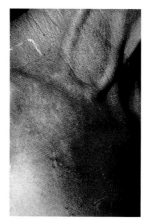

Fig. 1 **Jugular vein thrombophlebitis with thrombosis.**

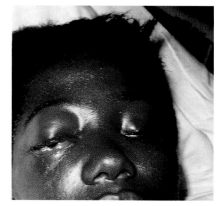

Fig. 2 **Cavernous sinus thrombosis with periorbital swelling obscuring 3rd, 4th and 6th nerve paralyses.**

Table 1 **Suppurative thrombophlebitis**					
Classification	**Causative organism**	**Clinical features**	**Confirmatory tests**	**Chemotherapy**	**Control**
Superficial	*S. aureus*, GNRs, anaerobes	Pus, local signs	M&C of pus, blood cultures	Flucloxacillin and excision	Asepsis
Pelvic	Streptococci, anaerobes	Systemic signs, lung abscess	Blood cultures, CT, imaging	Broad spectrum, drain, ligate	Prevent cause
Portal ('pylephlebitis')	Enteric GNRs, anaerobes	Systemic signs, liver abscess	Blood cultures, CT, imaging	Broad spectrum, drain, excise	Prevent cause
Intracranial	*S. aureus*, respiratory flora	Orbital oedema, cranial nerve and cerebral lesions Fits and coma	Blood cultures, CT, imaging	Flucloxacillin and metronidazole Surgery for cause, drain	Prevent cause

Table 2 **Infective lymphadenitis**

Classification	Causative organism	Clinical features	Confirmatory laboratory tests	Chemotherapy	Control
Bacterial					
Pyogenic	S. pyogenes	Cervical, regional	Throat, wound culture	Penicillin	Avoidance
Vincent's angina	Anaerobes	Cervical	M&C, anaerobic	Penicillin	Mouth care
Diphtheria	C. diphtheriae	Cervical	Specific culture	Penicillin	Immunise
TB	M. tuberculosis	Cervical	AFB M&C of pus	Triple	BCG
Chancroid	H. ducreyi	Inguinal	Special culture	Ceftriaxone	Safer sex
Plague	Y. pestis	Inguinal	Gram stain	Gentamicin and tetracycline	Rats + fleas
Syphilis 1	T. pallidum	Inguinal	Dark field micro	Penicillin	Safer sex
LGV	C. trachomatis	Inguinal	Serology	Azithromycin	Safer sex
Anthrax	B. anthracis	Regional	M&C	Penicillin	Of zoonosis
Listeriosis	L. monocytogenes	Regional	M&C, motility	Penicillin	Food hygiene
Rat-bite fever	S. moniliformis	Regional	Culture	Penicillin	Avoid rats
	S. minor	Regional	Dark field micro	Penicillin	Avoid rats
Tularaemia	F. tularensis	Regional	Serology	Streptomycin or gentamicin	Rodents/ticks
Brucella	Brucella spp.	General	Serology, culture	Streptomycin and tetracycline	Of zoonosis
Leptospirosis	Leptospira spp.	General	Serology	Penicillin	Rat control
Melioidosis	B. pseudomallei	General	Culture	Ceftazidime + meropenem	Wound care
Miliary TB	M. tuberculosis	General	CXR, Mantoux, AFB	Triple	BCG
Syphilis 2°	T. pallidum	General	Serology	Penicillin	Safer sex
Rickettsia					
Rickettsialpox	R. akari	Regional	Serology	Tetracycline	Mice control
Scrub typhus	R. tsutsugamushi	General	Serology (OX-K)	Tetra or chloramphenicol	Mite control
Fungi					
Histoplasmosis	H. capsulatum	General	Serology, CXR	AmB, ketoconazole	No bird faeces
Paracoccidioidomycosis	P. brasiliensis	Regional	M&C, histo, serology	Itraconazole, amB	None known
Parasites					
Filariasis	W. bancrofti	General/local	Blood film	Di-ethyl carbamazine	Mosquito control
Kala-azar	L. donovani	General	Bone marrow	Antimony	Sandfly control
Toxoplasmosis	T. gondii	General	Serology (histo)	Sulpha + pyrimethamine	Avoid hosts
Trypanosomiasis	Trypanosoma spp.	Local/general	Micro, serology	Suramin, melarsoprol	Tsetse control

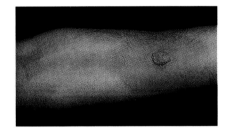

Fig. 3 **Streptococcal infection of a Mantoux test, with lymphangitis.**

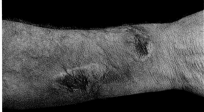

Fig. 4 **Nocardial lymphangitis and nodules in a gardener.**

Clinical features

Acute lymphangitis is characterised by a red streak (Fig. 3) from the primary site of infection towards the enlarged, tender regional lymph nodes. The onset is usually very abrupt with a rigor and high fever before the local infection appears. Recurrent episodes occur if scarring results, and are common in filariasis with chronic oedema, due either to streptococci or the parasite itself.

Chronic lymphangitis follows a granuloma or ulcer at the site of implantation by trauma from plants, wood or soil in sporotrichosis or nocardiosis, from swimming pools or aquaria in M. marinum. Reddish nodules appear and may ulcerate along the proximal lymphatics, palpable as a thickened cord.

Confirmatory tests

- In acute infection, Gram stain and culture of the local lesion, and blood cultures are needed. Nocturnal blood films are more helpful than serology in filariasis. Biopsy is rarely necessary.
- In chronic infection, specific fungal and mycobacterial stains and cultures are done.

Chemotherapy

- In acute infection intravenous penicillin G is needed, or flucloxacillin if staphylococci are likely. In filariasis, di-ethyl carbamazine is given in addition.

- In sporotrichosis, potassium iodide is used.
- In M. marinum infections, rifampicin plus ethambutol, or clarithromycin or co-trimoxazole have all been used with some success, as has surgical excision.

Control and prevention

This depends on avoidance of penetrating injury, or mosquitoes in filarial areas.

Lymphadenitis

Lymphadenitis is infection of lymphatic glands, while lymphadenopathy is enlarged lymph glands from any disease, infectious or non-infectious. Lymphadenitis is not a disease of itself, but a manifestation of many infections: the causative organisms, clinical features, confirmatory laboratory tests, chemotherapy, and control are summarised in Table 2, and detailed on the relevant pages.

Suppurative thrombophlebitis / Lymphangitis / Lymphadenitis

- *Suppurative thrombophlebitis* is bacterial infection of veins with thrombosis; the four major sites (superficial, pelvic, portal and intracranial) determine its features, treatment and control.
- Lymphangitis is inflammation of the lymphatics. Acute bacterial lymphangitis is usually streptococcal, while chronic lymphangitis is usually fungal, parasitic or mycobacterial.
- *Lymphadenitis* (infected lymphatic glands) is cervical, inguinal, regional or general, from a wide variety of bacterial, rickettsial, fungal and parasitic infections, of which streptococcal and tuberculous infections are common and important.

Myocarditis, pericarditis and rheumatic fever

Infections of the heart are classified by the anatomical areas affected (Fig. 1).

Myocarditis

Myocarditis is inflammation, usually caused by infection, of cardiac muscle. Infectious causes are classified by the causative organism into bacterial (rare), viral (commonest) and parasitic. The major infections are:

- Chagas' disease
- Diphtheria
- Lyme disease
- Viral myocarditis.

In addition, rheumatic fever produces a pancarditis, including myocarditis.

Clinical features. Myocarditis of any type produces chest discomfort; cardiac failure causes dyspnoea and oedema. Cardiomegaly causes functional mitral or tricuspid incompetence. Conduction system involvement causes arrhythmias. Arrhythmias and cardiac failure must be treated. If fatal, the heart is dilated with abnormal myocardium (Fig. 2).

Chagas' disease

Chagas' disease is caused by *Trypanosoma cruzi* (p. 83), a flagellated protozoan transmitted by reduviid bugs.

Clinically, the disease has two phases:

- acute infection, often in childhood, causes mild fever, malaise, an indurated red 'chagoma' at the site of infection with regional lymphadenopathy, or periorbital oedema (Romana's sign) from conjunctival infection. Myocarditis is rare but may be fatal.
- chronic Chagas' disease, years or decades later, causes cardiac arrhythmias, thromboembolism or cardiac failure, often right-sided. It may also cause mega-oesophagus or megacolon.

Confirmatory tests in acute disease are microscopic examination of fresh blood or blood films, while chronic disease is diagnosed serologically.

Chemotherapy and control. Benznidazole is most useful in the acute stage. Control and prevention is by insecticides and better housing.

Diphtheria

Diphtheria is caused by *Corynebacterium diphtheriae*. Systemic spread of the toxin results in damage to the heart 1–2 weeks

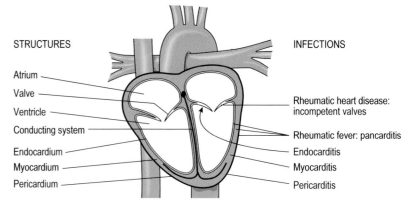

STRUCTURES — Atrium, Valve, Ventricle, Conducting system, Endocardium, Myocardium, Pericardium

INFECTIONS — Rheumatic heart disease: incompetent valves; Rheumatic fever: pancarditis; Endocarditis; Myocarditis; Pericarditis

Fig. 1 **The infections of the heart.**

after infection. Diphtheria (p. 120–121) is treated with penicillin and antitoxin. Vaccination has a major role in prevention.

Lyme disease

Lyme disease is caused by *Borrelia burgdorferi* (p. 58–59), a spirochaete transmitted by ticks. An initial rash occurs at the site of infection; disseminated disease (p. 154) can cause meningitis and arthritis as well as myocarditis. The diagnosis is clinical and serological. Oral doxycycline or amoxicillin is given for 10–21 days for mild myocarditis, with i.v. penicillin or ceftriaxone for 10–21 days for severe myocarditis.

Viral myocarditis

Myocarditis is most commonly caused by viruses, including Coxsackie group B (less often A), other enteroviruses, mumps, influenza and congenital rubella; it can cause acute heart failure or chronic cardiomyopathy. There is no specific treatment.

Pericarditis

Inflammation of the pericardium is classified into purulent, tuberculous, viral, amoebic, fungal and non-infectious causes. Pericarditis of any type produces chest discomfort, usually with fever. Dyspnoea can occur from co-existent myocarditis, from cardiac tamponade (when cardiac function is impaired by pericardial fluid), or later from constriction by fibrosed or calcified pericardium. Unlike myocarditis, oedema and arrhythmias are usually absent.

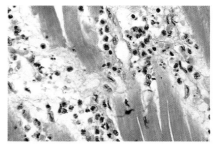

Fig. 2 **Myocarditis.**

Purulent pericarditis

Purulent pericarditis was classically due to spread from pneumococcal pneumonia; it is now more commonly due to staphylococci, enteric flora or other organisms after surgery or septicaemia.

Clinical features include high fever, severe chest pain and signs of sepsis. Urgent chest x-ray, echocardiograph or CT scan define the anatomical changes. Gram stain and culture of the pericardial aspirate define the microbial cause.

Chemotherapy is guided by the Gram stain, then sensitivity tests; initial empiric therapy may be flucloxacillin plus gentamicin. Prevention is by asepsis and treatment of septicaemia.

Tuberculous pericarditis

M. tuberculosis, the cause of tuberculosis (p. 60, 132), can infect the heart by local spread, usually from lung or glands. Clinically, the pericarditis may be acute with little effusion, but it is usually chronic, often with tamponade. Chronic constrictive pericarditis is very characteristic (Fig. 3). The extent of disease and the pathogen are defined as for purulent pericarditis but using AFB stain and cul-

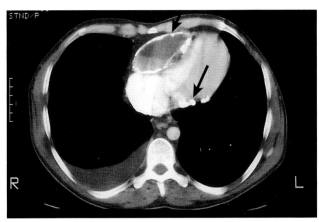

Fig. 3 **Constrictive pericarditis: CT scan.**

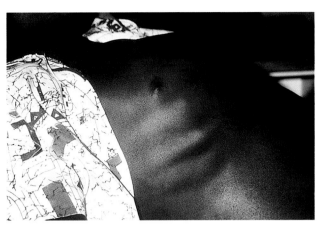

Fig. 5 **Rheumatic fever: chest deformity.**

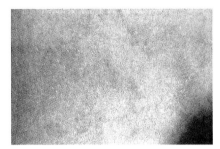

Fig. 4 **Rheumatic heart disease: erythema marginata.**

Table 1 **Modified Jones criteria for diagnosis of acute rheumatic fever: two major criteria or one major plus two minor criteria and evidence of group A streptococcal infection are required**	
Criteria	**Characteristics**
Major criteria	
Carditis	Pancarditis; common
Polyarthritis	Migratory around large joints; common
Erythema marginata	Faint fleeting rare rash (Fig. 4) with red irregular margins moving in minutes or hours like 'smoke rings'
Subcutaneous nodules	Rare; felt over bony prominences or tendons and last 1–2 weeks
Sydenham's chorea (St Vitus's dance)	Rare; rapid involuntary jerking of limbs, face or body
Minor criteria	
Previous ARF or RHD	
Arthralgia	
Fever	
Acute phase reactants	Erythrocyte sedimentation rate, C-reactive protein, white cell count
Evidence of infection	Anti-streptolysin O titre raised, DNAase B raised, positive culture, recent scarlet fever

ARF, acute rheumatic fever; RHD rheumatic heart disease.

ture. Anti-tuberculous triple therapy is required for at least 9 months. Surgery is essential for constriction.

Viral pericarditis

Viral pericarditis (the commonest form) is usually caused by Coxsackie group B (less often A), other enteroviruses, mumps, influenza or varicella. Clinically, there is mild fever and precordial discomfort, sometimes preceded by respiratory or gastrointestinal illness. Infection usually resolves in 2–6 weeks without specific therapy.

Rheumatic fever

Rheumatic fever follows streptococcal (*S. pyogenes*) infection, being a post-infectious complication that results from the immune response. Streptococcal cell wall antigens stimulate antibodies that also react with cardiac sarcolemma, joint and other tissues. The Jones criteria are diagnostic indicators for acute rheumatic fever (ARF, Table 1), which occurs 2–4 weeks after a streptococcal throat infection. Chronic rheumatic heart disease (RHD) results from repeated attacks of *S. pyogenes* with different M antigen types; it remains common in developing countries.

Clinical features. The diagnostic criteria have distinct features (Table 1, Fig. 4).

Complications of rheumatic fever include heart block and cardiac failure acutely, or later rheumatic heart disease, with stenosis or incompetence of aortic, mitral, tricuspid or pulmonary valves. Untreated, cardiac failure, cardiomegaly and even chest deformity follow (Fig. 5), prevented by timely prosthetic valve replacement.

Confirmatory tests. Because of the complications, children with fever and a sore throat should have a throat swab tested for streptococci (p. 36). A rising antibody titre to streptococci is also indicative. ECG often shows prolongation of the P-R interval or, sometimes, higher degrees of block.

Management. Penicillin is given for 10 days with anti-inflammatory drugs (especially aspirin and corticosteroids), bed rest and treatment of cardiac failure and arrhythmias. Penicillin treatment of streptococcal pharyngo-tonsillitis is preventative. Long-term penicillin prophylaxis is given after rheumatic fever; the duration is debated – to age 25, or 30, or lifelong?

Myocarditis, pericarditis and rheumatic fever

- Myocarditis is usually viral, but may be caused by Chagas' disease, diphtheria, Lyme disease or acute rheumatic fever. Rarer causes are toxoplasmosis, trichinellosis and trypanosomiasis. The infection and any resulting arrhythmias or cardiac failure must be treated.

- Pericarditis is also usually viral but may be purulent, tuberculous, amoebic, fungal or rheumatic. The cause is identified by culture, serology, imaging, aspiration and/or surgery.

- Acute rheumatic fever comprises pancarditis, migrating polyarthropathy, chorea and other specific, rare signs. It occurs after group A streptococcal infection, which it is important to confirm by laboratory tests. Chemotherapy with penicillin must be accompanied by anti-inflammatory drugs, and cardiac failure therapy as necessary. Long-term prophylactic penicillin is usually needed to prevent repeat attacks, which lead to rheumatic heart disease.

- The pathogens causing cardiac disease have distinct geographical locations.

Infective endocarditis

Endocarditis is infection of the cardiac valves, or sometimes the mural endothelium. Rarely, a similar clinical picture is due to infective aortitis or an infected coarctation of the aorta or patent ductus arteriosus.

Endocarditis has been **classified** by three major factors:

1. Severity and rapidity of infection (imprecise but useful in early management)
   - acute, developing in days, (often 3–6)
   - subacute, in weeks, (often 3–6)
   - chronic, over months (often 3 or more)
2. Valve type
   - native valve of the patient
   - prosthetic valve
3. Cause of bacteraemia, if known
   - **d**ental, medical or surgical procedures
   - **d**rugs: injecting drug use (IDU or IVDU)
   - **d**evices, e.g. intravascular catheters
   - **d**isease elsewhere, e.g. abscesses.

Endocarditis is further **described** by:

- the infecting microorganism, usually bacterial
- the infected valve(s), usually mitral or aortic, rarely tricuspid valve from IVDU.

The commonest type has been streptococcal subacute bacterial endocarditis (SBE) on native mitral or aortic valves (Fig. 1).

Causative organisms

There are two major causative **factors**:

- Firstly, an abnormal heart valve or endocardium, from congenital, rheumatic or other heart disease, or a prosthesis. All can lead to platelet-fibrin deposition, called non-bacterial thrombotic endocarditis (NBTE).
- Secondly, bacteraemia (or fungaemia) from procedures, drugs (IVDU), devices or disease.

There are five major groups of **pathogens**:

- oral streptococci, and enterococci
- *S. aureus*
- coagulase-negative staphylococci
- enteric Gram-negative rods (GNRs)
- fungi, mainly *Candida* spp.

However almost any microbe can cause endocarditis, including the 'HACEK' group of *Haemophilus aphrophilus* (p. 44), *Actinobacillus* (now *Haemophilus*) *actinomycetemcomitans*, *Cardiobacterium hominis*,

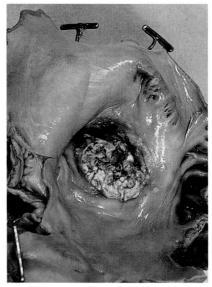

Fig. 1 **Infected 'native' valve.**

Eikenella corrodens (p. 53), and *Kingella kingae* (p. 43), anaerobes (p. 54), *C. psittaci* (p. 65), and *Coxiella burneti* (p. 67).

Pathogenesis

Clinical features are very varied but are basically the result of four mechanisms.

Valve infection produces proliferative 'vegetations', destruction and incompetence, while local spread can give septal abscesses, heart block and, rarely, septal rupture.

Bacteraemia produces fever and systemic symptoms, while metastatic spread can give abscesses in, e.g., the brain or kidney.

Embolisation, especially in Gram-positive and fungal infection, produces distal infarction in the periphery [splinter haemorrhages under finger or toe nails (Fig. 2), or skin or conjunctival petechiae] or in vascular organs, including the spleen (Fig. 3), kidney or brain. Embolisation also causes mycotic aneurysms in arteries (Fig. 4) or distal abscesses including micro abscesses ('Janeway lesions').

Immune complex deposition causes glomerulonephritis commonly, and Osler's nodes rarely; the latter are small painful red lumps in fingertips, palms or soles.

Clinical features

Patients fall into one of five groups:

Acute bacterial endocarditis is commonly due to *S. aureus* (80%), enteric GNRs or *P. aeruginosa*. It causes high fever, sepsis and rapid valve destruction.

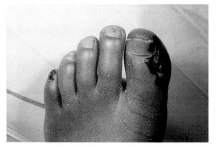

Fig. 2 **'Splinters' and infarcts produced by embolisation.**

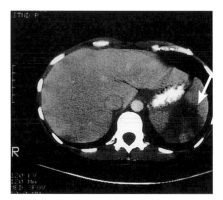

Fig. 3 **Splenic infarct (dark wedge) on CT scan.**

Subacute bacterial endocarditis is commonly due to viridans streptococci, enterococci, staphylococci or unusual Gram-negative rods. It causes weeks of fever, emboli, immunologic phenomena and cardiac murmur(s).

Chronic endocarditis (rare) is due to fungi, Q fever or coagulase-negative staphylococci. It causes months of fever, splenomegaly and murmur(s).

Prosthetic endocarditis occurs either *early* after operation usually due to staphylococci or enteric GNRs, or *late*, 2 months or more after operation, usually due to oral streptococci, enterococci or coagulase-negative staphylococci. Fever, bacteraemia and a new murmur occur earlier than emboli. Perivalvular leaks are serious; an occluded valve is rapidly fatal.

IVDU endocarditis is commonly due to *S. aureus*, streptococci, enteric GNRs, *P. aeruginosa* or *Candida* spp. Fever occurs for 1–2 weeks with tricuspid valve infection and *pulmonary* emboli.

Criteria for diagnosis

As the diagnosis is proven only by surgery or autopsy, various clinical diagnostic criteria have been used. Von Reyn's group proposed detailed criteria and categories. Echocardiograms, especially transoesophageal, so improved diagnosis that the Duke Endocarditis Service proposed new major and minor criteria, since modified (Table 1) which define three diagnostic categories:

1. DEFINITE (positive tissue microbiology, OR positive tissue histopathology OR 2 major criteria OR 1 major plus 3 minor, OR 5 minor criteria),
2. POSSIBLE (1 major plus 1 minor, OR 3 minor alone) or
3. REJECTED (alternate diagnosis, OR response to 4 days' antibiotics, OR negative pathology).

These correlate well with surgical or autopsy confirmation.

Blood cultures are essential to confirm bacteraemia; two urgently are usually sufficient in acute disease, while three or four in 12 hours are usual in subacute disease. Media must be rich with possible supplementation for fastidious organisms. Sensitivity testing with MIC and MBC (p. 240) is needed as body defences in cardiac valves are minimal, so bactericidal drugs are essential. The organism should be stored for 3 months in case of relapse.

Echocardiography is essential to show vegetations or valve dysfunction. Transoesophageal echocardiography (TOE) is needed if transthoracic examination is not diagnostic. Anaemia, neutrophilia or thrombocytopenia are common, and acute phase reactants are high. Serum biochemistry detects renal and/or hepatic impairment.

Management

Appropriate bactericidal antibiotics are given intravenously in high dose for 4–6 weeks, though uncomplicated patients with very sensitive organisms may have shorter courses, with the latter part orally and/or at home. Table 2 shows the usual antibiotics for major pathogens.

Response to therapy is monitored by resolution of fever and fall in acute phase reactants. Serum levels of gentamicin and vancomycin should be monitored.

Surgery is usually needed for prosthetic valve endocarditis (Fig. 5), chronic infection (including fungal endocarditis), culture-negative endocarditis and uncontrolled embolisation. It is essential for uncontrolled infection, any abscess, or uncontrolled cardiac failure.

Control and prevention. Prophylaxis before dental and other procedures likely to cause bacteraemia has not been proven effective, but logical regimens before risky procedures are widely advocated in patients at risk:

- High-risk patients include those with a prosthetic valve or previous endocarditis.
- High-risk procedures are those highly likely to cause bacteraemia, including dental extractions and periodontal, gastrointestinal and genitourinary procedures.
- Oral amoxicillin is usually advocated for lower-risk patients and procedures, replaced by clindamycin if the patient is hypersensitive to, or on long-term, penicillin.
- Intravenous ampi/amoxicillin plus gentamicin is usually advocated for high-risk patients and/or procedures; vancomycin replaces ampi/amoxicillin if the patient is hypersensitive to, or on long-term, penicillin.

Table 1 Duke Endocarditis Service Modified diagnostic criteria (abbreviated)

Major criteria	Typical blood culture
	Positive echocardiogram
	New valvular regurgitation
	Positive Q fever serology
Minor criteria	Predisposition
	Fever
	Vascular phenomena
	Immune phenomena
	Suggestive microbiology/serology
	Positive PCR on blood or tissue (suggested)
	New cardiac failure or conduction defects (suggested)

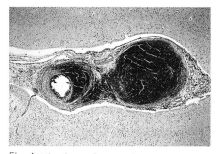

Fig. 4 **Histology of a mycotic aneurysm.**

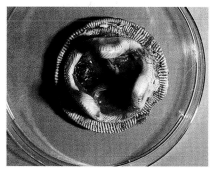

Fig. 5 **Infected prosthetic valve.**

Table 2 Antibiotic treatment

Microbe	Primary antibiotic[a]	Duration	Low dose gentamicin
Sensitive streptococci	Benzylpenicillin	2–4 weeks	2 weeks
Relatively resistant streptococci	Benzylpenicillin	6 weeks	4–6 weeks
Enterococci	Ampi- or amoxicillin	6 weeks	4–6 weeks
Staphylococci	Flucloxacillin	6 weeks	1–2 weeks
Gram-negative rods	Third generation cephalosporin	6 weeks	4–6 weeks
Fungal endocarditis	Amphotericin B	6 weeks or more	An azole
Other organisms	According to sensitivity tests		
Culture negative	Initially benzylpenicillin with gentamicin, then according to most likely organism(s)		

[a] Patients hypersensitive to penicillins may be de-sensitised, or treated with a cephalosporin or vancomycin.

Infective endocarditis

- Endocarditis is infection of the cardiac valves or mural endocardium. It is usually bacterial, sometimes fungal.
- The two causative factors are 'soil' and 'seed': platelet-fibrin deposition on abnormal endothelium or valve; bacteraemia.
- The major causative organisms are oral streptococci, staphylococci, enterococci, Gram-negative rods and *Candida* spp.
- The clinical features result from four mechanisms: valve and heart damage, systemic bacteraemia (with fever and distant abscesses), emboli (causing distant infarcts and aneurysms) and immune complex deposition (causing, e.g., glomerulonephritis).
- Endocarditis on prosthetic valves or in intravenous drug users has special additional features.
- Confirmation is mainly by blood cultures and echocardiogram (see criteria).
- Management involves high-dose, long-term treatment with (a) suitable antibiotic(s).
- Surgery is needed for uncontrolled infection or cardiac failure.
- Prophylaxis, usually with amoxicillin, is given to those with valve disease before procedures likely to cause bacteraemia.

Bacteraemia, septicaemia and fungaemia

1. Bacteraemia or fungaemia are characterised by live organisms in the blood, shown by a positive blood culture. These two terms do *not* describe the clinical condition, which varies from asymptomatic to mildly unwell to seriously ill.
2. Septicaemia (called 'sepsis', or 'the septic syndrome' in some countries), in contrast, is a *clinical* description meaning severe infection with fever, rigors ('shaking chills'), tachycardia and severe systemic symptoms. Bacteraemia is usually found.
3. Septic shock means septicaemia plus low blood pressure, vascular collapse, and decreased organ perfusion, so oliguria

with renal, cardiac and other organ failure result, with high mortality. Septic shock occurs through widespread immune responses to endotoxins and other pathogen components (p. 32).

One useful **classification** (Table 1) divides bacteraemias into:

- focal source found on clinical examination
- no focal source found, hence the epidemiologic *setting* guides investigation and empirical therapy.

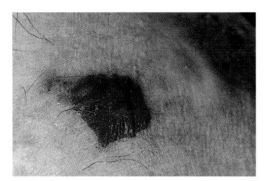

Fig. 1 **Septic embolus in *S. aureus* septicaemia. Diameter 2 cm, on arm.**

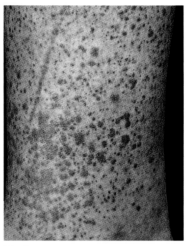

Fig. 2 **Vasculitis in *S. aureus* septicaemia.**

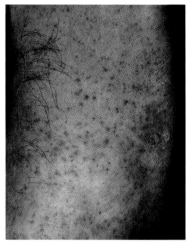

Fig. 3 **Haemorrhagic rash in meningococcal septicaemia.**

Table 1 **Classification and characteristics of septicaemia**

Classification	Causative organism (commonest only)	Clinical features	Chemotherapy (typical)	Control
With focal source		**Specific**		
Skin	Staphylococci	Furuncles	Flucloxacillin	Early treatment
	S. pyogenes	Erysipelas	Penicillin	Early treatment
CNS	N. meningitidis	Meningitis	Penicillin	Immunise some groups
	S. pneumoniae	Abscess (Fig. 5)	Penicillin	Immunise some groups
Ear or sinus	S. pneumoniae	Otitis media	Penicillin	Early treatment and immunise some groups
	H. influenzae	Sinusitis	Ceftriaxone	
Lungs	S. pneumoniae	Pneumonia	Penicillin	Immunise some groups
	H. influenzae	Abscess	Ceftriaxone	Immunise some groups
Heart	Streptococci	Endocarditis	Penicillin	Chemoprophylaxis
	Staphylococci		Fluclox ± Gent	Early treatment
Intravascular device	Staphylococci, resistant GNR	None, or local pus	Vanco + Gent	Asepsis
Abdomen	Aerobic GNR	Peritonitis	Ampi + Gent + Metro	Early treatment
	Anaerobes	Abscess	Ampi + Gent + Metro	
Bone or joint	Staphylococci	Osteomyelitis	Flucloxacillin	Early treatment
	H. influenzae	Septic arthritis	Ceftriaxone	
No focal source		**Non-specific**		
AIDS	S. pneumoniae	Dyspnoea	Timentin + Gent	Immunise
Cardiac valve disease	Streptococci,	Murmur	Penicillin	Chemoprophylaxis
	Staphylococci	Emboli	Fluclox ± Gent	Early treatment
Community acquired	GPC, GNR	None specific	Cefazolin + Gent	Immunise
Hospital acquired	GPC, GNR, P. aeruginosa	Wound, UTI, pneumonia	Timentin + Gent	Asepsis
Neonatal	Group B streptococci, GNR, Listeria sp.	Often none localising	Ampi + Gent	Asepsis
Neutropenia	GPC, resistant GNR	Often none localising	Timentin + Gent	Asepsis, chemoprophylaxis
Splenectomy	S. pneumoniae, H. influenzae	Often none localising	Penicillin, Ceftriaxone	Immunise

Ampi, ampicillin; Fluclox, flucloxacillin; Gent, gentamicin; Metro, metronidazole; Vanco, vancomycin; GNR, Gram-negative rods; GPC, Gram-positive cocci.

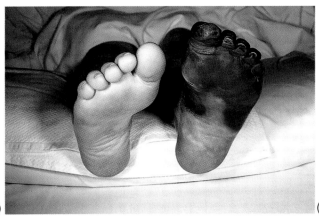 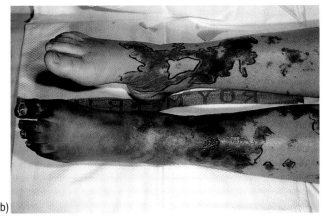

(a) (b)

Fig. 4 **Infarcted toes and forefoot with severe haemorrhagic rash in meningococcal septicaemia.**

Causative organisms

The pathogen depends on the *source* and the *setting* (Table 1). In general, staphylococci and streptococci are commoner than Gram-negative rods, while anaerobes, fungi and other organisms are uncommon.

Clinical features

Clinical features fall into four groups:

- general features of sepsis are found in all septicaemic patients: fever, headache, rigors ('shaking chills'), malaise, tachycardia and hypotension with pale, cold extremities
- specific clues are found in some patients:
  - a splenectomy scar
  - septic emboli, especially in staphylococcal sepsis (Fig. 1), which may also show vasculitis (Fig. 2)
  - meningococcal haemorrhagic rash with petechiae (Fig. 3), larger haemorrhages, and even digital or forefoot infarction (Fig. 4)
- focal sources of infection, if present, show their own distinctive clinical features (Table 1)
- epidemiologic *setting* may be vital (Table 1).

Confirmatory tests

Blood cultures, and microscopy and culture from likely sites, are always needed to find the organism. PCR may help. Chest x-ray, CT and other imaging are often needed to find the site. Serology is rarely useful in time.

Chemotherapy

This obviously depends mainly on the pathogen and the severity of disease, and to a lesser degree on the source, if known. Initial treatment is usually broad spectrum, with modification when the pathogen and source are found (Table 1). Surgery to drain abscesses and remove necrotic tissue is essential. Circulatory, respiratory and renal support is essential in sepsis and septic shock.

Control

Immunisation or chemoprophylaxis may be feasible to protect those with predisposing factors such as valve lesions, neutropenia or splenectomy. Aseptic technique is essential for hospital procedures, including intravascular device insertion and maintenance. Early treatment prevents progression to septicaemia.

> **Bacteraemia, septicaemia and fungaemia**
>
> - Viable bacteria or fungi in the blood are known respectively as bacteraemia or fungaemia.
> - Septicaemia is the clinical syndrome resulting from bacteraemia (or fungaemia). It can have a known focal source or be without an obvious cause, when the epidemiological setting is important.
> - Septic shock is septicaemia with hypotension and impaired tissue and organ perfusion.
> - Clinical features to be sought are:
>   - general signs of sepsis: fever, rigors and tachycardia
>   - specific signs giving clues to cause, e.g. meningococcal rash
>   - specific focal source
>   - epidemiologic setting.
> - Chemotherapy initially is usually broad spectrum, with modification when the pathogen and site are found.
> - Corrective surgery is necessary for abscesses and infarcts.
> - Circulatory, respiratory and renal support is essential in sepsis and septic shock.
> - Chemoprophylaxis, immunisation and aseptic technique reduce the risk of bacteraemia in predisposed groups of patients.

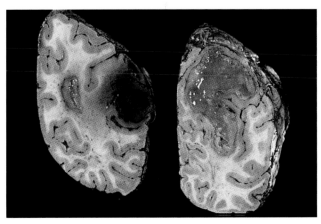

Fig. 5 **Multiple cerebral abscesses in cyanotic heart disease.**

Viral systemic infections

VIRAL INFECTIONS OF MOTHER, FETUS AND NEONATE

These are summarised in Table 1.

Non-viral infections of mother, fetus and neonate
See p. 214–215.

CHILDHOOD AND YOUTH

Cytomegalovirus (CMV) infections

Characteristics. CMV causes a range of infections at all ages characterised by latency, so immunosuppression causes re-activation.

Causative agent is human CMV, an enveloped double-stranded DNA herpes virus with only one serotype. Replication is described in p. 16–17 – mRNA is both (uniquely) brought into the host cell by the virus and also transcribed by host cell RNA polymerase, then translated into early non-structural proteins including DNA polymerase in the cytoplasm. This viral DNA polymerase then replicates genome DNA and late struc-

tural proteins, which are transported to the nucleus for viral assembly, then coated with envelope on exiting from the nucleus. *Transmission* is transplacental or by breast milk, saliva, sex and blood.

Clinical features vary with the host:
- In the fetus and neonates, CMV causes the **congenital CMV syndrome** in 20%, with microcephaly, fits, mental retardation, hepatosplenomegaly and jaundice (Table 1).
- In the immunocompetent, infection is often **asymptomatic**, or causes a **glandular fever-like** disease – see below.
- In the immunocompromised, it causes **severe organ disease** in eyes, brain and gut particularly – see HIV/AIDS (p. 149–151).

Confirmatory tests include PCR on body fluids or tissues, or serology for IgG and IgM, or stains for inclusion bodies in urine or tissues.

Chemotherapy is with i.v. ganciclovir or oral valganciclovir, which inhibit DNA polymerase. Foscarnet or cidofovir is used for resistant strains.

Control and prevention is by serology and amniotic fluid testing in pregnancy, and by chemoprophylaxis during known immunosuppression.

Epstein–Barr virus (EBV) infections

Characteristics. EBV is a herpesvirus like CMV, characterised by latency, re-activation with immune impairment, but also associated with neoplasia.

Causative agent is EBV, structurally identical with other herpesviruses but antigenically distinct with a viral capsid antigen (VCA), early antigens (EA) and nuclear antigen (EBNA), all used in diagnostic tests. Replication is like CMV, but mainly in B lymphocytes. Transmission is mainly by saliva.

Clinical features vary:
- **Asymptomatic** infection is usual and widespread in childhood.
- **Glandular fever** or **infectious mononucleosis** is due to first infection in youth or adulthood. Fever, pharyngitis, lethargy and lymphadenopathy occur, often with splenomegaly and rash, even purpura. Hepatitis or encephalitis is rarer. Total clinical recovery is usual but may take months. Causes of this syndrome include **C**MV, **H**IV seroconversion, **E**BV, **S**econdary syphilis and **T**oxoplasmosis (author's mnemonic).

Table 1 Possible effects of viral infections in pregnancy, to neonates, and in childhood

Organism	Mother in pregnancy	Fetus	Neonate vertical	Neonate post-natal	Child and youth
Cytomegalovirus	Investigate	Congenital CMV syndrome	Congenital CMV	Pneumonitis, hepatitis, haemolysis	Subclinical or glandular fever-like
Enterovirus					
Polio	Abortion, prematurity	No embryopathy	Flaccid paralysis	Polio in 5%	Vaccine prevents
Echo	Fever, coryza, gut symptoms	No embryopathy	Moderate & recover, or severe 'sepsis' & die	Usually mild, rarely organ infections	Rarely rash, meningitis, or myocarditis, as adults
Coxsackie	Stillbirth	Possible embryopathy	Mild in 50%, rarely fulminant	Often myocarditis, meningitis, other organs, 'sepsis'	Rarely rash, meningitis, or myocarditis, as adults
Hepatitis A	Usually none	No embryopathy	Hepatitis rare	Usually mild (hazard to others)	Usual mild hepatitis
Hepatitis B	Premature labour	No embryopathy Infection depends on maternal Ag	Mother eAg–, 20% infected Mother eAg+, 80% infected	Chronic carriage in 90% if infected in 1st month	New infection if IVDU Chronic carriage persists
Hepatitis C	Usually none	6% infected if mother RNA PCR+ (45% if also HIV+)	Hepatitis at fetal rate	Infection rare with care	As adult
HIV	Premature labour in 20%	No embryopathy Infection risk high if mother untreated	HIV and opportunistic infections and organ lesions	Rare with care	30% worsen rapidly
Herpes simplex	Usually none	5% of neonatal HSV Brain, eye, skin	85% of total. Local skin or eye, or disseminated (70% die) or pneumonia, or meningoencephalitis	10% of total. As vertical (local, or disseminated, or organ infection)	As adult
Measles	Abortion, premature labour	No embryopathy Rare isolated defects	Severe measles if mother has acute measles (no Ab)	Mild (modified by maternal antibody)	As adult
Mumps	Miscarriage	Possible embryopathy	Mild. Parotitis rare	Pneumonitis rare	Diabetes commoner
Papilloma virus	Warts worsen	Unaffected	Laryngeal papillomata	Laryngeal papilloma	Genital lesions (?abuse)
Parvovirus	Anaemia	Anaemia, hydrops, fetal death	Marrow suppression, hepatitis, myocarditis	Rare, mild, non-specific	'Slapped cheek' = Erythema infectiosum
Rubella	Usually none	Congenital rubella	Congenital rubella	Very mild	Usual mild disease
Varicella zoster virus	Usually none	Congenital varicella syndrome	Congenital varicella syndrome	Mild to fatal if mother has active infection at birth	1st infection, varicella. If re-activation, zoster

- X-linked lymphoproliferative syndrome in a rare congenital immune deficiency causes fatal infectious mononucleosis.
- **Burkitt's lymphoma** in Africa, nasopharyngeal carcinoma and some thymic carcinomas contain EBV and/or EBV DNA or EBNA, but the mechanism of carcinogenesis is still unclear.
- **Hairy leukoplakia** is a non-malignant white lingual lesion in AIDS (p. 150).

Confirmatory tests are FBE showing atypical lymphocytes, Paul Bunnell or similar test for heterophile antibodies (which agglutinate sheep red cells) from host-cell antigen modified by EBV. Tests for VCA (IgM in early illness, IgG shows prior infection) and EBNA help diagnostic difficulties.

Chemotherapy is usually unnecessary; i.v. aciclovir may help overwhelming infection.

Control and prevention is rarely feasible. No vaccine exists.

Measles (Rubeola)

Characteristics are conjunctivitis, coryza, Koplik's spots, cough, and confluent rash.

Causative agent is the measles virus, a single-stranded RNA virus having an envelope with haemagglutinin and fusion protein spikes. Replication uses a RNA polymerase to transcribe the negative polarity genome into mRNA. Transmission is by respiratory droplets, with high attack rates and severe disease unless immune.

Clinical features are as above. Koplik's spots are diagnostic, small white dots with a bright red rim on the oral mucosa. The rash soon follows, first face, then all over (Fig. 1).

Complications include pneumonia or otitis media commonly, encephalitis rarely, and SSPE very rarely (p. 96–97, 100).

Confirmatory tests are usually unnecessary, though PCR and serology are available.

Chemotherapy is not available.

Control and prevention is by vaccine, usually live attenuated, given with mumps and rubella as 'MMR'. Usually given after 15 months of age, plus a booster.

Mumps

Characteristics are mild systemic symptoms and parotitis, though about 30% of infections are asymptomatic.

Causative agent is the mumps virus, a paramyxovirus (Fig. 2) like measles, with similar replication and transmission.

Clinical features are fever and malaise followed by uni- or bilateral parotitis.

Complications are benign 'aseptic' meningitis (p. 94–95) and orchitis, which if bilateral in post-pubertal men can cause sterility.

Confirmatory tests are rarely needed, but IgM and IgG serology is reliable.

Chemotherapy is not available.

Control and prevention is with the live attenuated MMR vaccine.

Parvovirus (Erythrovirus) B19 infection

Characteristics depend on the time of infection.

Causative agent is the only single-stranded DNA virus infecting humans. Replication (and assembly) is in the nucleus of host endothelial cells and immature RBCs. The viral DNA has hairpin loops at each end making double-stranded areas for the cellular DNA polymerase for genome synthesis, and cellular RNA polymerase for mRNA synthesis. Transmission is intra-uterine or by inhalation.

Clinical features vary (Table 1):
- **Mild anaemia, arthritis or no symptoms** in pregnancy
- **FDIU** (fetal death in utero) in the first trimester, or **hydrops fetalis** (gross oedema from heart failure from anaemia) in the second trimester
- **Erythema infectiosum (slapped cheek disease, fifth disease)**, of childhood exanthemata after measles, rubella, scarlet fever and roseola) in childhood, with mild fever, coryza and bright red cheek rash, with fine lacy body rash (Fig. 3), soon recovering completely
- **Arthritis** from immune complexes, as in hepatitis B and rubella
- **Aplastic crises** in those with chronic anaemias such as thalassaemia
- **Chronic B19 infection** in the immunocompromised, with anaemia, leucopenia or pancytopenia.

Confirmatory tests are IgM and IgG serology, or PCR on blood or amniotic fluid.

Chemotherapy is not available, though pooled immune globulin is used in immunodeficiency.

Control and prevention is by isolation.

Rubella

Characteristics. Rubella in childhood is a mild disease characterised by rash and lymphadenopathy.

Causative agent is the rubella virus, a single-stranded enveloped RNA virus of the Togavirus family. Replication: The RNA is positive polarity so needs no viral polymerase for mRNA, translating directly into proteins including a RNA polymerase for genome replication in the cytoplasm, the envelope forming from the cell outer membrane. Transmission is by inhalation of droplets, or intra-uterine.

Clinical features are:
- **Congenital rubella syndrome** with malformations of eye (cataract), brain (mental retardation and deafness) and heart from maternal infection in the 1st trimester.

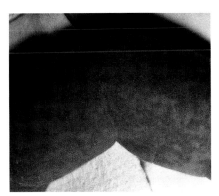

Fig. 1 **Measles: severe in a neonate, with little normal skin.**

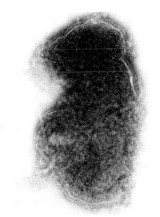

Fig. 2 **Paramyxoviruses cause mumps and measles.**

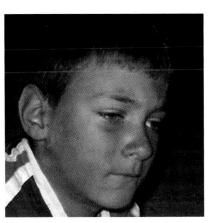

Fig. 3 **Parvovirus infection with slapped cheek.**

- **Rubella** in post-natal infections, with mild fever, macular face and trunk rash for 3 days, and posterior auricular lymphadenopathy.

Confirmatory tests are IgM for recent infection, and IgG for past infection by HI or ELISA on serum, and PCR on fluids or swabs.

Chemotherapy is not available.

Control and prevention is by vaccine, usually live attenuated, given with measles and mumps as 'MMR'.

Varicella zoster

Characteristics Varicella-zoster virus, like other herpesviruses, causes a range of infections at all ages, characterised by latency and hence re-activation with immunosuppression.

Causative agent is one virus, causing all three clinical syndromes. Replication is like CMV and HSV. Transmission is by inhalation of droplets, or intra-uterine.

Clinical features are:

- **Congenital varicella syndrome** of skin scars, limb hypoplasia and chorioretinitis from maternal infection in the 1st four months.
- **Varicella (chickenpox)** in post-natal primary infections, varying from mild

(Fig. 4) to very severe, with fever, malaise, and macular to papular to vesicular itchy centripetal rash. **Complications** include secondary bacterial skin infection (common), purpura, and organ infection, particularly pneumonia, especially in older or immuno-compromised patients.

- **Herpes zoster (shingles)** is due to re-activation years after varicella, with pain then vesicular rash in one or more unilateral dermatomes. It may be ophthalmic (often with keratitis or uveitis), or followed by postherpetic neuralgia (PHN) for weeks or months, or be recurrent, chronic or bilateral in the severely immunosuppressed, e.g. AIDS.

Confirmatory tests are seldom needed, but PCR on swabs or fluids gives rapid specific diagnosis, and IgM and IgG by EIA is also available.

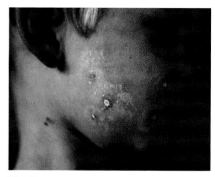

Fig. 4 **Chickenpox rash on face.** All four siblings were infected.

Chemotherapy. High-dose i.v. aciclovir or oral fam- or valaciclovir is useful if given early.

Control and prevention. Passive protection is available with Zoster Immune Globulin (ZIG), and a live attenuated vaccine is now widely available.

> ### Viral systemic infections of the young
>
> - Viral systemic infections of the young can be intra-uterine, intra- or post-partum from mother, in-hospital (neonatal) from staff, visitors or equipment, or in childhood or youth (see Table 1).
> - The 'childhood exanthemata' including measles, rubella, chickenpox, roseola and parvovirus all have fever, rash (of characteristic type) and constitutional symptoms.
> - Hepatitis B and C, HIV and the Herpes family are characterised by latent and/or chronic disease.
> - Passive protection with specific immunoglobulin is most useful in varicella.
> - Vaccines prevent measles, mumps, rubella, polio, varicella and hepatitis A & B, and now papillomavirus.

ALL AGES

Arboviral infections

Many systemic viral infections are from one of over 125 human **arbo**viruses ('**arthrop**od **bo**rne'), while a few are **robo**viruses (**ro**dent **bo**rne). In addition, many arboviruses have a rodent reservoir. 'Arbovirus' denotes the transmission mode, and is not a family – indeed it contains numerous members from five families. Most arboviruses have a defined geographic location. They cause four major clinical syndromes, though numerous individual viruses cause more than one syndrome (Table 1):

- Encephalitis (Fig. 1 and p. 96–97, 100–101)
- Arthritis with rash
- Fever with myalgia – see also Dengue below
- Viral haemorrhagic fever (VHF, including dengue HF), with three sub-types:
  – VHF with jaundice (particularly yellow fever)

  – VHF with pulmonary syndrome (Sin Nombre virus)
  – VHF with renal syndrome = HFRS (bunyaviruses).

VHF is also caused by *non*-arboviruses of the Arenavirus and Filovirus families, infecting directly from rodent reservoirs or infected humans with no known arthropod vector.

Arthritis with rash

The commonest arboviruses causing this syndrome are Chikungunya, O'nyong-nyong and Sindbis in Africa, and Barmah Forest and Ross River fever in Australia. In addition to the usual systemic symptoms of headache, lethargy and myalgia, a macular rash is prominent in 50%, and acute polyarthritis, often migratory, in up to 90%. Partial recovery often takes 2 months, and full recovery a year. There is no specific antiviral drug.

Dengue

Classification. Dengue is a systemic arboviral infection characterised by severe bone pain, and usually rash.

Causative agent is a flavivirus (Fig. 1) with four serotypes, transmitted by

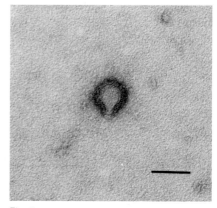

Fig. 1 **The Flavivirus group can cause encephalitis, haemorrhagic fever or dengue.** Bar represents 100 nm

Table 1 **Selected systemic virus infections**

Family	Genus/group	Encephalitis (E)	Haemorrhagic fever (HF)	Myalgia & fever	Rash & arthritis
Arenaviridae	Old world complex	Lymphocytic choriomeningitis (LCM)	Lassa fever	LCM	
	New world complex		South American HF (Machupo, Junin, etc.)		
Bunyaviridae	Bunya virus	California encephalitis group		Bunyamwera Oropouche	
	Phlebovirus	Rift Valley fever (RVF)	RVF	RVF Sandfly fever	
	Nairovirus		Crimean-Congo HF		
	Hantavirus		Hantaan (renal) Sin Nombre (pulmonary)		
Filoviridae	Filovirus		Ebola, Marburg disease		
Flaviviridae	Flavivirus (mosquito borne)	St Louis, Japanese, Murray Valley, West Nile	Yellow fever, dengue HF	Dengue	
	Flavivirus (tick borne)	Central European TBE, Russian spring-summer E	Kyasanur Forest disease, Omsk HF		
Reoviridae	Coltivirus	Colorado Tick fever (CTF)		CTF	
	Orbivirus	Kemerova		Kemerova	
Rhabdoviridae	Vesiculovirus			Vesicular stomatitis	
Togaviridae	Alphavirus	Eastern, Western and Venezuelan equine encephalitis			Chikungunya, O'nyong-nyong Barmah Forest, Ross River, Sindbis

Note: All but arenaviruses and filoviruses are arboviruses.
Viral zoonoses *not* listed in Table 1 include: monkey pox, tana pox, avian influenza, BSE, Foot and mouth disease, rabies, SARS (q.v.).

Aedes aegypti mosquitoes directly from infected humans, with a possible monkey reservoir.

Clinical features. It begins with fever, chills, nausea and vomiting but is characterised by severe and widespread pain – retro-orbital pain, headache, myalgia, plus rash in 60% (Fig. 2). After 5 days, fever remits for 3–4 days then returns ('saddleback fever') with arthralgia and bone pain (one popular name is 'breakbone fever') and dengue is a corruption of 'dandy' because of the delicate gait from pain. Recovery is usual in 2–3 weeks.

Confirmatory tests are either serology – new IgM, or 4-fold rise in total antibody, or PCR on serum.

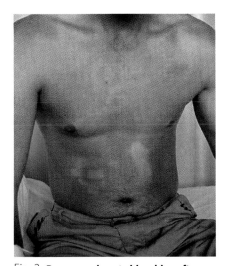

Fig. 2 **Dengue rash: note blanching after hand pressure.**

Chemotherapy is not available so treatment is symptomatic.

Complications. Dengue haemorrhagic fever (DHF) or dengue shock syndrome (DSS) are feared complications occurring with further attacks from different serotypes (see below).

Control and prevention depends on mosquito control, and avoidance of bites.

Fever with myalgia

This non-specific syndrome of fever, myalgia, headache, malaise, nausea and often vomiting is common with many arboviruses (Table 1), and is similar to dengue apart from the lack of bone pain. Rash and arthralgia occur sometimes, but haemorrhage and shock by definition do not. Again there is no specific treatment, and control and prevention depends on vector (mosquito, sandfly or tick) and reservoir (rodent, other vertebrates) control, and avoidance of bites or close contact with rodents (aerosols).

Haemorrhagic fevers

Classification. These systemic infections initially have general systemic flu-like symptoms, then develop haemorrhages in skin and from internal organs, with high mortality. Infection can be subclinical, shown only by later serology.

Causative agents. The viruses causing VHF are from two arbovirus families (bunya- and flaviviruses) plus two non-arbovirus families (arena- and filoviruses) (Table 1). Other non-arboviral causes in

endemic areas include bacteria (meningococcal, staphylococcal or streptococcal, leptospires, rickettsiae), *T. rhodesiense*, and rubella, enterovirus or herpesvirus infections.

Clinical features are summarised as:

- Usual initial flu-like illness with fever, headache, malaise, myalgia, nausea
- Skin and internal haemorrhages
- Specific symptoms in some: retinitis, encephalitis, conjunctivitis, bone pain.

Details are in Table 2.

Confirmatory tests may not be done in epidemics in endemic areas, diagnosis being clinical. Laboratory tests are dangerous, being virus isolation in tissue culture (or mosquitoes or mice), RNA detection by PCR, or serology for IgM then IgG.

Chemotherapy. Ribavirin is active against arena- and bunyaviruses. There is no specific treatment for Filo- or Flavivirus infections, being supportive with i.v. fluids.

Control and prevention is difficult before hospitalisation. Strict isolation, infection control, and stringent laboratory techniques are then essential.

Haemorrhagic fever with pulmonary syndrome

This is due to the Sin Nombre and other hantaviruses of the Bunyavirid family and also an arenavirus, Whitewater Arroyo virus in USA.

Table 2 Viral haemorrhagic fevers

Disease	Incubation period (days)	Initial symptoms	VHF symptoms	Duration (days)	Mortality
Bunyaviruses					
Rift Valley fever	2–6	Usual* + retinitis 1%, encephalitis 1%	In 1%, plus hepatitis with jaundice	Varies	Minimal except 50% in VHF
Crimean-Congo HF	1–3	Usual*	Severe, shock, DIC, bleeding, hepatitis	Short	20–50%
Flaviviruses					
Yellow fever	3–6	Usual*	Jaundice from day 3, gut bleeding, renal failure	Short, death day 3 onwards	20%
Dengue HF and dengue shock syndrome (DSS)	5–11	Usual* plus pain	Bleed days 5–10	Medium, 5–10	Low in DHF, 50% in DSS
Arenaviruses					
South American	7–12 usual, ±3	Usual* but insidious Rash and conjunctivitis	Vascular: oedema, bleeding, shock	Medium, 14	15–30%
Lassa fever	7–21	Usual* plus arthralgia, pharyngitis	Oedema + bleeding Diarrhoea + vomiting Confusion + lymph nodes	Medium 7–14	20% or more in pregnancy
Filoviruses					
Ebola Zaire fever } Marburg Disease }	3–7	Usual* + conjunctivitis	Diarrhoea,+ vomiting Conjunctivitis, slow pulse Bleed day 6. Rash sometimes	Medium, 7–16	50–80%

*Usual = headache, fever, malaise, myalgia and nausea.

The disease begins like other VHF with a flu-like illness of fever and myalgia, but in 4–5 days cough and dyspnoea develop, and may progress to pulmonary oedema and respiratory failure with 50% mortality. There is no specific treatment.

Haemorrhagic fever with renal syndrome
This is due to the Hantaan, Dobrara, Seoul or Puumala hantaviruses in Asia or Europe, with four characteristic phases:

- Toxic (4–7 days), with fever, headache, back pain, often blurred vision, petechiae and thrombocytopenia with leucocytosis
- Hypotensive, with clinical shock
- Oliguric (3–10 days) from acute interstitial nephritis, then
- Polyuric, with recovery.

Ribavirin is specific treatment, and supportive treatment of shock, renal failure, hypertension and complications is essential. Mortality is 5% in Asian forms, 1% with milder European disease.

Yellow fever
Yellow fever differs from other haemorrhagic fevers because it has been known for over 120 years, hepatitis is so prominent, haemorrhage is from internal organs rather than skin petechiae, and this life-threatening disease is vaccine-preventable.

It begins suddenly with, as usual, fever, headache and myalgia; but soon prostration, shock, jaundice and haematemesis follow, with hepatic and cardiac failure and death. Milder cases occur without jaundice and bleeding, so overall fatality rate is 20%.

The epidemiology is interesting, with two distinct cycles:

- Jungle yellow fever with monkeys as the permanent reservoir, transmission by tree-top *Haemagogus* spp. mosquitoes, and humans as accidental hosts.
- Urban yellow fever with humans as the permanent reservoir, and transmission by *Aedes aegypti* mosquitoes breeding in stagnant water.

Pox virus infections

Molluscum contagiosum, milkers' nodes, monkey pox, orf and **tanapox** are localised pox diseases described on p. 201.

Smallpox
Fortunately this terrible infection is eradicated from humanity, but is a bio-terrorism threat from the inhumane.

Causative organism is the smallpox or variola virus, an Orthopox virus (with Vaccinia) in the Poxviridae family of very large, enveloped, brick-shaped, complex, double-stranded DNA viruses. There are two strains, variola major causing classical smallpox with mortality of 10–50%, and variola minor causing the much milder alastrim, mortality < 1%.

Clinical features begin after an incubation period of 7–10 days, with sudden onset of fever and malaise, then in a few days progressive prostration and the characteristic centrifugal rash, worst on face and limbs, evolving through macules, papules, vesicles, pustules to crusts and scars if the patient survives.

Confirmatory tests are usually unnecessary, but viral antigens can be detected by immunofluorescence in vesicle fluid, or electron microscopy.

Chemotherapy was unsatisfactory, though methisazone and rifampicin have some activity.

Control and prevention has been achieved by widespread use of vaccination, surveillance and containment, with the last natural case in October 1977.

> *Viral systemic infections of all ages*
>
> - Arbovirus infections are arthropod borne, and cause four syndromes: arthritis with rash, encephalitis, fever with myalgia (including dengue), and viral haemorrhagic fevers (VHF), including those with jaundice (yellow fever), with pulmonary syndrome (especially Hantavirus), and with renal syndrome (bunyaviruses).
> - VHF is also caused by non-arboviruses called arenaviruses and filoviruses.
> - Poxviruses cause minor infections like molluscum contagiosum, monkeypox and orf, and the major infection smallpox, a bio-terrorism risk.

HIV and AIDS

Classification

The family Retroviridae contains three sub-families:

- Oncovirinae, including Human T-cell Lymphotropic Virus type I (HTLV-I) causing two different diseases – adult T-cell leukaemia/lymphoma (ATL) and Tropical Spastic Paraparesis (TSP) (p. 100–101). HTLV-II appears to cause these also, and was found in T hairy-cell leukaemia. HTLV-IV infects T-cells without killing them, and with no disease.
- Lentivirinae causing 'slow' infections, including the Human Immunodeficiency Virus (HIV, initially called HTLV-III) causing AIDS, the Acquired Immune Deficiency Syndrome. HIV-1 is much commoner than HIV-2 which occurs in Africa and has only 40% homology with HIV-1. It is much less transmissible.
- Spumavirinae, not known to cause any human disease.

Causative agent

This is HIV, usually HIV-1, as above.

Structure

Structure of all retroviruses is an enveloped virus about 100nm in diameter, with a diploid genome of two identical molecules of single-stranded positive-polarity RNA associated with a special enzyme, reverse transcriptase (RT) which is an RNA-dependent DNA polymerase.

In HIV, the RNA and RT with protein p7 are surrounded by a rectangular nucleocapsid of p24 protein, then the matrix protein p17, then the envelope with a transmembrane component gp41 and the external envelope glycoprotein gp120 (Fig. 1). The genome has three structural genes: *gag* codes for internal proteins, *pol* for 4 enzymes including RT, protease and integrase, while *env* codes for the external envelope. There are two regulatory genes for replication (*tat* for transcription and *rev* for late mRNA transport) and four accessory regulatory genes not required for replication.

Replication of retroviruses is unique, and as the name suggests, is the reverse of other RNA viruses, as retroviruses produce viral RNA from a *DNA* copy of the virion RNA.

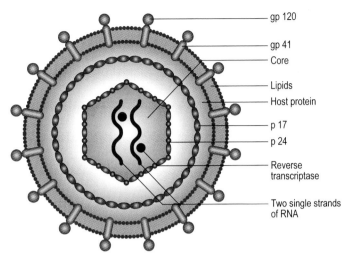

Fig. 1 **Structure of HIV.**

- gp 120
- gp 41
- Core
- Lipids
- Host protein
- p 17
- p 24
- Reverse transcriptase
- Two single strands of RNA

Attachment of HIV is by gp120 first to the CD4 molecule of T-helper lymphocytes, macrophages and other cells, then to a second receptor, a chemokine protein.

Entry is by gp41-mediated fusion of the two membranes, followed by Uncoating. Transcription of the RNA genome is by *RT* to double-stranded DNA. This enters the cell nucleus and is spliced (integrated) as provirus into the host DNA, giving permanent latent infection. This becomes productive when viral mRNA is transcribed from the provirus by host RNA polymerase, then translated in the cytoplasm into large polyproteins. These with new genomic RNA form into immature virions, then are cleaved by viral or cellular proteases as the virion buds from the cell wall.

Note that different anti-retroviral drugs (p. 234–235) target the initial fusion (Fusion Inhibitors), RT (Reverse Transcriptase Inhibitors, RTIs) or the proteases (Protease Inhibitors, PIs). Integrase is the target for a new fourth group.

Transmission is by body fluids or tissues, so may be:

- intra-uterine, intra- or post-partum from infected mother to fetus (vertical transmission)
- intravenous by transfusion, injecting drug use or 'sharps' injuries including needle-sticks
- intercourse is easily the commonest transmission mode. Genital ulceration from, e.g., syphilis or chancroid increases transmission.

Clinical features

These can follow five stages after initial exposure, though WHO, British and US classifications have fewer categories, differ in details, and one or more stages may be missed:

1. Seroconversion illness. Recognised in only 10–50%, this occurs 2–4 weeks after exposure, and is usually like glandular fever (p. 144–145) though aseptic meningitis, encephalitis or ascending polyneuropathy alone occur. All usually resolve without treatment. Initial serology by ELISA and even Western Blot may be negative (the 'window period'), but plasma proviral DNA, or RNA 'viral load', is usually positive. The highest viral load during this time is called the 'set point' for that patient, and indicates prognosis.

2. Asymptomatic. This stage often lasts for years. The virus however is not latent, multiplying actively in cells but with little or none in blood.

3. Persistent generalised lymphadenopathy (PGL). This is painless, usually symmetrical, in about 25% of those otherwise asymptomatic. It appears to have no influence on prognosis, but lymphoma must be excluded.

4. AIDS-related features or complex (ARC), not diagnostic of AIDS. These include oral or vaginal candidiasis, cervical dysplasia or carcinoma-in-situ, constitutional symptoms, chronic non-specific diarrhoea and bacillary angiomatosis. CD4 count must be above 200/microlitre.

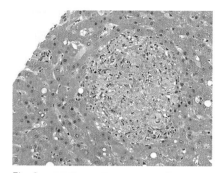

Fig. 2 **MAC: characteristic rounded granuloma in liver.**

Table 1 **AIDS-defining illnesses (ADIs) summarised**

Viral	Bacterial	Fungal	Parasitic	Other (infective basis)
CMV[a]	M. avium[b]	Candidiasis[a]	Cryptosporidiosis[c]	Cervical cancer, invasive 93*
Herpes simplex[a]	M. kansasii[b]	Coccidioidomycosis[b]	Isosporiasis[c]	Dementia / HIV encephalopathy
Kaposi's sarcoma	M. tuberculosis 93*	Cryptococcosis[b]	Toxoplasmosis[a]	Lymphoma[d]
PML	Salmonellosis[d]	Histoplasmosis[b]		Lymphoid interstitial pneumonia[e]
	Recurrent or multiple bacterial infections[e]	Pneumocystis jirovecii pneumonia (PCP)		Pulmonary lymphoid hyperplasia[e]
	Recurrent pneumonia[d] 93*			Wasting syndrome from HIV

PCP = Pneumocystis Pneumonia; PML = progressive multifocal leucoencephalopathy.
[a]Specific organ infections. [b]Extra-pulmonary or disseminated. [c]Chronic > 1 month. [d]Qualifications concerning site, type, or recurrence. [e]In child < 12 years old. *93 = Added in 1993 for > 12 years old.

Fig. 3 **PCP retinitis showing numerous discrete lesions** (contrast with CMV, Fig. 5, below).

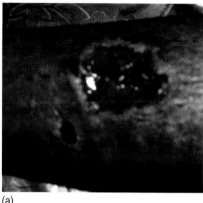

(a)

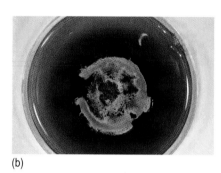

(b)

Fig. 4 *Penicillium marneffei.* **(a)** Ulcerating infection of the arm. **(b)** Culture showing typical colony and red pigment in medium.

5. AIDS. There are approximately 20 AIDS defining illnesses (ADIs), mainly infections where cell mediated immunity (CMI) is important, plus HIV encephalopathy and HIV wasting disease (Table 1). CD4 count of < 200 is diagnostic. All are less common and less severe with effective anti-retroviral drugs, but all need rapid diagnosis and expert treatment. Brief notes follow on the most important (5A–5D) (see other pages in Part IV – p. 94–223).

5A. Opportunistic infections (OIs)

Bacterial

M. avium **complex** causes fever and generalised infection diagnosed with special blood cultures and treated with specific multiple antibiotics (Fig. 2).

Tuberculosis is often rapidly progressive and may be multi-resistant.

Recurrent bacterial pneumonia – p. 128–129.

Fungal

Candidiasis affects deep tissues including oesophagus and lower respiratory tract, and needs systemic treatment.

Coccidioidomycosis and **histoplasmosis** – p. 70–73.

Cryptococcosis presents as cryptococcaemia or brain cysts – p. 98, 103.

Pneumocystis jirovecii pneumonia (PCP) causes fever, cough and dyspnoea with characteristic 'ground-glass' lungs on x-ray. Spread to retina (Fig. 3) or other tissues occurs. Treatment is co-trimoxazole or pentamidine.

Penicillium marneffei **infection** in SE Asia is systemic with fever, weight loss, anaemia and organ infections including skin (Fig. 4a), mucosa, lymph nodes and liver. Diagnosis is by blood and local cultures showing characteristic microscopy and colonies (Fig. 4b). Treatment with amphotercin B or itraconazole succeeds in 60–75% of cases.

Viral

CMV especially retinitis (Fig. 5), oesophagitis, colitis and cerebral infection.

EBV especially oral hairy leukoplakia and cerebral lymphoma.

VZV especially multi-dermatomal zoster, described on p. 146 (Fig. 6).

HSV especially of oesophagus or lung or liver – p. 201.

HHV8 (Human Herpes Virus 8) is the cause of Kaposi's sarcoma, a vascular tumour of skin, gut (Fig. 7) and lungs.

Anti-retroviral therapy may cause regression, otherwise use liquid nitrogen, radiation or anti-tumour agents.

PML causes unremitting dementia and death, with no useful treatment (p. 100).

Parasitic

Cryptosporidiosis causes chronic diarrhoea and bile duct disease (Fig. 8), treated with nitazoxanide, or paromomycin plus azithromycin.

Toxoplasmosis (p. 98, 103, 112) usually presents as brain cysts or retinitis, treated with sulphadiazine plus pyrimethamine.

Other

Lymphoid interstitial pneumonia (or pulmonary lymphoid hyperplasia) is recurrent pneumonia in children with distinctive histology, possibly from EBV.

5B. Malignancy

Cervical cancer (invasive) has become an ADI.

Lymphoma, especially cerebral, often from EBV (Figs 1 & 2, p. 92).

Fig. 5 **Cytomegalovirus (CMV) retinitis, showing yellow streaks of infected retina.**

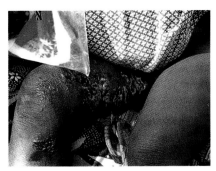

Fig. 6 **Herpes zoster in Rwandan child with HIV.**

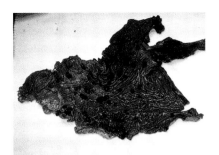

Fig.7 **Kaposi's sarcoma of stomach.**

5C. Dementia/HIV encephalopathy

Dementia/HIV encephalopathy with worsening cognition due to HIV replication in cerebral macrophages, capillary endothelium and glial cells causing cerebral atrophy and dilated ventricles on CT/MRI. Anti-retroviral drugs are the essential therapy.

5D. Wasting syndrome

Wasting syndrome from HIV is loss of > 10% body weight with fever and diarrhoea with no specific cause, and is particularly noted in Africa, probably because investigation for specific causes is limited.

Confirmatory tests

- **ELISA** for HIV antibody. Widely available, cheap, very sensitive, very reliable with few false-negative (after 3–4 weeks) or false-positive results. Rapid simple immunoassays are becoming available, plus antigen detection in combination assays.
- **Western blot** for viral proteins by polyacrylamide gel electrophoresis (PAGE), blotted onto nitrocellulose paper, reacted with the patient's serum, and shown by colour reaction with enzymatically labelled anti-human IgG. This is the 'gold standard' confirmation.
- **Viral load** in plasma (usually by PCR) measures the amount (number of copies) of viral RNA, very useful in monitoring treatment.
- **Plasma proviral DNA and viral culture** are specialised tests, useful, e.g., in early diagnosis when ELISA is negative.

Management

Chemotherapy, chemoprophylaxis against opportunistic infections, and **health maintenance** (both general and sexual) are the three management principles:

- **Highly active anti-retroviral therapy (HAART)** is triple therapy with drugs from at least two classes, usually two NRTIs and an NNRTI, or two NRTIs and a PI – see p. 234–235 for explanation and details, which are complex and specialised, especially in infected children, pregnant women, health workers and patients co-infected with Hepatitis B and/or C.
- **Chemoprophylaxis** is particularly against cryptococcal, MAC and toxoplasmal infections, TB and PCP.
- **Health maintenance** includes advice on diet, exercise, drugs, vaccination and travel.

Control and prevention

This depends on safer sex including condoms or continence, drug abuse programs including safe equipment and disposal, safe blood supplies, and strict infection control practices.

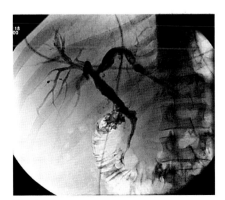

Fig. 8 **Cryptosporidium infection of bile duct showing classical 'beading'.**

HIV and AIDS

- The acquired immunodeficiency syndrome is caused by the Human Immunodeficiency Virus, a single-stranded RNA retrovirus.

- Replication of retroviruses is unique, with reverse transcriptase acting on virion RNA to produce a DNA copy which is integrated into host cell DNA, and subsequently gives viral genomic RNA and proteins to form new virions.

- Transmission is by intercourse, intravenously, inter-uterine or intra/post-partum.

- Infection progresses from a seroconversion illness to an asymptomatic stage (± lymphadenopathy) to AIDS-related infections to fully-developed AIDS with opportunistic infections (bacterial, viral, fungal ± parasitic), specific tumours, HIV encephalopathy and/or HIV wasting syndrome.

- Treatment is by at least three anti-retroviral drugs, with prophylaxis against common opportunistic infections when CD4 count is below 200.

- Adverse effects, drug interactions, resistance, adherence to life-long treatment and cost are often major problems.

- Control and prevention depends on safer sex, drug abuse programmes, safe blood supplies, and strict infection control.

Tropical systemic infections

Four major vector-borne systemic infections, mainly found in developing countries and the tropics, are described. Other systemic infections particularly found in the tropics are filariasis (p. 205), rickettsioses (p. 66–67), yaws (p. 203) and the zoonoses (p. 56–57, 212–213).

Table 1 **_Leishmania_ spp. and their clinical diseases**

Major species	Distribution	Disease
L. donovani complex including _L. infantum_	S. Asia, Africa, Mediterranean	Kala azar (visceral)
L. tropica complex including _L. major_	S. Asia, Africa, Mediterranean	Cutaneous 'Old World'
L. mexicana complex	Central and South America	Cutaneous 'New World'
L. braziliensis complex	Central and South America	Cutaneous and mucocutaneous

Kala azar

Leishmania (p. 82) are flagellated protozoa transmitted from animal reservoirs by biting flies. The genus is divided into four groups called complexes, and _L. braziliensis_ contains the sub-genus _viannia_. Visceral leishmaniasis is caused by a member of the _L. donovani_ complex, usually _L. donovani_ itself. It is transmitted by _Phlebotomus_ sandflies, either from canines or infected humans.

Leishmaniasis is classified into four types (Table 1) of which three are cutaneous (p. 205) and the fourth is kala azar or visceral leishmaniasis, where the parasite develops in the spleen and liver.

Clinical features
This chronic illness begins with fever and mild systemic symptoms, followed by wasting and, months or years later, by massive splenomegaly (Fig. 1), with anaemia, grey-black skin pigmentation ('kala azar' means black fever) and hepatomegaly. The patient looks and feels surprisingly well until the terminal stage. Skin lesions can appear weeks, months or years after kala azar; this is called post-kala azar leishmaniasis.

Confirmatory tests
The formol-gel test for very high serum immunoglobulins is simple but non-specific. Specific diagnosis is by seeing the amastigote stage of the parasite (Leishman-Donovan bodies) in bone marrow, splenic aspirate or liver biopsy. Culture and serology are less useful.

Chemotherapy
First choice drugs are parenteral pentavalent antimony compounds such as sodium stibogluconate or meglumine antimonate, given slowly because of toxicity. Reserve drugs are amphotericin B and pentamidine.

Control and prevention
Bed nets with insecticide are protective. Unlike the cutaneous forms, immunity does not develop in kala azar, so a vaccine is unlikely.

Malaria

Malaria is caused by a protozoan parasite, _Plasmodium_ spp. (p. 78), which is transmitted by the bite of the female anopheline mosquito, so is restricted to areas where these breed. Only the most dangerous, _P. falciparum_, has no hypnozoites ('sleeping parasites') in the liver; these cause relapses even years later.

Clinical features
Malaria is a very common, potentially fatal disease characterised by fever, headache and prostration, and often serious com-

Table 2 **Malaria**

Species	Areas	Asexual blood cycle	Relapses	Complications
P. falciparum	All malarious	48 hours (tertian)	None	Cerebral, renal, frequently fatal
P. vivax	Not W. Africa	48 hours (tertian)	Over 3 years	None
P. ovale	Tropical Africa	48 hours (tertian)	Over 20 years	None
P. malariae	Africa, South and Southeast Asia	72 hours (quartan)	Uncommon	Nephrotic syndrome

plications. It is classified by the interval between fever attacks (initiated by waves of release of parasites into the blood) and the causative parasite (Table 2). With each attack of fever (which may initially be daily with _P. falciparum_), the patient is first shivering cold, then hot and dry, then drenched with sweat. Headache is usually severe, with myalgia, leading at times to the tragic misdiagnosis of 'only influenza'. All malaria causes red cell destruction, with anaemia and splenomegaly in chronic disease. Falciparum malaria causes red cell sludging and cytokine release, causing cerebral malaria with convulsions and coma owing to capillary plugging; even with treatment, death is common.

Immune glomerulonephritis is common; nephrotic syndrome occurs especially in _P. malariae_ infections; 'black water fever' with haematuria and renal failure is another feared complication, which can occur after quinine treatment.

Confirmatory tests
Thick and thin blood films show the various forms of the parasites (Fig. 2). Antigen tests are improving. Occasionally bone marrow films are needed.

Chemotherapy
This is specialised and must change with drug resistance in various areas. Chloroquine is usual for non-falciparum strains,

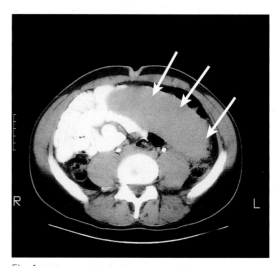

Fig. 1 **Kala azar: CT of spleen (upper right) into pelvis (shown by two white crescents of bone inferiorly).**

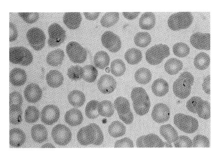

Fig. 2 **Malaria: blood film showing 'signet rings' of** *P. falciparum*.

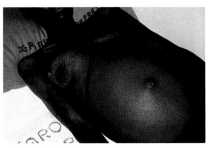

Fig. 3 **Schistosomiasis with hepatosplenomegaly and ascites.**

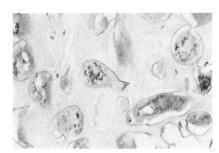

Fig. 4 *Schistosoma haematobium* **eggs in bladder biopsy.**

and artesunate, atovaquone-proguanil, quinine or mefloquin particularly for *P. falciparum*. Other artemisinin derivatives and lumefantrine are promising but resistance is already emerging. Primaquine is used to eradicate the liver 'hypnozoites'.

Control and prevention

Eradication is not possible because of resistance of mosquitoes to insecticides, and of many parasite strains to drugs. Control depends on insect repellents, bed-nets and imperfect chemo-prophylaxis with chloroquine, mefloquin or doxycycline until the many difficulties in developing malaria vaccines are overcome.

Schistosomiasis

Schistosomiasis is caused by *Schistosoma* spp. (p. 91). The vector is a snail, and the fluke larvae (cercariae) penetrate through human skin after release from the snail.

Clinical features

Schistosomiasis is <u>characterised</u> by urinary or bowel granuloma formation and haemorrhage, portal hypertension, and haemorrhage from oesophageal varices (thin-walled dilated veins).

It is <u>classified</u> into urinary schistosomiasis from S. *haematobium* (which causes haematuria), or intestinal from S. *mansoni*, S. *japonicum* or S. *mekongi*. All species cause lesions related to the parasitic development stages:

1. Skin penetration by cercariae from the aquatic snail host causes itch.
2. Migration causes allergic symptoms.
3. Maturation in the liver causes hepatitis.
4. Egg production in the vesical or mesenteric veins causes granuloma formation and haemorrhage.
5. Egg release causes portal hypertension, ascites, hepato-splenomegaly (Fig. 3) and oesophageal varices and haemorrhage.
6. Egg overflow into the systemic circulation causes pulmonary, cerebral and spinal cord granulomata.
7. Chronic S. *haematobium* infection causes bladder polyps and cancer.

Confirmatory tests

The distinctive eggs are found by stool or urine microscopy, or by bladder (Fig. 4) or rectal biopsy.

Chemotherapy

Praziquantel is effective in early infections, but extensive tissue damage is irreversible.

Control and prevention

Control and prevention is difficult and depends on education, sanitation, mass treatment or the use of molluscicides against the snails in some circumstances. A vaccine is not yet developed.

Trypanosomiasis

Trypanosomiasis is caused by *Trypanosoma* spp. (p. 83) which are blood and tissue flagellated protozoa. There are two forms of disease:

- African trypanosomiasis: caused by variants of *T. brucei* and transmitted by the tsetse fly. Infection has a local, a systemic and an encephalitic (sleeping sickness) phase, and is finally fatal unless treated early (p. 105)
- South American (Chagas' disease): caused by *T. cruzi*. Infection is initially acute but major chronic cardiac and intestinal disease can occur years later as a result of continued parasitic activity (p. 138).

Confirmatory tests

Microscopy and specific staining (Giemsa) detects amastigotes in anti-coagulated blood, blood films or lymph node aspirates. Chronic Chagas' disease is confirmed serologically.

Chemotherapy

Suramin is the drug of choice for early *T. brucei* infections, the alternative being pentamidine. Toxic organic arsenicals such as melarsoprol are needed for CNS infection. Benznidazole is most useful in the acute stage of *T. cruzi* infection.

Control and prevention

Control and prevention depends on tsetse fly/reduviid bug control, particularly around houses, protection from biting, and treatment of infected humans.

Tropical systemic infections

- Kala azar is visceral leishmaniasis; initial fever and wasting is followed by splenomegaly, anaemia and hepatomegaly.

- Malaria is caused by *Plasmodium* spp. in areas where anopheline mosquitoes breed. It causes fever, headache and prostration, with life-threatening cerebral and renal complications.

- Schistosomiasis is caused by the flukes *Schistosoma* spp. and is characterised by urinary or liver damage.

- Trypanosomes are transmitted by tsetse flies (African sleeping sickness) and reduviid bugs (South American Chagas' disease). Both diseases begin with fever and local changes at the site of the bite. African trypanosomiasis progresses to encephalitis, while Chagas' disease can have an interval of years before chronic disease develops with cardiac and intestinal damage.

Rarer systemic infections

Some rarer systemic infections are discussed here; others are on pages 152, 203, 205, 212–213.

Kawasaki disease

Characteristics of this childhood disease are fever, rash and lymphadenopathy (hence the previous name of mucocutaneous lymph node syndrome, MCLS), with variable multisystem involvement. The causative organism is uncertain.

Clinical features are in three phases:

- acute phase of 1–2 weeks of fever (100%); redness of conjunctivae, lips and oral mucosa with 'strawberry tongue' (90%); polymorphous rash (80%); red palms and soles with oedema of hands and feet (75%); and cervical lymphadenopathy (60%).
- subacute phase of about 3 weeks of desquamation, arthralgia or arthritis in 40%, and cardiovascular disease (including myocarditis, arrhythmias, mitral incompetence or aneurysms) in 20%, with 2% mortality. There may be hepatic, renal, urethral, eye or meningeal involvement.
- convalescent phase until recovery after 6–10 weeks of illness.

Confirmatory tests are not diagnostic and may include neutrophilia, thrombocytosis, elevated ESR, pyuria, elevated transaminases and mild CSF lymphocytosis.

Chemotherapy is not helpful, but i.v. gamma globulin and aspirin reduce aneurysm incidence by 80%.

Control and prevention is not yet feasible.

Listeriosis

Listeriosis is caused by *Listeria monocytogenes*, a motile β-haemolytic (Fig. 1) Gram-positive rod (p. 38) which can grow at domestic refrigerator temperatures. It is found in many animals and plants, and infects adult humans directly or through unpasteurised milk or cheese, or uncooked vegetables or meat.

Clinical features vary:

- adult disease varies from asymptomatic carriage through mild 'influenza' to meningitis (particularly in the immunocompromised)
- intra-uterine infection from mild bacteraemia in a pregnant woman causes abortion or fetal death
- neonatal infection causes septicaemia, pneumonia or meningitis.

Fig. 1 *Listeria monocytogenes* colonies on blood agar showing beta haemolysis.

Confirmatory tests. Microscopy and culture of blood, CSF or other infected sites yield *L. monocytogenes* with tumbling motility.

Chemotherapy is penicillin or ampicillin ± gentamicin.

Control and prevention is imperfect, with no vaccine. Pregnant women should avoid risky foods including unpasteurised milk or cheese, or uncooked vegetables or meat.

Lyme disease

Lyme disease is caused by the *Borrelia burgdorferi* group (p. 58). The reservoir hosts are deer and mice, and the vectors are hard-shelled *Ixodes* ticks. The disease has a patchy distribution on most continents.

Clinical features:

- acute fever, systemic symptoms and the distinctive skin rash (erythema chronicum migrans, ECM); the rash has an enlarging red border with central clearing, and occurs initially at the site of the tick bite, with later transient lesions elsewhere
- subacute cardiac (myopericarditis, heart block, p. 138) and neurological (encephalitis, meningitis, peripheral neuritis, p. 99) lesions follow weeks or months later
- chronic arthralgias or arthritis, at times with neuropsychiatric manifestations, occur months or years later.

Confirmatory tests. These are usually serological, as borreliae are rarely seen or cultured from skin biopsies.

Chemotherapy for acute disease is doxycycline, or amoxicillin for children and pregnant women. In cardiac, neurological or joint disease, i.v. penicillin or ceftriaxone seems more effective.

Control and prevention in the absence of a vaccine depends on avoiding tick bites.

Relapsing fever

Relapsing fever (RF), caused by spirochaetes of *Borrelia* spp. (p. 59), is characterised by alternating febrile and afebrile periods. The repeated fevers result from antigenic variation in the infecting bacteria. There are two types of RF:

- epidemic louse-borne RF is caused by *B. recurrentis* and is spread person-to-person by *Pediculus humanus* (Fig. 2).
- endemic tick-borne RF is caused by numerous *Borrelia* species; it is spread by soft *Ornithodorus* ticks from reservoirs in rodents.

Clinical features are similar in both endemic and epidemic RF: sudden fever, rigors, headache and myalgia, then hepatosplenomegaly. One week of bacteraemia alternates with 1 week without fever, repeated 3–13 times. Epidemic RF is similar to but usually more severe than endemic RF, with up to 10 times higher mortality.

Confirmatory tests. Microscopy of Giemsa-stained blood films shows the typical spiral bacteria; culture is used if films are negative. Serology is of little use.

Chemotherapy is by tetracycline, except for children or pregnant women. Chloramphenicol is an alternative.

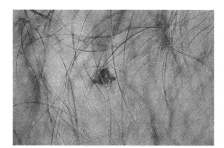

Fig. 2 **Louse and scratches.**

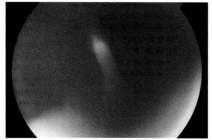

Fig. 3 ***Toxocara* eye infestation: scar and adhesion.**

amphenicol are used depending on sensitivity tests. Haemorrhage, perforation and other complications obviously need specific management.

Control and prevention depends on personal hygiene, safe food and water, and good sewage disposal facilities to control endemic disease. Carrier detection and treatment help to control outbreaks, and killed or oral live vaccine will protect travellers.

Control and prevention is by avoidance of ticks and lice.

Toxocariasis and visceral larval migrans

Infection with the dog or cat nematode ascarid worms (*Toxocara canis, T. cati,* p. 87) occurs especially in children. The eggs are ingested accidentally from soil, and the resultant larvae migrate via the bloodstream to numerous tissues, but cannot develop to the adult worms and so die. Their presence causes granulomata, tissue damage and necrosis. The most serious effects occur when the larvae infect the CNS or eye.

Clinical features include eosinophilia, cough and fever during the migration phase. Fits, retinitis with tumour-like masses then scarring (Fig. 3), or other organ damage, e.g. hepatitis, result from tissue invasion.

Confirmatory tests. Eosinophilia is indicative, and serology by fluorescent antibody detection confirms infection. Infected pets are found by stool tests.

Chemotherapy is by albendazole.

Control is by protecting children from dog and cat faeces, by treatment of pets, and proper disposal of animal faeces.

Typhoid fever (enteric fever)

Typhoid fever is caused by *Salmonella typhi* (p. 48). Paratyphoid fever is a milder illness caused by *S. paratyphi* A, B or C. Unlike other salmonellae, these four have no animal host, so transmission is person to person, usually via food or water.

Characteristics of this serious disease are high fever with systemic illness, constipation, increasing prostration, and sometimes a faint rash, intestinal haemorrhage or perforation.

Clinical features correlate with the four pathogenic stages:

■ invasion of the small intestine through Peyer's patches, and multiplication within macrophages during the 10-day incubation period
■ spread by bacteraemia to the reticulo-endothelial system (liver, spleen, bone marrow), where further multiplication occurs, causing 1–2 weeks of fever, malaise, generalised aches, hepatosplenomegaly, neutropenia and sometimes faint red 'rose spots' on the skin
■ re-invasion of the bloodstream and infection of other organs including the kidney and Peyer's patches again, causing apparent relapse in the third week with higher fever, gut haemorrhage or perforation, 'toxaemia' with myocarditis, renal or hepatic impairment, and other organ infection including osteomyelitis or endocarditis
■ a chronic asymptomatic carrier state persists in 1–2%.

Confirmatory tests. These follow from the above points. Positive blood cultures occur in the first 2 weeks, then positive urine and faecal cultures are obtained. Widal serology is most helpful in the unvaccinated, in non-endemic areas and when paired acute and convalescent samples are compared.

Chemotherapy is usually by ciprofloxacin, unless contraindicated (children), not tolerated or unavailable, when ceftriaxone, ampicillin, co-trimoxazole or chlor-

Yaws

Yaws is caused by *Treponema pallidum* subspecies *pertenue*; this variant is visually and serologically identical with other human treponemes but is not yet cultured in vitro (p. 58). Infection follows contact of abraded skin with exudate from surface erosions.

Clinically, like the other treponematoses, there are three stages:

■ a primary lesion which is a painless papule that becomes papillomatous with surface erosions, and then slowly heals
■ a secondary stage with similar but multiple papillomata which heal but may relapse; lymphadenopathy and osteitis may occur
■ a tertiary stage with multiple skin lesions of many types (plaques, nodules and especially ulcers), and gummata (chronic destructive ulcers) of bones, especially tibia, skull and nose (p. 203).

Confirmatory tests. Clinical diagnosis may be confirmed by dark ground microscopy (DGM) of exudates, or serology (VDRL, RPR, or EIA, and TPPA).

Chemotherapy is extraordinarily effective; one injection of benzathine benzylpenicillin is curative. Mass treatment with penicillin controls spread.

Rarer systemic infections

■ Kawasaki disease is mucocutaneous lymph node syndrome, of unknown cause treated with i.v. gamma globulin.
■ Listeriosis is acquired from food and is particularly hazardous in the immunocompromised and the fetus; it causes meningitis, fetal death or neonatal sepsis.
■ Lyme disease from *B. burgdorferi* transmitted by ticks has a distinctive rash and cardiac, neurological and joint sequelae.
■ Relapsing fever is caused by borreliae; it is endemic tick-borne or epidemic louse-borne, and is marked by relapses of fever, with myalgia and hepatosplenomegaly.
■ Toxocariasis occurs after the ingestion of larvae of *Toxocara* spp., migrating then dying in tissues to cause granulomata, particularly serious in the eye and brain.
■ Typhoid fever is caused by *S. typhi* transmitted person to person, and is marked by fever, prostration and sometimes a 'rose spot' rash, gut haemorrhage or perforation.
■ Yaws is a treponematosis caused by *T. pallidum* subspecies *pertenue*; it has a primary papule, secondary papillomata, and tertiary plaques and gummata.

Pyrexia of unknown origin (PUO)

Fever is generally defined as a temperature greater than 38.3°C (101°F) on several occasions. Classically, pyrexia of unknown origin (PUO) was defined as fever present for 3 weeks for which no cause had been found. Now, because of new diseases, new treatments and new prophylaxis, this 'classical PUO' is joined, particularly in hospital, by three new types of PUO: nosocomial PUO, neutropenic PUO and HIV-associated PUO. Further, outside hospitals, the general practitioner sees PUO as a 4–8-day fever (acute PUO) (p. 222). In nosocomial neutropenic, HIV-associated PUO and in returned travellers or recent immigrants, diagnosis cannot wait 3 weeks. Table 1 gives the main features of the six different types of PUO.

True fever must be distinguished from factitious fever, produced by the malingering or psychotic patient. The mechanism of production of fever is described on page 32.

Causes

Acute PUO is caused by infections in 75% of patients. Chronic PUO has over 100 causes (Table 2). Classical PUO has five major groups of causes:

- infections (20–40%)
- neoplasia, especially lymphomas and leukaemias (10–30%)
- collagen-vascular diseases (10–20%)
- miscellaneous (10–20%)
- undiagnosable, even after prolonged investigation (10–20%).

Investigation of PUO

Because there is such a wide range of possible causes of PUO, determining the cause is best undertaken in seven steps.

1. Full history. This must be taken carefully. All types of PUO can be initiated by drugs; travel history is an important factor because many of the zoonoses or vector-borne diseases have a distinct geographic distribution. In particular:

- classical: hobbies, occupation, travel, contacts, animals, family history
- nosocomial: procedures, devices, anatomical factors, drugs
- neutropenic: underlying disease, chemotherapy, drugs
- HIV-associated: drug use, travel, contacts, duration and control of HIV, infections, lymphoma

---

Table 1   **Six major types of PUO**

Classical PUO
- Fever on several occasions or over 3 weeks' duration
- Diagnosis uncertain despite investigations as an outpatient or during at least 3 days in hospital

Nosocomial PUO
- Fever on several occasions while receiving acute care
- No sign of infection on admission
- Diagnosis uncertain after 3 days despite investigations, including microbiological cultures incubating for 2 days

Neutropenic PUO
- Fever on several occasions
- Neutrophil levels in blood below 500 mm^3 or expected to fall below this in 1–2 days
- Diagnosis uncertain after 3 days despite investigation, including microbiological cultures incubating for 2 days

HIV-associated PUO
- Fever on several occasions for 3 weeks as OP or 3 days as IP
- Confirmed positive serology for HIV infection
- Diagnosis uncertain after 3 days' investigation, including microbiological cultures incubating for at least 2 days

Fever in general practice
- 4–8-day fever

Fever in returned traveller, recent immigrant or in the tropics
- Requires rapid diagnosis, particularly to exclude malaria

Table 2   **The AEIOU and A to Z of causes of five groups of PUO**

Classical PUO

1. Infections	**A**bscesses (especially intra-abdominal), **E**nteric fever, **I**nfective endocarditis, **O**steomyelitis, **U**rinary tract infections
	Biliary tract infections, brucellosis, borreliosis, (Numerous others: Psittacosis, Q fever, Relapsing and rat bite fevers, Salmonellosis, Tuberculosis and Viruses)
2. Miscellaneous	**C**NS disease: pontine or hypothalamic
	Drugs (dozens)
	Emboli, especially pulmonary
	Factitious fever
	Granulomatous diseases: Crohn's disease, hepatitis, sarcoidosis, temporal arteritis
	Habitual hyperthermia with no disease
	Inherited diseases: Familial Mediterranean fever, and others; **J**ob's syndrome; **K**ikuchi-Fujimoto disease (necrotising lymphadenitis)
3. Malignancies	**L**ymphomas: Hodgkin's and non-Hodgkin's; **L**eukaemias; **L**iver, kidney carcinomas
4. Collagen-vascular diseases	**M**ixed connective tissue disease, **N**ecrotising vasculitis, **O**ther vasculitis (allergic, drugs) **P**olyarteritis nodosa, **Q**uery Rheumatoid, **S**ystemic lupus erythematosus, **T**hromboses
5. Undiagnosed	**U**ndiagnosable; **V**iral infections? **W**er**Y XZ**ceptionally, rarities.

Nosocomial PUO (p. 218–219)

1. Underlying disease(s)	
2. Drugs	
3. Easy-to-diagnose infections	Pneumonia, skin, urinary tract, wound
4. Concealed infections	Occult device-related infections, e.g. sinusitis in intubated patient; pancreatitis or acalculous cholecystitis; Systemic candidiasis
	Transfusion-related infections, especially CMV, hepatitis C
	Vascular line-related infections

Neutropenic PUO (p. 220)

1. Underlying disease/condition	Organ transplants, leukaemia, lymphomas
2. Drugs	Anti-mitotics, cytotoxics, numerous others
3. Infection (causes 80–90% but confirmed in about 30%)	Early, bacterial: bacteraemia, i.v. lines, mouth, peri-anal, pneumonia, skin, soft tissue Later, fungal (*Candida*, aspergillosis) and viral: CMV, HSV

HIV-associated PUO (p. 149–151)

1. Underlying disease	Duration and control (viral load)
2. Drugs	Antivirals, antibiotics, numerous others
3. Infection	Mycobacteria: *M. avium* complex (MAC), TB, other
	Uncommon presentations of common infections in these patients, e.g. *P. jirovecii* pneumonia (PCP), cryptococcaemia or toxoplasmosis with fever alone
	CMV, HSV or other viral infections
	Intracellular infections: *Listeria, Salmonella, Histoplasma* spp., etc.
	Life-style related, e.g. endocarditis, syphilis
4. AIDS-associated tumours	Lymphomas etc.

Travellers/Immigrants PUO (p. 216–217)	Malaria, typhoid, dengue, hepatitis, etc.

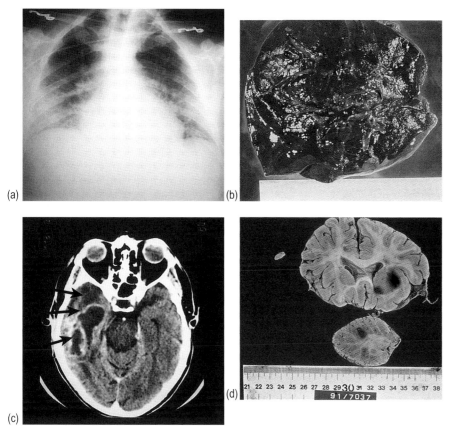

Fig. 1 **Aspergillosis. (a)** Chest x-ray showing widespread but non-specific opacities in a febrile patient with Hodgkin's disease. **(b)** Autopsy showed disseminated aspergillosis in lung. **(c)** CT showing brain abscesses. **(d)** Autopsy confirming aspergillosis in brain also.

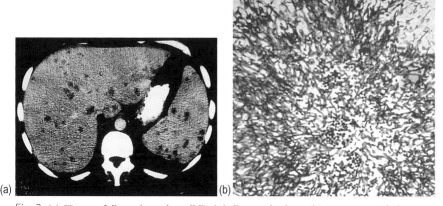

Fig. 2 **(a) CT scan of disseminated candidiasis in liver and spleen. (b) Autopsy proof of disseminated candidiasis.**

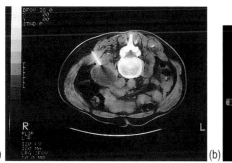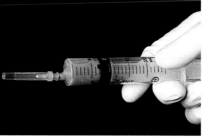

Fig. 3 **Tuberculous psoas abscess. (a)** CT scan showing psoas abscess, with needle. **(b)** The resultant pus, which was AFB smear positive and, later, culture positive for tuberculosis.

- travel associated (p. 152–155, 216–217): malarial areas, zoonoses, vector-borne disease.

2. Full examination. The presence of a fever should be confirmed. The abdomen, liver, spleen, peri-anal area, lymph nodes, eyes, joints, muscles, lungs and heart should be particular areas of concern. Any wounds or i.v. devices should be checked.

3. Non-invasive investigations. Routine blood tests and chest x-rays (Fig. 1a) should be supplemented with other imaging techniques, e.g. CT scan (Fig. 1c, 2a) and aspiration of abscesses (Fig. 3)

4. Review history. Further questions may be indicated.

5. Repeat examination. Some physical signs may be transient, e.g. rashes.

6. Invasive investigations. Biopsies of liver, bone marrow and, possibly, skin, lymph nodes, etc. may be necessary.

7. Therapeutic trial. Empirical treatment can begin if the diagnosis is probable but cannot be confirmed (e.g. culture-negative TB or endocarditis), or in AIDS and neutropenic patients, as infections progress very rapidly. If a non-infectious cause is suspected, corticosteroids or prostaglandin inhibitors may be used.

Management

Treatment depends on the eventual diagnosis; empirical treatment in rapidly progressive disease is required while test results are awaited. Neutropenic PUO requires rapid diagnosis. Mortality is highest in HIV-associated PUO, lowest in neutropenic PUO.

Pyrexia of unknown origin

- Classical PUO is now separated from nosocomial PUO, neutropenic PUO and HIV-associated PUO in hospital practice, plus fever in general practice and returned travellers/immigrants/in tropics.

- Classical PUO is caused by infections, malignancies, collagen-vascular diseases, miscellaneous conditions, and undiagnosable illness.

- Nosocomial PUO, neutropenic PUO and HIV-associated PUO are usually the result of the underlying disease, or infections or drugs (or AIDS-associated tumours).

- Diagnosis depends on history, examination, non-invasive and invasive investigations.

- Treatment depends on the likely or proven diagnosis.

Diarrhoeal disease I: general features

A number of clinical syndromes arise from ingestion of pathogens. These can be confined to the gut, or can spread to cause, e.g., liver and intra-abdominal abscesses (p. 164). Diarrhoeal Disease I discusses general features and special syndromes. Diarrhoeal Disease II and III describe bacterial, viral, protozoal and worm infections in detail.

Infective diarrhoea (frequent and/or loose bowel motions) occurs in six clinical syndromes:

- **Food poisoning**: often used loosely to mean any gastrointestinal illness following (dubious) food; strictly it means disease caused by food containing pre-formed toxin.
- **Gastroenteritis**: this causes nausea, vomiting and diarrhoea. Abdominal discomfort, cramps and fever may occur. The commonest causes are *Campylobacter jejuni*, *E. coli*, *Salmonella* spp. and viruses including Rotavirus, caliciviruses (Norwalk = Norovirus) and astroviruses. Rarer causes are *Bacillus cereus*, *Clostridium perfringens*, *Vibrio parahaemolyticus* and *Yersinia enterocolitica*.
- **Dysentery**: diarrhoea with blood and mucus in the faeces. Abdominal pain, cramps and fever are common. The usual cause is invasive large bowel infection, especially by *Entamoeba histolytica* or *Shigella* spp.
- **Enterocolitis**: inflammation of both the small and large bowel.
- **Traveller's diarrhoea**: any diarrhoeal illness associated with travel (p. 217).

- **Cholera**: caused by *Vibrio cholerae* and characterised by massive fluid loss through watery stools (p. 161).

Pathogenesis

Gut pathogens cause disease by five mechanisms:

- **Pre-formed toxin** causes short-incubation illness with marked vomiting. This is true food poisoning, as the bacteria produce toxin while multiplying in the contaminated food; the bacteria may be destroyed by food preparation, the toxin is not (e.g. *C. botulinum* and *Staph. aureus*).
- **Toxin produced in the gut** by microbes multiplying there causes the symptoms, hence the longer incubation period and marked diarrhoea (e.g. *V. cholerae*, enterotoxigenic *E. coli*.) Toxin can also have distant effects.
- **Tissue invasion** by enteroinvasive pathogens (e.g. *Entamoeba histolytica*, *Salmonella* spp., enteroinvasive *E. coli*, viruses). Mucosal invasion often causes fever, cramps and blood and mucus in faeces. Deeper invasion can lead to disseminated infection.
- **Parasitism** (frequently called infection) by protozoa and worms may cause mild acute to chronic diarrhoea, and may cause disseminated disease.
- **Perforation** can result from infection (or trauma), and gut microbes can then cause intra-abdominal infections (p. 164–165) or systemic sepsis.

Some pathogens can cause disease by more than one mechanism; for example *Campylobacter* spp. produce toxin in the gut and are also tissue invasive (Table 1).

Clinical syndromes

The clinical features can be grouped according to the pathogenesis; within these groups different pathogens show typical disease characteristics (Table 1).

Sources of infection

Infection occurs by the faecal–oral route from food, fluid or fingers. There are three major sources of infection:

- animal reservoirs: *Campylobacter* spp., *C. perfringens*, *Salmonella* spp. and *Y. enterocolitica*
- water: *Campylobacter* spp., enterotoxigenic *E. coli* (ETEC), *E. histolytica*, *Salmonella* spp. and *V. cholerae*
- food: all the causative organisms.

Prevention of infection thus depends on safe food handling, safe water supplies and proper sewage disposal.

Confirmatory tests

Microscopy and cultures of food or stools, selective PCR and ELISA tests are used to identify the causative organisms, important for individuals and in outbreaks of disease.

Causative organisms

These may be grouped (Table 1 and p. 160–163) as:

Classification/causative organism	Incubation period	Duration	Diarrhoea	Vomiting	Fever	Other
Pre-formed toxin (short incubation, vomiting prominent)						
B. cereus (emetic form)	1–6 hours	12–24 hours	+/–	Severe	0	Cramps
C. botulinum (adult form)	8–36 hours	Weeks to months	In 25%	In 50%	0	Constipation, paralysis
Staph. aureus	2–8 hours	12–24 hours	Frequent	Severe	Rare	–
Toxin produced in gut (medium incubation, marked diarrhoea)						
B. cereus (diarrhoeal form)	8–12 hours	12–24 hours	Marked	In 10%	0	Cramps ++
C. botulinum (infant)	8–48 hours	Weeks to months	Early	In 50%	0	Constipation, paralysis
C. perfringens (2 types)	8–24 hours	12–24 hours	Marked	In 10%	0	Cramps ++
E. coli (enterotoxigenic, ETEC)	12–48 hours	2–4 days	Mild to marked	+/–	0	–
V. cholerae	24–72 hours	1–7 days	Massive, watery	+/–	0	Severe dehydration
Tissue invasion (longer incubation, fever, pain, dysentery)						
Campylobacter jejuni (also produces toxin)	2–10 days	4–20 days	Marked	–	Yes	Cramps ++
E. histolytica	2–10 days	Days to weeks	Dysenteric	+/–	+/–	Cramps ++
E. coli (enteroinvasive, EIEC)	2–4 days	2–10 days	Some blood	–	+/–	Cramps ++
Salmonella spp.	1–3 days	2–7 days	Marked	Yes	Yes	Cramps +
Shigella spp.	1–4 days	2–4 days	Dysenteric	–	Yes	Cramps +++, tenesmus ++
V. parahaemolyticus (also produce toxin)	1–2 days	2–3 days	Marked	Yes	Yes	Cramps
Y. enterocolitica (also produce toxin)	3–7 days	1–2 weeks	Marked	30%	Yes	Cramps ++ and mesenteric adenitis
Caliciviruses including Norovirus (Norwalk)	1–2 days	2–3 days	Moderate	Marked	Yes	Cramps (± CNS symptoms)
Rotavirus or Astrovirus	2–6 days	2–6 days	Watery	Yes	Yes	Coryza and cough precede

Table 1 **Clinical features of diarrhoeal disease**

- usual pathogens: bacteria, protozoa, worms, viruses
- unusual pathogens: e.g. those causing sexually transmitted diseases can cause bowel disease (see below)
- normal gut flora: antibiotic use can disturb normal bowel flora leading to disease (see below)
- bacterial overgrowth: occurs particularly in those with a predisposing abnormality (see below).

Some pathogens have a distinct geographic distribution, some are found in animals and humans, others are only human pathogens. Some parasites are particularly common in AIDS patients. These differences are important for diagnosis, and for control and prevention. The individual pathogens are described in Diarrhoeal Disease II and III.

Special syndromes

Gay bowel syndrome
Homosexually active men can acquire gut infections in three additional ways:

- anal intercourse: sexually transmitted disease of distal bowel (proctocolitis)
- anal trauma: tears, ulcers, abscesses or fistulae
- oro–anal contact: ingestion of gastrointestinal pathogens.

Proctocolitis. The STD pathogens *N. gonorrhoeae*, *C. trachomatis*, *T. pallidum*, *H. ducreyi* and Herpes simplex virus all cause ano-rectal pain and diarrhoea or dysentery. Ulceration may occur in syphilis, chancroid and herpes simplex.

Traumatic infections. Pyogenic infections from trauma usually involve Gram-negative rods and anaerobes. They cause ulcers, peri-anal and ischio-rectal abscesses and fistulae (Fig. 1) with haemoserous discharge, pain and fever.

Ingested gut pathogens. These cause diarrhoea, often with abdominal pain, cramps and nausea. A wide range of pathogens may be involved: *C. jejuni*, *Shigella* or *Salmonella* spp., *E. histolytica*, *Cryptosporidium* spp., *Giardia lamblia*, helminths, fungi or viruses, especially Hepatitis A.

Confirmatory tests. Stool, ulcer or abscess microscopy and culture with special stains and cultures are needed for the range of likely pathogens. Syphilis, hepatitis and HIV serology is essential.

Chemotherapy depends on the specific pathogens found. Safer sex, anti-retroviral drugs and better hygiene have decreased the incidence markedly.

Antibiotic-associated disease
Antibiotic-associated diarrhoea is the general term for diarrhoea following antibiotic use (usually oral), while pseudomembranous enterocolitis (PMEC) describes the specific colonoscopic appearance of severe cases with typical fibrinous pseudomembrane over inflamed mucosa. Symptoms vary from mild diarrhoea to severe dysentery with blood loss, griping abdominal pain, fever and severe dehydration.

Many antibiotics alter bowel flora and allow the multiplication of *Clostridium difficile*, an antibiotic-resistant member of normal bowel flora in many people; it can also be acquired by cross-infection from other patients. Its cytotoxin and enterotoxin both cause diarrhoea. *Staph. aureus* and *Candida albicans* rarely may contribute.

Confirmatory tests. These may be unnecessary in typical cases, but anaerobic stool culture on specific media detects *C. difficile* (so-named because difficult to grow), and toxin detection is, e.g., by ELISA.

Chemotherapy. Oral metronidazole is the treatment of choice. Oral vancomycin is also effective, but the emergence of vancomycin-resistant enterococci (VRE) should limit its use to relapses of pseudomembranous enterocolitis.

Control and prevention depends on limiting antibiotic use, and using narrow spectrum ones whenever possible.

Tropical sprue
Characteristics are mainly chronic diarrhoea, glossitis and malnutrition during or after residence in the tropics. The causative organisms are uncertain, though there is often coliform overgrowth in the small bowel.

Clinical features often begin with acute enteritis and diarrhoea, followed by chronic diarrhoea with abdominal discomfort, anorexia, weight loss, glossitis and malnutrition. Laboratory diagnosis is partly by excluding parasitic and other diseases, especially giardiasis. Small bowel biopsy shows characteristic abnormalities: broad villi with chronic inflammatory cell infiltrate.

Chemotherapy is usually with tetracycline, folic acid and vitamin B_{12}.

Control and prevention is not yet feasible.

Bacterial overgrowth syndromes
Characteristics of these include chronic diarrhoea and malnutrition, from bacterial overgrowth in the upper small bowel. Predisposing structural or functional causes include achlorhydria, a blind loop from surgery, or impaired motility from diabetes or scleroderma.

Causative organisms are usually mixed aerobic enteric Gram-negative rods, and anaerobes.

Clinical features are chronic bulky offensive fatty diarrhoea, fatigue, weakness and weight loss.

Confirmatory diagnosis is by the C^{14}-glycocholic acid breath test for bile salt deconjugation by bacteria. Megaloblastic anaemia from vitamin B_{12} deficiency is usual.

Chemotherapy is usually with tetracycline, fat-soluble vitamins and vitamin B_{12}.

Control and prevention is seldom feasible except by avoiding the surgical creation of blind loops.

Reiter's syndrome
See p. 180–181.

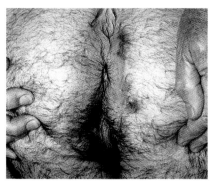

Fig. 1 **Fistulae from ischio-rectal abscesses.**

> *Diarrhoeal disease I*
> - Diarrhoeal disease is produced by three main mechanisms:
>   - pre-formed toxin is ingested in food and rapidly (hours) causes symptoms, including vomiting
>   - toxin produced in the gut by proliferating bacteria causes marked diarrhoea with a longer incubation time (hours to days)
>   - mucosal invasion causes disease after a number of days, often with fever, cramps and blood in faeces.
> - Sources of infection are food, water and, occasionally, person to person or directly from animals.
> - Gay bowel syndrome results from ingestion or ano-rectal implantation of organisms including those causing sexually transmitted diseases.
> - Antibiotic-associated diarrhoea and pseudomembranous colitis are caused by over-growth of *C. difficile* due to suppression of normal gut flora by oral antibiotics.
> - Bacterial overgrowth in the gut follows a structural or functional predisposition.

Diarrhoeal disease II: bacteria and viruses

Bacteria

Numerous bacterial pathogens cause diarrhoeal disease (Table 1); pathogenic mechanisms are on p. 158–159.

Bacillus cereus

B. cereus causes either short-incubation emetic illness from ingestion of pre-formed toxin, usually in rice, but also meats or vegetables, or longer-incubation diarrhoeal illness when ingested *B. cereus* produces toxin in the gut. Both illnesses are short in duration. Specific treatment is unnecessary. Food or stool culture may prove the cause.

Campylobacter spp.

These organisms, especially *C. jejuni*, are a common cause of gastroenteritis, often from chicken, other meats or milk. Toxin production and tissue invasion cause fever and marked cramps. Confirmatory diagnosis needs special stool culture (p. 50). Early oral erythromycin improves the slow recovery.

Clostridium botulinum

This is the second organism causing two distinct syndromes, either the adult form from pre-formed toxin in incorrectly preserved vegetables or fruits, or the *infant form* when ingested spores (usually in honey) produce toxin in the gut. In both, the toxin produces serious paralysis which may need respiratory support. Antitoxin treatment is unproven but usual.

C. perfringens

This is the third organism causing two distinct syndromes. The usual form is from food cooked sufficiently to kill vegetative cells but not enough to kill spores, which germinate and produce enterotoxin (α-toxin) which causes symptoms. The unusual 'pig-bel' (necrotising enteritis) occurs when spores of type C organisms are ingested (usually in pork). These produce β-toxin which survives in people whose gut is trypsin deficient from a protein-deficient diet. It especially occurs in New Guinea from an occasional feast. The β-toxin produces diarrhoea, haemorrhage and perforation with 50% mortality.

Escherichia coli

E. coli is normal gut flora; some **entero-pathogenic strains** (**EPEC**) have virulence factors causing diarrhoea and other gut damage.

Enterohaemorrhagic *E. coli* (EHEC). These strains (also named VTEC) produce Verotoxin, which binds to receptors on gut mucosa and the kidney causing mucosal damage and haemorrhage. Serotype O 157 causes **haemorrhagic colitis** (**HC**) and the **haemolytic-uraemic syndrome** (HUS) of haemolytic anaemia, thrombocytopenia and acute renal failure.

Enteroinvasive *E. coli* (EIEC). These invade gut mucosa, multiply, spread and destroy it, causing bloody diarrhoea.

Enteroadhesive *E. coli* (EAEC). These organisms adhere to and destroy the gut microvilli.

Enterotoxigenic *E. coli* (ETEC). These produce a heat-labile enterotoxin (LT) similar to cholera toxin, and/or several heat-stable toxins (STs). They cause fluid secretion and hence diarrhoea: the commonest cause in children in developing countries.

Confirmatory tests are specialised, except for an ELISA test of LT in ETEC. Chemotherapy is usually unnecessary.

Salmonella spp.

Salmonellae (apart from *S. typhi*) were the commonest cause of gastroenteritis in developed countries; now *Campylobacter* spp. are commoner. Diarrhoea results from invasion and inflammation of the small bowel mucosa, so fluid secretion increases. In rare patients with predisposing conditions [e.g. sickle cell anaemia, gastrectomy (Fig. 1) or cancer] salmonellae spread beyond the gut to cause septicaemia. Otherwise the illness is self-limiting, and antibiotics only prolong salmonellae excretion. Diagnosis is by stool culture and serotyping, important in tracing the source.

Control. From the large animal reservoirs, salmonellae are transmitted to humans by contaminated food (meat, eggs, dairy products), and can have secondary spread person to person. Control depends on food hygiene, pure water supplies and

Table 1 **Bacteria causing diarrhoeal disease**	
Organisms	**Mechanism**
Common in developed countries	
Campylobacter jejuni	Cytotoxin plus invasion
Clostridium perfringens	Enterotoxin plus β-toxin
Escherichia coli	Enterotoxin (ETEC); invasion (EIEC); verotoxin = haemorrhagic (EHEC)
Salmonella spp.	Invasion
Staph. aureus	Pre-formed toxin
Common in developing countries	
Escherichia coli	Enterotoxin (ETEC); invasion (EIEC); verotoxin = haemorrhagic (EHEC)
Salmonella spp.	Invasion
Shigella spp.	Invasion
Vibrio cholerae	Enterotoxin
Less common	
Clostridium botulinum	Pre-formed toxin in adults; enterotoxin in infants
Vibrio parahaemolyticus	Enterotoxin and invasion
Yersinia enterocolitica	Enterotoxin and/or invasion
Bacillus cereus	Pre-formed toxin or enterotoxin

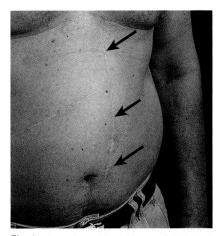

Fig. 1 **Two mouthfuls of take-away food resulted in severe salmonellal gastroenteritis and septicaemia in this man.** Note the gastrectomy scar. Other family members had only diarrhoea.

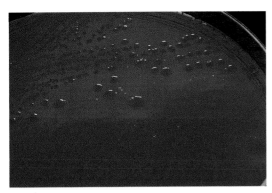

Fig. 2 *V. cholerae.* Golden yellow colonies on TCBS medium.

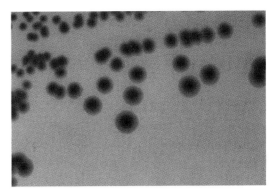

Fig. 3 *Vibrio parahaemolyticus* **(non-cholera Vibrio) green colonies.**

proper sewage disposal. People may continue to excrete organisms for several weeks after an infection so hand-washing before handling food is essential, and food handlers should not work until faecal cultures for salmonellae are negative.

Shigella spp.

Shigellae cause diarrhoeal disease of varying severity: mild (*S. sonnei*), more severe (*S. flexneri* and *S. boydii*), and severe **bacillary dysentery** with blood and mucus (*S. dysenteriae*). Shigellae cause diarrhoea by gut mucosal invasion; their enterotoxin is probably unimportant. Infection is common in children, in institutions and in developing countries because it is highly infectious (10–100 bacteria), so spread is person to person more commonly than by food or water. Diagnosis is by stool culture. Rehydration may be needed; antibiotics are only used for severe or systemic infection.

Staph. aureus

S. aureus causes sudden vomiting within 2–8 hours through pre-formed toxin, very like the emetic form of *B. cereus* disease. Culture of the causative food may, therefore, be negative, while latex agglutination test for toxin is positive.

Vibrio cholerae

Characteristically, classical **cholera** causes profuse watery diarrhoea, but milder infections also occur.

The causative organism is *Vibrio cholerae*, usually serotype 01, which has two biotypes, el tor and cholerae, and three serologic subgroups. The organism is now widely spread in Asian, African and American rivers, estuaries and coastal waters, and infection is by drinking infected water. Virulence factors protect the organism and allow it to adhere to the gut mucosa. Endotoxin production causes the disease (see Fig. 1, p. 50).

Clinical features are watery diarrhoea (up to 1 litre hourly), fever and dehydration, with tachycardia, hypotension, hypokalaemia and bicarbonate loss, then metabolic acidosis, renal failure and death in a few hours in severe untreated disease.

Confirmatory tests must not delay treatment. An experienced microscopist can find motile vibrios by dark-ground microscopy of faeces. Culture is best on a specific medium containing thiosulphate, citrate, bile and sucrose (TCBS agar, Figs 2 and 3).

Chemotherapy is less important than the essential prompt fluid and electrolyte replacement; oral replacement solutions minimise intravenous therapy. Antibiotics are not essential but tetracycline reduces the infective phase.

Control and prevention depends on water hygiene. There is no person-to-person spread. Current injectable vaccines give only partial protection for 6 months. New oral vaccines are promising.

Vibrio parahaemolyticus

This causes illness resembling *Salmonella* and *Shigella* spp. infections, but has a longer incubation period, with cramps and fever from invasion and toxin production in the gut. The organism is unusual in being a salt-loving vibrio, hence illness is from infected seafood or fish, and special culture media are needed (Fig. 3). Chemotherapy is usually unnecessary.

Yersinia enterocolitica

This is a rare cause of longer incubation illness marked by fever, pain, enterocolitis and mesenteric adenitis mimicking acute appendicitis. The organism grows at low temperatures (4°C, but prefers 22–25°C), so infection can occur even from refrigerated food, and is commoner in colder climates. Special cultures are required. Chemotherapy is unproven, but gentamicin and/or ceftriaxone are used in septicaemic patients.

Viruses

Rotavirus

This reovirus is the commonest cause of viral gastroenteritis in young children. Spread faeco–orally, it invades small bowel mucosa causing watery diarrhoea, nausea and vomiting. ELISA detects antigen in stool, and rehydration is the only treatment. Vaccine is now available (2007).

Caliciviruses including Norwalk (Norovirus)

Norovirus is a common cause of viral gastroenteritis in adults, often in groups. Spread faeco–orally and person-to-person, it invades small bowel mucosa causing marked vomiting with diarrhoea, fever and cramps. Diagnosis is clinical, or by PCR. Treatment is rehydration.

Astroviruses, **adenoviruses**, **picornaviruses** and **coronaviruses** rarely cause gastroenteritis.

Diarrhoeal disease III: protozoa and worms

Although many different protozoa and worms enter the bowel and may cause abdominal symptoms including diarrhoea (Table 1), many are rare or of restricted geographic distribution.

Protozoa

Balantidium coli (p. 81). This is a large ciliate parasite of pigs which infects humans by the faecal–oral or person-to-person routes. It invades colonic mucosa and is a rare cause of dysentery.

Cryptosporidium parvum (p. 79). This rarely causes disease in immunocompetent people but was a common cause of diarrhoea in AIDS patients before effective anti-retrovirals. Similar disease is rarely caused by *Isospora belli*, *Microsporidia* (including *Enterocytozoon* spp.) and *Cyclospora* spp. *Cryptosporidium* spp. are very resistant to disinfectants including chlorine, and infection is commonly water-borne, or person-to-person, including by sexual contact. Sometimes biliary tract infection causes cholangitis (p. 166–167), but the major infection is in the small bowel: diarrhoea is watery and profuse like cholera, causing dehydration and then malnutrition. Confirmation of diagnosis is by acid-fast stain of faeces (Fig. 1). Chemotherapy with nitazoxanide is probably better than paromomycin.

Dientamoeba fragilis (p. 81). This is not an amoeba but a motile flagellate. With no known cyst form, the delicate trophozoite is probably transported within *Enterobius vermicularis* (pin worm) eggs. It causes mild damage to colonic mucosa and rarely causes abdominal or diarrhoeal symptoms. Treatment is with doxycycline, metronidazole or iodoquine.

Entamoeba histolytica (p. 80). Infection occurs worldwide through ingestion of cysts in faecally contaminated food or water, rarely sexually. It causes **acute amoebic dysentery** with cramps and diarrhoea with blood and mucus. It also causes relapsing chronic amoebic dysentery, and amoebic abscesses in the liver (Fig. 2), lung and brain. Confirmation of

Table 1 **Intestinal parasitic infections**	
Causing diarrhoeal symptoms	**Causing systemic symptoms**
Protozoa	
*Giardia lamblia**	*Sarcocystis* spp.
*Cryptosporidium parvum**	*Toxoplasma gondii**
*Entamoeba histolytica**	
Isospora belli	
Dientamoeba fragilis	
Balantidium coli	
Nematodes	
*Ascaris lumbricoides**	*Dracunculus medinensis*
*Enterobius vermicularis**	*Toxocara canis* and *T. cati*
*Trichuris trichiura**	*Trichinella spiralis*
Ancylostoma duodenale[a]*	
Necator americanus[a]*	
Strongyloides stercoralis[a]*	
Cestodes	
Taenia saginata and *T. solium**	
Diphyllobothrium latum	*Echinococcus* spp.
Hymenolepis nana and *H. diminuta*	*Taenia solium*
Trematodes	
Fasciolopsis buski	*Fasciola hepatica*
Heterophyes heterophyes	*Opisthorchis sinensis*
Metagonimus yokogawai	*Paragonimus westermani*

[a] Transmission by skin penetration not ingestion.
*Common.

gut infection is by seeing the trophozoites in fresh warm stools. Metronidazole plus diloxanide have replaced less effective drugs.

Giardia lamblia (p. 81). Trophozoites from ingested cysts of this flagellate adhere to small intestinal mucosa; giardiasis varies from asymptomatic infection through acute watery diarrhoea to chronic intermittent diarrhoea with malabsorption. Confirmation may need small bowel content microscopy, as stool microscopy is often negative. Chemotherapy is by metronidazole, tinidazole or quinacrine; repeat courses may be needed. Cysts resist usual water chlorination levels.

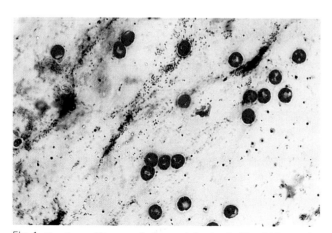

Fig. 1 ***Cryptosporidium* spp. in faeces stained red with acid-fast stain.**

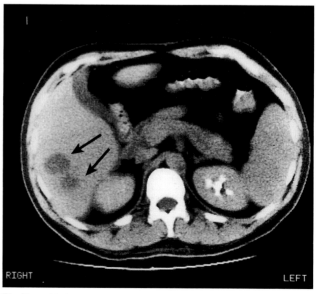

Fig. 2 **Multiple amoebic liver abscesses.**

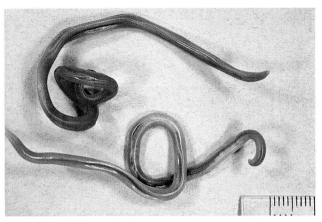

Fig. 3 **Roundworms.**

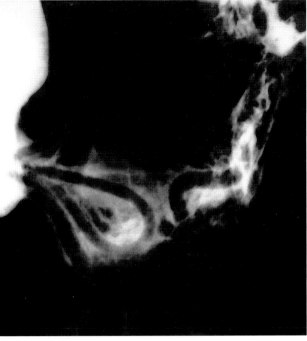

Fig. 4 **Round worms outlined by radio-opaque dye in the stomach.**

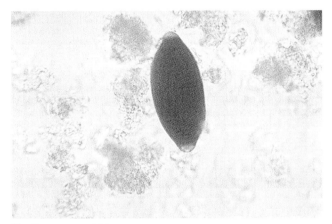

Fig. 5 *Trichuris trichiura* **egg.**

Intestinal helminths

Ascaris lumbricoides (p. 85). Round worm infections (Fig. 3) are very common. They may be asymptomatic or cause diarrhoea; however, abdominal discomfort is more common, and even bowel obstruction (Fig. 4), biliary obstruction or peritonitis can occur. Diagnosis is by stool microscopy, and chemotherapy is by mebendazole or pyrantel.

Enterobius vermicularis (p. 84). Pin- (= thread) worm infection is also common and also rarely causes diarrhoea. Peri-anal itch is typical, and diagnosis is by microscopy of adhesive tape after peri-anal application. Chemotherapy is by mebendazole or pyrantel for the whole family.

Trichuris trichiura (p. 84 and Fig. 5). Whipworm infection is less common; symptoms range from none through mild abdominal discomfort and bloody diarrhoea to rectal prolapse. Luminal worms in appendicitis may not be causal. Chemotherapy is by mebendazole or albendazole.

Ancylostoma duodenale, Necator americanus (**hookworms**) **and** *Strongyloides stercoralis* (p. 85). Unlike the three other helminths above, these infect by skin penetration. In the small intestine they can cause diarrhoea, but anaemia is the main effect of hookworm infection (Fig. 6); *S. stercoralis* causes systemic allergic symptoms, including rash and allergic pneumonitis. Treatment is by mebendazole or pyrantel for hookworm, while ivermectin or albendazole is better for *S. stercoralis*.

Cestodes. *Diphyllobothrium latum, Hymenolepis nana, Hymenolepis diminuta,* and *Taenia* spp. can all cause diarrhoea and other abdominal symptoms (p. 88–89).

Trematodes. *Fasciolopsis buski* and the rare *Heterophyes heterophyes* and *Metagonimus yokogawai* can also cause diarrhoea and other abdominal symptoms (p. 90–91).

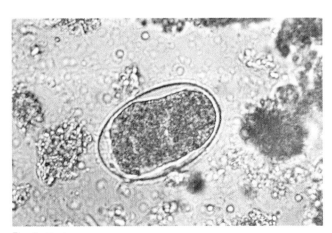

Fig. 6 **Hookworm egg.**

> ## *Diarrhoeal disease II and III: pathogens*
>
> - Many bacteria and viruses cause diarrhoeal disease; *Campylobacter* and *Salmonella* spp., *E. coli* and Rotavirus are frequent pathogens.
>
> - Protozoa can live in the gut and cause diarrhoeal disease, especially *E. histolytica, G. lamblia* and *Cryptosporidium* spp.
>
> - Nematodes, cestodes and trematodes are gut parasites that may also cause diarrhoeal disease.
>
> - Diarrhoeal disease is particularly threatening to the young, very old, malnourished and immunocompromised. Public health measures to prevent infection are vital to reduce disease.

Peritonitis and intra-abdominal abscesses

Peritonitis is <u>diffuse</u> infection in the peritoneal cavity, while intra-abdominal abscesses are <u>localised</u> collections of pus in the peritoneal cavity or abdominal organs. Peritonitis may localise to form one or more abscesses; conversely abscesses may rupture to cause peritonitis.

Peritonitis

Peritonitis is characterised by diffuse inflammation of the peritoneum. It is chemical or infective in origin.

Chemical peritonitis. This occurs when gastric, duodenal or bowel contents are released into the peritoneum when a peptic ulcer, gallbladder, or bowel perforates or is incised.

Infective peritonitis. This may be <u>primary</u> (**spontaneous bacterial peritonitis, SBP**), in individuals with predisposing conditions, e.g. cirrhosis or nephrosis, or in childhood.

<u>Secondary</u> peritonitis follows intra-abdominal infection from any cause:

- perforation of a viscus by traumatic, ulcerative or ischaemic rupture
- surgical leaks
- pelvic inflammatory disease (PID)
- peritoneal dialysis (PD) including continuous ambulatory peritoneal dialysis (CAPD)
- intra-abdominal infections or abscesses.

Causative organisms

Primary peritonitis in children and nephrotic patients is almost always caused by pneumococci and other streptococci. In cirrhosis, it can also be caused by bowel flora: enteric Gram-negative rods (GNRs), enterococci, and anaerobes especially *Clostridium* spp.

Secondary peritonitis is usually caused by bowel flora, hence it is a mixed infection from enteric aerobic GNRs, enterococci, and anaerobes, especially *Bacteroides fragilis*. In peritoneal dialysis, coagulase-negative staphylococci (CNS) are common. Rarely, abdominal tuberculosis or actinomycosis causes peritonitis.

Clinical features

These are three-fold:

- the features of peritonitis – fever, severe abdominal pain ('like the kick of a horse' on perforation, 'agonising' if diagnosed late), tenderness, rigidity

and guarding, diminished or absent bowel sounds, plus
- systemic signs of sepsis (p. 143) – superimposed on
- the features of the predisposing or underlying cause.

Confirmatory tests

Neutrophilia suggests infection; abnormal liver function tests suggest hepatic or perihepatic involvement. Gas under the diaphragm (without previous surgery) confirms a ruptured viscus, but only aspiration of peritoneal fluid (by needle, peritoneal dialysis catheter or laparoscopy) or surgical operation can prove peritonitis through subsequent microscopy and culture.

Management

- Empirical chemotherapy must cover the wide range of probable causative organisms, and hence is often triple therapy 'AGM' with ampicillin (for enterococci), gentamicin (for aerobic GNRs) and metronidazole (for anaerobes). Other possible drugs in severely ill patients include ticarcillin-clavulanate, piperacillin-tazobactam or imi/meropenem. Supplementary surgery is essential for perforation, leaks or abscesses and lavage may help cleanse the abdomen.

- In peritoneal dialysis peritonitis, intra-peritoneal vancomycin is usual empirical initial therapy.
- In primary peritonitis in childhood or nephrosis, penicillin or a third-generation cephalosporin is used until the organism is known.

Intra-abdominal abscesses

Intra-abdominal abscesses are characterised by a localised collection of pus. They are classified by their site and by their mode of origin (Table 1 and Fig. 1, as with abscesses in the chest; p. 130–131). Infections adjacent to an organ are termed para- or peri-, e.g. para-appendiceal abscesses. Diverticula are out-pouchings from the lower large bowel (Fig. 2) by which infections often occur.

Table 1 **Types of intra-abdominal abscess**	
General area	**Specific type**
1. Within viscera	Hepatic, pancreatic, splenic
2. Adjacent to bowel	Para-appendiceal, diverticular
3. Dependent peritoneal spaces	Subphrenic, paracolic, pelvic
4. Retroperitoneal	Perinephric, psoas

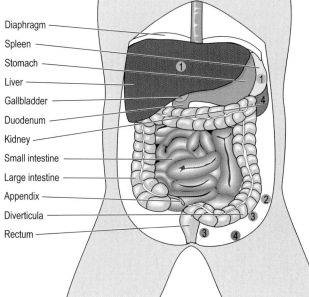

Diaphragm
Spleen
Stomach
Liver
Gallbladder
Duodenum
Kidney
Small intestine
Large intestine
Appendix
Diverticula
Rectum

1. Within viscera by trauma or septicaemia

2. Local spread from bowel

3. Dependent peritoneal spaces by distant spread

4. Retroperitoneal (perinephric and psoas) by local spread

Fig. 1 **Origin and types of intra-abdominal abscess.**

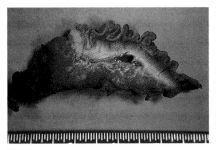

Fig. 2 **Diverticulitis, showing the dark opening of one large diverticulum on the mucosal surface. The abscess on the outer surface is hidden in this view.**

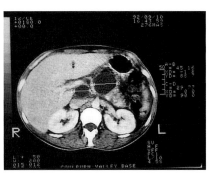

Fig. 3 **CT scan showing two large pancreatic abscesses (marked).**

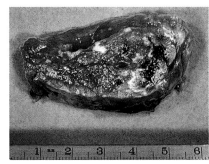

Fig. 4 **Acute pancreatitis: autopsy specimen showing necrosis and early abscess formation.**

Causative organisms

- The causative organisms are usually bowel flora in bowel-related abscesses – appendiceal, diverticular and pancreatic abscesses (Fig. 3) – and in most subphrenic, paracolic and pelvic abscesses.
- Hepatic abscesses (p. 168–169) are special, for they can arise from the upper bowel via the bile duct (cholangitis, p. 166), from the whole bowel by the portal vein (pylephlebitis, p. 167), from the bloodstream by the hepatic artery, or from trauma. As a result bowel flora, amoebae, hydatids, septicaemic organisms and skin or soil organisms can be involved (p. 168–169).
- Psoas and retroperitoneal abscesses usually arise either from the kidney, hence contain uro-pathogens as does a perinephric abscess (p. 176), or from the spine, hence often caused by S. *aureus* or M. *tuberculosis* (p. 208–209).
- Splenic abscesses usually result from septicaemia, caused by enteric GNRs, staphylococci, streptococci, salmonellae or anaerobes (about 20% each).

Clinical features

Though modified by the site and the underlying pathology, abscesses in general are marked by a swinging temperature, continuing longer than expected after, e.g., appendicitis, diverticulitis or pancreatitis (Fig. 4). Paralytic ileus with constipation and diminished or absent bowel sounds is common. In contrast to peritonitis, pain is not prominent early because the abscess is often separated from the sensitive peritoneum by the 'abdominal policeman', the omentum. A mass usually occurs late.

Confirmatory tests

While plain x-ray may be helpful, especially for gas in subphrenic abscesses (Fig. 5a), the CT scan has revolutionised the diagnosis of many abscesses (Fig. 5b), though small or multiple abscesses may not be visualised separately from bowel. Indium scans using the patient's labelled white cells are quicker and more specific than gallium scans. The causative organisms are diagnosed by Gram stain with aerobic and anaerobic culture of the abscess pus.

Management

Once visualised, the abscess(es) must be drained, under CT scan (Fig. 5b) or by surgery. For bowel-related abscesses, triple therapy 'AGM' (as for peritonitis, above) is still appropriate, but other regimens of similar broad spectrum can be used. Psoas, retroperitoneal, hepatic and splenic abscesses need specific chemotherapy for the pathogen.

Control and prevention

This depends on early surgery for appendicitis or diverticulitis, and early recognition and treatment of septicaemia and bowel, urinary and spinal infections.

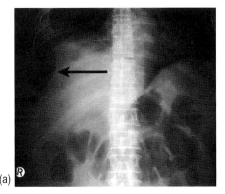

(a)

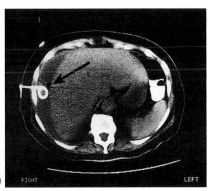

(b)

Fig. 5 **Subphrenic abscess. (a)** On abdominal x-ray (often seen best on chest x-ray). **(b)** On CT scan with 'pig-tail' drain inserted.

Peritonitis

- Chemical peritonitis is caused by leakage of gut contents or bile through trauma or perforation.
- Primary peritonitis occurs in childhood or in nephrosis (pneumococcal or streptococcal) or cirrhosis (bowel flora).
- Secondary peritonitis is usually caused by bowel flora following damage to the gut. Coagulase-negative staphylococci are common in peritonitis secondary to peritoneal dialysis.
- Clinical features are pain, guarding and rigidity, plus systemic evidence of sepsis.
- Initial chemotherapy for peritonitis must cover all likely pathogens, e.g. ampicillin, gentamicin, and metronidazole. Perforation and other anatomical defects need surgical cure.

Intra-abdominal abscesses

- Intra-abdominal abscesses are collections of pus that arise by traumatic implantation, local spread, distant spread or by septicaemia.
- Clinically, fever and systemic features are more prominent than pain or a mass until late.
- Confirmatory tests are CT or other imaging, and microscopy and culture when essential drainage is done. Chemotherapy is initially empiric against likely organisms, then specific.

Biliary infections

Cholecystitis

Cholecystitis is inflammation of the gallbladder, classified into acute (with or without calculi) and chronic. The latter usually follows acute attacks, and infection plays a small part so it is not further described.

Acute cholecystitis

Acute cholecystitis is acalculous ('without calculi') in about 15% of patients, occurring particularly in debilitated hospitalised patients; acute microvascular damage is probably mediated by endotoxin and activated Hageman factor XII.

Acute cholecystitis in over 85% of patients results from gallstones, usually obstructing the cystic duct, which leads to distension and inflammation (Fig. 1). Complications include:

- Arterial damage causing ischaemia, necrosis, gangrene, perforation and peritonitis, with *Clostridium perfringens* producing gas in the wall (emphysematous cholecystitis)
- Bacterial complications
  - local progression of infection with pus in the gallbladder ('empyaema', Fig. 2)
  - local spread to a pericholecystic collection, or to the common bile duct causing cholangitis (see below)
  - distant spread causing septicaemia
- Contiguous complications: lymphadenitis, pancreatitis (often with cholangitis) and peritonitis.

Causative organisms. These are bowel flora, including enterococci, aerobic Gram-negative rods, and anaerobes including *Bacteroides fragilis* and *C. perfringens*.

Clinical features. Pain is usual anteriorly in the right upper quadrant (RUQ) of the abdomen, commonly in the back also. Nausea, vomiting, fever and tenderness over the gallbladder are usual, but rigors, jaundice or hypotension suggest complications such as ascending cholangitis (see below).

Confirmatory tests. Ultrasound (Fig. 3) shows a dilated gallbladder and may show a dilated common bile duct. The HIDA scan shows no gallbladder in acute infection if the cystic duct is blocked; non-visualisation also occurs in early scans in over 50% of chronic cholecystitis patients. All operative specimens must be cultured.

Management. Debate continues whether chemotherapy should be given to all, or only to elderly or severely ill patients and/or those with complications (including cholangitis, emphysematous cholecystitis, perforation and peritonitis). Empiric therapy is against bowel flora, often triple 'AGM' (ampicillin, gentamicin and metronidazole). Early laparoscopic cholecystectomy is safer than delayed surgery, and is imperative in complicated disease.

Cholangitis

Cholangitis is infection in the bile ducts, a feared complication of biliary, pancreatic or bowel disease. A stone in the common bile duct is the commonest cause. Causative organisms are usually bowel flora, but may be parasites: *Ascaris lumbricoides, Clonorchis sinensis, Cryptosporidium* spp. (see AIDS cholangiopathy below) and *Fasciola hepatica*.

Clinical syndrome. In 85% of patients, Charcot's triad – fever, rigors and jaundice – occurs, which progresses to shock and liver failure.

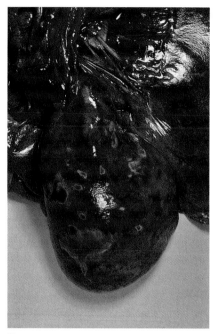

Fig. 1 **Acute cholecystitis, showing red, inflamed gallbladder with patchy necrosis.**

Confirmatory tests. Ultrasound and HIDA scans have diminished the need for percutaneous transhepatic cholangiography (Fig. 4). Blood and bile cultures are essential.

Management. Triple 'AGM' therapy as above is usual, but surgery to remove obstruction is essential. Control and prevention is by early treatment of precipitating factors, e.g. gallstones.

AIDS Cholangiopathy

This is a convenient label for a syndrome in AIDS patients characterised by persistent disabling pain and low-grade fever, in contrast to the acute course and high fever of bacterial cholangitis (above).

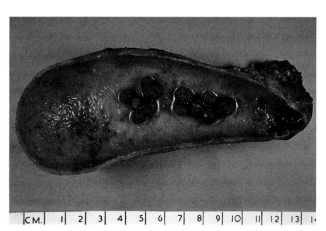

Fig. 2 **Empyaema of the gallbladder.**

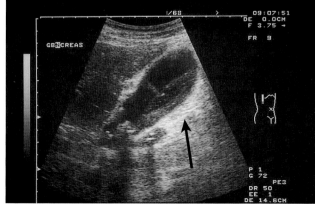

Fig. 3 **Ultrasound showing thick-walled gallbladder.**

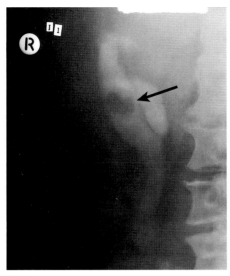

Fig. 4 **Dilated common bile duct (white dye) with large obstructing stone (dark gap).**

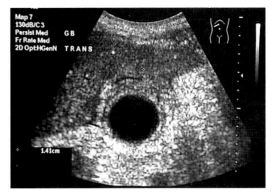

Fig. 5 **Ultrasound showing thick-walled gallbladder (transverse view) in cryptosporidiosis.**

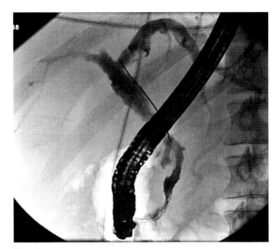

Fig. 6 **'Beading' of the common bile duct in AIDS cholangiopathy from cryptosporidiosis.**

Causative organisms are usually viruses particularly CMV, mycobacteria particularly *M. avium*, or parasites particularly *Cryptosporidium* spp. and Microsporidia. At times no infectious cause is found, and neoplasia (lymphoma, Kaposi's sarcoma) can present similarly.

Clinical syndrome. Persistent disabling RUQ pain and low-grade fever are usual, and chronic diarrhoea and weight loss common, but jaundice rare.

Confirmatory tests. LFTs are commonly 'obstructive' with very high alkaline phosphatase (ALP). Ultrasound (or CT) may show an enlarged gallbladder (Fig. 5). Retrograde cholangiography may show papillary stenosis, distal bile duct stricture or sclerosing cholangitis with both strictures and dilatation; 'beading' is characteristic (Fig. 6). AFB stains, microscopy for parasites, and PCR are often all needed.

Chemotherapy. This is useful for *M. avium* and CMV, but otherwise disappointing. Endoscopic sphincterotomy often relieves the pain though LFTs may worsen.

Control and prevention is by effective treatment of AIDS.

Portal pylephlebitis

Portal pylephlebitis is septic thrombophlebitis (venous infection with thrombosis – p. 136) of the portal vein. It arises from intra-abdominal, often appendiceal, infection. It can spread locally to the liver, or distantly by bacteraemia to the lung. As expected, bowel flora are the dominant pathogens.

Clinical features. Persistent high fever and signs of sepsis follow appendicitis or other intra-abdominal infection. If not diagnosed and treated, septic emboli lead to liver abscesses (p. 169), with right upper quadrant pain and enlarging liver.

Confirmatory tests. CT scanning can show the intra-abdominal cause and the resultant liver abscesses; it rarely shows the portal pylephlebitis, though FDG Positron Emission Tomography can. Blood cultures are essential. Chest x-ray may show lung abscesses and pleural fluid. Abscess pus must be aspirated or drained, and cultured aerobically and anaerobically.

Management. Pylephlebitis needs appropriate antibiotics against gut flora, such as 'AGM', plus removal of the cause and drainage of any abscesses.

Biliary infections

Biliary tract infections
- Acute cholecystitis, inflammation of the gallbladder, usually results from obstruction by gallstones. It causes fever and RUQ pain. Infection is usually by bowel flora, which are treated by broad-spectrum antibiotics, often 'AGM', preferably with early surgery.
- Cholangitis is infection of the bile ducts, usually by bowel flora. It causes fever, rigors and jaundice, often with shock. It is diagnosed clinically and by imaging, and is treated with broad-spectrum antibiotics and urgent surgery, because it is lethal.
- AIDS cholangiopathy has numerous causes including CMV, cryptosporidiosis and *M. avium* complex. 'Beading' on cholangiography is frequent, and medical treatment without HAART treatment of AIDS is unsatisfactory.
- Portal pylephlebitis is infection of the portal vein, usually by bowel flora from appendicitis or other abdominal infection. It causes liver abscesses, septicaemia and lung abscesses. It is treated by broad-spectrum antibiotics, removal of the cause, and drainage of abscesses.

Hepatic non-viral infections

Liver infections, abscesses and cysts

- Diffuse liver infections occur in kala-azar, malaria and schistosomiasis (p. 152–153), and viral hepatitis (p. 170–172). In addition, the liver is damaged in cholangitis (see above) and many systemic infections (p. 140–157).
- Disseminated liver infections occur in granulomatous hepatitis (p. 173), and in infections by mycobacteria (e.g., *M. tuberculosis* in miliary tuberculosis, p. 132–133, and *M. avium* in AIDS, p. 150, Fig. 2), by fungi (e.g., hepatosplenic candidiasis in disseminated candidiasis, Figs 2a and 2b, p. 157) and by other organisms (e.g., hepatic pneumocystosis, Fig. 1).
- Localised liver abscesses and cysts occur in a number of infections; three important ones follow.

Amoebic liver abscess

Amoebic abscesses are a complication of *Entamoeba histolytica* infection that can occur years after intestinal amoebiasis. Over 60% of patients are unaware of the preceding bowel infection. The abscesses arise by spread of the trophozoites up the portal vein and are often multiple and in the right lobe, but may be single or left-sided. They may spread to serous spaces (pleura, peritoneum or pericardium) or the lung, then brain. The lysis of liver tissue (*E. histo-lytica*) actually produces necrosis, 'like anchovy sauce', not a true pus-containing abscess.

Clinical features. Right upper quadrant pain and tenderness with fever are usual; only 25% have active amoebic dysentery. Systemic features including weight loss are prominent. Referred shoulder tip pain, pleural fluid and a raised right hemi-diaphragm occur with abscesses near the diaphragm while a superficial lateral abscess can even give visible bulging of the soft ribs in children (Fig. 2).

Confirmatory tests. Neutrophilia is usual, not eosinophilia. Ultrasound (Fig. 3) or CT scan show the abscess(es) (see Fig. 3, p. 162). Stool microscopy for amoebae is usually negative unless diarrhoea is present. Drainage is rarely needed now with better chemotherapy. Amoebae are not often seen in the aspirate, being found chiefly in the wall of the 'abscess'. Conversely, serology is usually positive.

Chemotherapy. Metronidazole has replaced emetine or chloroquine, and pain relief is usually rapid. Diloxanide furoate is used to treat intestinal infection. Emetine is sometimes used with metronidazole for complications such as peritonitis or pericarditis after rupture of an abscess.

Control and prevention depends on food hygiene, and effective treatment of intestinal amoebiasis.

Pyogenic liver abscess

Hepatic abscesses arise in four ways:

- from the upper bowel via the bile duct (cholangitis, p. 166)
- from any part of the bowel via the portal vein (pylephlebitis, p. 167)
- from the bloodstream via the hepatic artery
- from outside by a wound.

Causative organisms are therefore bowel flora, septicaemic organisms, or skin or soil organisms, depending on the source and route as above.

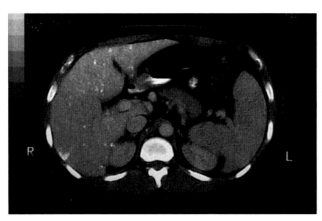

Fig. 1 **Hepatic pneumocystosis from *Pneumocystis jirovecii*, on CT showing numerous disseminated white lesions.**

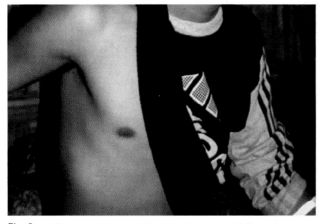

Fig. 2 **Visible lateral chest wall bulging from amoebic liver abscess.**

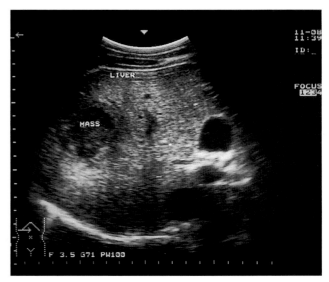

Fig. 3 **Amoebic liver abscess: ultrasound shows large single abscess ('mass').**

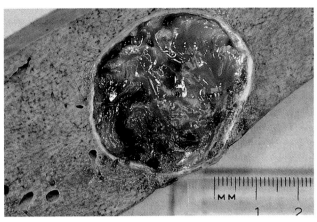

Fig. 4 **Hydatid cyst of liver: dead and inspissated.**

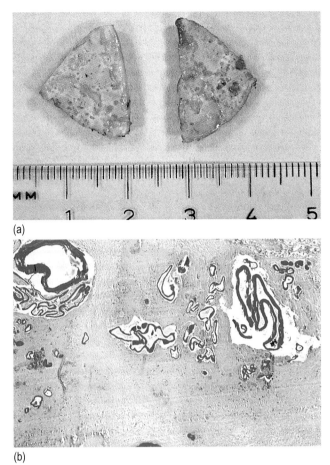

(a)

(b)

Fig. 5 *E. multilocularis* **infection, with many locules infiltrating the liver: (a) liver specimen; (b) microscopy.**

Clinical features arise from:

- the liver abscess itself: fever, right upper quadrant pain and tenderness (not with deep abscesses) and enlarging liver
- the source: rigors and jaundice with cholangitis, right lower abdominal pain and tenderness with appendicitis, rigors and shock with septicaemia.

Confirmatory tests. Imaging by ultrasound or CT shows the abscess (as with amoebic abscesses, Fig. 3), and often the source. Blood cultures and culture of the abscess pus show the causative organism(s).

Chemotherapy. Therapy depends on the cause; broad-spectrum empiric therapy such as 'AGM' (ampicillin plus gentamicin plus metronidazole) is used initially for bowel sources or septicaemia.

Hydatid cysts

Hydatid disease of the liver is usually cystic (Fig. 4) resulting from *Echinococcus granulosus* (p. 89), but rarely it is invasive caused by *E. multilocularis* spreading like a malignancy (Fig. 5). Cysts are usually single and in the right lobe, but may be multiple or in any part of the liver. Humans are infected with the encysted larvae of *Echinococcus* spp. in canine faeces. The intermediate hosts are herbivores, especially sheep and cattle (p. 88).

Clinical features. Cysts may be asymptomatic, or found through pressure on local structures, particularly the bile ducts, causing jaundice or cholangitis. Rarely spontaneous rupture or secondary infection occur. Cysts elsewhere may be found in life or at autopsy, especially in lung or brain (p. 103, 134). Old liver cysts calcify.

Confirmatory tests. Serology, particularly for arc 5 in a gel immunodiffusion test, is highly specific; other serology including latex agglutination is used for screening or supplementary testing. X-rays, CT and liver and brain scans are used for localisation.

Management. Albendazole is the drug of choice. Cysts can be aspirated under CT control in experienced units, but surgery may still be necessary, being very careful not to spill the infective cyst contents.

Control and prevention includes treating adult worms in farm herbivores, preventing dogs from eating raw infected animal (e.g. sheep) viscera, and hand-washing after dog or soil contact.

Hepatic infections

Diffuse liver infections occur in systemic tropical infections and viral hepatitis. The liver is damaged in cholangitis and many systemic infections. **Disseminated liver infection** occurs in granulomatous hepatitis, and in mycobacterial, fungal and parasitic infections.

Liver abscesses and cysts
- Amoebic liver abscess is characterised by past or present residence in an endemic area for *E. histolytica*, and by pain and fever, seldom by simultaneous dysentery. It is diagnosed by ultrasound or CT scan, and treated by metronidazole.

- Pyogenic liver abscess follows cholangitis, portal vein bacteraemia from abdominal sepsis, septicaemia or an external wound. Symptoms are local pain, fever and tenderness, plus symptoms from the source. Surgery may be needed for both the source and the abscess, and chemotherapy is essential.

- Hydatid cysts occur in endemic areas and often cause few symptoms. They are shown by imaging, may be confirmed by serology, and may respond to albendazole, although drainage or surgery are still often needed.

Viral hepatitis

Hepatitis from viral infection is of two types:

- primary liver infection with variable other organ involvement, particularly by Hepatitis A, B, C, D, E or G virus, or
- liver infection in systemic viral infections like EBV (glandular fever), CMV, HSV (Fig. 1) or yellow fever (Table 1 and see p. 144–148).

Hepatitis A

Classification. Previously called infectious hepatitis, it is transmitted faeco–orally.

Causative agent is Hepatitis A virus (HAV) which is Enterovirus 72, a picornavirus (Fig. 2), and so has a single-stranded RNA genome in a non-enveloped icosahedral nucleocapsid (p. 92–93). Incubation period is short, 3–4 weeks.

Clinical features are absent in most infections, which are asymptomatic, detected by IgG antibody. They are almost the same for all symptomatic viral hepatitis – anorexia, nausea, vomiting, fever and jaundice, with dark urine and pale stools. Rash is absent, and bleeding rare.

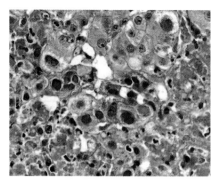

Fig. 1 **Herpes simplex hepatitis.** Liver biopsy shows haemorrhage, Cowdry type A inclusion, and a multi-nucleated giant cell. This young pregnant woman unfortunately soon died of liver failure.

Confirmatory tests are raised transaminase levels and development of IgM antibody.

Chemotherapy is not available, but fortunately recovery takes only 2–4 weeks, and there are *no* chronic sequelae – no carriers, no chronic hepatitis, no cirrhosis, no liver cancer.

Control and prevention is by active immunisation with inactivated vaccine (which is available combined with hepatitis B vaccine), by passive protection

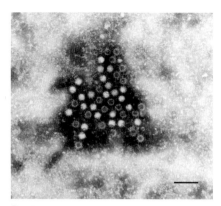

Fig. 2 **Hepatitis A virus.**

with immune globulin for close contacts, and by sewage disposal and hand-washing after defaecation.

Hepatitis B

Classification. Previously called serum hepatitis, it is transmitted by infected body fluids especially blood, and hence by injecting drug use, by needlestick or sharps injury, by untested blood transfusion, by sexual intercourse, transplacentally, and probably by birth canal secretions and breast feeding.

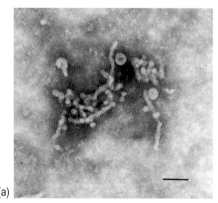

(a)

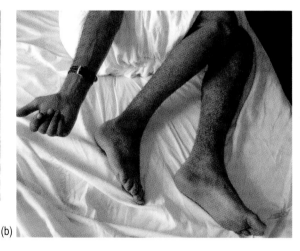

Fig. 3 **(a) Hepatitis B virus. (b) Acute hepatitis B with rash, fever and jaundice.**

(b)

Table 1 **Viral hepatitis**							
Virus	Abbreviation	Family	Genome	Transmission	Carriers	Laboratory tests	Vaccine and ImGlobulin use
Hepatitis A	HAV	Picornavirus	ssRNA	Faecal–oral	No	IgM	Yes/Yes
Hepatitis E	HEV	Calicivirus	ssRNA	Faecal–oral	No	Antibody	No/No
Hepatitis B	HBV	Hepadnavirus	dsDNA	Blood, sexual, birth-related	Yes	Surface Ag & Ab, Core IgM Ab	Yes/Yes
Hepatitis D	HDV	Deltavirus	ssRNA	Blood (sexual)	Yes	Delta Ag or Ab	No/No
Hepatitis C	HCV	Flavivirus	ssRNA	Blood (sexual)	Yes	HC AB, Viral RNA	No/No
Yellow fever	YF	Flavivirus	ssRNA	Mosquito	No	Antibody	Yes/No
EBV, CMV, HSV	EBV,	Herpesviruses	dsDNA	Saliva	Yes	IgG, IgM, EBNA Ab	No/No
	CMV,	Herpesviruses	dsDNA	Saliva, Placenta, Sex	Yes	PCR, IgG, IgM	No/No
	HSV	Herpesviruses	dsDNA	Saliva, Sex	Yes	PCR, IgG, IgM	No/No

Causative agent is Hepatitis B virus (HBV, Fig. 3a), a hepadnavirus which has a partly double-stranded circular DNA genome in a 42nm enveloped icosahedral nucleocapsid. The nucleocapsid contains the core antigen (HBcAg) and the e antigen (HBeAg), and the envelope contains the protein surface antigen (HBsAg) which can also exist as unique free 22nm spheres and filaments.

Each antigen stimulates production of a corresponding antibody:

- HBcAb particularly in natural infection, long-lasting but not protective as it cannot reach the internal core antigen
- HBeAb, an indicator of low transmissibility (as HBeAg indicates high transmissibility)
- HBsAb, found also after vaccination, and protective as it binds to HBsAg preventing viral infection of the liver cell.

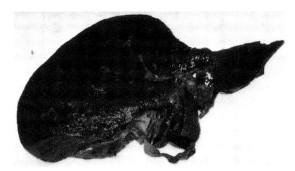

Fig. 4 **Acute on chronic hepatitis B infected liver with fibrosis.**

'Silent' Hepatitis B mutants can cause Non-ABCDE hepatitis with negative immuno-serology but positive HBsAg in liver cells and positive serum HBV RNA by PCR.

Clinical features initially are similar to hepatitis A, with many asymptomatic infections (recognised by HBsAb and HBcAb production), and some symptomatic; there are also differences – illness is often more severe, even life-threatening, and Ag-Ab immune complexes can cause urticaria, rash (Fig. 3b), arthritis, vasculitis and glomerulonephritis. Chronic sequelae are important – chronic carriage (defined as HBsAg in blood for over 6 months, though often life-long) in 5%, fibrosis (Fig. 4), cirrhosis, and hepatocellular carcinoma.

Confirmatory tests are abnormal Liver Function Tests, and in order of appearance (Fig. 5) HBsAg, HBeAg, HBcAb, HBeAb, then following a 'window period' after HBsAg normally disappears, HBsAb appears.

Chemotherapy is evolving, with pegylated interferon (alpha-2a) often combined with lamivudine, adefovir or other antivirals.

Control and prevention is either with vaccine for active protection, or HBIG (immune globulin) for passive protection to neonates or needlestick/sharps injuries. Donor blood must be tested, and needles never shared, recapped or discarded carelessly. Those with HBV-cirrhosis must be monitored to detect early liver cancer.

Hepatitis C

Causative agent is a enveloped flavivirus, with a single-stranded RNA genome, and no virion polymerase. There are at least six genotypes of HCV and many sub-genotypes from genetic variation causing a hypervariable region in the envelope glycoprotein, and multiple sub-species at any one time in the blood of an infected person.

Transmission is like hepatitis B, by infected body fluids; being 90% less infectious, the three important modes are injecting drug use, untested blood transfusion and needlestick injuries, while sexual or mother–child transmission are uncommon. It is the most prevalent blood-borne infection in 'developed' countries.

Clinical features resemble hepatitis B: most acute infections are asymptomatic, and clinical hepatitis uncommon (though usually less severe than hepatitis B), with similar autoimmune reactions – urticaria, arthritis, vasculitis, glomerulonephritis plus cryoglobulinaemia.

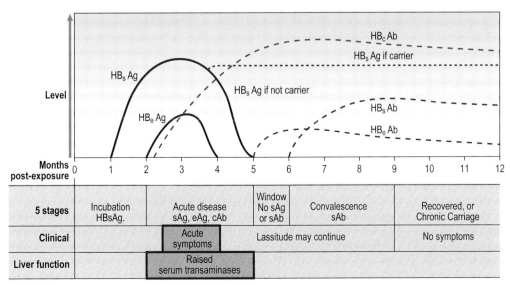

Fig. 5 **Hepatitis B: five stages with antigen and antibody levels.**

Chronic carriage is even commoner than in hepatitis B (in 75% for 1 year), with similar chronic sequelae in 10% – chronic active hepatitis, fibrosis, cirrhosis and hepatocellular carcinoma. Alcoholism greatly increases the risk of liver cancer.

Super-infection with Hepatitis A increases the risk of fulminant hepatitis and death. Co-infection with Hepatitis B increases the risk of cirrhosis and liver cancer. Co-infection with HIV leads to clinical complications, deterioration in disease, and troubles with therapy of both infections.

Confirmatory tests are non-specific Liver Function Tests (LFTs), and specific serology – firstly Hepatitis C antibody (combined IgG and IgM) by ELISA, and secondly confirmation with RIBA (recombinant immuno-blot assay). Thirdly, PCR test for viral RNA in serum indicates active disease if detectable for 6 months.

Chemotherapy. Interferon-alpha or pegylated interferon, with ribavirin if tolerated for chronic infection, eradicate HCV in 40–80% depending on the genotype.

Control and prevention is unsatisfactory. There is no vaccine or effective immune globulin. Donor blood must be tested, and needles never shared, recapped or discarded carelessly. Those with HCV-cirrhosis must be monitored to detect early liver cancer.

Hepatitis D

Classification. Also called Delta hepatitis, it is transmitted by infected body fluids.

Causative agent is unusual, being a defective virus without the genes to make an envelope protein around its single-stranded RNA genome, which encodes only the core protein, called delta antigen. Amazingly it uses the surface antigen of Hepatitis **B** (HBsAg) as its envelope, so can only replicate in cells also infected with HBV.

Clinical features in those co-infected with HBV and HDV simultaneously are, not surprisingly, more severe than hepatitis B alone, but chronic sequelae are similar. However, if a hepatitis B carrier is then super-infected with HDV, the resulting hepatitis is very severe, and if not fatal the sequelae of chronic hepatitis and cirrhosis are more common and more severe.

Confirmatory tests are again non-specific LFTs and specific serology for delta antigen or its IgM antibody.

Chemotherapy. Interferon-alpha improves but does not cure the infection.

Control and prevention. There is no HDV vaccine, but hepatitis B vaccine protects as HDV cannot replicate without HBV. Donor blood must be tested, and needles never shared, recapped or discarded carelessly. Those with cirrhosis must be monitored to detect early liver cancer.

Hepatitis E

Classification. Hepatitis E virus (HEV, no common name) is spread faeco–orally, commonly by water in epidemics in India, Africa and Central America, and hence in returning travellers.

Causative agent is a non-enveloped single-stranded RNA virus, probably a Calicivirus.

Clinical features are like hepatitis A except for severe disease and high mortality in pregnant women. Like hepatitis A, there is no chronic carriage nor other chronic sequelae.

Confirmatory tests are again non-specific LFTs, and specific serology for IgM antibody in acute disease or IgG for past exposure.

Chemotherapy is unavailable.

Control and prevention depends on good hand, food and water hygiene, and proper sewage disposal. There is no vaccine, nor specific immunoglobulin.

Hepatitis F

This does not exist. Clinical cases with no discoverable known virus were described, but no new virus found.

Hepatitis G

Causative agent is HGV, also called GBV-C, a single-stranded RNA virus distantly related to HCV. It is easily transmitted by body fluids including by blood transfusion, sexually and transplacentally.

Clinical features are strikingly absent in spite of persistent viraemia!

Confirmatory tests are by PCR on serum for viral RNA (showing active infection), or immuno-assay for antibody to envelope protein E2 (showing past infection).

Chemotherapy is unnecessary as there is no proven disease.

Control and prevention appears unnecessary.

Transfusion transmissible virus (TTV) and SEN-virus

These are both blood-borne, non-enveloped single-stranded DNA viruses found in normal people, in hepatitis patients, and particularly after blood transfusions, but neither is proven to cause hepatitis.

Viral hepatitis

- **Hepatitis A and E** are both transmitted faeco–orally, cause acute mild hepatitis (except for severe hepatitis E in pregnancy) which usually soon resolves completely.

- **Hepatitis B and C** are both transmitted by infected body fluids, as is the defective **Hepatitis D virus** which needs co-existing HBV infection to replicate. They often cause chronic infection, with chronic sequelae including fibrosis, cirrhosis and liver cancer.

- **Hepatitis F virus** has never been found, and **HGV, TTV and SEN-V** appear to cause no clinical infection.

Tropical and rare abdominal infections

Cholera is described on page 161. Worms and parasites causing abdominal disease in the tropics are described on pages 162–163.

Fitz-Hugh Curtis syndrome

This is a rare condition involving inflammation of the serous membrane covering the liver: perihepatitis. Causative organisms are either *N. gonorrhoeae* or *C. trachomatis*. Clinical features are right upper quadrant pain, tenderness and guarding, plus fever. Symptoms of the primary salpingitis, cervicitis, urethritis, or general peritonitis may be present. Confirmatory tests are microscopy, culture and PCR of cervix and urethra swabs. Laparoscopy can show adhesions like violin strings (Fig. 1). Chemotherapy is ceftriaxone and/or doxycycline. Division of the 'violin strings' can abolish chronic pain. Control and prevention is by safer sex to decrease genital gonorrhoea and chlamydial infection.

Granulomatous hepatitis

Granulomatous hepatitis is an uncommon condition with infectious and non-infectious causes; in idiopathic cases no cause can be found. Hepatic granulomata are collections of

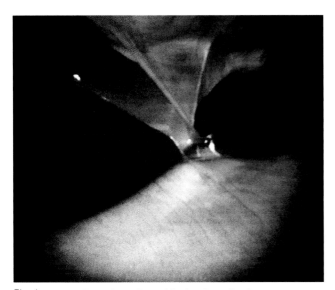

Fig. 1 **Fitz-Hugh Curtis perihepatitis showing adhesions at laparoscopy.**

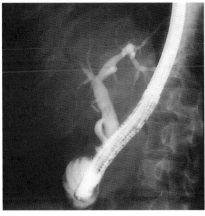

Fig. 2 **Clonorchiasis of the common bile duct.**

macrophages transformed into epithelioid cells, often with multinucleate giant cells, and sometimes with central 'cheesy' necrosis (caseation).

Causative organisms include: intracellular bacteria e.g. *M. tuberculosis, M. leprae, M. avium-intracellulare* complex, *Brucella abortus* and *T. pallidum*; fungi including *Histoplasma capsulatum*; viruses including CMV; parasites e.g. *Schistosoma* spp., and rickettsiae (including *C. burneti*: Q fever). Sarcoidosis, hypersensitivity and allergic diseases, and lymphomas are the commonest non-infectious causes.

Clinical features vary with the cause, but fever, malaise and weight loss are usual.

Confirmatory tests are liver biopsy to confirm granulomatous hepatitis, and Mantoux/Quantiferon test, chest x-ray, microscopy with special stains, cultures and serology to find the cause.

Chemotherapy depends on the cause, but anti-tuberculosis therapy must be given before steroids if no cause can be found. Control and prevention in contacts depends on the cause.

Yersinosis (abdominal)

Gastrointestinal infection with *Yersinia enterocolitica* or *Y. pseudotuberculosis* (p. 56–57) can uncommonly cause **enterocolitis** or **mesenteric adenitis** (infected mesenteric lymph glands). Yersiniae are found in many domestic and wild animals (i.e., these infections are zoonoses). *Y. enterocolitica* causes enterocolitis (p. 161) with diarrhoea, pain and fever; it also causes mesenteric adenitis, which mimics appendicitis, and, rarely, arthritis or erythema nodosum. *Y. pseudotuberculosis* causes abdominal pseudotuberculosis, i.e. mesenteric adenitis. Confirmatory tests are faecal cultures after 28 days of cold (4°C) enrichment, or cultures from lymph nodes or blood at 25°C. Serology is of limited use. Chemotherapy is not well established, but gentamicin or third-generation cephalosporins are active against both species. Control and prevention depends on food and water hygiene, and avoiding infected animals.

Fluke infections (p. 90)

Fasciolopsiasis is common in Southeast Asia. It is caused by *Fasciolopsis buski*, which attaches to the intestine causing diarrhoea with possible bleeding and ulceration. Later, the face, legs and abdomen may swell. The flukes *Clonorchis sinensis* and *Opisthorchis viverrini* also occur in Southeast Asia. They attach in the bile duct (Fig. 2) and so cause cholangitis (p. 164). Flukes are treated with praziquantel.

> ### Tropical and rare abdominal infections
>
> - Cholera is water-borne and widespread; it causes water and electrolyte loss through mild to overwhelming diarrhoea.
> - Fitz-Hugh Curtis syndrome is perihepatitis caused by gonorrhoeal or chlamydial infection.
> - Granulomatous hepatitis has both non-infectious and infectious causes, especially mycobacterial infection.
> - *Yersinia enterocolitica* and *Y. pseudotuberculosis* both cause mesenteric adenitis mimicking appendicitis.
> - Fluke infections cause gastrointestinal symptoms and cholangitis. *F. buski, C. sinensis* and *O. viverrini* are found in Southeast Asia.

Urinary tract infections: cystitis and pyelonephritis

Urinary tract infections (UTI) are classified into lower and upper tract infections.

Lower urinary tract infections include:

- *urethritis*: infection of the urethra, usually a sexually transmitted disease (p. 180–181)
- *cystitis*: infection of the bladder, often loosely called lower UTI, because it is so common
- *trigonitis*: localised cystitis of the triangle between the urethral and two ureteric orifices
- *the urethral syndrome*: dysuria and frequency without cystitis
- *prostatitis*: infection of the prostate (p. 176–177).

Upper urinary tract infections include:

- *ureteritis*: infection of the ureter; this is rare, usually caused by renal tuberculosis and is not discussed further
- *pyelitis*: infection of the pelvis of the kidney; it probably does not occur alone, without some renal infection, hence pyelonephritis
- *acute pyelonephritis*: infection of the renal pelvis and some of the renal tissue; it is the commonest upper UTI
- *chronic pyelonephritis*: diffuse interstitial nephritis with inflammatory changes; infection is difficult or impossible to prove, therefore it is not considered further.

Bacterial infection

Infection is usually acquired by the ascending route so faecal flora are common pathogens.

Bacteriuria is the presence of bacteria in urine. It is found in symptomatic UTI but it may also be asymptomatic.

Significant bacteriuria, the criterion of UTI, has been considered to be 10^5 (100 000) or more bacteria per ml of voided mid-stream urine. Less than 10^5 usually mean a contaminated specimen, not infection. However, with dysuria and pyuria, 10^3 to 10^4 bacteria per ml can signify infection.

Uncomplicated UTI is cystitis in the adult non-pregnant woman.

Complicated UTIs are infections in pregnancy, in children, in men, in sites other than the bladder, or with structural or functional defects. Complicated infections may be mixed, with two or more bacterial genera.

Recurrence is re-appearance of symptoms or infected urine after treatment or spontaneous improvement. It is either a relapse with the same organism, or a re-infection with a different organism. Re-infection means poor perineal hygiene or a persisting structural or functional defect, while relapse means such a defect, or inappropriate antimicrobial treatment.

Pathogenesis

The fundamental determining factors are the virulence and numbers of the infecting organism balanced against normal host defences and predisposing factors.

Predisposing factors either disrupt the flow of urine, or make the access and persistence of pathogens easier:

- urethra length: shorter in females
- presence or increased numbers of pathogens: poor perineal hygiene, sexual activity
- obstruction to complete bladder emptying: pregnancy, prostatic hypertrophy (Fig. 1), congenital abnormalities, neurological disease, tumours, etc.
- foreign bodies: calculi, catheters, etc.
- vesicoureteric reflux: congenital, pregnancy.

Obstruction, foreign bodies or reflux lead to stasis, residual bladder urine and loss of the normal flushing defences.

Cystitis

The bladder is usually infected from the perineum and urethra, especially when sexual activity or poor perineal hygiene cause faecal contamination.

Causative organisms

As most uro-pathogens come from faecal flora, the commonest is *E. coli*, causing 80% of community-acquired and 40% of hospital-acquired infections; pathogens in descending order of frequency are:

- *E. coli*
- faecal Gram-negative rods, *Klebsiella, Enterobacter, Serratia, Proteus* spp. and *Pseudomonas aeruginosa* (particularly in hospital-acquired UTI)
- coagulase-negative *Staphylococcus saprophyticus* (especially in sexually active young women)
- Gram-positive cocci including enterococci
- other organisms including *M. tuberculosis* and *Candida* spp.

Clinical syndromes

- Dysuria (pain on passing urine), urinary urgency, frequency and nocturia, suprapubic pain and tenderness, and low-grade fever are common.

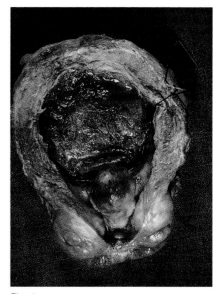

Fig. 1   **Cystitis, showing red, inflamed mucosa and greatly thickened wall, from prostatic obstruction.**

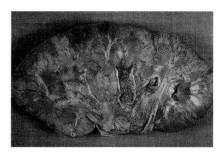

Fig. 2   **Pyelonephritis with intrarenal abscess.**

- High fever with loin and renal angle pain and tenderness may occur, particularly with obstruction. Because there is much overlap in symptoms and signs between lower and upper UTIs, it is impossible to distinguish them clinically with certainty.
- Conversely, particularly in the elderly, UTI can be present without symptoms.
- The prostate must be examined in men with cystitis.
- The **urethral syndrome** is dysuria and frequency without cystitis; it can be caused by urethritis, vaginitis, prostatitis, herpes genitalis or pathogens that are difficult to detect, e.g. chlamydiae.
- Complications of cystitis are rare.

Confirmatory tests

Microscopy and culture of a mid-stream urine specimen confirm a UTI, while ultrasound and/or IVP (intravenous pyelography) are needed to localise the site in women with recurrent infections and in men. Cystoscopy, biopsy and special stains and cultures are rarely needed. Micturating cysto-urethrography (MCU) is used to show reflux.

Chemotherapy

Similar cure rates in uncomplicated cystitis are found with numerous oral antimicrobials, e.g., trimethoprim, amoxicillin-clavulanate or cephalexin. Nitrofurantoin is an alternative to trimethoprim in pregnancy. Norfloxacin should be reserved for resistant infections.

Single-dose or short course (3-day) therapy is effective in uncomplicated infections in non-pregnant women. Complicated or recurrent infections should be treated according to sensitivity test, for 7–10 days. Intravenous therapy is

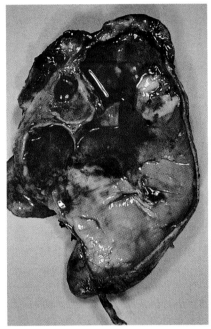

Fig. 3 **Pyonephrosis, showing destroyed kidney filled with pus.**

rarely needed. Predisposing factors should be removed if possible.

Control and prevention

Education in perineal and sexual hygiene, and removal of anatomical or functional defects are necessary; nightly or postcoital antibacterials are needed if the above fail or are not feasible. Triple micturition (urinating three times in succession with 1–3 minute intervals) minimises residual urine in patients with vesicoureteric reflux.

Pyelonephritis

Only acute pyelonephritis is discussed here. The routes are ascending infection as in cystitis, or (rarely) haematogenous in endocarditis, bacteraemia or septicaemia, especially caused by *Staph. aureus*.

Determining factors are the same as in cystitis: virulence and numbers of the organism versus host defences and predisposing factors.

Causative organisms

These are similar to those in cystitis. *Proteus mirabilis* is particularly associated with calculi (urinary stones), probably because its urease produces ammonia and alkaline urine, favouring stone formation.

Clinical features

Dysuria (pain on passing urine), urinary urgency, frequency and nocturia, and high fever with vomiting, loin and renal angle pain and tenderness are common. As with cystitis there is much overlap in symptoms and signs between lower and upper UTIs, so it is impossible to distinguish them clinically with certainty.

Complications

Complications of pyelonephritis are:

- local destruction, causing renal abscesses (p. 176), or papillary necrosis (particularly in diabetes, sickle cell disease or analgesic abuse), which can produce further obstruction (Fig. 2) or pyonephrosis (Fig. 3)
- local spread, causing perinephric abscess (p. 176)
- distant spread, causing bacteraemia (p. 142).

Confirmatory tests

As with cystitis, microscopy and culture of a mid-stream urine specimen confirm a UTI, while ultrasound and/or IVP are needed to confirm the renal site and show renal size, calculi and other abnormalities, e.g. staghorn calculus with pyonephrosis (Fig. 4). Cystoscopy, biopsy and special stains and cultures are rarely needed in acute infection.

Chemotherapy

Intravenous therapy is often needed initially, for example ampicillin and gentamicin. This may be replaced by oral amoxicillin-clavulanate or cephalexin according to sensitivity tests in community-acquired infections, but severe disease and/or resistant hospital-acquired organisms may need continuing intravenous reserve drugs. Rehydration and pain relief are important.

Control and prevention

Careful catheter and operative techniques minimise hospital-acquired infection, while removal of underlying urologic abnormalities prevents recurrence.

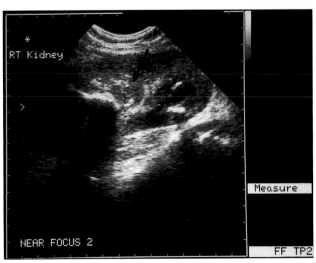

Fig. 4 **Pyonephrosis resulting from staghorn calculus (ultrasound).**

Cystitis and pyelonephritis

- Infection is usually ascending up the urethra by faecal flora.
- Infection occurs when the virulence and numbers of organisms exceed host defences.
- Host defences are impaired by poor perineal hygiene or anatomical or functional abnormalities, especially foreign bodies, obstruction or vesicoureteric reflux.
- Dysuria, frequency, fever, suprapubic and loin pain and tenderness are common in both lower and upper UTI.
- Urine microscopy and culture confirm infection, while renal ultrasound and/or IVP show renal abnormalities.
- Empiric treatment is followed by specific treatment after antibiotic sensitivity tests.
- Prevention depends on education and correction of defects more than on antibacterials.

Renal and perinephric abscesses/prostatitis

These three infections, adjacent to the urinary stream, are alike because they:

- may cause dysuria and frequency, mimicking a UTI
- often have negative or ambiguous urine culture and microscopy results
- are undiagnosable without specific investigation
- are serious if undiagnosed
- need specific treatment, which may be operative.

Intrarenal abscess

Renal abscesses are characterised by collections of pus *within* kidney tissue. They are classified by their causative mechanisms:

- ascending infection in pyelonephritis, especially with obstruction; this is the commonest mechanism, usually causing multiple abscesses (Fig. 1)
- haematogenous infection in bacteraemia, also usually multiple
- infection of a renal cyst, by bacteraemia or an operative procedure; usually single.

Causative organisms

Ascending infection is by the usual uro-pathogens: *E. coli, Klebsiella* spp. and other faecal pathogens. Haematogenous or operative infection is often with *Staph. aureus.*

Clinical features

Dysuria and frequency occur when abscesses communicate with the collecting system, but otherwise are absent. The important features are fever with loin or flank pain and tenderness which *persist* for 3 days or more after treatment starts for a UTI or bacteraemia. A palpable mass is rare.

Confirmatory tests

Urine biochemistry, microscopy and culture show proteinuria, haematuria, pyuria and bacteriuria in abscesses which communicate with the collecting system, but these tests are often negative or equivocal in abscesses from bacteraemia or infected cysts. Blood cultures are positive in one-third. The diagnostic tests are ultrasound and/or CT scanning (Fig. 2) to confirm the diagnosis and show the number and position of the abscesses.

Management

Initial broad-spectrum empiric therapy with, for example, ampicillin and gentamicin, or an anti-staphylococcal beta-lactam, is replaced by specific therapy after positive urine or blood cultures, usually continued for 6 weeks or more. Percutaneous drainage under CT control has largely replaced open surgery when drainage is needed for large or unresponsive abscesses. Therapy is needed for the underlying defect e.g. obstructive uropathy, papillary necrosis (Fig. 3) or endocarditis.

Control and prevention depends on early recognition and treatment of pyelonephritis, urinary obstruction and bacteraemia.

Perinephric abscess

Perinephric abscesses are collections of pus *next to* the kidney (Fig. 4). They can be classified by their cause:

- local spread in pyelonephritis or renal abscess, especially with obstruction
- haematogenous infection in bacteraemia; this is rare.

Causative organisms

Spread from pyelonephritis involves the usual uro-pathogens. Haematogenous infection is often with *Staph. aureus.*

Clinical features

Dysuria and frequency occur from pyelonephritis but otherwise are absent. Like a renal abscess, the important features are fever with loin or flank pain and tenderness which *persist* for 3 days or more after treatment starts for a UTI or bacteraemia. A mass develops if diagnosis is delayed.

Confirmatory tests

The tests used are the same as those described for intrarenal abscesses. Blood cultures are often positive. The diagnostic tests are ultrasound and/or CT scanning.

Management

Treatment for pyelonephritis or bacteraemia is initiated empirically and is then directed by urine or blood cultures. Drainage is essential, usually percutaneous under CT control (Fig. 5). Surgery is needed only for very large or unresponsive abscesses.

Control and prevention, as in renal abscesses, depends on early recognition and treatment of pyelonephritis, urinary obstruction and bacteraemia.

Prostatitis

Prostatitis is characterised by diffuse prostatic infection, which may progress to prostatic abscess. Prostatitis is classified as:

1. acute bacterial prostatitis,
2. chronic bacterial prostatitis or
3. chronic 'non-bacterial' prostatitis ('prostatosis').

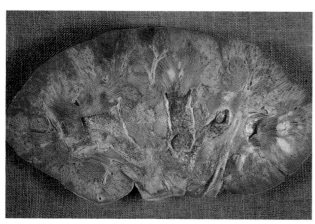

Fig. 1 **Intrarenal abscesses from acute pyelonephritis.**

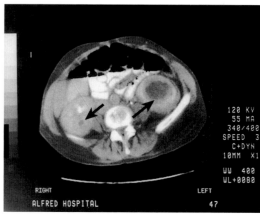

Fig. 2 **Intrarenal abscesses on CT.**

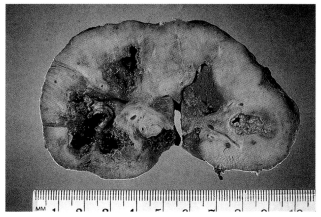

Fig. 3 **Intrarenal abscesses with diabetic papillary necrosis.**

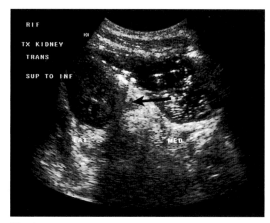

Fig. 4 **Perinephric abscess on ultrasound.**

Prostatitis is usually caused by ascending infection from the urinary tract, either from a UTI (cystitis or pyelonephritis) or from a sexually transmitted disease (usually urethritis). Haematogenous infection or lymphogenous spread from the rectum rarely occurs.

Causative organisms

Pathogens causing prostatitis are usually:

- uro-pathogens: *E. coli*, *Klebsiella* spp., other faecal Gram-negative rods or enterococci, from a UTI, or
- sexually transmitted pathogens: *N. gonorrhoeae* or *C. trachomatis*.

By definition, routine cultures are negative in 'non-bacterial' prostatitis, which may be caused by *C. trachomatis* or ureaplasma.

Clinical syndromes

1. In acute prostatitis, fever and perineal pain are usual, and symptoms of a lower UTI (dysuria and frequency) or of urethritis (dysuria and discharge) are frequent.
2. In chronic bacterial prostatitis, symptoms range from none (asymptomatic bacteriuria), to perineal or low back pain, to recurrent UTIs only temporarily responsive to antibacterials.
3. In chronic 'non-bacterial' prostatitis, symptoms again range from none to low back or perineal pain (the '**Chronic Pelvic Pain Syndrome**') to recurrent UTIs.

Confirmatory tests

1. In acute prostatitis, urethral swabs, urine microscopy and culture or PCR for *Chlamydia* and gonorrhoea usually show the pathogen, and acute prostatic tenderness is present rectally.
2. In chronic bacterial prostatitis the above tests are often negative, so localisation studies are needed:
   - Urethral urine is voided first (VB1), then a mid-stream (bladder) urine (VB2), then expressed prostatic secretions (EPS) during rectal prostatic massage, then a third voided urine (VB3). Positive microscopy and culture on VB1 indicates urethritis, on VB2 indicates cystitis, while positive EPS and/or VB3 indicate prostatitis.
   - Seminal ejaculate is more often culture positive than EPS.
   - Ultrasound may show an abnormal prostate.
   - Biopsy is the final arbiter.

3. In chronic 'non-bacterial' prostatitis all the above tests are negative except EPS show more than 10 white blood cells per HPF, and ultrasound may be positive. Routine cultures, by definition, are negative.

Chemotherapy

1. Acute prostatitis usually responds well to oral norfloxacin or co-trimoxazole for 2–4 weeks. For severe cases, intravenous broad-spectrum beta-lactams and/or gentamicin may be needed initially.
2. Chronic bacterial prostatitis usually only responds to a few drugs which penetrate into the non-acutely-inflamed prostate: norfloxacin or ciprofloxacin alone or with rifampicin, or co-trimoxazole for 6–12 weeks.
3. Chronic non-bacterial prostatitis responds poorly, but azithromycin or erythromycin for 2–4 weeks is worth a trial, and aspirin helps pain relief.

Control and prevention

This depends on early diagnosis and treatment of UTIs and urethritis.

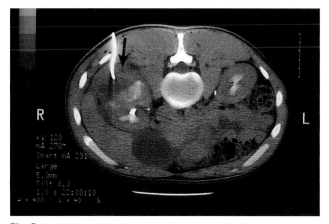

Fig. 5 **Perinephric abscess on CT, with catheter drain.**

Renal and perinephric abscesses/prostatitis

- These three infections, adjacent to the urinary stream, all may cause dysuria and frequency like a UTI, but usually have negative or ambiguous urine test results and, therefore, may be undiagnosed without specific investigation.

- Renal and perinephric abscesses typically show persistent fever and loin or flank pain that *persists* after apparently appropriate treatment for a UTI has started. They need urine and blood cultures, ultrasound or CT scans and continuing antibiotics. Perinephric abscesses usually need CT-directed drainage, rarely needed for renal abscesses.

- Prostatitis ranges from acute symptomatic to chronic asymptomatic with recurrent UTIs. Treatment may have to be empiric with norfloxacin or co-trimoxazole, or with azithromycin if *C. trachomatis* is suspected.

Tropical and rare urinary infections

Acute glomerulonephritis (AGN)

Unlike acute pyelonephritis, bacteria are *not* found in the urine and kidney when infection causes acute glomerulonephritis. The disease is caused by deposition of immune complexes (antibody with bacterial antigens or bacteria) onto the glomerular basement membrane. These complexes arise as a result of a distant infection (e.g. streptococcal impetigo). The immune complexes activate the complement and coagulation systems (p. 27–30) causing inflammation, with clotting, increased permeability, endothelial cell damage and mesangial proliferation (Fig. 1). Numerous other types of glomerulonephritis, not caused by infection, are not considered here.

Causative organisms

The commonest cause is *Streptococcus pyogenes*; acute glomerulonephritis is more common after a streptococcal skin infection than after streptococcal pharyngitis. The nephritogenic types are four or five of the 65 M types of *S. pyogenes*. Other organisms causing acute glomerulonephritic immune complexes are:

- *Plasmodium* species, especially *P. malariae*, then *P. falciparum*
- streptococci or coagulase-negative staphylococci (rarely other organisms) in bacteraemia resulting from endocarditis or infected intravascular shunts (Fig. 1b)
- viruses, including Epstein–Barr and Hepatitis B.

Clinical features

Post-streptococcal AGN follows 10–14 days after streptococcal pharyngitis (especially with group A, serotype M12) or after pyoderma or infected scabies (especially with group A, serotype M49). Rarely group C streptococci are responsible. Inflammation from the immune complexes causes haematuria and proteinuria, oedema and hypertension with headache. Nephritis from *P. malariae* often progresses to the nephrotic syndrome with persisting oedema and massive proteinuria. Focal or diffuse AGN in bacteraemia causes haematuria, proteinuria and renal impairment.

Confirmatory tests

In all cases, urine examination shows haematuria, proteinuria and hyaline casts, urine culture is sterile, and serum electrolytes, creatinine and urea show renal impairment. In streptococcal infection, throat or skin swabs are usually positive before therapy, and antistreptolysin O and DNAase B tests usually become positive in 1–2 weeks. In acute malaria with nephritis, thick and thin blood films are positive, but they are usually negative in malarial nephrotic syndrome, though antibody is positive.

Blood cultures and other tests in endocarditis are discussed on page 141.

Management

Penicillin for at least 10 days is given to eradicate causative streptococci. Because only 6–8% of *S. pyogenes* M types cause AGN, repeat attacks are rare (in contrast to rheumatic fever), so penicillin prophylaxis is not given after post-streptococcal AGN. Malaria and endocarditis are treated as described (p. 141, 157).

Hydatid disease

Larvae of the tapeworms *Echinococcus* spp. (p. 88–89) may be carried to any organ, where they encyst, forming a hydatid cyst. They occasionally lodge in the kidney, producing a space-occupying lesion (Fig. 2). Drugs often do not penetrate well, so treatment is operative removal, of the cyst only if possible.

Schistosomiasis

The eggs of the blood flukes (*Schistosoma* spp., usually *S. haematobium*, p. 91) can deposit in the bladder. Early there is

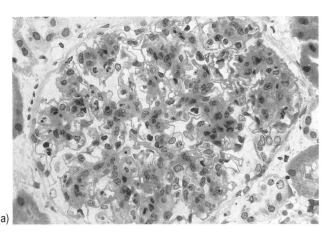

(a)

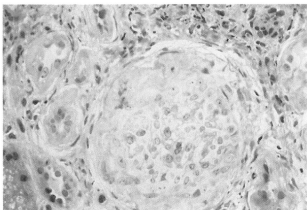

(b)

Fig. 1 **Glomerulonephritis. (a)** Acute post-streptococcal glomerulonephritis. **(b)** 'Shunt' glomerulonephritis.

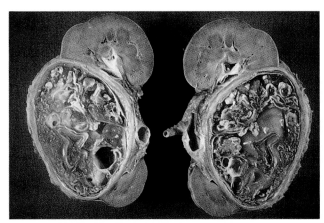

Fig. 2 **Hydatid of the kidney.**

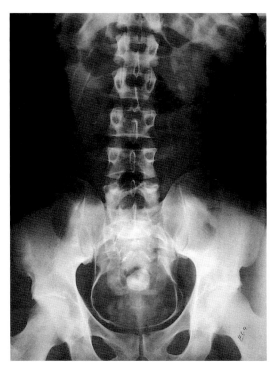

Fig. 3 **Schistosomiasis causing calcified bladder wall.**

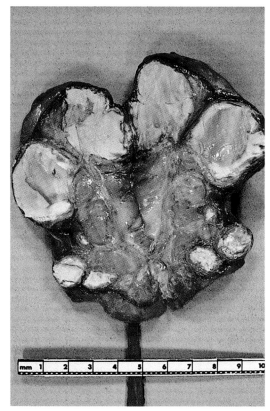

Fig. 4 **Renal TB showing massive destruction with caseation.**

cystitis with haematuria, then hepatosplenomegaly with portal hypertension (p. 153). Later there may be bladder calcification (Fig. 3). Treatment is with praziquantel.

Tuberculosis

Urinary tract tuberculosis, usually renal (Fig. 4), is secondary to haematogenous spread from a primary focus elsewhere – usually pulmonary, rarely gut. It is characterised by caseating destruction and heals with fibrosis, which often causes obstruction and bacterial UTIs. Spread may also have involved bone, joint, adrenal (Fig. 5), epididymis or other uro-genital organs.

Causative organism

This is *M. tuberculosis*, usually a human strain by inhalation causing primary pulmonary TB, occasionally bovine *M. tuberculosis* by ingestion, causing gastrointestinal TB (p. 60).

Clinical features

UTI symptoms of dysuria, frequency and loin or back pain are common, but fever and systemic symptoms are surprisingly uncommon.

Confirmatory tests

Urine examination often shows haematuria and proteinuria, but characteristically shows 'sterile pyuria' i.e. pyuria with usual cultures sterile. Urine cultures are positive in 80–90% when three successive early morning urine (EMU) specimens are cultured on specific mycobacterial media. Urine microscopy for acid-fast bacilli is unreliable because false positives occur from saprophytic mycobacteria (e.g. *M. smegmatis*) in healthy people. Chest x-ray shows pulmonary TB, often inactive, in over 70%. Renal ultrasound is often suggestive, while CT (or intravenous pyelography) is usually diagnostic.

Management

Triple therapy including isoniazid and rifampicin is usually needed for 9–12 months, longer in complicated or relapsed patients. Surgery is now used only for complications, including stricture or failed medical therapy. Control and prevention depends on BCG, and early, effective treatment of TB elsewhere.

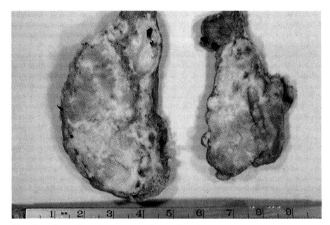

Fig. 5 **Adrenal TB showing typical tubercles**

> ### Tropical and rare urinary infections
>
> ■ Acute glomerulonephritis related to infection is an immune complex disease, with haematuria, proteinuria, oedema and hypertension. Treatment depends on the cause, usually streptococcal infection, malaria or endocarditis.
>
> ■ Renal tuberculosis is blood borne, usually from pulmonary TB. Sterile pyuria is usual, and special urine cultures are essential. Specific long-term anti-tuberculous therapy including isoniazid and rifampicin is needed.
>
> ■ Helminth parasites (tapeworms and flukes) can deposit in the pelvic veins, bladder and kidney causing characteristic lesions.

Urethritis

Urethritis is inflammation of the male or female urethra. It may be:

- chemical, e.g. from local disinfectants or anaesthetics
- mechanical, e.g. from catheters or other foreign bodies, or from a worried man 'stripping', i.e. digitally milking, his urethra on several days for signs of sexually transmitted disease (STD; also called venereal disease or VD)
- infective, the most common cause, often as a STD.

The two major types of infective urethritis are **gonorrhoea** and so-called **non-specific urethritis** (NSU) or **non-gonorrhoeal urethritis** (NGU).

Causative organisms

1. **Gonorrhoea** is caused by infection with *Neisseria gonorrhoeae* (p. 42). This pathogen only infects humans and is spread person to person, usually by sexual contact. It survives poorly outside the human host.
2. **NGU** has two major causes: *Chlamydia trachomatis* and *Mycoplasma genitalium* (p. 63, 64). It can also be caused, less commonly, by *Ureaplasma urealyticum*, *Trichomonas vaginalis* or *Herpes simplex*, and rarely by *Gardnerella vaginalis* or yeasts.
3. In addition to these sexually transmitted diseases, **bacterial urethritis** (*Escherichia coli*, *Klebsiella* spp., *Staphylococcus aureus*, etc.) occurs with catheters, strictures and urinary infections including prostatitis (Table 1).

The relative incidence of these causes varies with:

- **gender**: *C. trachomatis* in women causes cervicitis (p. 182–183) more commonly than symptomatic urethritis

- **sexual orientation**: gonorrhoea predominates in homosexual men, *C. trachomatis* in heterosexual men
- **clinical presentation**: clinical features vary with the cause (Table 2).

Clinical features

The two cardinal symptoms are discharge and dysuria. Discharge from the urethra varies from a scanty, clear or mucopurulent discharge, particularly in NGU, to copious yellow or yellow-green pus, particularly in gonorrhoea.

Dysuria means pain on passing urine and results directly from urethral infection and inflammation. It varies from mild (particularly in NGU) to extremely severe, 'like passing razor blades', particularly in gonococcal infections. It is often accompanied by urgency and frequency of micturition, and by nocturia, i.e. the (unusual) passage of urine during the night.

Systemic symptoms including fever and malaise may occur in gonorrhoea but are absent in NGU.

Signs include urethral tenderness and the discharge, which may only be visible after 'milking' the urethra from penile base towards the glans. Inguinal lymph nodes may be enlarged in gonorrhoea. The rectum and throat, and in men the testes, epididymis and prostate, or, in females, the cervix, Fallopian tubes and pelvis (cervicitis and pelvic inflammatory disease, p. 182–185), should be examined for local spread or co-existent infection. The skin and joints may show disseminated infection.

Complications of gonorrhoea

Complications of gonorrhoea are infrequent unless treatment is delayed or inadequate.

Local spread. This causes periurethral abscesses, urethral stricture, epididymitis or prostatitis, salpingitis and PID.

Distant spread. This causes gonococcaemia with skin or joint infection. It is rare in men, but occurs in 1–3% of women, particularly if there is unrecognised, asymptomatic cervicitis (p. 182).

Co-existent infection. The rectum and pharynx can be infected by direct contact with infectious discharge, usually urethral, and the pharyngitis is often asymptomatic. The proctitis (infection of the rectum) may be asymptomatic but more often causes pain and anal discharge.

Postgonococcal urethritis (**PGU**). This is the persistence of symptoms of urethritis after treatment for gonorrhoea. It is caused by gonococci resistant to the antibiotic chosen, by re-infection, by co-existing chlamydial infection (the commonest cause) or co-existing ureaplasmal infection.

Complications of NGU

Local spread. Acute epididymitis (Fig. 1) and prostatitis are not uncommon with chlamydial infection but are rare in ureaplasmal infection.

Reiter's syndrome. This is the triad of urethritis, arthritis and conjunctivitis. Additionally, 50% of patients have unusual skin or mucous membrane lesions (with even more unusual names): kera-

Table 2 **Clinical presentation of non-gonorrhoeal urethritis**			
	Non-gonorrhoeal urethritis (%)		
	Acute	Persistent	Recurrent
C. trachomatis	50	0	5
Mycoplasma/ Ureaplasma	30	50	20
Other infections	20	50	75

Table 1 **Characteristics of urethritis (infective)**						
Classification	Causative organism	Clinical features		Confirmatory tests	Chemotherapy	Control
		Discharge	Dysuria			
Gonorrhoea	*N. gonorrhoeae*	Purulent, severe	Moderate to gross	Gram-negative diplococci in pus cells	Ceftriaxone or ciprofloxacin	Treat partners
Non-gonococcal urethritis (NGU)	*Chlamydia trachomatis*	Mucoid to thin pus	Mild to moderate	PCR or EIA	Azithromycin	Treat partners
	Mycoplasma genitalium	Ditto	Ditto	Special culture	Azithromycin	Treat partners
	Ureaplasma urealyticum	Ditto	Ditto	Special culture	Azithromycin (erythromycin)	Treat partners
	Trichomonas vaginalis	Minimal or none	Minimal or none	Wet mount microscopy	Metronidazole	Treat partners
	Herpes simplex	Minimal or none	Minimal or none	PCR	A/Fam/Valaciclovir	Treat partners
	Rarer causes	Minimal or none	Minimal or none	Special M&C	Specific	Treat partners
Bacterial urethritis	*S. aureus* or enteric GNR	Purulent, moderate	Moderate to severe	Gram stain and culture	Flucloxacillin or gentamicin	Remove cause

M&C, microscopy and culture; GNR, Gram-negative rods; PCR, polymerase chain reaction; EIA, enzyme immuno assay.

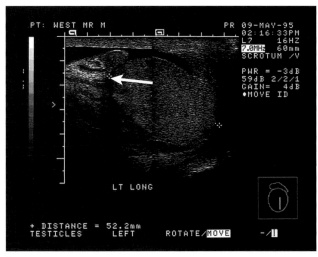

Fig. 1 **Chlamydial epididymitis with hydrocoele on ultrasound.**

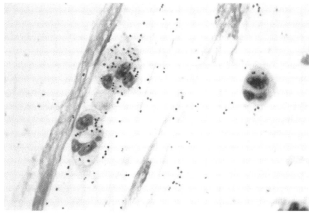

Fig. 2 **N. gonorrhoeae on Gram stain.**

todermia blennorrhagica (hard skin papules with a waxy yellow centre), circinate balanitis (rash with circular outline on penile skin), circinate or ulcerative vulvitis, iritis, pharyngitis or glossitis. Reiter's syndrome is most often caused by genital chlamydial infection but may also be post-dysenteric, i.e. following bacterial gastroenteritis caused by *Salmonella*, *Shigella*, *Campylobacter* or *Yersinia* spp. (p. 159).

Confusing conditions

In men, while prostatitis, cystitis or an upper urinary tract infection may need to be considered, the symptoms of urethritis are usually clear-cut, and only the causative organism is unclear.

In women, however, dysuria, urgency, frequency, and nocturia, with or without urethral discharge, may also be caused by:

■ bacterial cystitis: infection of the urinary bladder, with pyuria [i.e. polymorphonuclear leucocytes (PMNs) in the centrifuged deposit] and > 100 000 bacteria per ml
■ 'the urethral syndrome': most often urethritis caused by gonococcal or chlamydial infection but may be an atypical cystitis, or urethral trichomoniasis
■ vulvo-vaginitis, usually candidal, less often associated with *Gardnerella vaginalis*.

Confirmatory tests

Microscopy of the smear from a urethral swab showing increased numbers of pus cells, some containing Gram-negative intracellular diplococci, is almost pathognomonic ('certainly diagnostic') for gon-

orrhoea (Fig. 2). A special small calcium alginate swab must be used, as routine swabs are too large, and cotton inhibits fastidious pathogens like the gonococcus.

PCR on urethral swab or first-pass urine is necessary to diagnose chlamydial infection.

Culture (preferably by direct 'bed-side' inoculation) on special non-selective media (chocolate agar) and selective media (e.g. modified Thayer-Martin) in CO_2 is necessary to grow the fastidious gonococcus. Identification is by a positive oxidase reaction and by sugar fermentation. Chlamydial culture is out-dated.

Antibiotic sensitivity testing of gonococci is necessary in most countries, where resistance is common and often unpredictable. Serology is useless for gonorrhoea, and seldom used to diagnose chlamydial infection.

Chemotherapy

As negative investigations do not exclude infection, and double infections are so common, all patients with urethritis should be treated for **both** gonorrhoea and chlamydiae.

Penicillin cures uncomplicated gonorrhoeal urethritis caused by sensitive strains but has been largely replaced by ceftriaxone as penicillinase- or chromosomally-mediated resistance is common. Ciprofloxacin is effective for sensitive strains.

Azithromycin is used for chlamydial infection, and a second dose may be needed. Erythromycin is used in pregnancy, and for resistant *Ureaplasma* infections.

Control and prevention

Asymptomatic infected people, particularly women, form a reservoir for the gonococcus and for chlamydiae. As there are no vaccines, and chemoprophylaxis is not feasible, control depends on education, safer sexual practices, and rapid exact diagnosis with effective treatment of patients and their sexual partners.

Urethritis

■ Urethritis may be chemical or mechanical but is usually infective, particularly as a STD.

■ Gonorrhoea and non-gonorrhoeal urethritis (NGU, or NSU), usually caused by *C. trachomatis*, are most common.

■ Usual symptoms are discharge and dysuria. Co-existent cervical, rectal or pharyngeal disease is common and often asymptomatic.

■ Spread locally causes epididymitis, prostatitis, salpingitis and PID. Disseminated disease is rare. Reiter's syndrome can be a sequel of genital chlamydial infection.

■ Diagnosis depends on the urethral smear, Gram stain, PCR and culture.

■ Treatment is usually ceftriaxone for gonorrhoea, and azithromycin for chlamydial infection.

■ Control depends on education, safer sex, and rapid exact diagnosis with effective treatment of patients and their sexual contacts.

Cervical infections

Cervical infections can be classified into human papillomavirus infections and cervicitis.

Human papillomavirus infections

Human papillomaviruses are non-enveloped with a double-stranded circular DNA genome and icosahedral nucleocapsid (p. 92–93). They cause four different genital tract abnormalities:

- genital warts, usually by types 6 and 11, in men and women (see Fig. 5, p. 189), treated locally by cryotherapy, podophyllotoxin or imiquimod
- low-grade cervical dysplasia by both non-oncogenic and oncogenic types
- high-grade dysplasia by oncogenic types only, and hence pre-malignant
- cervical cancer, by oncogenic types, particularly by HPV-16 and HPV-18.

Diagnosis and treatment of dysplasia and cancer is outside the scope of this book.

Cervicitis

Cervicitis is inflammation of the uterine cervix, usually caused by infection. The important causes are:

- *Neisseria gonorrhoeae*
- *Chlamydia trachomatis*
- Herpes simplex virus.
  Less commonly, cervicitis may be:
- granulomatous: resulting from TB, anaerobes, schistosomiasis (Fig. 1)
- non-infectious.

Causative organisms

Gonorrhoea is caused by the Gram-negative diplococcus *N. gonorrhoeae* (p. 42), while *C. trachomatis* (p. 64) is the other common cause of endocervical infection. They commonly co-exist.

Gonococci have no exotoxin, and inflammatory responses cause tissue damage.

Intracellular chlamydiae destroy cells directly, aided by the host inflammatory response.

Herpes simplex virus causes infection and ulceration of the ectocervix. Granulomatous cervicitis caused by *Mycobacterium tuberculosis*, anaerobes such as *Bacteroides* and *Fusobacterium* spp., and schistosomal infections are all rare and not further discussed (Table 1).

Clinical features

Many infections are asymptomatic and only discovered when a sexual partner is found to be infected. When symptoms occur they include:

- vaginal discharge
- dysuria if urethritis (p. 180) co-exists
- abdominal pain and fever if local spread causes salpingitis or pelvic inflammatory disease (PID)
- further symptoms from distant spread (see below).

The diagnostic sign is cervical discharge, varying from purulent to clear, and from profuse to inconspicuous.

Differential diagnosis of uncomplicated cervicitis is mainly from vaginitis (p. 187).

Complications of gonorrhoeal cervicitis

Local spread. The gonococcus moves like the knight in chess, infecting urethra not vagina, cervix not uterus, fallopian tube not fimbriae (primarily), ovary not posterior abdominal wall. Salpingitis (Fallopian tube infection) leads to tubal blockage, tubo-ovarian abscesses (Fig. 2) and PID in about 15% of patients.

Distant spread. Gonococcaemia is rare, causing skin or joint infections. It occurs in 1–3% of women from unrecognised asymptomatic cervicitis. Disseminated infection is characterised by fever, headache and prostration (which may progress to septic shock, p. 32), a pustular skin rash, migratory arthralgias and then suppurative ('septic') arthritis in large joints, especially knees, wrists and ankles.

Congenital infection. Infection can be transmitted vertically to the child during childbirth (Fig. 3 and p. 215).

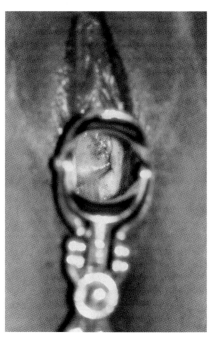

Fig. 1 **Cervicitis associated with schistosomiasis.**

Co-existent infection. The pharynx and rectum can be infected by direct contact with infectious discharge, usually urethral. Pharyngitis is often asymptomatic. Proctitis (rectal infection) may be asymptomatic but can cause severe anal pain and discharge.

Post-gonococcal cervicitis (PGC). This is the persistence of symptoms of cervicitis after treatment for gonorrhoea. It is caused by gonococci resistant to the antibiotic given, or reinfection, or co-existent chlamydial infection (the commonest cause).

Complications of chlamydial cervicitis

Local spread. Bartholinitis (infection of the duct of Bartholin's gland in the labia beside the vaginal entrance) is troublesome, but acute salpingitis (in 10%), and consequent tubal obstruction, ectopic pregnancy, infertility and PID are serious consequences.

Table 1 **Characteristics of cervicitis (infective)**					
Classification	**Causative organism**	**Clinical features**		**Confirmatory tests**	**Chemotherapy**
		Discharge	**Dysuria**		
Gonorrhoeal	*N. gonorrhoeae*	Purulent, severe	Moderate to gross	Gram-negative diplococci in pus cells	Ceftriaxone or ciprofloxacin
Chlamydial	*Chlamydia trachomatis*	Mucoid to thin pus	Mild to moderate	PCR or EIA	Azithromycin
Herpetic	Herpes simplex	Mucoid to thin pus	Nil to mild	PCR	A/Fam/Valaciclovir
Granulomatous	*M. tuberculosis*	Mucoid to thin pus	Nil to mild	Microscopy and culture	Specific triple
	Anaerobes	Mucoid to thin pus	Nil to mild	Anaerobic culture	Metronidazole usually
	Schistosomes	Mucoid to thin pus	Nil to mild	Microscopy, biopsy	Specific

In all cases, treat sexual partners.

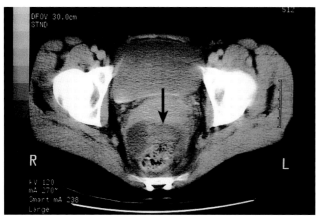

Fig. 2 **Infective cervicitis and salpingitis led to this pelvic tubo-ovarian abscess.**

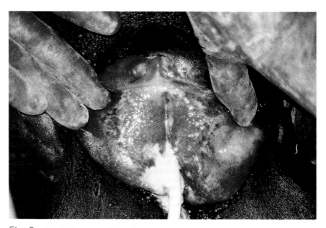

Fig. 3 **Cervical gonorrhoea in pregnancy.**

Distant spread. This may cause peritonitis and, rarely, perihepatitis with peritoneal adhesions like violin strings: the Fitz-Hugh Curtis syndrome (p. 173).

Co-existent infection. Chlamydial urethritis is present in over 50% of women with chlamydial cervicitis, and gonorrhoea also commonly co-exists at either site.

Cervical cytologic metaplasia. This often regresses after treatment of chlamydial infection. While cervical cytologic atypia and dysplasia (intraepithelial neoplasia) are statistically associated with chlamydial infection, the human papillomavirus (HPV) is the causal agent (see above).

Congenital infection. Infants born through an infected cervix usually become infected and often develop neonatal chlamydial pneumonia (p. 126).

Confirmatory tests

Microscopy of the smear from an endocervical swab showing increased numbers of pus cells, some containing Gram-negative intracellular diplococci, is pathognomonic for gonorrhoea. A special calcium alginate swab must be used, as cotton inhibits the fastidious gonococcus.

PCR tests on cervical swabs and first-pass urine diagnose chlamydial infection.

Culture (preferably by direct 'bed-side' inoculation) on special non-selective media (chocolate agar) and selective media (e.g. modified Thayer-Martin) in CO_2 is necessary to grow the fastidious gonococcus (Fig. 4). Identification is by a positive oxidase reaction and sugar fermentation.

Antibiotic sensitivity testing of gonococci is necessary in most countries, as resistance is common and often unpredictable.

Serology is useless for gonorrhoea, and is seldom used to diagnose chlamydial infection.

Chemotherapy

As negative investigations do not exclude infection, and double infections are so common, all patients with cervicitis should be treated for **both** gonorrhoea and chlamydiae.

Penicillin cures uncomplicated gonorrhoeal cervicitis caused by sensitive strains. This has been replaced by ceftriaxone where penicillinase- or chromosomally-mediated resistance is common. Ciprofloxacin is effective for sensitive strains.

Azithromycin is used for chlamydial infection, and a second dose may be needed. Erythromycin is used in pregnancy.

Control and prevention

As there are no vaccines, and chemoprophylaxis is not feasible, control depends on education, safer sexual practices, and rapid exact diagnosis and effective treatment of patients and their sexual contacts.

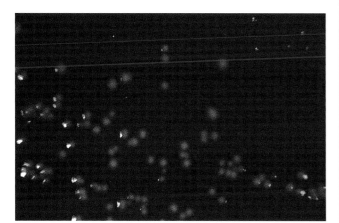

Fig. 4 **Culture plate of N. gonorrhoea.**

Cervical infections

Human papillomavirus infection
- The numerous types cause genital warts, low-grade cervical dysplasia, high-grade dysplasia and (particularly by types 16 and 18) cervical cancer.

Cervicitis
- Cervicitis is usually infective, particularly as a STD.
- The commonest causes are *N. gonorrhoeae* and *C. trachomatis*.
- Vaginal discharge, abdominal pain and dysuria are the usual symptoms. Co-existent urethral, rectal or pharyngeal disease is common and often asymptomatic.
- Spread locally causes bartholinitis, salpingitis and PID (p. 184). Peritonitis, perihepatitis, disseminated disease and Reiter's syndrome are all rare. Infants are infected by vaginal delivery through an infected cervix.
- Diagnosis depends on the endocervical smear, Gram stain, PCR and culture.
- Treatment is usually ceftriaxone for gonorrhoea, and azithromycin for chlamydial infection.
- Control depends on education, safer sex, and rapid exact diagnosis with effective treatment of patients and their sexual contacts.

Salpingitis and pelvic inflammatory disease

The term 'pelvic inflammatory disease' (PID) is unfortunately used in two different ways. A narrow (sensu stricto) use, especially by gynaecologists, means only acute salpingitis (Fallopian tube infection). A broader usage (sensu lato) includes endometritis, salpingitis, salpingo-oophoritis, tubo-ovarian abscess, inflammation of the adnexal ('adjacent') tissues and inflammatory 'pelvic mass', pelvic abscess, and peritonitis. This broader usage is convenient, for these conditions are a continuum, extending into each other, and clinically it is often impossible to tell either the exact anatomical extent or the pathological stage (Table 1).

Causative organisms

These conditions are usually polymicrobial, i.e. caused by a number of microbial species in a mixture, not by a single species. The most important causes are:

- *Neisseria gonorrhoeae* (p. 42), as a STD, particularly causing salpingitis and ascending infection
- *Chlamydia trachomatis* (p. 64) as a STD, also causing salpingitis and ascending infection
- anaerobic or mixed anaerobic and aerobic bacteria, particularly in endogenous postabortal, postpartum or postoperative endometritis (and endomyometritis when uterine muscle is infected)
- *Clostridium perfringens* (p. 40), as a life-threatening pathogen, especially where illegal abortions are done without aseptic technique
- *Actinomyces* spp. (p. 62), important in IUD-related infections
- *Mycoplasma hominis* (p. 63) is less important; *Ureaplasma* spp. and viruses, including HSV and CMV, are uncommon.

Clinical syndromes

The clinical features vary in severity and extent, depending on the cause, organism, site and extent of disease.

Endometritis. PV bleeding and fever are prominent, often with some pelvic pain and uterine tenderness.

Urethritis. If co-existing (p. 180), it causes dysuria.

Salpingitis, salpingo-oophoritis and adjacent tissue infection. The classic triad of vaginal discharge, pelvic pain and fever is only present in about 25% of patients. Tubal tenderness is common. Pain on moving ('rocking') the cervix and adnexal tenderness in the fornices are usual on vaginal examination. A pelvic mass may be present from swollen infected tissues without actual abscess formation. Systemic symptoms develop.

Table 1 **Characteristics of salpingitis and PID**

Classification	Causative organisms	Clinical features	Confirmatory tests	Chemotherapy*
Endometritis	MAA, CP	PV bleeding, fever, uterine tenderness, pain	Cervical swab, M&C	Cefoxitin ± gentamicin
Salpingitis and salpingo-oophoritis	MAA, NG, CT	PV discharge, pelvic pain, fever, cervical tenderness	Cervical swab, culdocentesis	Ceftriaxone + azithromycin
Tubal and tubo-ovarian abscess	MAA, NG, CT	As salpingitis, plus tubal mass and systemic symptoms	Culdocentesis then operate	Cefoxitin, azithromycin, gentamicin
Pelvic abscess	MAA, NG, CT	As salpingitis, plus pelvic mass and systemic symptoms	Culdocentesis then drain	Cefoxitin, azithromycin, gentamicin
Peritonitis	MAA, NG, CT	Abdominal pain, guarding and rigidity, shock	Laparotomy, M&C	Cefoxitin, azithromycin, gentamicin

MAA, mixed anaerobic and aerobic organisms; NG, *N. gonorrhoeae*; CP, *Cl. perfringens*; CT, *C. trachomatis*; M&C, microscopy and culture.

*Ceftriaxone is used especially for gonococci, cefoxitin for anaerobes. In all STDs, treat sexual partners.

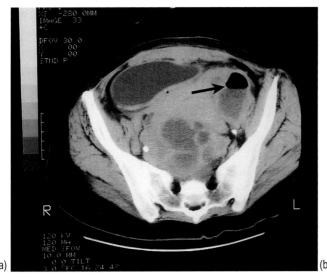
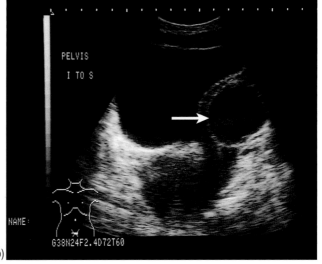

Fig. 1 **Tubo-ovarian abscess. (a)** CT scan. **(b)** Ultrasound. Both show fluid levels (different patients).

Tubo-ovarian abscess. A tubal mass develops (Fig. 1) and systemic symptoms with fever usually increase.

Pelvic abscess. A tender pelvic mass is present, and systemic symptoms with fever are prominent.

Local peritonitis. If present, this produces abdominal pain and tenderness.

Generalised peritonitis from rupture of a tubal or pelvic abscess. Both abdominal pain and fever increase, and abdominal muscle guarding and rebound tenderness appear, with paralysed bowel (called 'paralytic ileus'), vomiting, severe systemic symptoms and shock.

Confusing conditions

Differential diagnosis in mild cases includes vaginitis (p. 187) or cervicitis (p. 182), while more severe disease must be distinguished from acute appendicitis, endometriosis, ectopic pregnancy, or ovarian cyst rupture or haemorrhage.

Confirmatory tests

Useful specimens include endocervical swabs, pus from culdocentesis (aspiration through the posterior vaginal fornix for salpingitis or tubal abscess), and pus from laparotomy.

Laboratory tests for gonorrhoeal and chlamydial infections are outlined below:

- **Microscopy** of the smear from an endocervical swab showing increased numbers of pus cells, some containing Gram-negative intracellular diplococci, is almost pathognomonic ('certainly diagnostic') for gonorrhoea. A special calcium alginate swab must be used, as cotton inhibits fastidious pathogens like the gonococcus.
- **Polymerase chain reaction (PCR) testing** is used to diagnose chlamydial infection.
- **Culture** (preferably by direct 'bed-side' inoculation) on special non-selective media (chocolate agar) and selective media (e.g. modified Thayer-Martin) in CO_2 is necessary to grow the fastidious gonococcus. Identification is by a positive oxidase reaction, and sugar fermentation. Blood culture may be positive in peritonitis.
- **Antibiotic sensitivity testing** of gonococci is necessary in most countries, as resistance is common and often unpredictable.

- **Serology** is useless for gonorrhoea, and seldom used to diagnose chlamydial infection.
- **Imaging** by ultrasound and/or CT scan can show the site and extent of infection, including abscesses (Fig. 1).

Chemotherapy

Empiric chemotherapy usually combines a beta-lactam active against *N. gonorrhoeae* (usually ceftriaxone) and anaerobes (often cefoxitin), with azithromycin for chlamydial infection, or an aminoglycoside for Gram-negative aerobes. For infections probably acquired sexually, give ceftriaxone (or cefoxitin) plus azithromycin for gonorrhoea and chlamydial infection (or amoxicillin/clavulanate plus azithromycin orally for mild infection). For postabortal, postpartum and postoperative infections, cefoxitin plus gentamicin, clindamycin plus gentamicin, or ampicillin plus metronidazole plus gentamicin are all effective. Benzylpenicillin and/or metronidazole must be used for suspected or proved clostridial infections

Mild cases may be treated orally as out-patients, but intravenous therapy for at least 4 days in hospital is needed in **p**regnancy, **p**resence of IUD, **p**elvic or tubal abscess, **p**eritonitis, **p**ossible other diagnosis, or **p**revious failed oral treatment.

Chemotherapy alone is insufficient in five situations:

- foreign bodies such as IUDs or retained products of conception must be removed
- unruptured abscesses must be drained
- intra-abdominal ruptured abscess with peritonitis needs immediate abdominal surgery
- clostridial infections need surgery and often hyperbaric oxygen
- extensive infection with destroyed organ function needs excision (Fig. 2).

Control and prevention

- For sexually acquired infections, control depends on education, safer sexual practices and rapid exact diagnosis and effective treatment of patients and their sexual contacts.
- For postabortal, postpartum and postoperative infections, control depends on chemoprophylaxis when relevant, aseptic procedural technique and rapid exact diagnosis and treatment.

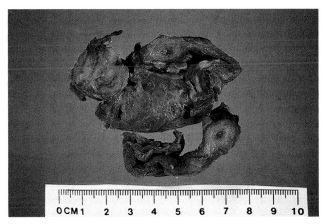

Fig. 2 **PID: pathological specimen of uterus and both tubes.**

> ### Salpingitis and PID
>
> - PID can include endometritis, salpingitis, salpingo-oophoritis, tubo-ovarian abscess, inflammation of the adnexal ('adjacent') tissues and inflammatory 'pelvic mass', pelvic abscess, and/or peritonitis.
> - PID is either sexually acquired or else follows abortion, birth, an IUD or gynaecologic surgery.
> - Most infections are polymicrobial: the commonest organisms are *N. gonorrhoeae, C. trachomatis,* or mixed anaerobic and aerobic organisms.
> - Vaginal discharge, pelvic pain and fever are the usual symptoms, but spread of infection causes abdominal pain, tubal and pelvic masses, signs of peritonitis, paralytic ileus and shock.
> - Diagnosis depends on the endocervical smear and special stains and cultures on aspirated pus. Serology is of little use. Imaging shows the site and extent of abscess formation.

Epididymitis, orchitis and balanitis

Epididymitis

Epididymitis is inflammation of the epididymis, usually caused by infection, rarely by trauma. Infection from a STD or from the urethra, bladder or prostate ascends via the vas deferens. It can also result from local or blood-borne spread in systemic disease.

Causative organisms

Ascending infection from the bladder occurs in children, infancy and older men. In the latter, prostatic hypertrophy, catheterisation or instrumentation can cause partial obstruction which predisposes to ascending infection. The usual organisms are *E. coli* and *Klebsiella* spp.

In sexually active men infection is usually sexually acquired – gonococcal or chlamydial – but it can involve *E. coli* from an unrecognised structural abnormality or anal intercourse.

In children, septicaemia can cause epididymitis, involving, for example, *Neisseria meningitidis* or *Haemophilus influenzae*.

Rarely epididymitis can occur as the result of systemic disease, such as TB (Fig. 1), blastomycosis, coccidioidomycosis, brucellosis or schistosomiasis.

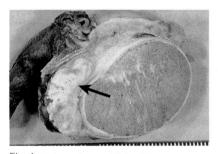

Fig. 1 **Tuberculous epididymitis.**

Clinical features

From the urinary and epididymal infection there is urethral discharge (which may be minimal), dysuria, frequency and nocturia. In addition, the scrotum is painful and swollen with redness and tenderness of the epididymis, progressing to hydrocoele, orchitis and fever.

Complications

Complications include chronic epididymitis, with or without a chronic sinus, and epididymo-orchitis, which may progress to testicular abscess, testicular infarction or infertility.

Confusing conditions

This includes torsion, infarction, abscess, traumatic rupture, or tumour of the testis, or torsion of the appendages.

Confirmatory tests

These are microscopy, culture and PCR of urine and urethral discharge for specific pathogens. Ultrasound is useful to exclude testicular torsion. Aspiration of the epididymis is used in complicated cases. Cystoscopy, intravenous pyelography and micturating cysto-urethrography are used to define structural abnormalities of the urinary tract.

Chemotherapy

For sexually acquired infections, ceftriaxone or ciprofloxacin (depending on local resistance patterns) plus azithromycin are given. For ascending infections from bacteriuria, a broad-spectrum penicillin or cephalosporin is usual until sensitivity results are available. Scrotal support and analgesia are helpful, and surgery may be needed for complications.

Control and prevention

This depends on the origin of the infection. For STDs, sexual partners should be traced and treated. For ascending infections from bacteriuria, predisposing obstruction or stasis must be remedied.

Orchitis

Orchitis is inflammation of the testis, commonly caused by viral disease such as mumps, less commonly by spread from epididymitis (see above) and, rarely, from metastatic, blood-borne spread. Causative organisms, therefore, are gonococci, chlamydiae, uro-pathogens such as *E. coli* or *Klebsiella* spp., or systemic infections including TB (Fig. 2). Clinical features are high fever, nausea and vomiting with acute testicular pain, swelling and tenderness. Confirmatory laboratory tests are urethral and urine microscopy, culture and PCR. Ultrasound differentiates from epididymitis. Management is like that for epididymitis.

Balanitis

Balanitis is inflammation of the glans, corona or shaft of the penis. It is usually caused by *Candida albicans* infection acquired from an infected sexual partner. Small vesicles develop into thrush-like patches with itching and burning. It may spread to scrotum, groins and perineum. Microscopy and culture confirm. It is cured with local nystatin or clotrimazole creams, and treatment of the sexual partner(s).

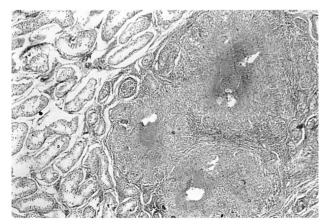

Fig. 2 **Tuberculous orchitis.**

Epididymitis, orchitis and balanitis

- **Epididymitis** is usually sexually acquired or an ascending infection from the urinary tract, but rarely it can arise from systemic disease.

- The common causes are gonorrhoea and chlamydial infections, or uro-pathogens such as *E. coli*.

- Local pain, swelling, redness and tenderness, urethral discharge and dysuria are the common symptoms.

- Spread locally causes hydrocoele and orchitis, which can progress to abscess and sinus formation.

- **Orchitis** (inflammation of the testes) is usually due to mumps, less often to spread from the epididymis. Severe pain and tenderness need analgesia and support.

- **Balanitis**, inflammation of the skin of the penis, is usually caused by *C. albicans* and treated by local creams.

Vaginitis and vulvo-vaginitis

Vaginitis is inflammation of the vagina; co-existent inflammation of the vagina and exterior vulva is called vulvo-vaginitis. A Bartholin's gland duct infection causes a vulval abscess (Fig. 1).

Differential diagnosis is from excessive physiological discharge, non-infectious vaginitis (e.g. chemical), and from cervicitis (p. 182).

There are four common infectious causes: candidiasis, trichomoniasis, bacterial vaginosis and Herpes genitalis.

Candidiasis

Candida infection (p. 68–69) is usually endogenous, and favoured by increased glycogen, altered normal bacterial flora (p. 22) and poor cell-mediated immunity (CMI) (p. 29), so predisposing factors include pregnancy or the 'pill', systemic antibiotics, diabetes, steroid treatment, or excessive warmth and moisture from synthetic underwear.

Candidiasis is marked by pruritus and a thick, white, cheesy discharge, adhering to the vaginal wall in white spots, looking like a thrush's breast (Fig. 2). Dyspareunia (pain on intercourse) and dysuria may occur.

Microscopy shows yeasts and pseudohyphae with a wet mount in 10% KOH (which incidentally destroys trichomonads).

Culture is easy on specific media but does not prove the diagnosis as *Candida* spp. are found in 40% of normal women.

Treatment is with local clotrimazole or miconazole. Oral azoles are reserved for chronic relapsing cases. Male sexual partners with balanitis should be treated (p. 186).

Predisposing factors should be controlled where possible.

Trichomoniasis

Trichomoniasis is caused by the protozoan flagellate *Trichomonas vaginalis*. Infection is acquired sexually.

Trichomoniasis may be asymptomatic, but often causes severe itching with a copious, purulent, frothy, foul discharge. The erythematous vaginal wall is reddened, but the distinctive 'strawberry cervix', friable with punctate haemorrhages, is rare.

Fresh vaginal discharge is examined in a saline wet mount to show motile trichomonads.

Patients and their sexual partners are treated with metronidazole. It is controlled like other STDs, by education, safer sex, and rapid diagnosis and treatment of patients and partners.

Bacterial vaginosis

Bacterial vaginosis is associated with *Gardnerella vaginalis*, probably acting with various anaerobes, including *Bacteroides* spp. and the curious curved *Mobiluncus* (Fig. 3). Infection is

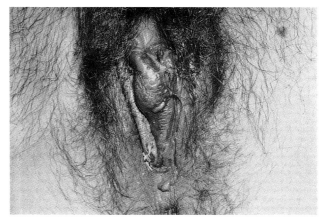

Fig. 1 **Vulval abscess.**

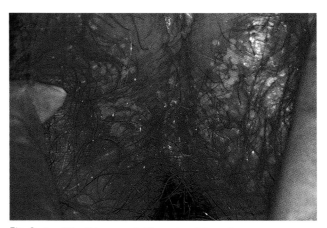

Fig. 2 *Candida albicans* **vaginitis: aceto-white stain.**

probably endogenous. Inflammation is surprisingly absent, so the previous name of 'non-specific vaginitis' is not now used.

Symptoms are absent or mild, with thin, frothy discharge and some vaginal odour.

Fresh vaginal discharge in a saline wet mount may show 'clue cells', which are squamous epithelial cells with their borders obscured by innumerable tiny coccobacilli.

Treatment is metronidazole. In pregnancy, ampicillin or clindamycin can be used.

Genital herpes

This is caused by Herpes simplex virus; the clinical features, confirmatory tests and chemotherapy are compared with other ulcerating STDs in Table 1 on p. 188.

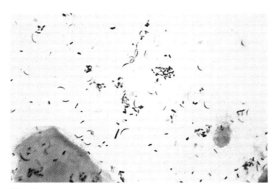

Fig. 3 *Mobiluncus* **sp. in bacterial vaginosis.**

> ### *Vaginitis and vulvo-vaginitis*
>
> ■ These are usually caused by candidiasis (from *C. albicans*), trichomoniasis (from *T. vaginalis*), bacterial vaginosis (from *G. vaginalis* and mixed anaerobes) or herpes simplex.
> ■ Clinical features are commonly vaginal discharge and vulval itch, sometimes with ulceration, dysuria or dyspareunia.
> ■ Diagnosis is by microscopy of a wet mount of fresh vaginal discharge, with culture or PCR if negative.
> ■ Treatment is an imidazole such as clotrimazole for candidiasis, metronidazole for trichomoniasis or bacterial vaginosis, and a/fam/valaciclovir for herpes.
> ■ Control is by reducing the predisposing factors, by education and safer sex, and early diagnosis and treatment of sexual partners.

Tropical and rare sexually transmitted diseases

Characterised by genital ulceration, four sexually transmitted diseases (STDs) are discussed here. Except for syphilis, they are rare in developed countries, but common in many developing countries. Table 1 compares their major features with herpes genitalis caused by Herpes simplex virus, the commonest ulcerative STD.

Differential diagnosis includes fixed drug eruption and traumatic ulcers. Other STDs discussed in this book include gonorrhoea and chlamydial infections, urethritis, cervical infections, salpingitis, pelvic inflammatory disease (PID), epididymitis, orchitis, balanitis and vaginitis (p. 180–187), lice and scabies (p. 77) and the 'gay bowel syndrome' (p. 159).

Confirmatory tests should be done whenever available, for clinical diagnosis even by experienced clinicians is wrong in 40% of patients! When testing is unavailable, 'syndromic management' treats the diseases most likely in each country or area.

Control of all STDs depends on education, safer sex, and rapid exact diagnosis and treatment of patients and their sexual partners.

Chancroid

Chancroid ('like a syphilitic chancre') is an ulcerating venereal disease also known as 'soft sore', describing two major differences from syphilis: the ulcer is soft, and sore. In Africa and other tropical areas it is frequently associated with HIV infection. The causative organism is Haemo-philus ducreyi (p. 44), a small Gram-negative cocco-bacillus.

The clinical features of a painful ulcer with ragged edges and a necrotic base, detailed in Table 1, help in differential diagnosis although clinical diagnosis can be unreliable. Autoinoculation, by contact of adjacent surfaces, can produce 'kissing' ulcers, while scarring during healing can produce a 'saxophone penis' (Fig. 1).

Confirmatory testing by culture on special media is difficult. Gram stain is unreliable because of numerous similar bacteria. Multiplex-PCR is excellent but expensive and rarely available.

Chemotherapy is by single-dose azithromycin, ciprofloxacin (1–3 days) or ceftriaxone, with rare failures.

Donovanosis

This has many synonyms, of which **'granuloma venereum'** is more accurate than **'granuloma inguinale'**, as this is the one ulcerative STD in which inguinal lymphadenopathy is not present; 'Donovanosis' is now usual.

It is spread by non-sexual trauma as well as sexually, and as vaginal and rectal lesions are often inconspicuous, sexual partners may appear uninfected. The causative organism is Klebsiella (was Calymmatobacterium) granulomatis, a Gram-negative bacterium (p. 53).

The clinical features of this painless destructive genital ulcer (Fig. 2) with pearly everted edges are summarised in Table 1.

Confirmatory tests are Giemsa stain of wet ulcer smears, or ulcer tissue crushed between two microscope slides, or histology. Bipolar-staining rods (Donovan bodies) are seen within macrophages. Culture is specialised.

Chemotherapy is by weekly azithromycin for 3 weeks or until fully healed. Doxycycline, erythromycin or ceftriaxone are probably inferior.

Lymphogranuloma venereum (LGV)

As the name describes, LGV is a STD characterised by inguinal lymphadenopathy; genital ulceration is inconspicuous. The causative organism is Chlamydia trachomatis, serotypes L1, L2 and L3 (p. 64), whereas urethritis, cervicitis and other chlamydial genital disease (p. 180–186) is caused by serotypes D–K.

Clinical syndromes

Genital infections have a *primary* phase with a self-healing often undiagnosed genital ulcer, a *secondary* phase with

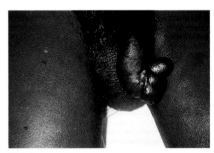

Fig. 1 **Chancroid: 'saxophone penis'.**

Table 1 **Comparison of rare and 'tropical' ulcerating STDs with herpes simplex**					
	Chancroid ('soft sore')	**Granuloma inguinale (Donovanosis)**	**Lymphogranuloma venereum**	**Syphilis**	**Herpes simplex**
Causative organism	Haemophilus ducreyi	Klebsiella granulomatis	Chlamydia trachomatis	Treponema pallidum	Herpes simplex virus
Clinical features					
Ulcer	**Marked, 1–10**	**Marked, 1 or more**	**Inconspicuous**	**Single**	**Clusters**
Border	Flat, ragged	Elevated, pearly	Flat	Rolled	Flat
Induration	Soft	Firm	Nil	Firm–hard	Soft
Pain	Marked	Minimal	None	None	Marked
Depth	Deep	Moderate	Shallow	Shallow	Shallow
Base	Necrotic, yellow	Granulomatous	Pink-red	Clean	Red
Secretion	Blood or pus	Sero-sanguineous	Serous	Serous	Serous
Progression	Progresses, coalesces	Progresses, coalesces	Heals	Heals	Heals
Lymph nodes	**Painful, enlarged**	**Nodes not enlarged**	**Painful, many enlarged, form sinuses**	**Painless, enlarged, 'rubbery'**	Mild pain
		Inguinal granuloma (pseudo-bubo)			
Systemic	Minimal	Usually none	Marked	Minimal	Minimal
Confirmatory tests					
Preferred	Special culture (PCR if available)	Swab or crushed tissue	PCR if available	Dark-field microscopy	PCR
Alternative	Gram stain	Histology	Serology	EIA/RPR/TPPA	Tzanck
Chemotherapy					
Preferred	Azithromycin	Azithromycin	Doxycycline	Penicillin	Famciclovir or valaciclovir
Alternative	Ceftriaxone or ciprofloxacin	Ceftriaxone or doxycycline	Erythromycin (?Azithromycin)	Tetracycline/Erythromycin	Aciclovir

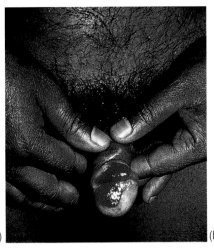 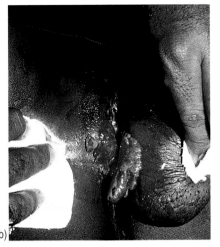 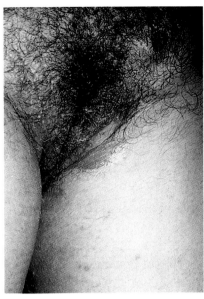

(a) (b)

Fig. 2 **Granuloma inguinale. (a)** Penile ulcer. **(b)** Vulval elephantiasis.

Fig. 3 **Secondary syphilis, mucous patch.**

systemic symptoms and marked inguinal and other lymphadenopathy that progresses to abscess, sinus and fistula formation, and a *tertiary* phase of fibrosis, stricture and lymphatic obstruction. By contrast, if the initial lesion is anorectal, the primary phase is marked by severe local symptoms (diarrhoea, anorectal pain and discharge) and systemic upset with fever.

Confirmatory tests are serology (immunofluorescence being preferable to complement fixation testing) or DIF or PCR of bubo (lymph node) aspirate for chlamydia.

Management

Chemotherapy is by tetracycline or erythromycin for at least 14 days. Azithromycin is unproven. Abscesses need aspiration through adjacent normal skin, and surgery may be needed for fistulae, strictures or elephantiasis from lymphatic obstruction.

Syphilis

A painless, indurated, infectious, self-healing genital ulcer called a chancre is the characteristic of the *primary* stage of syphilis. The *secondary* stage has systemic symptoms such as fever and myalgia, and may include lymphadenopathy, patchy alopecia, a highly variable but usually symmetrical rash including palms and soles, or painless, shallow, infectious ulcers ('mucous patches', Fig. 3) of mucous membranes and genitalia, and infectious condylomata lata ('flat warts') around the anus (Fig. 4). There is then a *latent* stage of many years before the *tertiary* stage of cardiovascular, CNS, bone, joint or skin involvement.

The causative organism is *Treponema pallidum*, a spirochaete that does not stain with Gram's or other routine stains and cannot be cultured on media (p. 58).

The differential diagnosis of genital syphilis includes chancroid, granuloma inguinale and sometimes LGV, as well as herpes simplex, venereal warts (Fig. 5) TB, and traumatic ulcers.

Confirmatory tests are dark-field microscopy for spirochaetes, and serology such as rapid plasma reagin (RPR) or EIA and *T. pallidum* particle agglutination (TPPA) tests, which are often negative in primary syphilis, but almost always positive in secondary syphilis. HIV antibody testing, after counselling and consent, is usually indicated.

Single-dose benzathine benzylpenicillin has been widely used for chemotherapy, but a 10-day course of procaine benzylpenicillin is probably superior. Doxycycline is used in penicillin hypersensitivity, and erythromycin in hypersensitivity in pregnancy. All sexual contacts within 90 days must be treated.

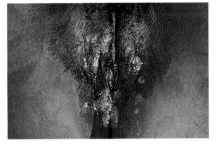

Fig. 4 **Secondary syphilis: condylomata lata.**

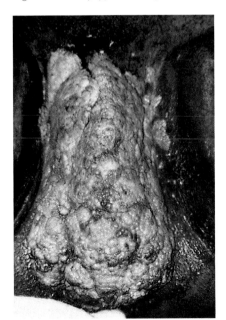

Fig. 5 **Massive vulval warts.**

Tropical and rare sexually transmitted diseases

- Chancroid is a soft ragged necrotic painful ulcer with painful inguinal lymphadenopathy; it is caused by *Haemophilus ducreyi* and is treated with azithromycin or alternatives.
- Granuloma inguinale has an ulcer with a firm, elevated pearly edge and granulomatous base, with little pain and some inguinal infiltration. Causative organism is *Klebsiella granulomatis*. Treatment is azithromycin, ceftriaxone or doxycycline.
- Lymphogranuloma venereum has an inconspicuous ulcer but marked painful lymphadenopathy, which forms abscesses, sinuses, fistulae, scars and strictures. Causative organism is *Chlamydia trachomatis*, serotypes L1, L2 and L3. Treatment is by doxycycline or erythromycin. Azithromycin is unproven.
- Syphilis has a primary chancre which is firm, painless, infectious and self-healing, and a secondary stage which includes infectious genital mucous patches and condylomata lata. Treatment is by penicillin if possible, otherwise tetracycline or erythromycin.
- Confirmatory tests of all are special stains, special culture, PCR and/or specific serology.
- Control of all STD involves education, safer sex, exact diagnosis, and rapid treatment of patients and their sexual partners.

Streptococcal skin and soft tissue infections

Local streptococcal infections of the skin and soft tissues occur at all levels (Fig. 1).

In addition, distant streptococcal infections affect the skin:

- erythema nodosum
- erythema marginata
- purpura fulminans
- scarlet fever.

Pyoderma is a confusing term used either generally to mean all superficial bacterial skin infections or specifically for impetigo.

The appearance of skin lesions is described clinically in several ways:

- colour
  - erythema: redness caused by vasodilatation
  - petechiae: tiny purplish discolorations from bleeding
  - purpura: large purplish discoloration from bleeding
- texture
  - macules: flat spots
  - papules: small raised lumps
  - nodules: larger firm lumps
  - plaques: large flat-topped palpable lesions
- contents
  - vesicles: small watery blisters
  - bullae: large watery blisters > 0.5 cm
  - pustules: blisters containing pus
- skin integrity
  - erosion: superficial loss of skin
  - ulcer: deeper hole, may bleed
  - crust: leakage of blood or serum drying on skin.

LOCAL INFECTIONS

Impetigo

Impetigo (Fig. 2) is a superficial infection caused by *Streptococcus pyogenes* (group A, p. 36), and may follow nasopharyngeal carriage or infection. Some strains are nephritogenic, so acute glomerulonephritis follows. In addition, *Staphylococcus aureus* (p. 34) often secondarily infects impetigo.

Clinical features. Impetigo begins, often on the face, with small papules or vesicles that ulcerate and ooze highly infectious, thin, sero-purulent fluid which dries in typical crusts that last up to 2 weeks and heal without scars. Usually there is no systemic illness. School children and other groups in close contact are commonly affected. Spread is typical, both to other parts of the body, and to other people (contacts). It must be distin-

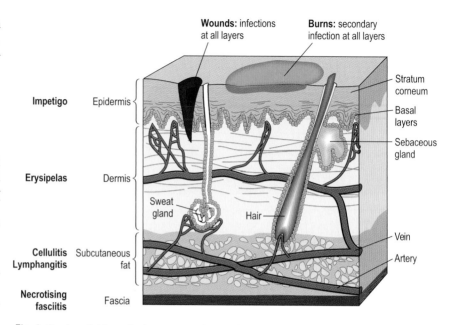

Fig. 1 **Section of skin and subcutaneous tissues, showing the levels affected by different streptococcal infections.**

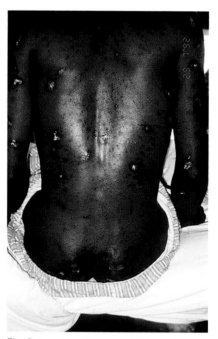

Fig. 2 **Impetigo.** Note superficiality, scabs or crusts, and serous discharge.

guished from bullous impetigo, with big (> 1 cm) bullae, caused by staphylococci (p. 192).

Confirmatory tests. Diagnosis is usually clinical, but swabs of the oozing fluid grow the streptococcus and show any secondary infection.

Chemotherapy. Systemic penicillin is effective, making the lesions non-infectious within 48 hours; obviously a penicillinase-resistant type is used if staphylococci are present. Local antiseptics may be used in conjunction with penicillin to

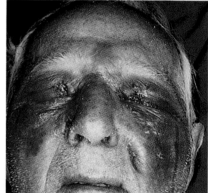

Fig. 3 **Erysipelas.** Note fiery red colour and sharply demarcated edge.

diminish infectivity but are ineffective alone.

Erysipelas

Unlike impetigo, which is troublesome but trivial, erysipelas is a serious and even life-threatening disease, with rapidly spreading infection in the dermis (Fig. 3). Erysipelas is also caused by *Strep. pyogenes* (group A), but sometimes by group B, C or G streptococci. Some patients suffer many episodes.

Clinical features. A bright red area, tingling more than painful, appears and spreads rapidly, with a raised sharply defined edge. The face is the classical site, so the diagnosis may be missed when a leg or other site is involved. Lymphangitis follows. Predisposing factors, both to the initial attack and to recurrence, are lymphatic obstruction, skin disease (which may be occult, e.g. tinea between the toes), injury or surgery.

Confirmatory tests. These are often unnecessary, and skin swabs or aspirate are usually negative without other skin disease. Throat cultures are positive in about 30% of patients, blood cultures in only 5%.

Chemotherapy. Systemic penicillin must be given immediately (use cephalothin if the patient is hypersensitive). Clindamycin decreases streptococcal toxin production.

Control and prevention. Recurrent attacks can be prevented or minimised by attention to the predisposing factor(s). If these cannot be removed, long-term penicillin can be used.

Wounds and burns

These may be infected by streptococci (p. 197).

Cellulitis and lymphangitis

While these can still be caused by *Strep. pyogenes* infection, they are now much more commonly caused by *Staph. aureus* or other organisms (p. 192–193).

Fig. 4 **Erythema marginata.** Note faint red-brown rash with distinctive irregular margin and central paler area.

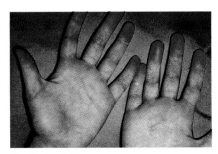

Fig. 5 **Scarlet fever.**

Necrotising fasciitis

This is now rarely caused by *Strep. pyogenes* (see gangrenous infections, p. 195).

SKIN MANIFESTATIONS OF DISTANT INFECTIONS

Erythema nodosum

Erythema nodosum (EN) is a condition characterised by red or red-purple lumps, often tender and often on the legs. It can be caused by a number of infections:

- mycobacterial infections (TB or leprosy, p. 104)
- streptococcal infections
- *Chlamydia trachomatis* (p. 189) (lymphogranuloma venereum)
- *Yersinia* infections (p. 56)
- systemic fungal infections (p. 68–73).

There are also numerous causes which are not proved to be infective. These include Crohn's disease, ulcerative colitis, sarcoidosis and systemic lupus erythematosus. Drugs (e.g. sulphonamides) also cause EN.

The lumps appear at the onset or during the course of the conditions listed above. They seldom ulcerate.

Confirmatory tests. Tests are directed at the underlying disease.

Management. This is directed at the underlying condition. Corticosteroids, if not otherwise contraindicated, may be used to hasten resolution and relieve pain.

Erythema marginata

This is a faint, widespread, migrating skin rash, with an irregular red-brown margin and a paler centre (Fig. 4). It is very rare but is pathognomonic of ('found only in') rheumatic fever.

Purpura fulminans

This is usually defined as symmetric peripheral gangrene, with distal ischaemic necrosis of two or more extremities without large vessel occlusion. It is an extremely serious sign of disseminated intravascular coagulation (DIC), occurring in streptococcal, meningococcal and other septicaemia, often heralding death.

Scarlet fever

Scarlet fever follows a streptococcal infection. Certain strains of *Strep. pyogenes* contain a lysogenic phage which codes for an erythrogenic toxin which has three effects:

- erythrogenic, giving the typical rash
- pyrogenic, giving fever
- endotoxic, giving shock.

Clinical syndrome. Scarlet fever has a number of features:

- the primary streptococcal infection, usually pharyngitis and tonsillitis, rarely a skin or wound infection
- diffuse red rash (Fig. 5), spreading from the chest over the whole body except for the face, palms and soles; it feels rough like sandpaper, then desquamates as the rash fades
- circum-oral pallor
- a coated 'white strawberry tongue' which becomes a beefy 'red strawberry tongue' when the coating disappears
- an enanthem of small red spots on the palate
- fever and prostration
- rarely, septicaemia, arthritis, jaundice, death.

The incubation period is about 3 days and the disease is most commonly seen in children under 10 years of age.

Confirmatory tests. Swabs from the portal of entry (throat, skin, wound or even uterus) grow the organism. Skin tests are no longer used.

Chemotherapy. Penicillin is the drug of choice, with supportive measures.

Control. Widespread use of penicillin to treat throat infections, and improved socioeconomic conditions, including less crowding and better ventilation, have greatly decreased the incidence of scarlet fever, rheumatic fever and acute glomerulonephritis in developed countries.

Streptococcal skin and soft tissue infections

- Local streptococcal infections include impetigo, erysipelas, cellulitis, necrotising fasciitis (depending on the level of tissue infected), wound infections, and secondary infections of burns.
- Distant streptococcal infections can cause erythema nodosum, erythema marginata, purpura fulminans and scarlet fever.
- Impetigo is superficial and has a serous ooze that is very infectious.
- Erysipelas is serious, with systemic symptoms, and needs urgent systemic penicillin.
- Cellulitis and fasciitis are now less commonly streptococcal.
- Erythema nodosum, erythema marginata and purpura fulminans can be important but rare signs of distant streptococcal infection.
- Scarlet fever with scarlet rash and strawberry tongue is caused by erythrogenic toxin-producing *Strep. pyogenes*.

Staphylococcal skin and soft tissue infections

<u>Local</u> staphylococcal infections, beginning with the most superficial, are:

1. bullous impetigo (in the epidermis)
2. paronychia (around nails)
3. folliculitis (in hair follicles)
4. furuncles (in epidermis and dermis)
5. carbuncles (in subcutaneous tissues)
6. cellulitis (in subcutaneous tissues).

Staphylococcal infections here, as elsewhere in the body, are <u>characterised</u> by:

- suppuration (pus formation)
- necrosis of local tissues
- abscess formation.

In addition, <u>distant</u> staphylococcal infections affect the skin (see opposite).

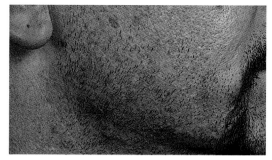

Fig. 1 **Folliculitis.** Note small yellow pustules around hair follicles, with little surrounding inflammation.

LOCAL INFECTIONS

Bullous impetigo

Bullous impetigo is caused by particular strains of *Staph. aureus* and is distinguished from streptococcal impetigo (p. 190) by large bullae (blisters) containing yellow pus and, of course, many staphylococci on Gram stain and culture.

Although these strains, like those causing the scalded skin syndrome (SSS), produce exfoliatin (the epidermolytic toxin), bullous impetigo differs from SSS in three ways: blister culture is positive, erythema is only local around the bullae, and Nikolsky's sign is negative. Bullous impetigo particularly infects infants and young children, is highly infectious by direct spread, and is controlled by stopping this spread and giving a penicillinase-resistant penicillin, e.g. flucloxacillin.

Paronychia

An <u>acute paronychia</u> is an infection next to a fingernail or toenail, characterised by quite severe pain and tenderness, redness, heat, swelling and pus formation. Surgical incision is usually necessary, plus an anti-staphylococcal antibiotic such as flucloxacillin.

<u>Chronic paronychiae</u> differ in the following ways:

- usually affect several fingers
- associated with repeated immersion in water
- less pain, swelling and pus formation
- causes include *Candida* spp. and other organisms
- medical therapy is difficult, but surgery is unnecessary.

Folliculitis

Folliculitis (Fig. 1) is a common but usually trivial infection localised to a hair fol-

licle, with a small bead of pus and some adjacent erythema. It often heals spontaneously but otherwise is cured by needling the apex and applying antiseptic. When it affects an eyelash it is called a **stye** or **hordeolum**, and removal of the lash plus local antibiotic are usually necessary. When it affects the beard area, it is called **sycosis barbae**, is more troublesome, and oral antibiotics and a dermatologist's care are usually necessary.

Furuncles (boils)

Boils are a common and more severe form of folliculitis, often affecting sebaceous and sweat glands. A boil is a painful, tender, elevated red-rimmed pustule (Fig. 2) that grows until it discharges or is opened with a sterile needle or blade.

There is usually no host abnormality apart from nasal carriage of the causative strain of *S. aureus*.

In contrast, there is often some host abnormality such as acne, diabetes or abnormal white cell function in:

- **furunculosis:** multiple boils
- **chronic furunculosis:** persistent or recurrent boils
- **hidradenitis suppurativa**, a deep suppurative infection of the sweat glands, usually in axilla or groin, for which skilled antibiotic therapy is often necessary.

Fever or chills, however, are uncommon with any of the above.

Carbuncles

Fusion of a number of furuncles causes a carbuncle, a very unpleasant but now uncommon condition, with extension deeply and widely in the subcutaneous tissues, and multiple but ineffective sinuses to the skin (see Fig. 4, p. 35); the back of the neck was a common site. Fever, chills and even bacteraemia can follow. High-dose parenteral anti-staphylococcal antibiotics are essential, and surgical removal

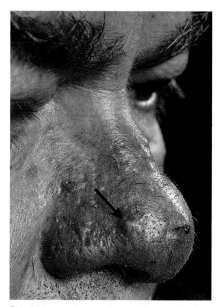

Fig. 2 **Furuncle.** Note larger collection of yellow pus, raised from skin surface with definite red inflamed edge.

of the central core of necrotic infected tissue is usually needed.

Cellulitis

What may be called '*simple*' cellulitis is an infection of the skin and subcutaneous tissues, characterised by redness, swelling and pain, with little or no skin or tissue necrosis. *Complicated* cellulitis (and deeper infections) characterised by necrosis (gangrene) and/or gas formation are discussed on p. 194–195.

Causative organisms. *S. aureus* and *Strep. pyogenes* are easily the commonest causes of cellulitis; less often, group B, C or G streptococci, *Aeromonas hydrophila* from fresh water (p. 196), *Erysipelothrix rhusiopathiae* from meat or fish (p. 39), enteric Gram-negative rods, or other organisms are responsible.

The clinical features are variable, depending on the organism, the host response and the route of infection, which can be from a skin abrasion, a traumatic or surgical wound, a furuncle

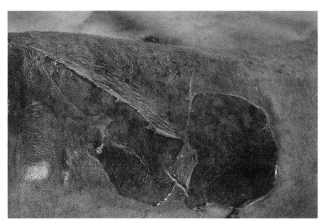

Fig. 3 **Scalded skin syndrome.**

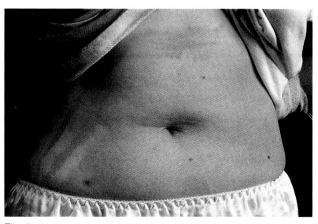

Fig. 4 **Toxic shock syndrome.** Note erythema with no local skin lesion.

or subcutaneous infection, or even blood-borne from septicaemia.

■ Streptococcal cellulitis has the brilliant red, hot, shiny skin of erysipelas but lacks the sharp raised edge, and there is greater swelling from the subcutaneous infection (see Fig. 1, p. 220). Lymphangitis and lymphadenopathy are prominent, but there is minimal pus without a prior wound. High fever and tachycardia characterise this serious infection, in which bacteraemia and shock can develop in 6–12 hours.

■ Staphylococcal cellulitis has less brilliant redness, but pain, tenderness and thick yellow pus are more prominent. Fever, malaise and regional lymphadenopathy usually develop more slowly than in streptococcal cellulitis. Local abscesses, skin necrosis, thrombophlebitis, bacteraemia and distant ('metastatic') abscesses follow if treatment is delayed or inadequate.

Confirmatory tests are made on pus using Gram stain and cultures; blood cultures are done if bacteraemia is possible. Swabs from unbroken skin are useless and may mislead.

Chemotherapy. Intravenous penicillin G is the treatment of choice for streptococcal cellulitis, but if *Staph. aureus* is the known or probable cause, a penicillinase-resistant penicillin such as flucloxacillin must be given. Pain relief and immobilisation in the acute stage are important, and pus must be drained.

Control and prevention.
Recurrent cellulitis occurs due to predisposing factors including:

■ lymphatic, venous or arterial insufficiency
■ scars or retained foreign bodies from injury or surgical operation
■ skin disease
■ immune deficiency or immunosuppression.

The predisposing factor(s) obviously should be treated or removed if possible.

Otherwise, suppression with the relevant oral penicillin or erythromycin may be necessary long term or even life long, as relapses have occurred when penicillin was stopped after 5 years' apparently successful control.

SKIN MANIFESTATIONS OF DISTANT INFECTIONS

Scalded skin syndrome

Staphylococcal scalded skin syndrome (SSS) is known in neonates as **Ritter's disease** or **pemphigus neonatorum**. It is caused by strains of *Staph. aureus* of phage group II; these produce toxins called exfoliatins which cause intraepidermal cleavage planes. **Staphylococcal scarlet fever** is a rare, milder disease with erythema but no exfoliation.

Clinical features. The three clinical characteristics are **e**rythema, **e**normous bullae and **e**xtensive exfoliation (desquamation). Fever and erythema develop, then bullae, then exfoliation, often in sheets and occurring initially in the face, axillae and groins. Nikolsky's sign is removal of the upper layers of the epidermis by gentle sliding movement of the examining finger! (Fig. 3).

Confirmatory tests. The distant causative infection (e.g. conjunctival, umbilical) is swabbed for Gram stain and culture, as the dramatic skin lesions do not contain the staphylococcus.

Chemotherapy. A penicillinase-resistant penicillin such as flucloxacillin is

given, and fluid replacement is usually necessary.

Control depends on early diagnosis and active treatment of all staphylococcal infections, especially in neonates and infants.

Toxic shock syndrome (TSS)

TSS is a serious systemic infection caused by *Staph. aureus* strains producing toxic shock syndrome toxin 1 (TSST-1). Predisposing factors include multiplication of the organisms and magnesium binding in certain high-absorbency tampons and a genetically ineffective antibody response. Skin or other tissues may be the primary site in men and non-menstruating women.

Clinical features. High fever, myalgia, vomiting and diarrhoea develop quickly. This is followed by a skin rash (Fig. 4) (which later exfoliates at a deeper level than in SSS), then shock, hypotension, and renal and often hepatic impairment within 36–48 hours.

Confirmatory tests. Treatment must precede laboratory results, but the primary site must be sampled for Gram stain and culture. Toxin detection is only available in special laboratories.

Chemotherapy. The primary site is removed or treated, and high-dose intravenous anti-staphylococcal penicillin is given, while shock and organ failure are treated appropriately. TSS is much less common since certain high-absorbency tampons were withdrawn from sale.

Staphylococcal skin and soft tissue infections

■ Local staphylococcal infections (*Staph. aureus*) are characterised by pus formation, necrosis of local tissues and abscess formation. They range from simple boils to cellulitis.
■ Management is with a penicillinase-resistant penicillin and appropriate surgical drainage.
■ Distant infections affect the skin through toxins produced by *Staph. aureus.*
■ Scalded skin syndrome is characterised by erythema, enormous bullae and extensive exfoliation (desquamation).
■ Toxic shock syndrome (TSS) is characterised by fever, skin rash and shock.

Gas-forming and gangrenous infections

Gas-forming and gangrenous (necrotising) infections are limb- and life-threatening conditions that occur at four tissue levels – A skin; B subcutaneous tissues; C fascia; D muscle.

Three necessary conditions are:

■ portal of entry: traumatic or surgical wound
■ anaerobic area: ischaemic tissue, foreign body
■ pathogen entry: faecal or soil contamination usually.

They are classified by **tissue level (ABCD), pathogen, necrosis, gas formation** and **host defences (E).**

AB1. Chancriform ulcers

A punched-out ulcer with skin and subcutaneous tissue necrosis, but no gas, rather like a syphilitic chancre, is characteristic, with little adjacent cellulitis initially.

Infectious causes include chancroid, cutaneous diphtheria, mycobacterial infections, syphilis, tularaemia (p. 213), ecthyma (see below) and anthrax (p. 39 also).

Cutaneous anthrax, very rare in developed countries, progresses from a painless papule through a vesicular 'malignant pustule' to a black necrotic ulcer with extensive red non-pitting oedema. The patient becomes very ill with high fever and bacteraemia. Gram stains of the lesion and blood culture show distinctive 'bamboo-like' chains of Gram-positive rods. High-dose intravenous penicillin is the drug of choice. The patient's occupation, or exposure to infected animals or their products, and lack of pain, are important diagnostic clues.

Pyoderma gangrenosum is a complication of diseases including ulcerative colitis. One or more nodules break down to deep necrotic coalescing ulcers, colonised by *Staphylococcus aureus*, streptococci and Gram-negative bacilli. Treatment includes steroids with antibiotics.

AB2. Synergistic gangrene

Rapidly progressive destruction of skin and subcutaneous tissue without gas (Fig. 1) is characteristic, caused by different bacteria acting synergistically. Other names are 'symbiotic gangrene' and 'progressive bacterial synergistic gangrene'.

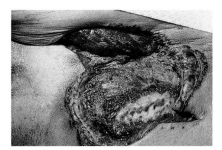

Fig. 1 **Synergistic gangrene.**

Meleney's gangrene is a related disease characterised by *synergistic gangrene plus* subcutaneous necrotic tracks to distant sinuses.

The causative organisms are always multiple; the classical pair are S. *aureus* and a micro-aerophilic or anaerobic streptococcus at the advancing edge, but other anaerobes and *Proteus* spp. are often found in the ulcer.

Clinically, this unusual necrosis typically complicates a contaminated wound, with expanding massive ulceration, and destruction of all tissue down to muscle (Fig. 1). There is often surprisingly little 'systemic toxicity'.

Confirmatory diagnosis is secondary to clinical diagnosis; ulcer cultures are misleading, but excised tissue should grow pathogens.

Management includes broad-spectrum antibiotics, e.g. flucloxacillin, gentamicin and metronidazole, but radical surgical excision of the advancing edge is almost always necessary, and rarely an old-fashioned diathermy 'firebreak' is needed.

B. Crepitant anaerobic cellulitis

Gradual onset of a crepitant, predominantly subcutaneous tissue infection around a wound is characteristic.

It is classified into clostridial and non-clostridial types. The former must be distinguished from clostridial **myo**necrosis (see below).

The causative organisms are *Clostridium perfringens* or other *Clostridia*, or mixed anaerobes, including *Bacteroides* spp. and *Peptostreptococci*, rarely *Escherichia coli* or *Klebsiella* spp. *Cl. septicum* is often associated with colonic cancer.

Clinically, there is gas causing bubbly crepitus on palpation beneath the wound, but little pain, tenderness, pus, skin involvement or toxaemia.

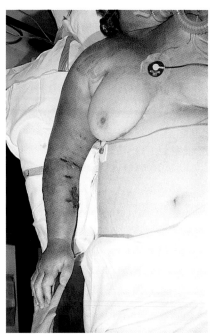

Fig. 2 **Fatal necrotising fasciitis (streptococcal) after elbow operation.** Note relatively small area of skin necrosis initially, yet even amputation did not save her life.

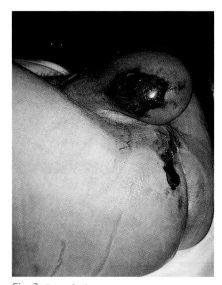

Fig. 3 **Fournier's gangrene.**

Confirmatory tests are Gram stain, and aerobic and anaerobic cultures, important to determine the causative organisms. X-ray shows gas bubbles in connective tissue, *not* muscle.

Chemotherapy must usually begin before culture results are available and should include penicillin and metronidazole.

Surgery is necessary to determine the extent of disease, drain any pus and remove necrotic subcutaneous tissue (not uninvolved muscle).

C. Necrotising fasciitis

Fulminant fascial necrosis is characteristic. It is now rarely caused by *Strep. pyogenes* group A (Fig. 2), being usually a mixed anaerobic infection. When affecting the male genitalia it is called **Fournier's gangrene** (Fig. 3).

Clinically, it is acute, with severe systemic toxicity and fever, but initially little skin involvement (Fig. 2). There is rapid extensive destruction of fascia with minimal gas, then skin necrosis; the muscle is surprisingly spared.

Skin swabs are unhelpful, but pus or tissue grows the causative organisms.

Intravenous high-dose penicillin plus metronidazole or imipenem is appropriate chemotherapy, but surgery is essential.

D1. Non-clostridial myonecrosis

Muscle necrosis and some gas are characteristic, with less subcutaneous and lesser skin involvement.

There are four subtypes:

1. Anaerobic streptococcal myositis. This rare acute infection is caused by anaerobic streptococci, often with Group A streptococci or *Staph. aureus*. There is red swollen skin and a 'sour' exudate. Muscle pain, gas and gangrene follow, then shock and death unless urgently treated with high-dose penicillin and surgical debridement.

2. Synergistic necrotising cellulitis (misnamed, actually **myositis**). This rare aggressive infection is caused by mixed anaerobes. There is marked local tenderness from muscle and subcutaneous tissue destruction, with some gas production, but little skin change except drainage of thin 'dishwater' pus from small ulcers. Systemic toxicity is marked, and urgent treatment with antibiotics, e.g. penicillin and metronidazole, and surgery is essential.

3. Infected vascular gangrene. This less aggressive infection is caused by mixed anaerobes (e.g. *Bacteroides* spp., anaerobic streptococci) and enteric aerobes in patients with arterial impairment, especially diabetics. There is muscle necrosis, gas and foul pus, but this is usually controlled by appropriate antibiotics and local excision of dead muscle.

4. Fulminant myonecrosis. See immunocompromised host below.

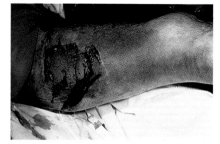

Fig. 4   **Gas gangrene.**

D2. Clostridial myonecrosis (gas gangrene)

Muscle necrosis and gas formation with consequent skin and subcutaneous tissue destruction and multisystem failure are characteristic of this rapidly fatal disease (Fig. 4). The causative organism is usually *Cl. perfringens*, rarely other *Clostridia*, e.g. *Cl. septicum*.

Clinically the onset is abrupt after an incubation period of 6–72 hours, with severe local pain, fever, pallor and sweats. Local skin oedema quickly leads to discoloration, blistering and necrosis, with crepitus and dirty blood-stained pus with a musty or mouse-like odour. If treatment is delayed, then shock, haemolytic anaemia, jaundice, renal failure and death follow from clostridial toxins attacking particularly muscle and blood.

Confirmatory laboratory diagnosis by urgent Gram stain must not delay treatment. If x-rayed on the way to theatre, there are bubbles and linear gas shadows in the muscles and soft tissues.

Urgent treatment combines high-dose intravenous penicillin and metronidazole or imipenem with surgical removal of all dead or dying muscle, even amputation, and, if available, hyperbaric oxygen.

Prevention depends on antibiotic prophylaxis and removal of ischaemic tissue and foreign bodies from pre-disposed wounds.

E1. Immunocompromised host

Unusual necrotising infections occur, in addition to the forms described

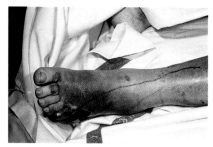

Fig. 5   **Diabetic foot infection with gangrene.**

above, worsened by impaired host response:

- *Aspergillus* spp. and the Phycomycetes (*Rhizopus*, *Mucor* and *Absidia* spp.) cause serious, often untreatable and hence fatal gangrenous cellulitis, with a black anaesthetic ulcer and a relentlessly advancing purplish oedematous edge.
- *Aeromonas hydrophila* causes a plaque, followed by a necrotic ulcer. It can also cause crepitant cellulitis.
- *Bacillus cereus* causes crepitant cellulitis.
- *Cryptococcus neoformans* causes a plaque, then a necrotic ulcer (see Fig. 4, p. 221).
- *Klebsiella* spp. or *Nocardia* spp. cause fulminant myonecrosis.
- *Pseudomonas aeruginosa* can cause a gangrenous cellulitis, or **ecthyma gangrenosum**, a black necrotic ulcer with surrounding erythema.

E2. Diabetic foot infections

Gangrene, particularly digital, in foot infections in diabetics is likely, because of vascular disease and the impaired host response (Fig. 5). Mixed infections with staphylococci, streptococci and anaerobes are common, with enteric Gram-negative colonisation. Pus and excised tissue should be cultured and appropriate chemotherapy given. Surgery should be conservative whenever possible, but underlying osteomyelitis must be sought and treated (p. 207).

Gas-forming and gangrenous infections

- Predisposing factors are a wound, an anaerobic area and contamination by pathogens.
- Infections are often mixed; anaerobes including *Clostridia* are prominent.
- Clinical classification depends on the **tissue level**, **pathogen**, **necrosis**, **gas formation** and **host defences.**
- Immunocompromised patients have special pathogens and unusual infections.
- Treatment with chemotherapy and surgery is urgent for rapidly progressive infections; identification of pathogens should occur as fast as possible.

Wound, bite and burn infections

Traumatic wound infections

These are best classified into infections from:

- skin flora
- a perforated viscus
- water or animals
- soil.

Wounds infected by skin flora

The causative organisms will usually be *Staphylococcus aureus* or *Streptococcus pyogenes*, and the resultant infections, depending on the level infected, will be erysipelas (uncommonly; p. 190), cellulitis (commonly; p. 192), or one of the rare infections described on pages 194–195.

Immobility, particularly in severely ill patients, can lead to bed sores, which can become infected (Fig. 1).

Wounds perforating a hollow viscus

The causative organisms obviously depend on the viscus perforated: most feared is colonic flora, with huge numbers of pathogenic aerobic and anaerobic Gram-negative and Gram-positive organisms. These cause peritonitis and local abscesses (p. 164–165), followed by septicaemia and distant infections if untreated (p. 142–143).

Small bowel, gastric and biliary wounds cause fewer infective problems initially, though chemical peritonitis from gastric acid or bile becomes secondarily infected if untreated.

Respiratory flora causes few infections at skin or subcutaneous levels, though the pleural cavity can become infected, called an empyaema (p. 131).

In all cases, management includes empiric antibiotics aimed at the likely flora, operative cultures, cleansing and closure of the perforation, drainage as necessary, maintenance of vital organ functions, and modification of antibiotic therapy if culture results and the clinical course so indicate.

Wounds infected from water or animals

Responsible organisms include:

Aeromonas hydrophila. This Gram-negative rod causes acute cellulitis around traumatic wounds sustained while swimming. Treatment can be ciprofloxacin, co-trimoxazole or a later cephalosporin.

Erysipelothrix rhusiopathiae. This Gram-positive rod causes **erysipeloid**, an uncommon occupational skin infection of those handling raw meat or fish. Usually confined to the fingers or hands, the lesion has a purplish-red raised edge and a centre fading as the lesion enlarges. Pus is uncommon, with burning rather than pain. Microbiologic confirmation of the diagnosis usually needs Gram stain and culture of biopsy of the edge of the lesion, surface swabs being negative (p. 37). Healing is accelerated by penicillin or cephalosporin treatment. Septicaemia is uncommon, but when it occurs, endocarditis often follows and is fatal in about 30% of patients.

Mycobacterium marinum. This atypical mycobacterium (p. 61) growing optimally at 25–32°C in water causes '**fish tank granuloma**' (= 'swimming pool granuloma') at the site of abrasions. The lesions are chronic, nodular or ulcerating, on the hands or over bony prominences, usually single, but rarely ascending like sporotrichosis. Biopsy is often necessary for diagnosis. Specialist referral is essential, for treatment is difficult, as the organism is relatively resistant. Early lesions may respond to long-term clarithromycin, co-trimoxazole, tetracycline or combined rifampicin-ethambutol, but excisional surgery and skin grafting may be necessary for advanced lesions.

Soil-contaminated wounds

The major causative organisms are:

- *Clostridium perfringens* and related clostridia (p. 40)
- *Cl. tetani*: tetanus (p. 41)
- *Cl. botulinum*: wound botulism (p. 41)
- *Mycobacterium ulcerans* (Bairnsdale or Buruli ulcer) (p. 202)
- *Cladosporium* spp. and other fungi: subcutaneous mycoses (p. 75, 204)
- *Sporothrix schenckii*: sporotrichosis (p. 204).

Surgical site infections

These are classified into superficial if above the deep fascia, and deep if below (Fig. 2). Gangrenous and gas-forming infections are considered on p. 194–195.

Causative organisms in surgical site infection include:

- *Staph. aureus* commonly (see Fig. 3, p. 23) and '*S. epidermidis*' rarely
- Streptococci, especially group A, and enterococci

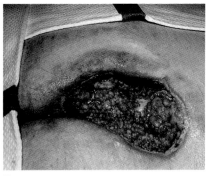
Fig. 1 **Infected bed sore.**

- enteric Gram-negative rods, e.g. *Escherichia coli, Klebsiella* spp.
- anaerobes, usually mixed
- *Pseudomonas aeruginosa*
- Clostridia, very rarely.

Infection can occur from four sources: the patient's own normal flora (usual), the theatre staff (uncommon but infamous), the environment, or equipment (unacceptable).

Clinical features. Redness, swelling, local pain and heat develop, and progress to a purulent discharge from the wound or around a suture ('stitch abscess') if untreated or if the infection is deep.

Confirmatory tests. Swabs of the discharge should always be Gram stained and cultured to isolate the pathogen, determine the antibiotic sensitivities and convince the surgeon.

Management. Pus must always be drained and foreign bodies removed. If cellulitis is established or spreading, antibiotics are needed. Initial empiric chemotherapy is aimed at the likely pathogens, e.g. flucloxacillin against *Staph. aureus* for many superficial operations; cephalosporin or gentamicin plus metronidazole against bowel flora after abdominal operations.

Control and prevention includes:
- good surgical technique
- prophylactic antibiotics immediately before and during operation
  - if postoperative infection likely, e.g. colonic surgery
  - if consequences of infection are devastating, e.g. valve replacement
  - chosen for likely pathogens.

Animal and human bite infections

Bite injuries vary in degree and in the likely infecting pathogens. They can be classified into:

- human bite injuries
- human fist injuries
- animal bites by different species
- specific pathogens causing specific diseases.

Causative organisms

The important organisms likely to infect these injuries are:

- *Pasteurella multocida* (p. 57)
- *Eikenella corrodens* (p. 53)
- 'mixed anaerobes' (p. 54; *Bacteroides, Fusobacterium*, etc.)
- *Capnocytophaga canimorsus* (previously called DF2); rare but kills if untreated (Fig. 1, p. 212).
- *Staph. aureus* and streptococci ('viridans', group A) (p. 34–37).

Clinically, the bite injury is very variable, and deep injury should be sought, especially tendon or joint in fist injuries. Gram stain and culture only help if infection is uncontrolled.

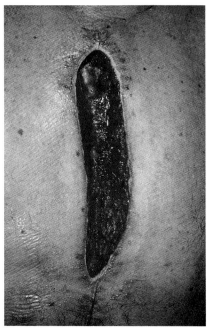

Fig. 2 **Infected sternal wound.**

Chemotherapy should be immediate and broad spectrum, including (for clostridial and *Eikenella* spp.) amoxicillin or ticarcillin with clavulanate. Surgery is important to remove dead tissue and repair deep structures, but because of the high risk of infection the wound should not be sutured except for potentially disfiguring facial wounds. Tetanus prophylaxis should be given, and rabies considered.

Seal finger is a curiosity, similar to erysipeloid but following a seal bite. The causative organism is unknown, but tetracycline treatment is effective.

Specific pathogens transmitted by bites include:

- *Clostridium tetani* (p. 41)
- rabies virus (p. 96–97)
- *Streptobacillus moniliformis* and *Spirillum minor* (p. 53): rat bite fever
- *Bartonella* spp., especially *B. henselae*: cat scratch disease.

Rat bite fever. This is an acute illness with high recurrent fever, chills, rash and, with *S. minor*, lymphangitis and lymphadenopathy, with *S. moniliformis* myalgia, arthralgia and arthritis. Laboratory diagnosis is specialised (p. 53). Penicillin is the treatment of choice.

Cat scratch disease. The skin lesion is only a small papule or pustule but impressive regional lymphadenopathy persists for 3–6 months. Internal organ infection (peliosis) occurs in AIDS. Culture is difficult, but PCR or histology is usually diagnostic. Treatment is usually a macrolide, ciprofloxacin or co-trimoxazole.

Infected burns

Infection has been a major cause of morbidity and mortality in burns, as any burn damages or removes the first line of defence (the skin), and extensive burns impair other host defences also.

Causative organisms include *Staph. aureus, Strep. pyogenes* (now fortunately rare), enteric Gram-negative rods (*Escherichia coli, Klebsiella* spp., etc.) and *Pseudomonas aeruginosa*. The sources are as for wound infections: the patient, the staff, equipment and the environment.

Clinical features are usually confined to pus, fever, and skin graft loss (Fig. 3) but spread into deeper tissue layers can cause septicaemia.

Confirmatory diagnosis by Gram stain and culture is important to determine the pathogens and their antibiotic sensitivities, hence the appropriate antibiotic therapy.

Control rests on four principles:

- primary early burn wound therapy to remove necrotic tissue and cover the area by skin grafts or other materials
- cross-infection control
- topical antibacterial use, usually silver sulphadiazine (SSD)
- prophylactic antibiotics used only at times of decreased host resistance and microbial contamination, e.g. the immediate 3 days after the burn injury, or before excision or grafts.

Infections of pre-existing skin conditions

Any eczematous or ulcerating skin disease can become infected, for example:

- **a**cne conglabata
- **b**ullous and vesicular eruptions
- **c**hronic ulcers
- **d**ermatophytosis and intertrigo
- **e**czematous or exfoliative conditions.

The causative organisms are usually those infecting burns (see above) and pus is the predominant sign. Gram stain and culture should be done, and appropriate antibiotics given.

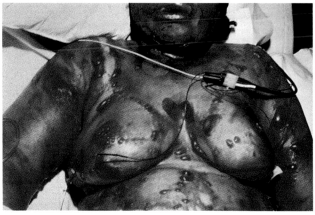

Fig. 3 **Infected burns.**

> ### Wound, bite and burn infections
>
> - Wounds can be traumatic, surgical, bites or rupture of the skin defences by burns or pre-existing disease.
>
> - Infection of wounds comes from skin flora (patient or staff), perforated viscera, environment (contaminating foreign bodies, water, animals, soil or air), or equipment.
>
> - Management involves drainage of pus, removal of foreign bodies and necrotic tissue, and antibiotics, chosen empirically against likely pathogens until confirmatory tests prove the pathogen(s).

Fungal infections of the skin, hair or nails

Superficial mycoses

Superficial mycoses are characterised by infection of the outermost layers of skin and hair, hence there is no host response. Four are recognised (see also p. 74).

Tinea versicolor (pityriasis versicolor)

Tinea versicolor is caused by *Malassezia furfur* (*Pityrosporum orbiculare*) and is found worldwide. Clinically, the two major characteristics are hypopigmentation and scaling. Initially perifollicular, the hypopigmentation spreads and coalesces. It is asymptomatic, or mildly itchy. Diagnosis is confirmed by a KOH preparation of skin scales showing clusters of yeasts with short hyphal fragments, so-called 'spaghetti and meatballs'. Treatment is by selenium sulphide or a topical azole.

Tinea nigra

Tinea nigra is caused by *Exophiala werneckii* and is characterised by dark brown or black macules (Fig. 1). It is particularly common in warm countries. Clinically, the asymptomatic lesions are usually on the palms or soles and enlarge peripherally. The differential diagnosis from malignant melanoma is most important, made by finding the characteristic dark two-celled oval yeasts and short hyphae in KOH mounts. Treatment is to remove the stratum corneum by scraping, by adhesive tape or by a keratolytic such as Whitfield's ointment.

Black piedra

Black piedra is caused by *Piedraia hortae* infection forming hard black nodules along the hair shaft. The diagnosis is easily confirmed by microscopy. Cutting or shaving the hair usually avoids topical antifungal agents.

White piedra

White piedra is caused by *Trichosporon beigelii* infection forming soft cream-white sleeves around the hair shafts. Differential diagnosis includes the harder more adherent 'nits' of pediculosis (see Fig. 1, p. 77), distinguished by microscopy. Treatment is also by cutting or shaving the hair.

Cutaneous mycoses (dermatophytoses)

Cutaneous mycoses (tinea or 'ringworm') are characterised by infection of

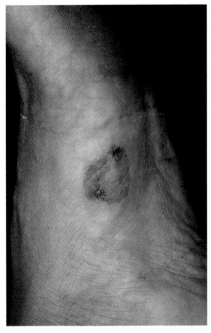

Fig. 1 **Tinea nigra.**

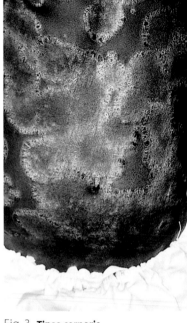

Fig. 3 **Tinea corporis.**

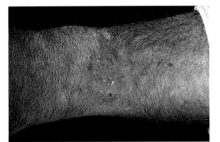

Fig. 2 ***M. gypseum* geophilic infection from soil contact in drain worker.**

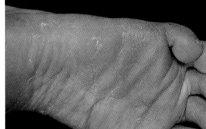

Fig. 4 **Tinea pedis.**

the keratinised layer of the skin, hair or nails. The clinical disease depends on the specific infecting fungus and on the host response. The clinical classification depends on the body area involved:

- skin: tinea corporis (of the body), tinea cruris (groins), tinea manuum (hand), tinea pedis (feet)
- hair: tinea capitis (scalp), tinea barbae (beard)
- nails: tinea unguium.

Tinea of the skin

The causative organisms are commonly *T. rubrum*, *T. mentagrophytes*, *E. floccosum* and, on the body, *M. canis*, but any of the other species of dermatophytes (p. 74–75) can infect (Fig. 2). Predisposing factors include warmth and moisture, so shoes, tight underclothes and obesity can be causative factors.

The clinical features vary. On the body, groins and hands, the common lesion is a round or irregular ('gyrate') scaly area

with a red edge and a healing or scaling centre (Fig. 3). Other forms are vesicular, pustular, granulomatous or, very rarely, mycetoma.

Tinea pedis (Fig. 4) is commonly inter-digital (intertriginous) with red scaling and white macerated fissuring, but may be hyperkeratotic or vesicopustular.

The differential diagnosis is wide, and includes seborrhoeic dermatitis, lichen planus, candidiasis and psoriasis. Confirmatory diagnosis is by KOH mount and culture.

Chemotherapy is usually by a topical antifungal, commonly an imidazole such as clotrimazole. Oral terbinafine is replacing griseofulvin for extensive disease. Control and prevention aims at removing predisposing factors, and preventing reinfection from self or others.

Tinea of the hair (capitis, barbae)

Mycoses of the hair are either non-inflammatory or inflammatory. The causative organisms are from the genera *Trichophyton* or *Microsporum*.

Clinical syndromes are scaling and alopecia, with short broken hairs in ectothrix ('outside the hair') infections, and 'black spots' where a hair has broken off at follicular level in endothrix ('inside the hair') infections. The inflammatory types begin as pustular folliculitis, which can progress to wide-spread suppuration under a fluctuant scalp (**kerion**), with malaise, fever and local lymphadenopathy. Scarring and alopecia may then be permanent. In the principal differential diagnosis, bacterial folliculitis, alopecia is extremely uncommon.

Confirmation is by showing fluorescent endothrix-infected hairs with a Wood's light, by microscopy of KOH-treated hairs and scales, and by culture.

Chemotherapy with terbinafine (preferred) or griseofulvin is essential, as topical medications are not curative. Griseo-

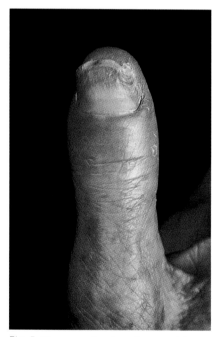

Fig. 5 **Tinea unguium (onychomycosis).**

fulvin is usually given for a period of 6–8 weeks, but a single large (3g) dose cures 80% of children with ectothrix infections. Control and prevention is by avoiding overcrowding and by good hygiene, including avoiding shared contaminated combs.

Tinea of the nails (unguium)

The causative organisms of onychomycosis are usually *Trichophyton* species, most commonly *T. rubrum* or *T. mentagrophytes*. Some other fungi including *Aspergillus*, *Candida* (Fig. 6) and *Fusarium* spp., can infect the nails. Clinically, white discoloration that is **distal with subungual** hyperkeratosis giving a thickened discoloured nail separated from the nail bed is most common (Fig. 5), though sometimes **proximal** leuconychia or **superficial** (white nail) infection occurs. Co-existent tinea pedis or corporis is common.

Confirmatory diagnosis depends on culture from the infected subungual, proximal or superficial areas.

Chemotherapy, except for superficial disease, is by terbinafine (6–12 weeks) or griseofulvin for 4 months for finger-nails, and 6, 9 or even 12 months for the slower growing toe-nails.

Cutaneous candidiasis

The cutaneous manifestations of *Candida* infection include:

- local infection in the normal host
- immunocompromised host infection
- local sign of disseminated disease.

Normal host

Intertrigo (in skin folds), napkin rash, balanitis, folliculitis and vulval, peri-anal and interdigital *Candida* infections are all similar, with initial vesicles or pustules which break to leave spreading red, moist, itchy areas with irregular white borders. There is often co-existing vaginal or rectal infection. Species other than *C. albicans* are unusual. Diagnosis is confirmed by Gram stain and culture, and local antifungal therapy (e.g. with clotrimazole) is usually curative. Prevention and control of recurrences depends on attacking predisposing factors such as moisture, obesity and diabetes, and any vaginal or rectal source.

Paronychia (Fig. 6 and p. 192), and **onychomycosis** (see above) also occur.

Immunocompromised host

Chronic mucocutaneous candidiasis (**CMC**) is a severe chronic disease in those, usually children, whose T-cells fail to respond to *Candida* antigen in vitro or in vivo. Clinically, oral thrush is usually followed by nail then skin infections of variable severity but unremitting chronicity. In addition, about half have an endocrinopathy, e.g. hypoparathyroidism or Addison's disease, often with autoimmune antibodies.

Confirmatory diagnosis depends on T-cell function tests, Gram stain and culture, and appropriate endocrine function tests. Treatment is difficult and disappointing.

Local sign of disseminated disease

Macronodular candidiasis is a useful diagnostic sign in some patients with disseminated candidiasis, when scattered pink-red maculopapular lesions appear over the scalp and body. Histopathology stains on punch biopsy are more reliable than culture. Treatment is for disseminated candidiasis (p. 69).

Subcutaneous mycoses

See page 204.

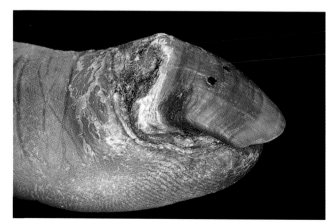

Fig. 6 *Candida* **infection of nail, with paronychia.**

> ### *Fungal infections of the skin, hair or nails*
>
> - Superficial mycoses affect the hair (piedra) and outer layer of the skin (tinea versicolor or tinea nigra).
>
> - Cutaneous mycoses affect various areas of the body including hair and nails. The success of treatment depends upon the region infected.
>
> - Candidiasis occurs in the skin and nails of immunocompetent hosts. Chronic mucocutaneous candidiasis and disseminated disease can occur if immune function is compromised.

Viral infections of skin, mucosa and soft tissues

Enterovirus infections

Enteroviruses cause skin, mucous membrane and soft tissue infections plus asymptomatic infections and many disease syndromes which are described here for convenience.

Classification. Enteroviruses are classified into:

- Polio virus (p. 96–97)
- Coxsackie viruses, divided into Groups A and B by mouse pathogenicity
- ECHO viruses (**E**nteric **C**ytopathic **H**uman **O**rphan, because discovered in faeces before any associated diseases were known)
- Numbered simply as Enterovirus 70, 71 etc., because of difficulties with classification. Enterovirus 72 causes hepatitis A.

Causative organisms. All are Pico*rna*viruses, 20–30nm (Pico = small) non-enveloped RNA viruses.

Replication (Table 1, p. 17) is in the cytoplasm, and after uncoating the single-stranded RNA genome acts directly as mRNA for translation to a large polypeptide, which is cleaved to form both structural proteins for progeny capsids, and RNA polymerase to synthesise progeny genomes. After assembly, release occurs.

Transmission is usually faecal–oral, sometimes by respiratory aerosols.

Clinical features:

1. **Prenatal and neonatal infections** are on p. 144–145.
2. **Myo-mucocutaneous:**
    - **Enteroviral rash,** a non-specific maculopapular rash, occurs often just with fever, from numerous Coxsackie or ECHO viruses, and recovers spontaneously in a few days.
    - **Epidemic myalgia = Pleurodynia** ('painful pleura') = **Bornholm Disease** (Danish island) from Coxsackie B virus has fever and severe pleuritic chest pain needing pain relief, but with no serious tissue damage and complete recovery.
    - **Haemorrhagic conjunctivitis** is a very infectious acute infection, usually by Enterovirus 70, with bulbar petechiae, but recovering completely without treatment.
    - **Hand, foot and mouth disease,** usually from Coxsackie A5 or A6 or Enterovirus 71, has a painful vesicular stomatitis with vesicular rash on

hands and feet, lasting about a week, and quite infectious.
    - **Herpangina** due to 7 types of Coxsackie A viruses has acute fever and sore throat from vesicles which ulcerate and heal in 4–6 days.

3. **Organ infections:**
    - '**Aseptic' meningitis** (p. 94–95) or **meningoencephalitis** (p. 96) is commonly due to ECHO, Coxsackie A or B, or Enterovirus 70 or 71. Any of the five mucocutaneous clinical features above may be associated. It is seldom severe, and recovers without specific treatment in 10–14 days. **Paralysis** like polio may occur with Coxsackie A7 or Enterovirus 70 or 71.
    - **Hepatitis** or **diarrhoeal disease** is sometimes due to enteroviruses.
    - **Myocarditis and pericarditis** are commonly due to Coxsackie B viruses. Severe or fatal in neonates or infants, they are usually milder in adults, with 'URTI', fever, chest pain, arrhythmias, pericardial rub and sometimes cardiac failure. Recovery is usual.
    - **Post-viral chronic fatigue syndrome** with months of muscle weakness, fatigue and poor concentration may be sometimes due to Coxsackie B viruses.
    - **Respiratory infections** including colds, 'pseudo-influenza', bronchitis and pneumonia can be due to ECHO viruses, Coxsackie A21 or B, or enterovirus 68.

Herpes simplex virus infections

Although Herpes simplex virus can cause deep infections, it particularly causes infections of skin and mucous membranes, so is described here.

Other Herpesvirus infections are by CMV, EBV, HHV 6 and VZV, described on p. 144–145, and by HHV8, described on p. 150.

Classification is into Herpes simplex virus Types 1 and 2 (HSV-1, HSV-2) by antigenic and genomic DNA differences.

Causative agents are HSV-1 and HSV-2. They are enveloped double-stranded DNA herpesviruses.

Replication is initially in skin or mucous membrane, then virus migrates to the trigeminal ganglion (HSV-1) or lum-

bar and sacral ganglia (HSV-2). Details are on p. 16–17.

Asymptomatic infection is common, revealed only by subsequent serology.

Latency is a feature, like all herpesviruses, with multiple copies of DNA in the cytoplasm of infected neurons with minimal transcription and no translation, until **recurrence** after re-activation by, e.g., sunlight, trauma, hormones, fever or immunodeficiency.

Transmission. HSV-1 is commonly transmitted by saliva in early life, while HSV-2 is mainly transmitted sexually.

Clinical features of HSV-1 are primary and recurrent lesions:

- **Gingivo-stomatitis** in infancy or childhood with fever, irritability, and blisters and ulceration of mouth and lips, healing in 15–20 days. It recurs as: **Herpes labialis,** 'cold sores of the lips' with one or more painful blisters, usually at the same site, healing in 5–10 days. In adults, HSV-2 can be the cause.
- **Herpetic whitlow** is a purulent blister on finger (Fig. 1) or hand, usually from direct contact.
- **Kerato-conjunctivitis** is potentially serious and needs urgent treatment to prevent corneal scarring and even blindness.
- **Encephalitis** may be primary or a recurrence. Unusually, it particularly affects one temporal lobe, with fever, headache, fits, confusion, and if untreated stupor, coma and death. LP shows lymphocytosis, elevated protein, and HSV on PCR. CT or MRI show the infected area. High-dose i.v. aciclovir is given urgently.

Clinical features of HSV-2 are primary and recurrent lesions:

- **Genital herpes** (Herpes genitalis) arises from sexual contact with asymptomatic or active infection. It can affect

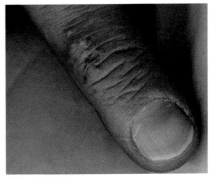

Fig. 1 **Herpetic whitlow.**

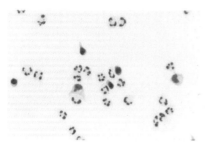

Fig. 2 **Mollaret's meningitis.** Note tail on lymphocyte (towards top left), and three nuclei like 'footprints'.

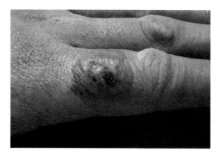

Fig. 3 **Orf on a shepherd's finger.**

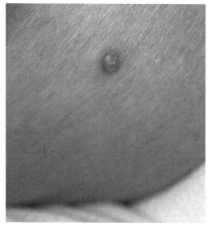

Fig. 4 **Molluscum contagiosum pearly nodule.**

urethra, cervix, rectum or external genitalia and anal area with painful blisters. Primary attacks are more severe with fever and inguinal lymphadenopathy. Details are in Table 1, p. 188. HSV-1 is less common.

■ **Congenital herpes** from primary infection and viraemia in pregnancy is a rare cause of skin, eye or brain lesions in the fetus.

■ **Neonatal herpes** can occur if vaginal delivery occurs through even asymptomatic genital herpes, but is worst with maternal primary infection. It can cause superficial skin, mouth or eye infections, or serious pneumonia, meningoencephalitis or disseminated infection. It is prevented by caesarean section, and treated with aciclovir. See also Table 1, p. 144.

■ **Aseptic meningitis** in adults is usually mild. Recurrent 'Mollaret's meningitis' (Fig. 2) is probably usually due to HSV.

■ **Hepatitis** (Fig. 1, p. 170) and other organ infections occur with immunodeficiency.

Confirmatory tests are usually PCR on swabs or fluids. IgM and IgG, especially if type-specific, may indicate the diagnosis.

Chemotherapy is with i.v. aciclovir, or oral fam- or valaciclovir.

Control and prevention is by avoiding contact, by caesarean section as above, and at times by long-term suppression with a-, fam- or valaciclovir during immunosuppression.

Poxvirus infections

Classification. All belong to the Poxviridae family. The Orthopox genus contains smallpox virus, vaccinia (used in smallpox vaccination), and monkeypox virus. The Parapox genus contains the viruses causing milker's nodes and orf. Molluscum contagiosum virus is a Molluscipox, and Tanapox virus a Yatapox.

Causative agents. All pox viruses are very large and complex, without sym-

metry. The DNA genome is in the dumbbell shaped core with a core (inner) membrane, compressed by two lateral bodies within the outer membrane with surface tubules. Most virions stay cell-associated and have no envelope when released by cell death, while those otherwise released have an envelope of both host cell lipids and viral polypeptides. Enveloped or not, all are infectious.

Clinical features:

■ **Smallpox** see Viral systemic infections (p. 148).

■ **Milker's nodes** and **orf** (Fig. 3) are occupational diseases of cattle or sheep handlers. Milker's nodes are vascular papules or nodules, while orf progresses from vesicles to pustules to granulomatous, coalescing lesions taking weeks to heal.

■ **Molluscum contagiosum** forms pearly umbilicated papules over the body from viral multiplication in the epidermis. Benign and common in the normal host (Fig. 4), it may become severe and generalised in AIDS.

■ **Monkeypox** was recognised after the eradication of smallpox, as it is like mild smallpox. Recovery occurs in over 98%. Infected monkeys from west-central Africa have been imported into USA, infecting humans and prairie dogs.

■ **Tanapox** from monkeys is also like mild smallpox, in west and east Africa.

■ **Vaccinia virus** is derived from cowpox, and used for smallpox vaccination, causing a localised pustule which heals completely in about 3 weeks. Protection against smallpox is usually complete for 3 years and incomplete for up to 20 years. Complications are uncommon, but include generalised vaccinia.

Confirmatory tests are specialised, and include electron microscopy, virus culture, gel diffusion and PCR.

Chemotherapy is usually ineffective. Local measures are used for molluscum contagiosum.

Control and prevention. Vaccination with vaccinia protects against smallpox. The others depend on avoiding close contact with infected hosts.

Warts

Classification is into over 100 types by DNA restriction fragment analysis.

Causative agent is the human papillomavirus (HPV), a non-enveloped virus with circular double-stranded DNA and icosahedral capsid. Transmission is by close contact.

Clinical features are well-known – common skin or anogenital warts (see Fig. 5, p. 189). Some types cause cervical dysplasia and cervical cancer, see p. 182.

Confirmatory tests are seldom needed.

Chemotherapy is with podophyllum or imiquimod. Cryotherapy is often better.

Control and prevention is by avoiding close contact.

Viral infections of skin, mucosa and soft tissues

■ Enteroviruses are picornaviruses, and include polio, Coxsackie- and ECHO viruses. They cause polio, and congenital, neonatal and organ infections, as well as skin and muscle infections.

■ Herpes simplex virus is characterised by latency and reactivation. Type 1 particularly causes skin, mucosa and brain infections, while Type 2 usually causes genital and neonatal infections, rarely organ infection.

■ Poxviruses include smallpox, vaccinia, orf and molluscum contagiosum viruses. They cause skin nodules or vesicles, severe only in smallpox.

■ Papillomaviruses cause warts, cervical dysplasia and cervical cancer.

Tropical and rare bacterial skin and soft tissue infections

Erythrasma

Erythrasma is a superficial skin infection caused by *Corynebacterium minutissimum*, a Gram-positive filamentous diphtheroid identified by coral-red fluorescence under a Wood's light, and cocci and filaments up to 10μm long in KOH mounts. Pink or red-brown scales in intertriginous areas or toe-webs are treated with oral erythromycin for 5–21 days.

Mycetoma (madura foot)

Mycetomata are chronic infections of the subcutaneous tissues characterised by swelling, sinuses, and suppuration.

They are classified into:

- **Actinomycotic mycetomata** caused by various Actinomycetes (*bacteria*) including *Actinomyces*, *Nocardia* and *Actinomadura* spp. (p. 62) and
- **Eumycotic mycetomata**, caused by many *fungi* including *Madurella* and *Pseudallescheria* spp. (p. 75).

Clinically, after implantation of soil organisms, usually into the foot, there is massive swelling and deformity, with pus discharging through numerous sinuses. Pain is not prominent.

Culture and microscopy are essential to distinguish the actinomycete infections which often respond to antibacterials, from fungal infections needing antifungal drugs.

Chemotherapy is usually penicillin for *Actinomyces* spp., or sulphonamides and an aminoglycoside for *Nocardia* spp. Itraconazole orally often avoids excision or amputation for fungal mycetoma.

Mycobacterial infections

Tuberculosis

There are five forms of cutaneous tuberculosis caused by *Mycobacterium tuberculosis*. All but scrofuloderma are rare.

- **Scrofuloderma** is skin infection around sinuses draining from underlying tuberculous lymph nodes (see Fig. 2, p. 122).
- **Lupus vulgaris** (meaning 'common wolf') has 'apple-jelly-like' nodules that coalesce to (wolf-like) devour tissue.
- **Primary inoculation TB** in pathologists and embalmers from accidental inoculation leads to ulceration and lymphadenitis.
- **Tuberculosis verrucosa cutis** with warty plaques occurs also by inoculation, usually in young adults in tropical areas.
- **Tuberculides** are scattered papulonecrotic nodules denoting tuberculosis elsewhere in the body.

All are diagnosed and treated as tuberculosis elsewhere (p. 232)

Leprosy

The skin manifestations of leprosy range from the single anaesthetic hypopigmented *tuberculoid* plaque through *intermediate* forms to the numerous, large, deforming, destructive lesions of the *lepromatous* form (see p. 104).

Bairnsdale (Buruli) ulcer

The Bairnsdale ulcer (Fig. 1) is so named because *M. ulcerans* (p. 61) was first isolated from a patient from Bairnsdale in Australia, and the ulcer is now most commonly seen around Buruli in Africa.

Clinically, a subcutaneous nodule forms at the inoculation site. This breaks down

Table 1 **Summary of some tropical bacterial skin infections**

Category/ classification	Causative organism	Clinical features	Confirmatory diagnosis	Chemotherapy	Control and prophylaxis
Bacterial mycetoma	*Actinomyces* spp. *Nocardia* spp.	Swelling, suppuration, sinuses	Granules, Gram-positive clubs, granulomata	Penicillin or sulphonamides, surgery	Avoid soil inoculation
Mycobacteria					
Tuberculosis	*M. tuberculosis*	Chronicity, ulceration	AFB smear, biopsy, culture, PCR	Triple (including isoniazid and rifampicin)	BCG, isonicotinic acid hydrazide for contacts
Leprosy	*M. leprae*	Anaesthesia, pigmentation, ulceration, deformity	AFB smear, biopsy (snip), clinical	Triple (including dapsone and rifampicin)	BCG?, avoid close contact
Bairnsdale (Buruli) ulcer	*M. ulcerans*	Ulceration, undercut-edge	AFB smear, biopsy, PCR	Triple ARC, ?Excise and graft	BCG?, avoid soil, scratches
Fish tank granuloma	*M. marinum*	Ulceration, granuloma	AFB smear, biopsy	Co-trimoxazole or combined rifampicin-ethambutol	Avoid fish and trauma
Spirochaetal					
Yaws	*Treponema pallidum* ssp. *pertenue*	1. Painless papules 2. Generalised papillomata 3. Gummata, ulceration	Microscopy (dark ground), serology (late), clinical	Penicillin	Treatment (perhaps mass), avoid skin contact
Pinta	*T. carateum*	1. Pruritus, papules, pale areas 2. Pintides 3. Pale areas	As yaws	Penicillin	Treatment, avoid skin contact
Bejel (endemic syphilis)	*T. pallidum* ssp. *endemicum*	1. Mucous ulcer 2. Oropharyngeal 3. Gummata	As yaws	Penicillin	Avoid shared utensils
Syphilis	*T. pallidum* ssp. *pallidum*	1. Chancre 2. Rash (varies) 3. Gumma, CNS, etc	Microscopy (dark ground), serology	Penicillin	Control copulation
Tropical pyomyositis	*Staph. aureus* (*Strep. pyogenes*)	Pain, tenderness, swelling, fever	Gram stain, culture	Drainage, flucloxacillin, (Penicillin G)	None known
Tropical ulcer	Anaerobes Spirochetes	Deep ulcer	Microscopy, clinical	Penicillin	Avoid trauma

AFB, acid-fast bacilli; ARC, amikacin, rifampicin and clarithromycin (or ciprofloxacin).

to form a chronic ulcer with undercut edges, at times slowly healing on one side while continuing to destroy tissue on the opposite side of the ulcer. There are no systemic symptoms unless secondary infection occurs.

Clinical diagnosis is confirmed by culture (at 32°C) or histopathology, if smears for acid-fast bacilli from the ulcer are negative. Chemotherapy usually includes amikacin, rifampicin and clarithromycin, but excision and grafting may be needed.

Fish tank granuloma

M. marinum infections are described on page 196.

Spirochaetal infections

Yaws

The causative organism is *Treponema pallidum*, subspecies (ssp.) *pertenue* (p. 58), visually and serologically identical with other human treponemes and also not yet cultured in vitro. Yaws is a disease of the tropics. Infection follows contact of exudate with abraded skin. Clinically, like the other treponematoses, there are three stages:

- The *primary lesion* is a **p**ainless **p**apule that **p**rogresses, becomes **p**apillomatous with surface erosions then slowly heals.
- The *secondary stage* has similar but multiple papillomata that heal but may relapse. Lymphadenopathy and osteitis may occur.
- The *tertiary stage* has multiple skin lesions of many types (plaques, nodules

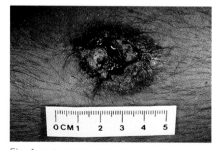

Fig. 1 **Bairnsdale or Buruli ulcer.** Note undermined edge.

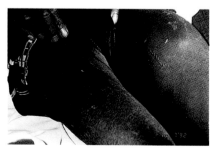

Fig. 2 **Tropical pyomyositis.** Note thigh swelling.

and especially ulcers) and **gummata** (chronic destructive ulcers) of bones, especially skull, nose and tibia.

Clinical diagnosis may be confirmed by dark ground microscopy (DGM) of exudates, or serology (EIA, RPR and TPPA). Chemotherapy is extraordinarily effective, one injection of benzathine benzylpenicillin being curative, and controlling spread.

Pinta

The causative organism is *T. carateum* (p. 58). Transmission is, like yaws, by infectious secretions onto broken skin.

Pinta (Spanish for 'blemish') is seen in dry rural areas of Central and South America. Clinically, the *primary* stage shows pruritic papules that merge, persist for months, then heal with hypopigmentation. The *secondary* lesions are small, multiple, pigmented papules called pintides. These persist or recur for years, until the *tertiary* stage occurs with multiple disfiguring hypopigmented areas.

Clinical diagnosis is confirmed by DGM or serology. Chemotherapy is by penicillin, and all stages should be treated to control transmission, though early stages respond best, and depigmented (achromic) lesions remain.

Bejel (endemic syphilis)

The causative organism is *T. pallidum*, ssp. *endemicum*. Transmission is person-to-person by direct contact, or via common cooking cauldrons and cutlery through the oral mucosa.

Clinically, the *primary* lesion is usually unseen, but uncommonly ulcerates. The *secondary* lesions can be oral mucous patches, peri-oral papules or peri-anal condylomata lata. *Tertiary* lesions are usually obvious gummata of skin or bone. Clinical diagnosis is again confirmed by DGM or serology. Chemotherapy and control is again long-acting penicillin.

Syphilis

The causative organism is *T. pallidum*, ssp. *pallidum* (p. 58). Transmission is virtually always venereal (p. 189), at times transplacental, almost never accidental (by needlestick) as the spirochaete is very

susceptible to drying and light, and soon dies outside the body.

- The *primary* stage is the classic chancre.
- The *secondary* stage includes a rash of astonishing variability, from macular to maculopapular to papular to pustular (pustular syphilids). It persists for many weeks and typically involves palms and soles, unusual in other diseases.
- *Tertiary* involvement of the skin is rare, either by local gumma (chronic destructive ulceration) or from bone disease.

Clinical diagnosis is usually confirmed by serology (sometimes unhelpful), or rarely by DGM or histopathology. Chemotherapy is by penicillin; dose and duration depend on the stage. Primary and secondary lesions resolve remarkably. Unlike most other tertiary syphilis, gummata also respond well.

Tropical pyomyositis

Obviously, this is a pus-forming infection of a patient's muscle in the tropics; the causative organism is usually *Staphylococcus aureus*. *Why* it occurs is less obvious – predisposing factors may be trauma or parasitic infestation.

Clinically, pain, swelling (Fig. 2) and tenderness develop over 2 or 3 days in a leg or trunk muscle, followed by fever, and local heat and erythema if subcutaneous spread occurs. Multiple abscesses are uncommon. Very acute onset suggests *Streptococcus pyogenes* as the cause. Diagnosis is by Gram stain and culture of operative pus. Chemotherapy with i.v. penicillinase-resistant penicillin is an adjunct to surgical drainage of all abscesses. *S. pyogenes* needs penicillin G treatment.

Tropical ulcer

This is a deep, chronic painful skin ulcer of uncertain aetiology, possibly anaerobes and/or spirochaetes (see Fig. 3, p. 217). Specific causes should be excluded. Most respond to penicillin, local care and improved nutrition.

> ## Tropical and rare bacterial skin and soft tissue infections
>
> - Mycetoma is easily diagnosed clinically, but culture is essential to distinguish bacterial infections, treated by antibacterials, from fungal infections needing antifungal drugs.
> - Mycobacterial infections are chronic, characteristic clinical conditions (e.g. leprosy), confirmed by special stains and/or culture, with specific long-term chemotherapy and limited special surgery.
> - Spirochaetal infections have primary, secondary and tertiary stages. The geographic area and clinical syndromes combine to give the diagnosis. Confirmation is usually by serology, rarely by microscopy, and never by culture. Chemotherapy is penicillin.
> - Tropical pyomyositis is also a clinical diagnosis, confirmed by microscopy and culture of pus at operation. *Staph. aureus* is treated with flucloxacillin, *Strep. pyogenes* with penicillin G.

Tropical and rare fungal and parasitic skin and soft tissue infections

Subcutaneous mycoses

Sporotrichosis

The cause is *Sporothrix schenckii* (p. 75). Clinically, there are three forms:

- **Lymphocutaneous infection** follows neglected implantation of the fungus from soil or vegetation. Slowly a painless papule appears, enlarges and ulcerates, then multiple painless nodules appear along draining lymphatics (not at lymph nodes) and also chronically ulcerate. Systemic symptoms are absent.
- **Cutaneous infection** occurs as a verrucous or ulcerated plaque.
- **Disseminated disease** to lungs, bones or brain is very rare.

Confirmatory diagnosis by culture of pus or tissue is not difficult. Histopathology shows granulomata, micro-abscesses and pseudo-epitheliomatous hyperplasia (excess of normal epithelial cells). Chemotherapy is by itraconazole, or potassium iodide.

Chromoblastomycosis (chromomycosis)

This is caused by the implantation of one of many melanin-containing 'dematiaceous' fungi, particularly *Fonsecaea* spp. (p. 75).

Clinically, early smooth papules become verrucous with age. Infection spreads proximally, so there are proximal smooth lesions and cauliflower-like distal ones. Pain, sinuses and systemic symptoms are absent without secondary bacterial infection.

Confirmatory diagnosis is by histopathology, showing pigmented fungi ('copper pennies', sclerotic or 'Medlar bodies'), and granulomata, micro-abscesses and pseudo-epitheliomatous hyperplasia. Culture is unreliable as the causative fungi are frequent contaminants.

Chemotherapy with itraconazole is used for extensive disease, while surgical excision is used for localised early disease.

Rare fungal infections

Phaeohyphomycosis (including phaeomycotic cyst). Over 40 dematiaceous fungi can be causal. Clinically, the lesions are single and slow growing. Histopathology shows brown septate hyphal fragments. Chemotherapy with

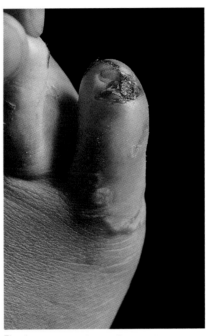

Fig. 1 **Cutaneous larva migrans.** Note elevated tracks of worms at base of toe.

itraconazole is uncertain, so excision is common. Unlike chromomycosis, dissemination causes brain and other abscesses.

Hyalohyphomycosis by hyaline (not dematiaceous) fungi is described with AIDS (p. 150).

Eumycotic mycetoma. This is described with actinomycotic mycetoma (p. 202).

Lobomycosis. This disease is geographically localised. The causative fungus, *Loboa loboi*, has never been cultured. Clinically, chronic warty, nodular, subcutaneous lumps form. Microscopy shows budding yeast-like fungi in chains. Treatment is excision.

Rhinosporidiosis. This is caused by *Rhinosporidium seeberi*, probably an aquatic protist, not a fungus! Clinically, there are large vascular friable warts or polyps, often involving the nasal mucosa. Diagnosis is confirmed by histopathology showing endospores within large spherules. Treatment is excision.

Parasitic infections

Cutaneous amoebiasis

Entamoeba histolytica skin infection is rare, occurring by extension from rectal

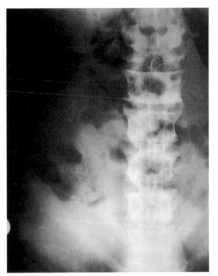

Fig. 2 **Guinea worm: x-ray showing calcification of dead worms above iliac crest.**

or anal infection, from a bowel fistula, or from anal or perhaps vaginal intercourse.

Clinically there is extending ulceration, pain and bleeding, which can mimic a carcinoma. It is therefore essential that diagnosis is confirmed by tissue smear or biopsy. Chemotherapy is with metronidazole; surgery can be harmful. Control and prevention depends on hygiene, and early treatment of intestinal and visceral infection.

Cutaneous larva migrans

This is characterised by red, itchy, snake-like tracks ('creeping eruption'), usually caused by migrating larvae of the dog and cat hookworm *Ancylostoma braziliense* (p. 87), less commonly by larvae of other animal or human hookworms including *Strongyloides stercoralis* (p. 85).

Clinically there is little to find except the multiple tracks (Fig. 1), but rarely there is pulmonary or systemic involvement. Clinical diagnosis may be confirmed by biopsy, though this rarely identifies the causative parasite.

Chemotherapy is albendazole or ivermectin. Control depends on avoiding contact with infected soil, and treating infected hosts.

Dracunculiasis (Guinea worm)

This is characterised by a chronic skin ulcer from which the causative worm *Dracunculus medinensis* (Fig. 2) partly

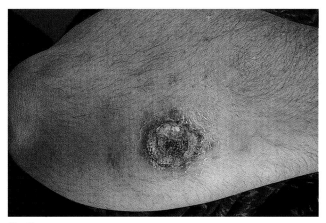

Fig. 3 **Leishmaniasis: ulcerated papule.**

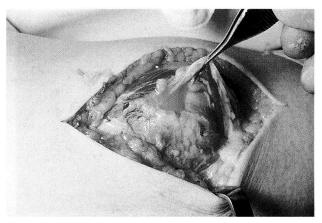

Fig. 4 **Hydatid of the thigh.**

protrudes. Infection results from drinking infected water (p. 86–87).

Clinically a painful papule, usually on the leg, ulcerates and the worm becomes visible. Systemic symptoms of itch, nausea, diarrhoea and dyspnoea may occur even before ulceration. The ulcers may be multiple and/or secondarily infected. Clinical diagnosis is easy, but may be confirmed by showing larvae in the ulcer fluid.

Chemotherapy is by niridazole or mebendazole, which reduce inflammation and allow the 60–100 cm worm to be removed by slowly winding it on to a matchstick over 4–7 days. Control depends on clean drinking water, by preventing contamination of wells and streams with larvae from ulcers.

Filariasis

This is characterised by acute lymphangitis and lymphadenitis, then chronic lymphatic obstruction. The causative organisms are *Wuchereria bancrofti*, *Brugia malayi* and *B. timori* (p. 86–87). Clinically, infection may be asymptomatic despite microfilaraemia, or there may be recurrent brief attacks of acute lymphatic inflammation including fever, headache and, for example, epididymitis.

Chronic lymphadenopathy may remain, then chronic lymphatic obstruction develops causing lymphoedema, hydrocoele and eventually elephantiasis (thick, fissured elephant-like skin). Clinical diagnosis may be confirmed by finding microfilaria in blood films, taken at midnight except in South Pacific infection. However, blood films are often negative even in active infection. Chemotherapy is unsatisfactory, as diethylcarbamazine or ivermectin kill microfilariae but may cause inflammation around adult worms. Control is by avoiding mosquito bites.

Cutaneous and mucocutaneous leishmaniasis

Animal hosts for these zoonoses (p. 82) include rodents and canines, while sandflies are the vectors. A simple classification (p. 152) is:

- **'Old World' disease** (single, multiple or diffuse) cutaneous infection caused by *Leishmania major* or *L. tropica*, occurring in the Middle East (Baghdad boil), India (Delhi boil), Africa and the Mediterranean (Bouton de Crete). Clinically either single or multiple papules ulcerate with a hard base or horn, then slowly heal (Fig. 3). In diffuse disease, many non-ulcerating papules appear.
- **'New World' disease** (single, multiple, diffuse) cutaneous or mucocutaneous infection caused by the *L. mexicana* complex or the *L. braziliensis* complex in Central and South America (Espundia, Chiclero's ear). Single, multiple and diffuse disease again show papules, ulceration and slow healing, though fungating and keloidal forms occur. All may be followed by disfiguring upper lip and nasal mucosal destruction ('tapir nose'), progressing

to buccal, oral and laryngeal involvement, aspiration pneumonia and death.

- **Post kala-azar dermal leishmaniasis** caused by *L. donovani*. In the Indian subcontinent and Africa a few patients develop cutaneous depigmentation (sometimes with nodules) weeks, months or years after kala-azar (p. 82, 152).

Clinical diagnosis of leishmaniasis is often simple but should be confirmed by Giemsa stains on tissue or ulcer scrapings, not surface swabs. The leishmanin test may assist, and serology is now helpful. Chemotherapy is specialised, based on pentavalent antimony compounds. Amphotericin B and pentamidine are second-line drugs. Control is difficult, depending on sandfly avoidance.

Onchocerciasis and loiasis

See these infections on pages 86–87 and 111.

Hydatid cysts

These may be found in soft tissue anywhere in the body (Fig. 4) (p. 88–89).

> ### Tropical and rare fungal and parasitic skin and soft tissue infections
>
> - Many different fungi and parasites cause skin disease.
> - The clinical presentation often suggests the causative parasite but rarely suggests the causative fungus, except in sporotrichosis.
> - Confirmatory diagnosis is necessary, by microscopy or histopathology with specific stains.
> - Chemotherapy is specialised and often unsatisfactory. Surgery is limited to excision of localised disease.
> - Control depends on avoiding, protecting or treating the source (soil, water, animal or human), or avoiding the insect vector.

Osteomyelitis

Osteomyelitis is infection of bone and bone marrow. Infection comes directly from a focus of infection (e.g. a compound fracture) or from circulating infection. Osteomyelitis is classified by numerous criteria; the Cierny–Mader (CM) staging uses four anatomic types (I–IV), with three host types (Normal, Immunocompromised or Untreatable). The classification here is by acuity plus a specific feature:

- acute
  - acute haematogenous osteomyelitis
  - acute contiguous-focus osteomyelitis
  - acute ischaemic-neuropathic osteomyelitis
- subacute
  - device-related osteomyelitis
  - vertebral body osteomyelitis
  - fungal osteomyelitis (rare)
- chronic
  - pyogenic ('bacterial') osteomyelitis
  - actinomycosis (rare)
  - brucellosis (rare)
  - tuberculous osteomyelitis.

Acute osteomyelitis and chronic pyogenic osteomyelitis are described here. All others are described on pages 208–209.

Acute haematogenous osteomyelitis (CM stage I)

Characteristic of this condition is infection in the metaphysis of a long bone, localised by slow blood flow in the unusual sinusoidal venous system, poor collateral circulation and few phagocytes. Infection arrives by bacteraemic spread from a primary source, often cutaneous but frequently inapparent.

Causative organism
This is usually *Staph. aureus*, sometimes streptococci or Gram-negative rods; *Haemophilus influenzae* is commoner in unvaccinated children.

Clinical features
Disease occurs in five clinical settings: neonates (p. 215), children, adults, sickle cell anaemia, and injecting drug users. Fever, severe deep 'bone' pain and acute local bony tenderness are hallmarks; limited movement is usual, while swelling, except in digits or neonates, is late. Systemic symptoms of bacteraemia (high fever, sweats, rigors) are commoner in children, and help to distinguish osteo-

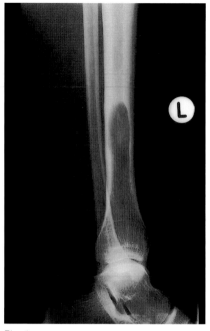

Fig. 1 **Extensive Brodie's abscess in lower third of tibia.**

myelitis from a sickle cell crisis. Injecting drug users often have infected injection sites.

Complications include:

- local destruction: causing dead bone called a **sequestrum**
- local spread in children: usually laterally because of the avascular epiphyseal plate, causing subperiosteal pus and, later, enveloping new-bone formation called an **involucrum**
- local spread in adults: usually through the vascular epiphysis into the adjacent joint, causing 'septic' arthritis
- distant spread: causing **bacteraemia**, septicaemia or sometimes endocarditis, especially in injecting drug users
- chronicity: causing a localised **Brodie's abscess** (Fig. 1) or widespread chronic osteomyelitis, see below.

Confirmatory tests
Blood cultures and bone scan are important, for x-rays are usually negative initially. White cell count (WCC), neutrophil count, erythrocyte sedimentation rate (ESR) and C-reactive protein (CRP) are all elevated. Ultrasound detects fluid in adjacent soft tissues or joints. Microbiologic examination of this fluid or aspirated pus from bone is diagnostic. Open biopsy with microscopy and culture is used when treatment response is poor or diagnosis uncertain.

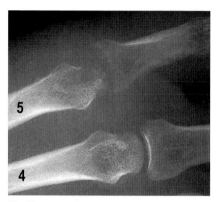

Fig. 2 **Contiguous osteomyelitis of phalangeal head of fifth finger from infective septic arthritis.** Compare with normal joint and bone of fourth finger.

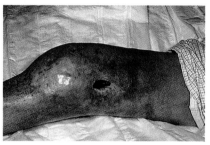

Fig. 3 **Chronic osteomyelitis.** Infection in femur of 68 years duration, showing **s**carlet **s**welling, **s**carring, **s**inus and **s**tiffness (ankylosed knee).

Management
Treatment is initially empirical with flucloxacillin, plus gentamicin if a Gram-negative rod is suspected (e.g. in drug users), or with ceftriaxone in children over 6 months of age. Specific therapy is given after positive culture and sensitivity testing. Pus must be drained, and sequestra removed surgically.

As antibiotics penetrate into bone relatively poorly:

- bactericidal drugs are preferred
- initial therapy is high-dose and intravenous for 2 weeks in adults, or 4–7 days in children
- subsequent oral therapy is high-dose, well-supervised, carefully monitored and continued for total treatment time of 4 weeks in children and 6 weeks in adults.

Control and prevention depends on early diagnosis and treatment of primary sources of bacteraemia, and education about safe equipment and techniques in injecting drug users.

Acute contiguous-focus osteomyelitis

Characteristic of acute contiguous infection is spread from an adjacent focus. The four major causes are:

- infective arthritis (Fig. 2)
- post-trauma infections (open fractures, bone surgery)
- soft tissue infections (skin wounds, pressure ulcers, sinus mucosa in sinusitis)
- puncture wounds (feet, animal bites).

The initial 'Osteitis' (infection of cortical bone only, because the infection begins *outside* the bone, 'CM Stage II, Superficial'), may progress to 'CM III, Localised Osteomyelitis'.

Causative organisms
Infections are often mixed and include:

- *S. aureus* and other staphylococci, especially postoperatively
- enteric Gram-negative rods, especially in mandible, pelvis and small bones
- *Pseudomonas aeruginosa*, especially in punctures through smelly 'sneakers' to the calcaneum
- *P. multocida*, especially after animal bites
- anaerobes, especially in facial, pelvic or sacral osteomyelitis, and in bite infections.

Clinical features
Symptoms are usually acute, with fever, pain, soft tissue swelling, redness and tenderness. Pus may form in any wound. The features may be subacute in sacral or skull infections, or in deep postoperative infections with less virulent pathogens like coagulase-negative staphylococci.

Confirmatory tests
These include culture of the adjacent focus and blood, bone scans, and x-ray, which is more likely to be positive as the history is longer. Sinus cultures are often misleading because of contaminating surface organisms.

Management
Successful treatment depends on adequate deep cultures; antibiotics according to sensitivity tests are needed for at least 4 weeks.

Pus must be drained, and necrotic tissue or sequestra removed surgically.

Control and prevention
Depends on early diagnosis and treatment of infections adjacent to bone.

Acute ischaemic-neuropathic osteomyelitis

Characteristically, ischaemic-neuropathic osteomyelitis occurs with arterial or nerve disease or in diabetic foot infections (p. 195), resulting from the impaired host response, neuropathic damage and vascular disease.

Causative organisms are usually mixed, with staphylococci, streptococci and anaerobes common, plus enteric Gram-negative rod colonisation.

Clinical features are predominantly local, with pain, swelling, redness, cellulitis, ulceration and pus. Impaired sensation and circulation are common, hence gangrene and offensive odour.

Confirmatory tests are appropriate cultures of pus and any available tissue, for surface swabs are usually misleading. Bacteraemia is uncommon, and the usual x-rays and technetium bone scans are difficult to interpret because of ischaemia, neuropathy, trauma and cellulitis. Indium and gallium scans can be more helpful.

Chemotherapy is directed by sensitivity tests on *deep* specimens. Surgery should be conservative whenever possible, but pus must be drained, and necrotic tissue and sequestra removed surgically.

Control and prevention depends on educating the at-risk patient with diabetes, neuropathy and/or ischaemia, plus early treatment of local infections.

Chronic osteomyelitis (pyogenic)

Chronic osteomyelitis is characterised by bone infection lasting months or years. It is caused by the usual pyogenic bacteria particularly staphylococci. Tuberculosis and other special chronic or subacute forms are described on pages 208–209.

Chronic pyogenic osteomyelitis sometimes presents as a late, localised Brodie's abscess (Fig. 1) without a history of acute osteomyelitis, or more usually as chronic osteomyelitis following unresolved acute osteomyelitis, of any of the above three types.

Clinical features
Symptoms are usually mild pain with swelling, which may be scarlet, with sinuses, scarring and stiffness if infection spreads to the adjacent joint (Fig. 3).

Confirmatory tests
Tests should include bone biopsy for the definitive organism(s), as secondary colonising organisms are usual and misleading in sinus and surface swabs. X-ray and CT scan define the extent and can show patchy destruction, sequestrum formation, a cloaca (hole in bone leading to a skin sinus), periosteal new bone formation and overall thickening with sclerosis. CM Stage IV is 'diffuse, circumferential and/or permeative'. ESR and CRP help assess progress during treatment.

Management
Treatment is usually with flucloxacillin, often plus rifampicin, for at least 6 months and, at times, for years. Surgery is needed to drain pus, remove devitalised and dead bone, and stabilise, both at the onset and during chemotherapy. Hyperbaric oxygen therapy and vascularised muscle flaps can improve the modest cure rate. Control and prevention depends on cure of acute osteomyelitis.

Osteomyelitis

- Osteomyelitis is infection of bone and bone marrow; it can be acute, subacute or chronic, and caused by local or haematogenous spread.

- Acute haematogenous disease occurs in the metaphysis of a long bone from bacteraemia; it causes fever and severe bone pain.

- Acute contiguous-focus disease is initiated by spread from an adjacent focus; it usually causes pain, fever and soft tissue swelling.

- Acute ischaemic-neuropathic disease is usually found in diabetics, and presents with pain, ulceration and cellulitis.

- Chronic pyogenic osteomyelitis lasts months or years and is usually caused by staphylococcal infection. It presents with mild pain and swelling, and often a sinus.

- Blood and deep cultures and bone scans direct treatment including long-term antibiotics and at times surgery for drainage, excision or replacement.

Special, tropical or rare bone infections

Acute and chronic pyogenic osteomyelitis are presented on pages 206–207. Here subacute and other chronic forms of the disease are described.

SUBACUTE OSTEOMYELITIS

Device-related osteomyelitis

Bone infection can present weeks or months after insertion of an orthopaedic device.

Classification

Classification is into infection around fixateurs, nails, pins, plates, rods, screws and other temporary devices which later can be removed, or around prosthetic joints, intended to be permanent.

Causative organisms

Usually S. aureus or coagulase-negative staphylococci: either can be meticillin sensitive or resistant. Streptococci, Gram-negative rods or other bacteria are less common.

Clinical features

Symptoms are mainly of wound breakdown and purulent discharge (Fig. 1). Fever is uncommon, and pain or loosening occur late.

Confirmatory tests

Early samples of the wound discharge for microscopy and culture are reliable but become misleading with time owing to secondary colonising bacteria; deep cultures at bone level are then needed. X-ray changes are late; bone scans are unhelpful due to the recent procedure. Erythrocyte sedimentation rate (ESR) is elevated and of use in following progress.

Chemotherapy and control

Chemotherapy depends on the organism isolated. Mixed infections are uncommon. Surgery is needed to drain pus and remove necrotic tissue. In infections around temporary devices, the device is removed when union occurs or the site is stable, and antibiotics are then continued for 6 weeks or longer. Infected prosthetic joints are a specialised problem: in brief, infection cannot be cured while the prosthesis is in situ, and while antibiotics may suppress the infection, for cure the prosthesis must be removed and either replaced or arthroplasty or arthrodesis done.

Control and prevention depend on rigorous operative asepsis and appropriate chemoprophylaxis.

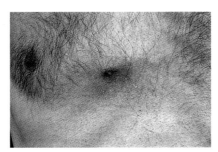

Fig. 1 **Infected total knee prosthesis, with discharging wound (disregard the snail-like suture dressings!).**

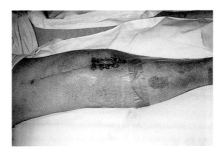

Fig. 2 **Tuberculous sinus from rib.**

Vertebral body osteomyelitis

Infection can occur in one or more vertebral bodies. The route is usually blood-borne but sometimes occurs directly from operation or procedure (see also vertebral disc infections, p. 211).

Causative organisms

Usually S. aureus, rarely with Gram-negative rods including Salmonella or Pseudomonas spp. Candida spp. can infect in drug addicts. Chronic spinal tuberculosis and brucellosis are described below.

Clinical features

Clinical features are persistent back pain, muscle spasm, referred pain (e.g. sciatica or hip pain) and later spinal cord compression with paraparesis or paraplegia (weakness or paralysis from the waist down). Fever is common with S. aureus, less prominent with other organisms.

Confirmatory tests

Tests are imaging by CT or MRI (see Fig. 4, p. 211) to identify the extent of disease, and microscopy and culture of vertebral body samples taken by needle aspiration or open operation to define the pathogen and exclude alternative diagnoses, including tumour.

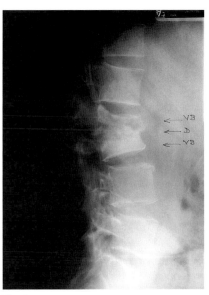

Fig. 3 **TB spine: radiograph showing typical disc destruction and wedge-shaped collapse of adjacent vertebral bodies.**

Chemotherapy and control

Chemotherapy depends on the pathogen and sensitivity tests (e.g. flucloxacillin for sensitive staphylococci). Control and prevention depends on treatment of any potential primary source, and procedural asepsis.

Fungal osteomyelitis

Characteristics of this rare infection are chronicity, osteolytic ('bone dissolving') lesions and eventually an overlying 'cold' abscess, i.e. it resembles tuberculosis. The route is usually blood-borne during disseminated fungal disease; rarely it occurs by direct inoculation in sporotrichosis. Immunosuppression by drugs or disease, and injecting drug use are predisposing factors.

Causative organisms

Usually Candida spp., but osteomyelitis occurs in systemic mycoses, aspergillosis, sporotrichosis and zygomycosis.

Clinical features are those of the underlying disease, plus fever, chronic bone pain, bony tenderness and failure to respond to antibacterial drugs. A cold abscess overlying superficial bones is a valuable clue. Infection can spread to adjacent joints.

Confirmatory tests are fungal blood cultures, bone scan, x-ray and CT scan with diagnostic aspiration for microscopy, special stains and fungal culture. Serology assists with systemic mycoses.

Management. Chemotherapy is classically with amphotericin B, but the newer potent azoles are less toxic and often effective. Control and prevention depends on early treatment of local and systemic fungal disease.

CHRONIC OSTEOMYELITIS

Actinomycosis

Actinomycosis is a very rare chronic bone infection from dental, sinus or lung actinomycosis. The causative organism is usually *A. israelii*, rarely other species (p. 62).

Clinical features are sinus formation, sulphur granules in the pus, scarring and slow progression across tissue planes. Pain and fever are not prominent.

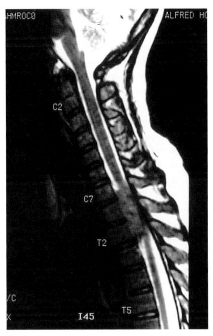

Fig. 4 **TB spine on MRI, showing cord dysfunction at T1–2.**

Confirmatory tests are imaging by x-ray, bone scan or CT as needed; sulphur granules from the pus and bone specimens are taken for microscopy (branching Gram-positive filaments) and anaerobic cultures for at least 10 days. Mixed 'associate' bacteria are not uncommon.

Chemotherapy is high-dose long-term penicillin, initially intravenous for 4–6 weeks, then oral for up to 12 months. Rarely other antibiotics are needed.

Control and prevention depends on treatment of potential primary sources.

Brucellosis

Brucellosis is a very rare infection in bone, as vertebral osteomyelitis following disc space infection during chronic localised brucellosis. The causative organism is usually *B. melitensis* (p. 56).

Clinical features are back pain, fever, malaise and lethargy. Splenomegaly and hepatomegaly if present are useful clues. Confirmatory tests are bone scan, CT and aspiration for microscopy and special prolonged culture in CO_2. Serology is helpful if positive but can be negative during active bone infection.

Management. Chemotherapy is usually with rifampicin plus doxycycline for 6 weeks; gentamicin for 2 weeks can be used instead of rifampicin. Co-trimoxazole is an alternative to doxycycline. Surgery is rarely needed. Control and prevention is by animal brucellosis eradication programmes, and prompt effective treatment of acute brucellosis.

Tuberculosis

Tuberculosis may affect the spine, other bones or joints. Characteristics are chronicity, bone and joint destruction, spread with adjacent 'cold' abscesses (i.e. without palpable heat, and minimal visible inflammation; see Fig. 1, p. 210) and TB elsewhere, often pulmonary or renal. The route is usually blood-borne, sometimes lymphatic, and rarely directly from a caseating node. The causative organism is usually *M. tuberculosis*, occasionally *M. bovis* from unpasteurised milk; rarely an 'atypical' mycobacterium can be involved (p. 60–61).

Clinical features

Clinical symptoms are relatively late, and include pain, deformity or swelling with little fever or systemic symptoms. A sinus develops from superficial bones (Fig. 2). Spinal TB often starts in the disc and spreads to adjacent vertebral bodies (Fig. 3); it can cause flexion deformity (kyphosis, **Pott's disease**), referred pain (e.g. sciatica or hip pain), and later spinal cord compression with paraparesis or paraplegia (weakness or paralysis from the waist down).

Confirmatory tests

- Mantoux, ESR (often useful in following progress) and FBE
- bone, other tissue, sputum and/or urine mycobacterial stains and specific culture and sensitivity tests
- chest x-rays often show the primary focus, which may now be inactive
- bone x-rays can show destruction and collapse (Fig. 3) and adjacent abscesses, while CT shows further detail, and MRI particularly shows disc, bone and CNS involvement (Fig. 4).

Management

Chemotherapy is triple therapy including isoniazid and rifampicin for 9–12 months. Surgery is needed to drain pus, remove necrotic tissue and correct deformity. If expert surgery is unavailable, simpler means can be effective (Fig. 5).

Control and prevention depends on BCG, and effective treatment of all active early TB.

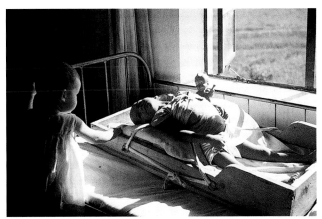

Fig. 5 **TB spine showing effective correction by simple means in Bangladesh.**

> ### Special, tropical or rare bone infections
>
> - Subacute bone infection can occur after insertion of an orthopaedic device and in vertebral bodies. Staphylococci are the commonest cause.
> - Fungal infection is a rare cause of subacute or chronic osteomyelitis, usually following disseminated disease in the immunocompromised.
> - Actinomycosis or brucellosis rarely spreads to infect bone.
> - Tuberculosis of bone can occur secondary to TB elsewhere; it causes bone destruction and 'cold' abscesses.

Joint infections

Infective arthritis

Characteristics

Infection in a joint is termed infective arthritis. Like osteomyelitis, because of the relatively avascular epiphyseal plate, the features in neonates and children differ from those in adults. It is classified clinically into:

- acute, usually from pyogenic bacteria ('septic arthritis'), or viruses
- chronic, usually tuberculous (Fig. 1), spirochaetal or fungal.

The *route* is usually blood spread from a primary focus: occasionally it is caused directly by trauma, surgery or animal or human bites.

Predisposing and risk factors are:

- existing joint damage, especially rheumatoid arthritis or gout
- immunosuppression, by disease or drugs
- injecting drug use
- joint surgery.

See also infected prosthetic joints, which are actually osteomyelitis at the prosthesis–bone interface (p. 208).

Causative organisms

The likely pathogen causing joint infection varies with the age and situation of the patient (Table 1).

Clinical features

A red, hot, swollen, tender, immobile joint is usual except in neonates, the immunosuppressed, viral infections and in deep joints like the hip. A primary focus should be sought, particularly in the skin, heart or genitalia. Skin rash is common in disseminated gonococcal, staphylococcal and streptococcal infections, early Lyme disease (erythema chronicum migrans) and

viral infections. Adjacent tenosynovitis strongly suggests gonorrhoea in the 15–40 age group, otherwise rheumatoid arthritis, gout or trauma.

Arthritis is common in arbovirus infections (especially Chikungunya, O'nyong-ngong, Ross River and Barmah Forest fevers), hepatitis B, mumps, parvovirus and rubella infections. Arthralgia alone occurs uncommonly in adenovirus, CMV, ECHO, HIV, measles, infectious mononucleosis and varicella.

Post-infectious 'reactive' arthritis occurs after chlamydial urethritis, and with some *Campylobacter*, *Shigella*, *Salmonella* and *Yersinia* spp. gut infections in HLA B27-positive patients (Reiter's syndrome, p. 180). Being immunologically mediated, the joint is sterile.

In rheumatoid arthritis or gout, differentiating between an acute exacerbation or supervening acute bacterial arthritis is often difficult, requiring careful investigation.

Confirmatory tests

First, the site of infection is located by clinical examination and ultrasound. Plain x-ray initially may be normal (Fig. 2a) or show only soft-tissue swelling and/or a distended joint; it

Table 1 **Major pathogens in joint infections**	
	Pathogen
Neonates	
Hospital-acquired	*S. aureus*, *Candida* spp., Gram-negative rods
Acquired from mother	Group B streptococci or gonococci (totalling 90%)
Children	*S. aureus*, *H. influenzae*, streptococci (totalling 70%)
Adults (15–40 years)	Gonococci (90% of cases)
Adults (40+ years)	*S. aureus* (70% of cases)
Less common	Mycobacteria, spirochaetes, fungi, viruses

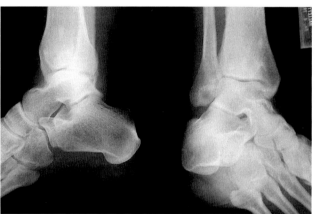

(a)

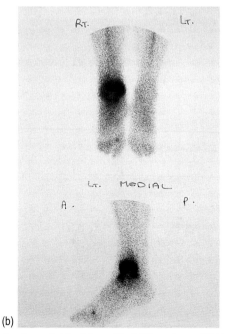

(b)

Fig. 2 **Infective arthritis of the ankle. (a)** Normal x-ray. **(b)** Abnormal 'hot' bone scan (same patient, same day).

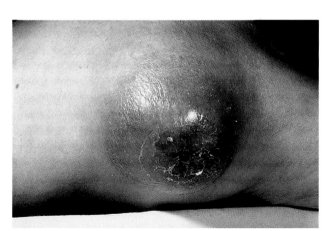

Fig. 1 **Tuberculosis of elbow joint, with overlying 'cold abscess'.**

Table 2 **Joint fluid examination**

Characteristic	Normal	Bacterial infection	Inflammatory[a]	Non-inflammatory[b]
Clarity	Clear	Opaque	Cloudy	Transparent
Colour	Clear	Purulent	Light yellow	Light yellow
WCC/mm^3	< 200	> 100 000	2000–80 000	200–2000
Neutrophils	< 25%	> 75%	50–75%	< 25%
Gram stain	Negative	Often positive	Negative	Negative
Culture	Negative	Often positive	Negative	Negative
Glucose	Same as in blood	Less than in blood	Much less than in blood	Same as in blood

[a]Inflammatory: rheumatoid arthritis, gout/pseudogout, Reiter's syndrome, rheumatic fever, viral infection.
[b]Non-inflammatory: osteoarthritis, trauma, neuropathy.

Table 3 **Gram stain guidance for initial antibiotics in septic arthritis**

Gram stain	Likely organisms	First choice	Alternatives
Gram-positive cocci	Staphylococci or streptococci	Flucloxacillin	Cephalothin
Gram-negative cocci	Gonococci	Ceftriaxone	Ciprofloxacin
Gram-negative cocco-bacilli	H. influenzae	Ceftriaxone	Amoxicillin-clavulanate
Gram-negative rods	E. coli or other enterics	Gentamicin	Ceftriaxone
No organism:			
Neonate	Various (see Table 1)	Ceftriaxone ± gentamicin	Ceftriaxone + flucloxacillin
Child	S. aureus, H. influenzae	Ceftriaxone	Amoxicillin-clavulanate
Adult to age 40	Gonococci	Ceftriaxone	Ciprofloxacin
Older adult	S. aureus, Gram-negative rods if risk factors	Flucloxacillin (± gentamicin if risk factors)	Ceftriaxone (± tobramycin if risk factors)

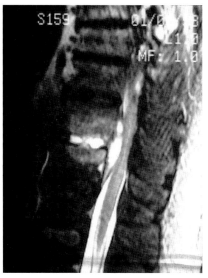

Fig. 4 **Infected disc (white, horizontal) from discography with contiguous vertebral osteomyelitis and intraspinal abscess (white, vertical), shown by MRI.**

excludes some possible diagnoses including fractures. Bone scans are unnecessary early unless adjacent osteomyelitis is suspected, or clinical examination is equivocal (Fig. 2b).

Secondly, the pathogen is identified by blood cultures and joint aspiration (Fig. 3) with microscopy and culture of the joint fluid. Joint fluid examination is helpful even if Gram stain shows no pathogen (Table 2). Sometimes open operation is needed, for example in deep joints like the hip.

Management

Therapy has three principles:

- hydration and nutrition of the patient
- surgery, either arthroscopic or open, to remove necrotic tissue, drain pus and lavage the joint

- initial empiric antibiotics, guided by the Gram stain if bacteria are seen (Table 3), then with specific antibiotics directed by culture and sensitivity tests.

Control and prevention

This depends on early diagnosis and treatment of possible primary foci.

Intervertebral disc infections

Infection within the vertebral discs differs from other joint infections because there is no joint space, and a poor blood supply in adults. Infection is either blood-borne (especially in children) or directly from surgery or discography (especially in adults). Spread is to the vertebral end plates, vertebral body (p. 208) and paraspinal abscesses.

Causative organisms

Pathogens are usually *S. aureus* (blood-borne), coagulase-negative staphylococci

after procedures, *M. tuberculosis*, Gram-negative rods or, rarely, fungi.

Clinical features

Symptoms include back pain, limited mobility and fever.

Confirmatory tests

Imaging confirms disc involvement, and needle aspiration provides samples for microscopy and culture. Open operation to provide culture material is necessary if aspiration fails. While bone scans and CT are useful, MRI is most precise in showing spinal canal or cord involvement (Fig. 4).

Chemotherapy and control

Chemotherapy is guided by vertebral disc culture, being usually flucloxacillin for sensitive staphylococci, vancomycin for meticillin-resistant staphylococci, ceftriaxone or gentamicin for Gram-negative rods, or anti-TB therapy.

Control and prevention

By treatment of potential primary sources, and procedural asepsis.

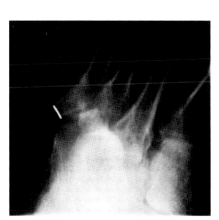

Fig. 3 **Gonococcal arthritis, showing marker for aspiration under x-ray control.**

> ### Joint infections
>
> - Infection of joints occurs usually from blood-borne pathogens but also directly by procedures or trauma.
> - Likely pathogens vary with the patient's age and predisposing risk factors.
> - Bacterial arthritis usually produces a hot swollen tender joint; antibiotics are initially empirical, then guided by sensitivity tests.
> - Intervertebral disc infections cause pain, fever and limited mobility. They result from blood-borne infections, surgery or procedures.

Zoonoses

Zoonoses are infectious diseases transmitted between vertebrate animals and humans in which the human infection is incidental, that is, not part of the pathogen's life cycle. Common sources are farm animals and domestic pets, therefore sufferers are often farmers, veterinarians, abattoir workers and pet-owners; research workers and those visiting or living in areas with infected wild animals may also be at risk (Table 1).

The clinical syndromes often follow logically from the route of infection:

- **i**nsect bites to bloodstream: often multi-organ or systemic disease
- **i**ncisors (animal bites): local or systemic disease (Fig. 1)
- **i**mplanted via wounds or abrasions: local or systemic disease
- **i**ngestion: gut or systemic disease
- **i**nhalation: pulmonary or systemic disease.

Arthropod-borne viral zoonoses are described on p. 92–93 and 146–148. Six non-viral zoonoses are described here.

Brucellosis

Brucellosis is caused by *Brucella* spp. (p. 56), which infect humans by contact with infected animals or their products (particularly milk and cheese):

- *B. abortus*: cattle
- *B. melitensis*: goats and sheep
- *B. suis*: pigs
- *B. canis*: dogs.

Animal infection is often asymptomatic, affecting particularly erythritol-rich tissues like uterus, placenta and breast, which explains the incidence of animal abortion, the risk to abattoir workers of air-borne infection from the placenta, and the high infectivity of milk and cheese. Human infection is usually by ingestion, but can be implanted through the skin, or by inhalation.

Clinical syndromes

- **Acute brucellosis** may be localised and suppurative, or systemic with multi-organ involvement and waves of fever ('undulant fever'). *B. abortus* and *B. canis* cause mild undulant fever, rarely suppuration; *B. suis* causes severe suppurative chronic disease, while the commonest, *B. melitensis*, causes acute severe complicated disease. Brucellae are intracellular pathogens of reticuloendothelial cells. This inaccessibility of the pathogen explains why the disease

persists, relapses are common, and chemotherapy is often ineffective.
- **Subacute brucellosis** causes intermittent fever with systemic symptoms, myalgia, arthralgia, cough and depression.
- **Chronic brucellosis** causes similar symptoms, and in addition can localise to various tissues including bone (p. 209).

Confirmatory tests

Special prolonged blood culture and serology are the most important.

Chemotherapy and control

Chemotherapy is usually with rifampicin plus doxycycline for 6 weeks. Gentamicin for 2 weeks can be used instead of rifampicin. Co-trimoxazole is an alternative to doxycycline. Surgery is rarely needed for localised disease. Control and prevention is by animal brucellosis eradication programmes, and prompt effective treatment of acute brucellosis.

Leptospirosis

Leptospirosis is characterised by human infection with *Leptospira interrogans* (p. 59) from the asymptomatic chronically infected kidneys of animals, usually livestock or rodents. Infection is by direct animal contact, or indirect contact with animal urine on vegetation (sugar cane) or in soil or water. *L. interrogans* has more than 200 serovars, previously called

Table 1 **Invasion by five routes**			
Invasion route	**Animal reservoir**	**Mechanism**	**Disease example**
Insect bite	Rodents	Flea bite	Plague
Incisors (animal bite)	Dog	Direct bite	*Capnocytophaga canimorsus* infection
Implanted through skin	Goats, sheep	Touching wool, skin	Anthrax
Ingestion	Cows, goats, etc.	Milk, cheese	Brucellosis
Inhalation	Birds	Droppings	Psittacosis

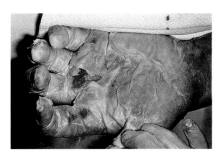

Fig. 1 **Zoonotic infection with *Capnocytophaga canimorsus* through a dog bite, with fatal outcome (p. 197).**

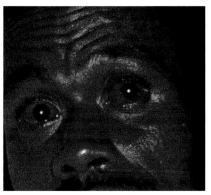

Fig. 2 **Leptospirosis: Weil's disease with jaundice and conjunctivitis.**

separate species. Humans are usually infected by serovar *canicola* from dogs, *icterohaemorrhagiae* from rats, *hardjo* from cattle, or *pomona* from pigs.

Clinical syndromes

Leptospirosis has four clinical syndromes:

- asymptomatic infection detected only by serology (common)
- acute flu-like illness with fever and myalgia (common)
- acute 'aseptic' meningitis (p. 94–95) (common)
- Weil's disease (leptospirosis icterohaemorrhagica) with fever, jaundice, haemorrhage and hepato-renal failure (Fig. 2) (rare).

Confirmatory tests

Serology by the Microscopic Agglutination Test (MAT) is usually diagnostic. Culture of blood or CSF in the first 10 days, then urine for some weeks is positive only on special media unavailable in most laboratories.

Chemotherapy and control

Penicillin or tetracycline probably shortens the course of the self-limiting flu-like or meningitic forms, and improves prognosis in Weil's disease. Control and prevention is by rodent control and prevention of occupational exposure.

Plague (the 'black death')

Plague is caused by *Yersinia pestis* (p. 57) which is transmitted animal to animal, and animal to human by flea bites; it exists in two epidemiological forms:

- sylvatic plague: wild mammals including rodents
- urban plague: rats and humans.

Three major clinical forms of plague are:

- **bubonic plague:** infection is via the skin from an infected flea, causing swollen regional lymph nodes called buboes; this form is not readily transmitted person to person
- **septicaemic plague:** fever, prostration, skin haemorrhages and rapid (black) death
- **pneumonic plague:** caused by bacteraemic spread in bubonic or septicaemic plague, or by inhalation; this form is highly infectious person to person by inhalation.

Less common clinical forms are cutaneous, tonsillar and meningeal.

Clinical syndromes

Bubonic plague is commonest, with fever, rash, swollen lymph nodes (buboes), then prostration from septicaemia and mortality up to 75% if untreated. Terminal pneumonia from the septicaemia can infect others by inhalation, causing overwhelming pneumonic plague, fatal in > 90% if untreated.

Confirmatory tests

Gram's or Wayson's stain of bubo aspirate show typical bipolar staining of Gram-negative rods (like safety pins) in over 50%, and blood cultures are positive in two-thirds (bubonic plague) to nearly 100% in pneumonic plague and septicaemia.

Chemotherapy and control

Either gentamicin or tetracycline is effective. Control and prevention is by rodent and flea control, avoidance of wild animals in endemic areas, and by vaccine in specific groups including laboratory workers.

Toxoplasmosis

Toxoplasmosis is characterised by human infections which vary with age (see Clinical syndromes). It is caused by *Toxoplasma gondii* (p. 78), which has its sexual life cycle in felines, predominantly domestic cats. Oocysts in cat faeces are the usual source, either directly via contaminated soil, or indirectly through cysts in the raw or undercooked meat (chicken, pork, beef or mutton) of another animal that has ingested the oocytes.

Clinical syndromes

There are five clinical syndromes:

- congenital infection of the fetus, usually from a primary maternal infection during pregnancy (p. 214–215)
- asymptomatic infection, usually in childhood
- primary systemic infection, giving a 'glandular fever' syndrome
- localised tissue cysts, especially in retina or brain (p. 112, 103)
- re-activation of asymptomatic infection in the immunocompromised, e.g. cerebral toxoplasmosis in transplant patients or AIDS (p. 150).

Confirmatory tests

Serology is the usual diagnostic method, with CT scans of brain in cerebral infections.

Chemotherapy and control

Pyrimethamine plus sulphadiazine (or clindamycin if intolerant) is the usual treatment for symptomatic disease. Control and prevention depends on avoiding cats and cat faeces in pregnancy, avoiding raw or undercooked meat, and chemoprophylaxis in the sero-positive immunocompromised patient.

Trichinosis

Trichinosis is characterised by the deposition in human striated muscle of larvae of *Trichinella spiralis* (p. 87). This is a nematode parasite of carnivores, including pigs and bears. Humans are a dead-end host, infected by eating raw or undercooked meat (e.g. pork) containing encysted larvae.

Clinical syndromes

These vary from abdominal distress, fever and 'flu' to severe myalgia and periorbital oedema. Rarely, myocarditis, pneumonitis or encephalitis are fatal.

Confirmatory tests

Clinical findings of eosinophilia, myalgia and periorbital oedema, with an appropriate food history, give a presumptive diagnosis. Cysts can be found in the infected meat. Definitive diagnosis by human muscle biopsy is seldom necessary.

Chemotherapy and control

Albendazole is used, with steroids to control marked allergic symptoms.

Control and prevention depends on freezing meat at –40°C, and proper cooking (not by microwave). Pigs or bears should not eat garbage, which may contain infected meat.

Tularaemia

Tularaemia is caused by *Francisella tularensis* (p. 57); infection is transmitted at least four ways to humans: **i**mplanted via the skin or conjunctiva when handling infected mammals, by **i**nsect or tick bite, by **i**ngestion of infected meat, or by **i**nhalation, especially in laboratories. *F. tularensis* is found in many reservoir hosts, including mammals (rabbits, rodents) and ticks, and in water. Hunters, trappers and campers in tick areas are therefore at risk.

Clinical syndromes

Clinical features depend on the portal of entry:

- ulceroglandular, with local ulcer at the tick-bite site, and regional lymphadenopathy (inguinal, axillary), in 80%
- typhoidal with systemic disease and pneumonia, from ingestion or inhalation, in 10%
- oculoglandular, oropharyngeal and glandular (without ulceration) are all rare.

Confirmatory tests

Microscopy is difficult and culture is dangerous, so serology is the method of choice.

Chemotherapy and control

Streptomycin is the usual chemotherapy, or gentamicin. Control and prevention depends on avoidance of ticks and infected or sick animals, especially rabbits. Gloves minimise skin contact.

Zoonoses

- Infections of humans by animal pathogens are called zoonoses.
- Infection occurs through incisors (animal bites), insect bites, ingestion, inhalation and implantation through skin injuries.
- Brucellosis is caught from infected animals and their products (milk, cheese).
- Brucellae are intracellular pathogens which cause acute and chronic disease.
- Plague is transmitted from rats by flea bites; the pneumonic form is infectious by inhalation.
- Toxoplasmosis is a common latent infection from cats; congenital disease is often fatal.

Maternal, fetal and neonatal infections

Infections of the mother and baby can be classified as occurring:

- before birth: called prenatal/antenatal in mother, prenatal/congenital in fetus
- during birth: puerperal or perinatal
- after birth: postnatal in mother, neonatal in newborn baby.

See also pages 144–146.

MATERNAL INFECTIONS

Prenatal infections

The hormonal, immunological and anatomical changes of pregnancy make maternal infections during pregnancy:

- more common, e.g. urinary tract infections (p. 174)
- more obvious, when latent viral infections re-activate, e.g. herpes simplex, CMV
- more severe, e.g. candidiasis, UTI, listeriosis, malaria, viral hepatitis, polio and influenza
- more serious, because of the effect on the fetus, see below.

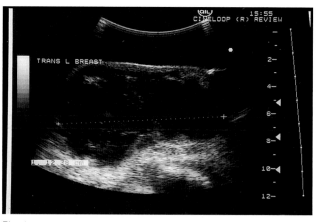

Fig. 1 **Breast abscess shown on ultrasound (between +.......+).**

Three new tissues appear which can be infected: the fetus, the placenta with membranes, and the lactating breast.

Perinatal infection

Puerperal sepsis

This is characterised by bacterial endometritis acquired in childbirth.

Causative organisms now are usually mixed aerobic and anaerobic bowel flora, rather than the fearsome *Streptococcus pyogenes* or *C. perfringens* of former years. The route is ascending, and predisposing factors are premature rupture of the membranes, prolonged labour, instrumentation and retained placenta or membrane fragments.

Clinical features. Clinically there is fever, offensive lochia (the vaginal blood and fluids post-delivery) and systemic upset, even septicaemia. Lower abdominal pain and a tender uterus develop.

Confirmatory tests are Gram stain and cultures of high vaginal swabs and of blood.

Management. Broad-spectrum antibiotics are required, such as ampicillin or ticarcillin with clavulanate, a later cephalosporin, or clindamycin with gentamicin. Penicillin is given for *S. pyogenes*. Surgery is necessary for myonecrosis or abscesses.

Control and prevention depends on chemoprophylaxis during prolonged rupture of the membranes, on handwashing and asepsis.

Postnatal breast infections

Breast infections are characterised by local inflammation and fever. They may occur soon after delivery from epidemic or endemic hospital-acquired staphylococci, or weeks later as sporadic mastitis from a combination of milk stasis and infection through cracked nipples.

Causative organisms are usually staphylococci, rarely beta-haemolytic streptococci or bowel flora.

Clinical features are local pain and tenderness, segmental redness and fever. Initial milk stasis progresses to cellulitis then abscess, with extreme localised tenderness and high fever.

Confirmatory tests are microscopy and culture of pus, from the nipple, from aspiration or from operation. Ultrasound is very helpful in abscess identification (Fig. 1).

Management. Chemotherapy is usually with flucloxacillin or a first-generation cephalosporin. Drainage is essential for an abscess.

Control and prevention depends on nipple hygiene, and massage to prevent milk stasis.

FETAL AND NEONATAL INFECTIONS

Prenatal (congenital)

Any severe bacteraemic or septicaemic infection in pregnancy can infect the fetus, usually killing it. Numerous viruses cause fetal infections, chiefly CMV, Hepatitis B, HIV, HSV, Rubella and VZV, see p. 144–146. Congenital infection (usually not fatal to the fetus) is also caused by four unusual intracellular organisms: a bacterium (congenital listeriosis), a mycobacterium (leprosy), a spirochaete (syphilis) and a parasite (toxoplasmosis).

Congenital listeriosis

Listeria monocytogenes, a beta-haemolytic Gram-positive rod (p. 38), causes a zoonosis from many animals including cattle, and infection is often from unpasteurised milk or cheese.

Clinically, maternal infection is often asymptomatic or like mild influenza, but it is bacteraemic and fetal infection is severe, causing death or premature birth, often with neonatal septicaemia, pneumonia and abscesses.

Confirmatory tests are blood, CSF, skin or abscess cultures.

Chemotherapy is by penicillin or ampicillin.

Control and prevention depends on animal and food hygiene, and avoiding products made from unpasteurised milk.

Congenital leprosy

Mycobacterium leprae can spread to the fetus during bacteraemia in maternal lepromatous leprosy. Clinically it is rare, but the child is born with leprosy (p. 104) and needs specialist treatment. Control depends on treatment of adults.

Congenital syphilis

Treponema pallidum infection of the fetus occurs in areas where routine antenatal serological screening for syphilis is not done.

Clinically an infant with congenital syphilis characteristically has rhinitis and a depressed nasal bridge with other cartilage and bone defects, skin rash and mucosal lesions, lymphadenopathy and hepatosplenomegaly. Subsequent dentition shows notched incisors called Hutchinson's teeth.

Confirmatory tests are positive serology in the mother and *T. pallidum*-specific IgM in the baby.

Chemotherapy is with penicillin for mother and child.

Control and prevention depends on antenatal screening and therapy before the fourth month.

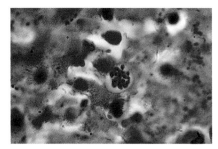
Fig. 2 **Toxoplasmosis showing tissue cyst (central) in the brain.**

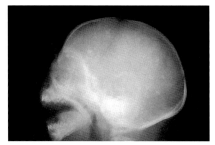
Fig. 4 **Congenital toxoplasmosis showing microcephaly and scattered calcification on skull radiograph.**

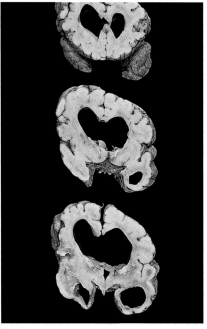
Fig. 3 **Congenital toxoplasmosis showing massive ventricles in hydrocephalus.**

Congenital toxoplasmosis

Toxoplasma gondii (Fig. 2) causes a zoonosis principally from cats (p. 78, 214–215).

Clinically, maternal infection is usually primary and asymptomatic (like listeriosis), but the fetus may die or become severely affected (often months after birth), with **c**onvulsions, **c**horioretinitis, **c**erebral atrophy and hepatosplenomeg-aly, with consequent **m**icrocephaly, **m**assive ventricles (Fig. 3) and **m**ental retardation.

Confirmatory tests are toxoplasma-specific IgM in cord blood, and positive maternal serology. Skull x-ray may show microcephaly and calcification (Fig. 4).

Chemotherapy is with sulphonamide and pyrimethamine.

Control and prevention is by avoiding cats and undercooked meat (with tissue cysts) during pregnancy.

Perinatal infections

Perinatal infections are acquired by the neonate during labour (mainly during prolonged rupture of the membranes) or during travel down an infected birth canal.

Causative organisms are:
- from maternal bacteraemia or viraemia (hepatitis B, HIV)
- bowel flora from the rectum
- specific pathogens from cervix or vagina, including group B streptococci, *N. gonorrhoeae*, *C. trachomatis*, *C. albicans* or viruses (including HSV and papilloma virus).

Clinical features vary with the pathogens:

- maternal bacteraemia is usually fatal to the baby
- inhaled bowel flora or group B streptococci cause severe pneumonia, septicaemia, meningitis or death
- gonococcal ophthalmia neonatorum ('eye infection of the newborn') is an acute purulent conjunctivitis and blepharitis, serious if untreated
- chlamydial ophthalmia neonatorum is less severe than gonorrhoeal but inhaled chlamydia cause a severe neonatal pneumonia
- neonatal candidal infection is mainly oral or peri-anal thrush.

Confirmatory tests include local eye, skin, blood, CSF and endotracheal microscopy, cultures and PCR as appropriate, with chest x-ray for pneumonia.

Chemotherapy depends on the cause and clinical features: penicillin or ceftriaxone for gonorrhoea; empiric broad-spectrum cover such as ceftriaxone and gentamicin for pneumonia, septicaemia and/or meningitis; nystatin or an azole for candidal infection.

Control and prevention depends on prophylactic antibiotics for labour involving prolonged rupture of the membranes and at-risk babies, with aseptic technique for delivery, and neonatal care.

Postnatal (neonatal) infections

Pneumonia, septicaemia, meningitis

Characteristically, these most serious neonatal infections commence at or before birth (see above) but may be postnatal. They are caused by inhaled bowel or vaginal flora or other pathogens; neonatal pneumonia (p. 126) and septicaemia can disseminate causing meningitis, infective arthritis (p. 210–211) or osteomyelitis (p. 206–207).

Clinically, early signs are often non-specific with listlessness, pallor, poor feeding and diarrhoea, while fever may be absent, and specific signs too late.

Confirmatory tests include local eye, skin, blood, CSF and endotracheal microscopy and cultures as appropriate, with chest x-ray for pneumonia.

Chemotherapy is initial empiric broad-spectrum cover such as ceftriaxone and gentamicin, then as directed by sensitivity tests.

Control and prevention depends on prophylactic antibiotics for prolonged rupture of the membranes or at-risk babies, with aseptic technique for delivery and neonatal care.

Umbilical stump infections

These are caused by unsterile dressings, including soil and manure; neonatal tetanus usually fatal. Prevention is by maternal immunisation during pregnancy and the use of sterile dressings, which also prevent staphylococcal and other umbilical infections.

Cross-infection from hospital staff or other babies

Cross-infection can involve staphylococci, streptococci, bowel flora and viruses, including Herpes simplex. Skin, eye and gut infections result. Control is by good infection control, particularly hand disinfection.

Infection from mother

Sometimes mothers infect their babies post-natally with viruses via maternal milk, blood or saliva.

Oral pathogens

Babies can ingest pathogens, usually in unsterile feeds; this occurs chiefly in developing areas when babies are not breast fed, and causes diarrhoeal disease (p. 156–163).

> ## Maternal, fetal and neonatal infections
>
> - Infections can be more severe or re-activate during pregnancy.
> - Many viral and non-viral infections can pass to the fetus causing congenital disease. The fetus may die or have serious postnatal illness or malformation.
> - Puerperal sepsis is bacterial endometritis acquired in childbirth, largely prevented by asepsis and chemoprophylaxis.
> - Neonates can be infected during labour, particularly if the birth canal is infected (e.g. in gonorrhoea), or may become infected after delivery (from the mother, hospital staff, equipment or food).

Travellers and recent immigrants

Travel often tilts the balance against host defences and in favour of microbial attack when unprepared host defences face new attacks from:

- unfamiliar microbes, e.g. parasites, fungi
- unfamiliar vectors, e.g. mosquitoes, ticks, bed-bugs
- unfamiliar vehicles, e.g. foods, drinks
- unfamiliar activities, e.g. casual sex, water sports.

The common results, therefore, are unfamiliar illness in travellers and recently returned travellers, or illness unfamiliar in industrial countries occurring in recent immigrants, particularly from developing countries. Some of these infections can be avoided by preparing host defences (e.g. immunisation). Once infection has occurred, diagnosis and treatment must follow.

Preparing host defences

Malaria prophylaxis

Intending travellers to areas with endemic malaria should institute three measures, though none is 100% effective:

1. Be aware of the risks, and that *early* diagnosis and treatment are vital.
2. Avoid mosquito bites, by using window and door screens, repellents containing DEET (diethyl toluamide), protective clothing and minimising outdoor after-dark activities, when most malarious mosquitoes bite.
3. Chemoprophylaxis. Chloroquine weekly is used where chloroquine-resistant *P. falciparum* is absent. For areas with chloroquine resistance, use mefloquine weekly (unless contraindicated or resistance known), doxycycline daily, or atovaquone-proguanil daily. As resistance is spreading, up-to-date advice is essential before travel to a particular area.

Food and drink precautions

'Peel it, boil it, or forget it' is the rule to minimise gut infection from food or drink, from infected animals, or from contamination with human faecal pathogens from the unwashed hands of infected food-handlers, or from faecally-contaminated soil or raw food. Specifically, avoid salads, vegetables, fruit, dairy products (including ice-cream), uncooked meat, unboiled or bottled water (even for teeth-brushing), uncarbonated soft drinks, ice, iced tea or coffee. The following are usually safe: cooked food while hot, boiled water, carbonated drinks, alcohol, hot tea or coffee.

Sexually transmitted disease precautions

There are four principles:

- **a**bstinence is absolutely safe
- **b**arrier contraceptives in women are *no* barrier contra (against) pathogens.
- **c**ondoms are compulsory in casual sex
- **p**rostitutes are perilous (over 70% are infected with HIV in some areas)

Skin, respiratory, ear and eye precautions

Bathing, swimming, diving and boating all give water exposure and the risk of skin injury. Hazards include water-borne skin infections (aeromonads, group A streptococci, *M. marinum*, schistosomiasis, vibrios), ear infections (especially pseudomonal), eye infections (including conjunctivitis) and gut infections (p. 158–163). Respiratory infections, especially viral, are common in travellers, but few precautions are useful except avoidance of the obviously infected.

Immunisation

There are three categories:

- **r**outine for all travellers: diphtheria, tetanus, pneumococcal and measles vaccination should be updated, plus polio and BCG for travel or residence in rural developing areas, and rubella for women of child-bearing age
- **required** for entry to some countries: yellow fever or meningococcal vax (Mecca pilgrims)
- **recommended**, depending on destination, duration and details of visit: cholera, hepatitis A and B, influenza, Japanese B encephalitis, meningococcal, plague, rabies, typhoid and yellow fever vaccines.

Check recent recommendations well before travel to allow multiple doses.

Special precautions

Infants and young children, the pregnant traveller, the immunocompromised traveller, and those with chronic disease all need specialised advice.

Personal medical kit

The need and contents depend on travel destinations and duration, so may include insect repellent and antimalarials, water purifier, rehydration salts, anti-diarrhoeal and anti-emetic tablets, anti-infectives (both systemic, and local for skin, eye and ears) and condoms, sunscreens and drugs for pre-existing disease and non-infectious hazards.

Diagnosing and treating infection

Illness in returned travellers and recent immigrants should always be considered in relation to the involved geographic areas. Fever characteristics can also be indicative (Table 1).

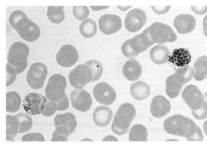

Fig. 1 **Blood film of *P. vivax* showing two schizonts and (centrally) one ring form.**

Table 1 **Fever in travellers**		
	Acute fevers (within 3 weeks)	**Chronic fevers (after 3 weeks)**
Major causes	Malaria, typhoid and paratyphoid fevers. Viral infections including dengue, hepatitis A, HIV, yellow fever, viral haemorrhagic fevers	Malaria, typhoid and paratyphoid fevers, amoebic liver abscess, filariasis, HIV, kala-azar, tuberculosis, viral hepatitis
Less common causes	Typhus, urinary tract infections, prostatitis, rickettsial infections, African trypanosomiasis, brucellosis	Sexually transmitted disease (syphilis), endocarditis, brucellosis, non-infectious causes (e.g. collagen diseases, drug fever, lymphoma)

Malaria and other fevers

Malaria must be diagnosed or excluded immediately, as delay can be fatal. Enteric fever (typhoid and paratyphoid) and viral haemorrhagic fevers are the other major infections needing rapid diagnosis and infection control. Causes of fever are many; the commonest are shown in Table 1 (see also p. 142–157). Clues to the cause include the pattern of fever:

- tertian: every third day (i.e. 48-hourly) in falciparum or vivax malaria is classical, but fever is often daily early in malaria
- persistent, always above normal: in typhoid and other bacteraemias
- intermittent, with afebrile hours: in kala-azar, TB and abscesses

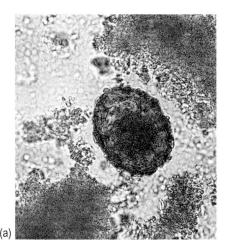

(a)

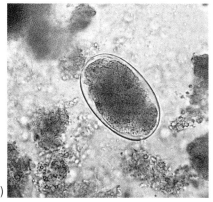

(b)

Fig. 2 **Stool microscopy showing (a)** *Ascaris lumbricoides* **egg and (b) hookworm egg.**

- relapsing, with afebrile days: in borrelioses, brucellosis, malaria, trypanosomiasis and viral infections like dengue.

Clinical clues also include:

- bleeding: haemorrhagic fevers
- chest signs: typhoid, TB
- jaundice: hepatitis, yellow fever
- liver tender or enlarged: amoebic abscess, hepatitis, kala-azar
- rash: rare in typhoid, common in typhus and viral infections
- spleen tender or enlarged: malaria, typhoid, kala-azar, brucellosis.

Confirmatory tests must include thick and thin blood films for malaria (Fig. 1 and p. 153); if negative, do blood culture and FBE with differential white blood cell count and film, urine and stool microscopy and cultures, liver function tests, chest x-ray, and imaging of any mass or unexplained tenderness. Serology is more useful in chronic fevers as two specimens two or more weeks apart are usually needed.

Chemotherapy obviously depends on the cause.

Diarrhoeal disease

There are many bacterial and viral causes of diarrhoeal disease (Table 1, p. 158) plus intestinal parasitic infestation (Table 1, p. 162). 'Traveller's diarrhoea', especially from enterotoxigenic *E. coli* (ETEC), is commonest during travel, while *Campylobacter*, *Salmonella*, *Shigella* and amoebic infection are more commonly found in returnees and immigrants. The characteristics of the symptoms are also indicative:

- pre-formed toxin: short incubation, vomiting prominent
- endotoxin made in gut: medium incubation, marked diarrhoea, no fever
- invasive pathogen: longer incubation, fever, pain, blood in faeces.

Other indicators are:

- possible exposure: developing country and particular area, shellfish, homosexual contact, immunocompromised

patient (especially HIV infected, p. 149–151)
- symptoms and signs: fever, abdominal pain, blood or mucus in the stools, and the character of the diarrhoea (acute, chronic, watery, foul).

Confirmatory tests are initially stool microscopy for cysts, ova and parasites (Fig. 2) plus stool culture. If negative, special stains, serology and other tests may be needed.

Chemotherapy depends on the cause. If none is found, symptomatic treatment may suffice, or empiric therapy with, for example, norfloxacin or metronidazole.

Sexually transmitted diseases

These usually present as genital discharge (p. 180–183) or genital ulceration (p. 188–189) and are investigated and treated accordingly. HIV infection is described on p. 149–151.

Skin infections

There are many bacterial (p. 202–203), fungal and parasitic skin infections (p. 204–205) particularly occurring in the tropics. These cause local disease or disseminated systemic symptoms. 'Tropical ulcer' is a progressive, offensive, destructive ulcer (Fig. 3), at times following skin trauma, in which anaerobes play an important role. It is usually responsive to penicillin and/or metronidazole.

Eye and ear infections

These are described on pages 106–107 and 110–111.

Respiratory infections

Tuberculosis and tropical respiratory infections are described on pages 132–135.

Immigrants

Recent immigrants may import many infections, which may be acute or chronic as above, or asymptomatic. Specific screening programmes are usually aimed at the major infections in their previous homeland.

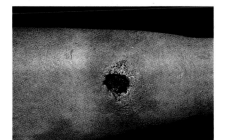

Fig. 3 **Tropical ulcer.**

> ### *Travellers and recent immigrants*
> - Travel precautions against microbial attack begin before travel, including education, immunisations, and prophylactic drugs.
> - Travel precautions continue during travel, including prophylactic drugs and behaviour modification towards food, drink, leisure and sex.
> - Travel-acquired infections may present after return, chiefly with fever (malaria, enteric fevers and haemorrhagic fevers), diarrhoea, sexually transmitted disease, or skin, eye, ear or respiratory infection.
> - All need skilled diagnosis and treatment.

Hospital-acquired infections

Hospital-acquired infection (= nosocomial infection) is characterised (obviously!) as any infection acquired in hospital. Community-acquired infections incubating on admission to hospital are excluded, though they may subsequently cause hospital infection in another patient. The following principles apply to all healthcare facilities including private medical practices. Greater attention is now given to the risks of hospital-acquired infections to staff as well as to patients.

Host–microbial relationships and the initiation of infection are described on pages 20–25; host defences are described on pages 26–31.

Classification

Nosocomial infections can be classified by four sequential steps:
1. **reservoirs** and sources of infection
2. **routes** of transmission
3. **rupture** of our host defences
4. **resultant** major infections.

Reservoirs and sources of infection

These are either endogenous (from the patient's own normal flora; p. 22–23) or exogenous. The latter derive from:
- *people* (hospital staff or another patient), usually directly
- *environment*, usually by indirect spread from sources such as air, dust, linen, food, water and other fluids, including disinfectants(!) and intravenous fluids
- *equipment* such as endoscopes and ventilators.

Some of these can be a *reservoir* (e.g. infected fluid) which contaminates *sources* (bottles or bowls), so eradication of the source is insufficient and the reservoir must also be found.

Route of transmission

Spread of infection can occur by:
- *direct contact*: person-to-person *cross-infection*, usually via the hands (sexually transmitted infection is rare, although the author has seen one youth with gonorrhoea after 7 weeks in hospital, in traction!)
- *indirect contact*: via some object, as above
- *common vehicle*: a special form of indirect contact in which one infected vehicle, commonly food or fluid, infects many
- *airborne spread*: either by *droplets* travelling 1–2 metres, or smaller *droplet nuclei* travelling a kilometre or more
- *vector-borne spread*: unusual but not unknown in hospitals.

Rupture of host defences

The *portals of entry* are the urogenital tract, skin, respiratory tract, the mouth and the gastrointestinal tract. High-risk patients have impaired host defences (see p. 220–221) from:
- age: the very young and the elderly
- antibody defects: lack of vaccination or previous exposure (chickenpox, CMV, hepatitis B)
- disease causing immune defects: e.g. HIV, diabetes, hepatic or renal impairment, cancer or lymphoma, especially with neutropenia
- drugs causing immune defects: e.g. cytotoxics, steroids or immunosuppressives (e.g. transplant patients)
- defective organs: e.g. pre-existing urinary, lung or skin disease
- defective skin or tissues: trauma, theatre (surgery), treatment or tubes; multitrauma and/or multiaccess result in multirisk (Fig. 1).

Resultant major infections

The four major types of infection are:
- urinary tract infections (about 40%)
- surgical site infections (about 25%) (Fig. 2)
- lower respiratory infections (about 10%)
- bacteraemias (about 5%).

Skin ulcer, pressure sore (Fig. 1, p. 196), gut and other infections make up the remaining 20%.

Causative organisms

The major pathogens are *S. aureus*, *E. coli* and other enteric Gram-negative rods and *P. aeruginosa*, though their relative importance differs (Table 1). Infrequent pathogens are enterococci, streptococci, coagulase-negative staphylococci, anaerobes and *Candida* spp. Multi-resistance is now common and important, including MRSA, VISA, VRE, ESBL-GNRs and ESCAPPMs – i.e. Meticillin-Resistant *Staph. aureus*; Vancomycin Intermediate *S. aureus*; Vancomycin-Resistant Enterococci; Extended Spectrum Beta-Lactamase (producing) GNRs; and *Enterobacter*, *Serratia*, *Citrobacter*, *Acinetobacter*, *Providentia*, *Proteus* and *Morganella* spp.

Clinical features

Urinary tract infections. Predisposing factors are catheters, stents, surgery or obstruction. Route of infection is usually ascending, with the usual uropathogens (p. 174). Symptoms and signs are often only cloudy offensive urine: fever is often absent or minimal, and dysuria only when there is no catheter.

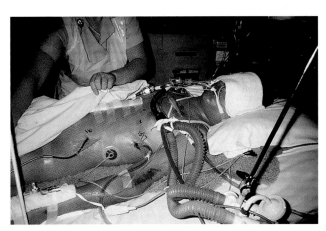

Fig. 1 **Multitrauma and multiaccess gives rise to a multirisk situation.**

Table 1 **Major pathogens in hospital-acquired infections**		
Category/classification	**Causative organism (%)**	**Chemotherapy**
Urinary	E. coli (40)	Gentamicin or directed
	Enteric GNRs (25)	by sensitivity tests
	Enterococci (15)	Ampicillin
	P. aeruginosa (10)	Tobramycin
Surgical site	S. aureus (20)	Flucloxacillin
	Enteric GNRs (15)	Gentamicin or directed by
	E. coli (12)	sensitivity tests
	Enterococci (12)	Ampicillin
Pneumonia/lower respiratory	Enteric GNRs (35)	Timentin
	S. aureus (15)	Flucloxacillin
	P. aeruginosa (15)	Tobramycin
	E. coli (10)	Gentamicin
Bacteraemia	Enteric GNRs (20)	Gentamicin
	S. aureus (12)	Flucloxacillin
	E. coli (12)	Gentamicin
	Coagulase-negative staphylococci (10)	Vancomycin

GNR, Gram-negative rods.

Surgical site infections. Redness, swelling, local pain and heat occur around the wound, progressing to purulent discharge (superficial infections) or deep abscesses (p. 196).

Lower respiratory infections (p. 126–129). Predisposing factors are recumbency, anaesthesia, other pulmonary disease or trauma, and mechanical ventilation. The route of infection is by inhalation. Symptoms and signs vary. In non-ventilated patients, fever and dyspnoea are common. Cough and sputum are less common in ventilator-associated pneumonia (VAP), where increasing difficulty in oxygenation with opacities on chest x-rays may overshadow fever and increasingly purulent tracheal aspirate.

Bacteraemias (p. 142–143). Predisposing factors are intravascular devices and infection elsewhere, causing bacteraemia or fungaemia. Route of infection is direct contact from imperfect aseptic technique, or blood-borne from infection elsewhere. Symptoms and signs are fever, then septicaemia. Search for a source elsewhere, and signs of infection at the device entry site.

Infected burns. Infected burns may be considered with surgical wounds in that the skin barrier is broken. In burns there are also abnormalities of immune response and loss of fluid. Although initially sterile, burns are quickly colonised by mixed bacterial flora including pathogens (p. 197).

Confirmatory tests

Tests vary with the site, but obviously include local microscopy and culture (urine, wound, sputum, burn, etc.) and blood cultures. Chest x-ray is needed in suspected pneumonia. Sources in, or spread to, other organs need specific imaging.

Chemotherapy

Antibiotic treatment varies with the site; initial empiric therapy is outlined in Table 1 and is replaced by directed therapy when the infecting organism and sensitivities are known.

THE PRINCIPLES OF INFECTION CONTROL

Sources
Sources of infection are diminished by providing sterile equipment, dressings, fluids and drugs, and clean food, drink, linen and environment. Hospital staff with communicable infections must not have patient contact, while staff with HIV/AIDS, hepatitis B or C need specific review, counselling and exclusion from procedures. Specific staff need hepatitis B, BCG and other immunisation.

Spread
Spread is diminished by:
- building design, air-conditioning and isolation of selected patients to limit airborne spread
- hand-washing, 'no-touch' and aseptic techniques, 'universal precautions' and careful placement of infected and susceptible patients in wards to limit contact spread
- educated staff behaviour to prevent contamination of equipment (Fig. 3) to limit indirect spread
- insect screens in tropical areas to limit spread by vectors.

Hand-washing or disinfection before touching an uninfected patient, and after touching an infected patient, are crucial in infection control.

'Universal precautions' mean that *all* blood and body substances of *all* patients are considered potentially infectious at *all* times; this is necessary because it is not feasible to detect all infectious patients, especially with HIV, hepatitis B and C. Previous 'source isolation' is now needed less for infectious patients, e.g. respiratory isolation to control airborne spread.

Susceptible patients
Susceptible patients need:

- **p**ortal **p**rotection
- **p**roper **p**rocedural techniques
- **p**rophylactic antibiotics when indicated
- **p**rotective isolation for immunocompromised patients.

For all patients, the major infection risks can be avoided by careful management:

Urinary infections. Aseptic technique is required for operations, procedures and catheterisation, with closed catheter drainage and aseptic catheter care. Chemoprophylaxis usually fails and is seldom indicated.

Surgical site infection. Procedural techniques and, when indicated, prophylactic antibiotics reduce infection rates (p. 196).

Respiratory infections. Pre-anaesthetic assessment, postoperative physiotherapy, plus tracheostomy and ventilator care including 'no-touch' during endotracheal aspiration all decrease infection risks.

Bacteraemia. Aseptic preparation of all fluids and equipment is essential as is care in insertion, additions and changes of intravascular devices and fluids (especially total parenteral nutrition). Potential sources elsewhere must be treated.

Staff
Staff need protection by education in Universal Precautions, in care with sharps and in needlestick prevention, and by immunisation when appropriate.

Surveillance
Surveillance helps control by monitoring the incidence of major infection risks, monitoring the observation of infection control measures, devising protocols for new equipment and procedures, and, when any of these fail, investigating outbreaks.

> ## Hospital-acquired infections
>
> - Sources are people (hospital staff or patients) or things (equipment, food, fluids, drugs or equipment).
> - Spread is by direct or indirect contact, common vehicle, airborne spread or vectors.
> - Susceptible patients include the very young and old and those with defects in immune defences or in organs.
> - Subsequent infections are chiefly urinary, surgical site, respiratory and bacteraemia.
> - Surveillance and infection control measures limit infection.

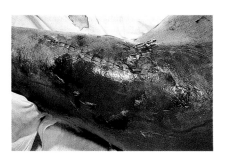

Fig. 2 **Necrotising fasciitis after hip surgery.**

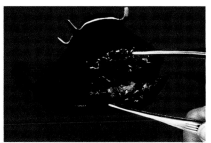

Fig. 3 **P. aeruginosa growing in an anaesthetic mask.**

Infections in compromised patients

Basic principles

Immune defences can be divided into two groups: non-specific and specific (p. 26–29).

Non-specific defences (innate, constitutive, p. 24–27) are:

- 1st line: skin and mucous membranes (especially against surface organisms)
- 2nd line: phagocytosis by neutrophils and macrophages, with complement and other chemicals (especially against pyogenic bacteria and GNRs).

Specific immune defences (inducible, adaptive, p. 28–29) are:

- 3rd line: antibodies from B-cells (especially against encapsulated bacteria and GNRs)
- 4th line: cell-mediated immunity (CMI) from T-cells (especially against intracellular organisms).

Any one (or more) of the four lines can be compromised, rarely by:

A. **Congenital** defects (primary immunodeficiency, rare), or by
B. **Acquired** (secondary, common) defects from disease, drugs, procedures or surgery.

Certain organisms are common pathogens in each compromised state. All need swift and specialised investigation and treatment; correction of the underlying defects is attempted when possible.

Control and prevention of infection (p. 219) depends on asepsis, hygiene, antimicrobials at times of greatest risk, removal of devices, and decrease or cessation of causative drugs or radiation; immunisation is only useful when the 3rd and/or 4th lines (B- and T-cell function) are intact.

Impaired immune defences result in:

- infection by organisms that would not normally be hazardous
- minor infections becoming life threatening
- the usual symptoms of infection being absent or minimal, so prompt diagnosis and treatment are vital.

Specific defects

Congenital skin disease

Several rare diseases such as **epidermolysis bullosa atrophica** cause excessively fragile skin, easily invaded by pyogenic bacteria, including staphylococci and streptococci, which cause severe infections, often fatal even with expert care.

Acquired breaches in the skin or mucous membranes

Acquired breaches are very common with many obvious causes. All enable surface organisms including staphylococci, streptococci (Fig. 1), *Pseudomonas aeruginosa*, enteric Gram-negative rods and fungi such as *Candida* to reach and infect deeper tissues. Resultant infections include:

- burns, surgical and other wound infections (p. 196–197)
- bacteraemia from intravascular devices (p. 142–143)
- prosthetic infections (p. 208)
- skin infections (p. 190–199)
- failure of clearance: urinary tract infections (p. 174), cystic fibrosis (p. 125).

Congenital phagocyte defects

The commonest (but still very rare) phagocyte deficiency is in **chronic granulomatous disease**, actually a group of disorders characterised by failure of the oxidative burst in neutrophil phagocytosis (p. 26). This results in recurrent pyogenic infections including dermatitis, adenitis, pneumonia, enteritis and colitis, all with characteristic abscesses. *S. aureus* and enteric Gram-negative rods, including salmonellae and *Serratia* spp., are common. Death is usual by age 10.

Acquired phagocyte defects

Acquired phagocyte defects are common, chiefly neutropenia from *leukaemia* (Fig. 2) or its treatment with cytotoxics, steroids or radiation before bone marrow transplantation. Pyrexia of unknown origin (p. 156–157), often with septicaemia, is common. Intravascular devices are a common source. Staphylococci and enteric Gram-negative rods are usual early in neutropenia, while fungi infect later. Tests and therapy must be swift and sure, or mortality is high.

Congenital complement defects

Deficiency of any component from C1 to C9 can occur. Because of the alternate pathway, defects in C1, C2 and C4 have little effect on infections, while defects in C3 or C5–8 cause repeated serious infections, usually with encapsulated bacteria such as pneumococci, meningococci, gonococci and *H. influenzae*.

Acquired complement defects

Acquired complement defects are uncommon alone but occur in combination with other immune defects in chronic diseases, e.g., systemic lupus erythematosus (SLE), some types of nephritis, sickle cell or liver disease and malnutrition (see below). They cause infections chiefly with encapsulated bacteria.

Congenital antibody defects

Many rare disorders are known in which either individual classes (IgG, IgA, IgM)

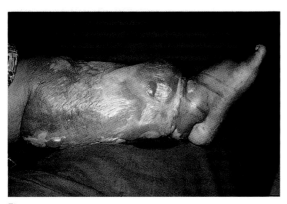

Fig. 1 **Acquired breach in skin during surgery, with resultant group A streptococcal cellulitis.**

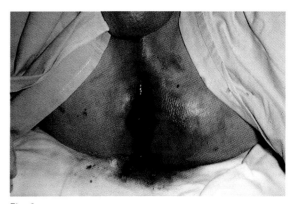

Fig. 2 **Acquired phagocyte defect: neutropenia caused by leukaemia, with resultant peri-anal spreading suppuration.**

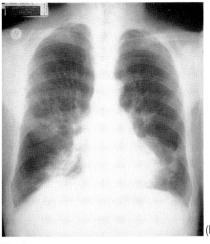
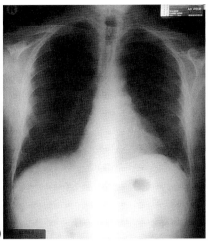

(a)   (b)

Fig. 3 **Antibodies are absent in agammaglobulinaemia, with resultant chest infection (a), which needed lung transplantation (b).**

of antibodies or all gammaglobulins are defective. They include **Bruton's agammaglobulinaemia** and '**common variable immunodeficiency**'. Patients are prone to infection, often with encapsulated bacteria, hence they often have ear, sinus or chest infections (Fig. 3). Auto-immune disease often co-exists.

Acquired antibody defects

Antibody defects are commonly acquired in lymphoid malignancies such as lymphoma, chronic lymphocytic leukaemia and multiple myeloma, with diminished or abnormal B-cell function and antibody synthesis. Other causes are splenectomy, which removes many B-cells (and diminishes clearance of intravascular organisms); burns, in which immuno-globulins are catabolised; and protein-losing enteropathy and nephrotic syndrome, in which immunoglobulins are lost. Infection with encapsulated bacteria or Gram-negative rods is common and can be catastrophic.

Congenital CMI defects

The **DiGeorge syndrome** of thymic hypoplasia and absent parathyroid glands is one of at least 10 rare syndromes with defects in CMI, and consequent life-threatening infections from a wide range of intracellular bacteria (mycobacteria, *Listeria*), fungi, parasites and viruses. In contrast, **chronic mucocutaneous candidiasis** shows selective failure of T-cell CMI against *C. albicans*, with re-current and progressive oral, nail and skin infections. Endocrinopathy and au-to-antibodies commonly co-exist. Life is unpleasant and short.

Acquired CMI defects

There are four major causes of acquired CMI defects:

- drugs and radiation
- infections, especially HIV
- malignancies
- malnutrition.

All have other effects on host defences so are discussed below.

Congenital combined defects

Severe combined immunodeficiency (SCID) has both B- and T-cell dysfunction, with consequent serious infections by encapsulated and intracellular bacteria, and fungi, parasites and viruses. Bone marrow transplantation offers hope of survival.

Acquired combined defects

Acquired combined defects are found in six common situations:

Drugs and radiation:

- steroids decrease numbers and function of lymphocytes, monocytes and eosinophils and decrease neutrophil accumulation in inflammation
- cytotoxics cause leucopenia, and impair both T- and B-cell function
- ciclosporin specifically suppresses T-cell function
- irradiation decreases lymphoid cell proliferation.

HIV infection causes major T-cell and CMI deficiency but also impairs B-cell function; neutropenia is common in AIDS.

Malignancies cause defects in neutrophil numbers and function, in antibody production and (particularly in lymphoid tumours, e.g. Hodgkin's disease) in CMI. In addition, drugs and irradiation (as above) further impair host defences, and skin and mucosal surfaces are often damaged by devices, disease or drugs.

Malnutrition (p. 33) can affect all host defences: in vitamin deficiencies and protein-energy malnutrition (PEM), skin and mucosal damage occurs, complement synthesis is severely decreased, neutrophil chemotaxis is slow, antibody formation and function are widely impaired, and T-cells are grossly decreased.

Systemic infections (p. 142–157) particularly TB, leprosy, brucellosis and viruses (including CMV, EBV and HIV) can impair host defences, especially CMI.

Transplantation involves major immunosuppressive drug use (see above) and causes widespread compromise of host defences, and a wide range of resultant infections (Fig. 4).

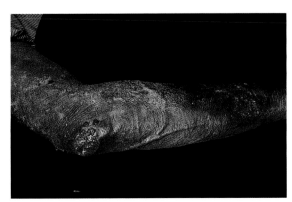

Fig. 4 **All defences breached after heart transplantation, with resultant cryptococcal skin infection.**

Infections in compromised patients

- Defects in any of the four lines of host defences can be congenital or acquired; defects of several lines may be combined.
- 1st line skin and mucous membrane defects result in infections by surface microbes: pyogenic bacteria, pseudomonads or common fungi.
- 2nd line neutrophil ('pus cell') defects result in infections with the pyogenic organisms, or Gram-negative rods (GNR).
- 2nd line complement defects result in infections with encapsulated bacteria, or *S. aureus*.
- 3rd line antibody defects also result in infections with encapsulated organisms, GNR, or some parasites.
- 4th line CMI defects result in infections with intracellular bacteria, fungi, parasites and viruses.
- All need swift and specialised tests and treatment, with correction of the underlying defects(s) when possible.

Infection in General Practice patients

Most infections in general practice are common, relatively easily diagnosed and treated, and seldom severe: these include otitis media, sinusitis, pharyngitis, gastroenteritis, urinary tract infections and tinea. Conversely in each organ system there is at least one important infection which is superficially similar but serious, which is rare but rapidly progressive, requiring rapid recognition, timely treatment and swift specialist supervision (Table 1). These include meningitis with meningococcaemia, where the early rash (Fig. 1) can appear like a common viral infection until rapid progression to gangrene (see Fig. 4, p. 143). Similarly, common acute conjunctivitis (Fig. 2) is superficially like iritis but note the localised limbal injection and irregular iris (Fig. 3).

Causative organisms

Most infections in general practice are caused by staphylococci, streptococci, *H. influenzae*, enteric Gram-negative rods (especially *E. coli*) and fungi, usually dermatophytes or *Candida albicans* (Table 2). Local sensitivity patterns should be obtained from the local laboratory. Penicillin and cephalosporin resistance in pneumococci is increasingly important.

Confirmatory tests

These are often unnecessary initially but are needed for recurrent or persistent infection (Table 2).

Chemotherapy

Each GP is familiar with a small range of antibiotics, including penicillin, flucloxacillin, erythromycin or roxithromycin, amoxicillin (± clavulanate), a first-generation cephalosporin, trimethoprim (± sulphamethoxazole), and an azole; rarely others are needed.

Control and prevention

The GP can advise the patient, household and contacts on immunisation, hygiene, and early diagnosis and treatment to limit the spread of infections.

Table 1 Common infections, and superficially similar serious infections		
Organ system	**Common infection**	**Superficially similar, serious infection**
CNS	Frontal sinusitis	Bacterial meningitis
Ear	Otitis media	Mastoiditis
Eye	Conjunctivitis	Keratitis, iritis
Respiratory	Sinusitis	Parameningeal abscess
	Pharyngitis,	Epiglottitis
	Viral URTI/LRTI	Pneumococcal pneumonia, TB
	Exacerbation COAD	TB
Systemic	'Viral infection', flu	Meningococcaemia, endocarditis
Gut	Gastroenteritis	Bacillary dysentery, appendicitis
Urinary	Uncomplicated UTI	Pyonephrosis, abscess
Genital	Vaginitis	Pelvic peritonitis
Skin	Tinea	Nocardiosis
	Bacterial skin/wound	Streptococcal cellulitis
Skeletal	Trauma, sprain, gout	Osteomyelitis, infective arthritis

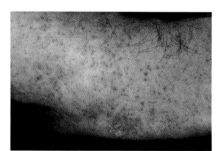

Fig. 1 **Early meningococcal rash.**

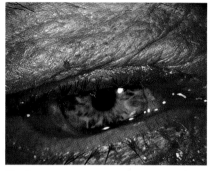

Fig. 2 **Acute staphylococcal conjunctivitis is common.**

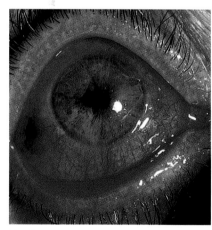

Fig. 3 **Iritis has limited limbal injection, and irregular pupil.**

Table 2 Common infections in general practice				
Category/ classification	**Causative organism**	**Clinical features**	**Confirmatory laboratory tests**	**Chemotherapy**
Skin	S. aureus	Boils	None, or	Flucloxacillin
	S. pyogenes	Impetigo	skin swab M&C	Penicillin
	Dermatophytes	Tinea		Azole
Respiratory	S. pyogenes	Pharyngitis	Throat swab	Penicillin
	S. pneumoniae	Otitis, sinusitis,	Nasal or ear M&C?	Amoxicillin, cefaclor,
	H. influenzae, viruses	Bronchitis	Sputum M&C	or augmentin
Gut	Campylobacter,	Gastroenteritis	None (stool M&C	None initially
	E. coli, Shigella spp.,		if persists or	(Erythromycin for
	viruses		traveller)	Campylobacter)
Urinary	E. coli, other GNRs,	Cystitis or	None initially, urine,	Augmentin or cephalexin
	S. saprophyticus	pyelonephritis	M&C if recurrent	or trimethoprim
Genital	C. albicans,	Vulvo-vaginitis	None initially, M&C	Azole
	Gardnerella		if recurrent	
	C. trachomatis,	Urethritis,	M&C, PCR	Ceftriaxone + azithromycin
	N. gonorrhoeae	cervicitis		

M&C, microscopy and culture; PCR, polymerase chain reaction.

> ### General practice patients
>
> - Common infections in general practice are relatively easily diagnosed and treated, and seldom severe, but the few important infections which are superficially similar but serious require rapid recognition.
> - Confirmatory tests are often unnecessary initially but are needed for recurrent or persistent infection.

Infections in elderly patients

Infections in elderly patients are more common, more serious and more difficult to treat, because of numerous predisposing and perpetuating factors, and numerous patho-physiological defects.

Predisposing and perpetuating factors

Impaired defences include:

- skin and mucous membrane defects: collagen ageing
- body fluids less bactericidal: gastric and prostatic vulnerability
- antibodies and CMI wane
- clearance mechanisms wane (urinary and respiratory tracts vulnerable).

Anatomic changes include:

- prostatomegaly causes urine stasis in men (Fig. 1)
- cystocoele causes urine stasis in women.

Co-existent disease. Diabetes mellitus, chronic lung disease, heart failure, strokes, mental impairment and fractures all impair structure and function.

Medication. Sedatives, hypnotics, etc. also impair function.

Patho-physiological defects

- fever is often absent or slight in infection
- immunisation, while recommended, gives lower, less prolonged antibody response
- co-existent disease of heart, lungs or kidneys makes complications of infection more likely and more serious

- renal impairment, often silent, alters drug excretion, especially of aminoglycosides, which require dosage modification.

Major infections

Urinary tract infections

UTIs (p. 174–177) are common in the elderly; they are often asymptomatic and usually associated with prostatomegaly and consequent obstruction in men (Fig. 1), or residual bladder urine and stasis in women. Causative organisms are the usual uro-pathogens, *E. coli* and other enteric bacteria. Clinical features may be absent, or infection may present simply with cloudy or offensive urine. Fever and dysuria are rarer. Confirmatory tests are urine microscopy and culture plus ultrasound to show prostate size and/or residual urine in recurrent infections. About 10% of renal function is lost each decade from age 30, and over 60% is lost before serum creatinine rises. Chemotherapy is guided by sensitivity testing, usually amoxicillin ± clavulanate, or cephalexin. If possible, causative conditions should be removed; chemoprophylaxis is only used for very frequent recurrences.

Lower respiratory infections

Characteristics of lower respiratory infections (p. 116–117, 124–129) include gradual or terminal illness with bronchopneumonia ('the old man's friend') or aspiration pneumonia; less often, acute illness may occur with pneumococcal

pneumonia. Causative organisms are the usual respiratory pathogens, chiefly *S. pneumoniae*, *H. influenzae*, *C. pneumoniae*, *M. pneumoniae* and viruses. Enteric Gram-negative rods are commonly found but are less commonly pathogenic, and *M. tuberculosis* must be remembered.

Clinical features vary from mild dyspnoea, cough and mucopurulent sputum with little or no fever to (rarely) high fever, marked cough and haemopurulent sputum. Confirmatory tests are sputum microscopy and culture with chest x-ray, noting that pulmonary opacities may result from collapse, infarction or heart failure rather than infection.

Chemotherapy is usually initially with penicillin or ceftriaxone, but metronidazole for aspiration, doxycycline for 'atypical' organisms, gentamicin for Gram-negative rods, or anti-tuberculous therapy is given when relevant. Control and prevention depends on removal or treatment of predisposing factors when possible.

Skin and soft tissue infections

Skin and soft tissue infections (p. 190–199) tend to be progressive because of ischaemia, oedema and/or diabetes. Causative organisms are streptococci, staphylococci, anaerobes including clostridia, and enteric Gram-negative rods. Clinical features are pus, putrid odour and progression (Fig. 2). Confirmatory tests are aerobic and anaerobic examinations of pus. Chemotherapy is with amoxicillin plus clavulanate, with metronidazole or, for example gentamicin, as clinical response and cultures indicate. Control and prevention depends on minimising predisposing factors. Diabetics should have prophylactic antibiotics including penicillin before lower limb surgery.

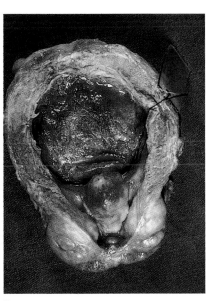

Fig. 1 **Cystitis, showing red, inflamed mucosa and greatly thickened wall, from prostatic obstruction.**

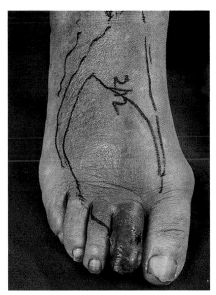

Fig. 2 **Diabetic with early gangrene and progressive cellulitis: inner line is 2nd December, outer line is 3rd December.**

Infections in elderly patients

- Infections in elderly patients are more common, more serious and more difficult to treat. Complications are common.
- Precipitating and perpetuating factors include impaired defences, anatomic changes, co-existent disease and medications.
- The three commonest infections are of urinary tract, lower respiratory tract and skin/soft tissues.
- Antibiotic dosage often needs modification, especially aminoglycosides, as silent severe renal impairment is common.

Sterilisation and disinfection

Health requires the absence of infection, so methods for killing or reducing the numbers of pathogenic microorganisms are important in reducing disease. Like much essential knowledge, this is boring but beneficial.

Definitions

Sterilisation kills all viable (able to multiply) microbes, including viruses, fungi, parasites and their cysts, bacteria and, particularly, bacterial spores. Prions survive conventional sterilisation.

Disinfection by a disinfectant substance or process is killing or removing most but not all viable microbes. It is divided into high-level, intermediate and low-level disinfection (Fig. 1).

Antisepsis is disinfection of the skin using an antiseptic. Skin cannot be sterilised and remain alive.

Asepsis is the absence of microorganisms and infection; hence aseptic methods in surgery and medical procedures aim to produce this aseptic state (p. 196, 219).

Pasteurisation is gentle disinfection by gentle heating.

Principles

1. 'Clean first, disinfect/sterilise next', i.e. reduce the *bio-burden* of organisms and organic material first, so the process is easier, shorter and reliable.
2. 'Strong enough for long enough', i.e. rate of kill is proportional to *time* multiplied by *concentration*.
3. 'Horses for courses', i.e. choose the appropriate process and details depending on the purpose and risk, hence the extent of microbial killing needed. Consider also the materials, risk of damage, toxicity, time, cost and resources available.
4. '*Control the process, not the product*': adhere to a known, proven and tested process rather than test for unsterile or dangerous equipment afterwards.

Classification by risk

There are three categories of items:
1. High risk (critical items). These contact tissues or blood. They include surgical instruments and arthroscopes. They must be sterilised.
2. Intermediate risk (semi-critical). These contact mucous membrane or non-intact skin. They include G-I endo-

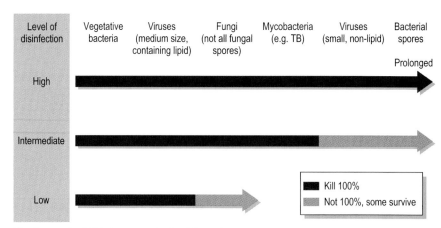

Fig. 1 **Levels of disinfection and microbial resistance.**

scopes and respiratory tubes. They need high-level disinfection.
3. Low risk (non-critical). These contact only intact skin. They include ward equipment and stethoscopes. Low-level disinfection is sufficient.

Sterilisation methods

There are four methods of sterilisation:
- irradiation
- filtration
- chemicals: 'liquid sterilants'
- heat: the most certain and widely used.

Irradiation
Irradiation can be by:
- ultraviolet light, used in laboratory safety cabinets; eyes must be shielded to prevent damage
- ionising radiation by electrons from cobalt-60 or a linear accelerator to sterilise heat-sensitive, pre-packed, single-use plastic items, including syringes and catheters.

Filtration
Filtration usually uses nitrocellulose membrane filters (Fig. 2), for sterilising heat-sensitive-liquids, including serum and antibiotics. However many filters labelled 'sterilising' only filter bacteria, so the filtered fluid may contain mycoplasmata, viruses or prions.

Chemicals
A few 'high-level' chemicals are sporicidal and viricidal and hence can sterilise. Use is limited by toxicity and irritation.

Formaldehyde is rarely used to disinfect empty rooms after very infectious patients.

Formalin is used to fix tissues for safety in laboratories, other than where it would inhibit desirable cell or microbial cultures.

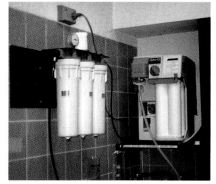

Fig. 2 **Filtration of water for microbiologic media.**

Glutaraldehyde, ortho-phthal-aldehyde (OPA), hydrogen peroxide and peracetic acid are used for invasive instruments which cannot otherwise be sterilised, for example bronchoscopes, cystoscopes, anaesthetic equipment and some plastics. The aldehydes need specially ventilated procedure rooms and operating theatres.

Ethylene oxide needs a special chamber, often called a 'bomb' as the gas is explosive in air! It diffuses well into materials and is used for heat-sensitive articles such as plastic, rubber and complex equipment.

Hydrogen peroxide gas plasma is newer, promising, and being evaluated.

Heat
This can be dry or moist heat.

Dry heat is used as:
- red heat: for metal loops during bacterial cultures
- flaming: for lighting microscope slides wetted by methylated spirit (!)
- hot air ovens: 160°C for 60 minutes for scalpels, scissors, and substances (oil, grease, wax) impermeable to moist heat
- infrared radiation: seldom used now.

Table 1 Disinfectants

Class	Chemical	Advantages	Disadvantages	Uses
Alcohols	Ethyl alcohol, isopropyl alcohol	Quick action, broad spectrum; can combine with others, e.g. chlorhexidine	Damage mucous membranes	Skin and surfaces
Aldehydes	Formalin (liquid, gasª)	Excellent spectrum	Very irritant	Preserve dead tissues (liquid), room fumigation (gas)
	Glutaraldehyde [Cidex, Aidal]	Excellent spectrum, less irritant	Expensive, needs exhausts	Endoscopes
	O-phthalaldehyde	Less toxic	Stains protein grey	As glutaraldehyde
Diguanides	Chlorhexidine	Broad activity, combines with alcohol, etc.	Easily inactivated	Surfaces, mucous membranes, hands
Halogens	Hypochlorites [Milton]	Spectrum includes viruses; organic material inactivates; cheap	Corrodes metal	Blood spills and soiling
	Iodine and iodophores	Sporicidal	Coloured	Skin disinfection
Heavy metals	Silver iodide plus biguanide [Surfacine]	Broad spectrum, persistent	Limited experience	Surfaces, hands, ?devices
Hexachlorophane replacements	Irgasan, triclosan [pHisohex]	Combine with soap, anti-staphylococcal	Poor killing of GNRs	Skin disinfection
Peracetic acid and/or hydrogen peroxide	Vary	High level, broad spectrum	Limited experience	Heat-sensitive immersible items
Phenolics	Numerous soluble	Wide activity	Not sporicidal	General purpose on surfaces
Quaternary ammoniums	Benzalkoniumª [zephiran]	Moderate spectrum, detergent activity	Poor killing GNRs, easily inactivated	Environmental cleaning
	Cetrimide [cetavlon]	Combine with chlorhexidine, detergent activity	Poor killing GNRs, easily activated	Wound cleansing, antiseptics

Trade names in [brackets]; GNR, Gram-negative rod.
ªSuperseded where better alternatives are available.

Moist heat is achieved by boiling water, or autoclaving. Boiling in water 'for 5, 10 or 20 minutes' kills non-sporing microbes but not necessarily all spores. Hence, boiling is unreliable for sterilisation, as the variable quoted times show.

Autoclaving is the most reliable and efficient sterilising process. It depends on steam under pressure, hence it is hotter than 100°C (e.g. 121°C for 15 minutes or 132°C for 3 minutes). These time–temperature combinations are proven to kill pathogenic spores. Six times longer is needed for prions, on high-risk equipment from high-risk patients.

Special autoclaves are used, often in central sterile supply units (CSSU), operating theatre suites or laboratories

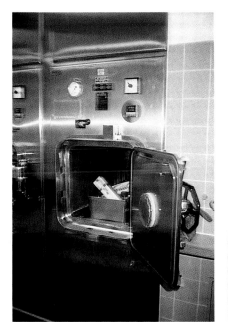

Fig. 3 **Autoclave.**

(Fig. 3). The load (instruments, drapes, dressings, etc.) is first cleaned to reduce the bio-burden of organisms (see above). The load is then carefully packed to ensure steam can penetrate throughout it, locked in the autoclave, air is exhausted, then steam under pressure admitted for the correct ('holding') time. Modern autoclaves then dry the load; pressure must reach atmospheric before opening the door.

When all steps are controlled and the correct temperature held for the correct time, sterility should be assured. In addition, the process is checked, preferably by culturing special spore strips of known heat resistance; autoclave tape, which changes colour, is less reliable.

Disinfection methods

Washing removes some surface microbes, so has some disinfectant action by itself. Detergents including soap make it more effective. In addition, this 'bio-burden' removal makes subsequent disinfection by heat or chemicals more effective.

Heat by boiling, as discussed above, disinfects but does not reliably sterilise.

Pasteurisation is a gentle disinfection by low-temperature heating (63°C for

30 minutes or 72°C for 20 seconds) of milk or other liquid foods which would be unpalatable after more vigorous disinfection such as boiling.

Chemicals are the usual disinfectants (Table 1). They are used especially on skin, surfaces and some instruments and supplies which cannot be sterilised.

Disinfectants

The success of a disinfectant depends on the:

- **T**ype, time and concentration of disinfectant
- **I**nactivation by minerals (hard water) or microbes
- **M**icrobial type, state (especially spores), and number
- **E**nvironmental pH, temperature and moisture
- **S**urface disinfected (skin, metal, porous materials).

Control of all these variables is difficult; the process recommended by the manufacturer and relevant authorities must be observed. 'In-use' tests by adding known organisms then culturing samples (after disinfectant dilution or neutralisation) can be done in hospitals, especially for Infection Control investigations.

Sterilisation and disinfection

- Sterilisation is killing *all* viable microbes, including their spores, while disinfection is killing or removing *most but not all* viable microbes.
- Four principles are: clean first, disinfect/sterilise next; the right process for the purpose; process must be controlled; strong enough for long enough.
- The four methods are irradiation or filtration (special purposes for each), chemicals (chiefly for disinfection) and heat (for sterilisation).

Antimicrobials: general properties

Throughout this book, the importance of control of sources of infection has been stressed; in some instances general environmental hygiene is effective, in others specific measures are required. However, once a pathogen has invaded and is causing disease, antimicrobial treatment may be needed to supplement host defences.

Firstly, empiric non-scientific medicine produced four important 'antimicrobials' (properly, 'antimicrobial drugs') before microbes were known to cause infections:

- emetine for amoebic dysentery in China from 500 BC
- quinine in cinchona bark for malaria in Peru before the 16th century
- mercury for syphilis by Paracelsus in Europe in 1530
- potassium iodide for syphilis in 1836.

Secondly, the scientific development of synthetic antimicrobials began with P. Ehrlich in Germany with methylene blue for malaria in 1891, the organic arsenicals 'atoxyl' (1902) and 'trypan red' (1904) for trypanosomiasis, and 'salvarsan 606' for syphilis (1909). Atebrin for malarial prophylaxis was made in 1932, and the first effective sulphonamide, prontosil red, by G. Domagk in 1935.

Thirdly, the great phase of antibiotics from living organisms began in 1928 when A. Fleming noted the anti-staphylococcal activity of 'penicillin', made by a contaminating fungus, *Penicillium notatum*. Penicillin was developed to clinical use by H. Florey and E. Chain, initiating a wonderful group of antibiotics. A second great group of antibiotics, aminoglycosides, was found in 1944 by S. Waksman, isolating streptomycin from *Streptomyces griseus*. A third group, cephalosporins, was developed from *Cephalosporium acremonium*, found by G. Brotzu in 1945.

Classification

Antimicrobials are classified by the pathogens targeted, e.g. antibacterials or antifungals. This grouping may be subdivided, e.g. antibacterials include urinary antiseptics and anti-mycobacterial drugs.

Antimicrobials, especially antibacterials, are strictly classified into chemotherapeutic agents (synthetic chemicals), and antibiotics, produced from living ('bios' = life) organisms, usually fungi. However, 'antibiotic' is often used loosely to mean all antibacterials.

Antibacterials can be further described by their:

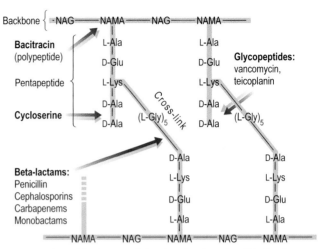

Fig. 1 **The structure of peptidoglycan and the site of action of antibiotics.** Structure varies slightly among species; this is the structure of *Staph. aureus*. NAG, N-acetylglucosamine; NAMA, N-acetylmuramic acid.

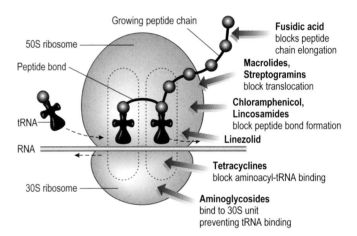

Fig. 2 **Specific site of action of antibacterials inhibiting protein synthesis.**

- chemical structure (penicillins, cephalosporins, etc.)
- effect on bacterial growth (bacteriostatic or bactericidal)
- target site (see below).

Target site classes

Cell wall synthesis inhibitors
(p. 228–230)

The cell wall synthesis inhibitors are bactericidal because they block synthesis of the rigid peptidoglycan component of the wall (Fig. 1), so growing cells lyse and die. They do not affect eucaryotic cells, nor microbes that lack peptidoglycan, or can prevent the antibiotic reaching their peptidoglycan. These antibiotics are:

- beta-lactams: penicillins, cephalosporins, carbapenems, monobactams
- glycopeptides: vancomycin, teicoplanin
- polypeptide: bacitracin
- cycloserine.

Protein synthesis inhibitors
(p. 230–231)

Protein synthesis inhibitors act on varying stages of protein synthesis (Fig. 2); if these are unique to bacteria (e.g. affect the bacterial 70S ribosome rather than the eucaryotic 80S ribosome) they are selectively toxic. However, eucaryotic mitochondrial protein synthesis occurs on 70S ribosomes and can be affected. This group includes:

- aminoglycosides: streptomycin, gentamicin, tobramycin, netilmicin, amikacin, spectinomycin, neomycin
- tetracyclines: tetracycline, doxycycline, minocycline
- linezolid
- chloramphenicol
- lincosamides: clindamycin, lincomycin
- macrolides: erythromycin, roxithromycin, azithromycin, clarithromycin, spiramycin
- streptogramins
- fusidic acid.

Aminoglycosides cause ineffective proteins to form and so are bactericidal. All the others in this group have a reversible (bacteriostatic) action and so protein synthesis begins again when antibiotic levels decrease.

Nucleic acid synthesis inhibitors
(p. 231–232)
Nucleic acids are made by all cells so the possibility of selective drugs toxic only for microbes is limited. Some pathways have distinct features that can be targeted, or some enzymes are sufficiently different for a selective effect to occur:

- Folic acid synthesis: a precursor of purines and pyrimidines is folic acid which microbes can only synthesise; humans obtain folic acid in food. Sulphonamides and trimethoprim interfere with folic acid synthesis.
- RNA polymerase: inhibited by rifamycins (rifampicin, rifabutin).
- DNA structure: disrupted by nitroimidazoles (e.g. metronidazole).
- topo-isomerase: blocked by quinolones (norfloxacin, ciprofloxacin and others).

Cell membrane function inhibitors
Drugs that destroy the selective permeability of membranes will kill both microbial and human cells. As a result, they will be relatively toxic if given systemically. Colistin acts like a detergent, disrupting the cell membrane phospholipid. The polyene antifungal drugs (e.g. amphotericin B and nystatin) act by damaging sterols in eucaryotic membranes; they are particularly toxic to fungi through their action (p. 232) on ergosterol but also affect human cells.

Uncertain targets
The target of some anti-mycobacterial drugs is uncertain: isoniazid may act on mycolic acid synthesis, which would explain its specific activity, while ethambutol may inhibit RNA synthesis (p. 232).

Characteristics

Physicochemical properties
These are important in relation to the effectiveness and mode of administration of a drug, particularly whether they are stable to gastric acid and are absorbed from the gut and hence can be given orally; if unstable or not absorbed, they need injection. Other important factors are whether the drug will cross barriers within the body – into cells, into the brain across the blood–brain barrier, into other protected tissues like prostate, or into cysts.

Spectrum and type of activity
- The spectrum of activity is the range of organisms against which an antimicrobial is usually active.

The minimal inhibitory concentration (MIC) is the smallest concentration of antimicrobial which is bacteriostatic, reversibly inhibiting bacterial growth, so re-growth occurs if the antimicrobial is removed by excretion or inactivation. By contrast, the minimal bactericidal (or fungicidal) concentration (MBC, MFC) is the smallest concentration irreversibly killing the microbes, so they do not regrow if the antimicrobial is removed.

Mechanisms of resistance
Some bacteria are innately resistant to certain antibiotics because they lack a target site or are impermeable to the antibiotic; **other bacteria acquire resistance, by one of three mechanisms:**

1. Altered target site. These may result in lower affinity for the antibiotic, or additional target enzymes may emerge unaffected by the drug.
2. Altered uptake. Effective drug concentration in the bacterial cell can be decreased either by decreasing permeability or by actively pumping the drug out of the bacterial cell.
3. Antibiotic-inactivating enzymes. These occur particularly against penicillins, cephalosporins and aminoglycosides.

Resistance spreads between bacteria in three genetic ways:

1. Chromosomal mutation, usually random, causes an altered protein, e.g. a ribosomal protein (streptomycin resistance) or altered enzyme (sulphonamides). Selection by the antibiotic after each cell division will result in a resistant population.
2. Transmissible plasmids are small circular DNA units replicating independently of the chromosome, and transmissible between cells. They have four advantages over chromosomal muta-

tion: transfer between bacteria is more rapid than cell division; resistance to numerous *individual* antibiotics can be carried at once; resistance to several *classes* of antibiotic can be carried at once; and one class of plasmid can enter numerous genera, e.g. TEM-1 beta-lactamase in enteric Gram-negative rods, in *N. gonorrhoeae* and in *H. influenzae*.
3. Transposons, called 'jumping genes', move from the security of the chromosome to the mobility of a plasmid, and from one plasmid to another.

Resistance spreads between bacteria in three physical ways:
1. Conjugation (by direct contact)
2. Transduction (by phages)
3. Transformation (uptake of free DNA).

Pharmacokinetics
The pharmacokinetics of a drug describe its behaviour in the body: absorption, distribution ('penetration'), protein binding, serum and tissue concentrations, serum half-life, metabolism and excretion. Important factors that will alter the effective half-life of the drug (and its toxicity) include the age of the patient, concurrent diseases particularly of organs which metabolise or excrete the drug (usually liver and kidney), genetic factors (slow and fast drug metabolism) and interaction with other drugs.

Side effects, toxicity
Even safe effective antibiotics like penicillins fall short of Ehrlich's ideal of a 'magic bullet' which would not affect humans yet would eradicate germs by a single 'dosa sterilisa magna' (great sterilising dose). Side effects and toxicity are often similar within a group of antibiotics, e.g. all aminoglycosides are ototoxic and nephrotoxic but vary in degree.

Clinical use
The indications, dosage and routes used for each antibiotic follow from all the above properties (see p. 228–235).

> ### Antimicrobials: general properties
> - Antimicrobials are classified by the type of pathogen targeted, the disease for which they are effective, and the mechanism of action.
> - True antibiotics are the products of living organisms, although the term is used loosely to include synthetic and semi-synthetic chemicals.
> - Antibacterials can act on cell wall, protein and nucleic acid synthesis, on the cell membrane or as antimetabolites blocking metabolic pathways.
> - Antibiotic resistance may be innate because bacteria lack the target site or are impermeable to the antibiotic, or may be acquired. Bacteria acquire resistance by one of three mechanisms: an altered target site, altered uptake or by antibiotic-inactivating enzymes.
> - Resistance spreads between bacteria in three genetic ways: chromosomal mutation, transmissible plasmids or transposons.
> - Important characteristics of an antimicrobial include its physicochemical properties, mode of action, spectrum of activity and resistance, pharmacokinetic properties, dose and route, side effects and toxicity and clinical indications.

Antimicrobials: specific antibacterials I

The detailed mechanisms of action of all antimicrobials are covered on pages 222–223 and 234–235. The specific characteristics of the antibacterials are described here and on pages 230–232.

Cell wall synthesis inhibitors

Action is bactericidal by blocking cross-linking of peptidoglycan chains in the dividing bacterial cell wall (Fig. 1, p. 226).

Penicillins

The penicillins all have a similar structure, differing side chains giving different drugs (Fig. 1). The side chains of the natural product can be modified chemically to give a wider spectrum of activity. A common bacterial drug resistance is via beta-lactamases (Fig. 2).

Pharmacokinetics. Some penicillins are stable to gastric acid and absorbable (penicillin V, ampi/amoxicillin, flucloxacillin) and so can be given orally. Others must be given by injection: penicillin G, ticarcillin and piperacillin. All penetrate widely, except poorly to CSF and brain; all have relatively short half-lives, are little metabolised and have renal excretion.

Spectrum/use. This varies and is shown in Tables 1 and 2.

Toxicity. This is minimal, almost limited to hypersensitivity, chiefly rash (Fig. 3) or fever, rarely anaphylaxis.

Cost. This is small except for flucloxacillin, ticarcillin and piperacillin.

Cephalosporins

Structure of cephalosporins differs from the penicillins in having a six-member ring attached to the beta-lactam ring (Fig. 1):

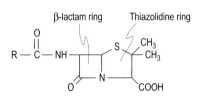

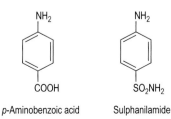

Fig. 1 **The structures of some antimicrobials.**

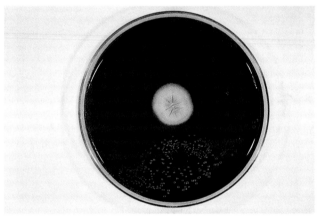

Fig. 2 *Penicillium notatum* (central, large, white), a source of penicillin, killing the (yellow-white) colonies of *Staphylococcus aureus*, except where protected by the beta-lactamase from a *Bacillus* (dark colony, lower quarter).

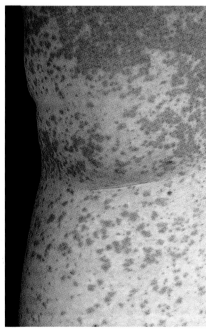

Fig. 3 **Penicillin rash.**

Table 1 The ABC of antibiotics

Antibiotic	Bacterial spectrum							Clinical uses
	AnO	Sta	Str	Enc	GNC	GNR	Ps	
Penicillins								
Flucloxacillin	++	3+	++	+	–	–	–	Staphylococcal infections (not MRSA)
Penicillin V, G	++	+	3+	++	++	+	–	Erysipelas, gas gangrene, endocarditis, meningitis, pharyngitis
Ampi/amoxicillin (improved by BLI)	++	+	++	3+	++	+	–	Bronchitis/sinusitis/otitis media; combined with gentamicin in abdominal and urinary infections
Ticar/piperacillin (improved by BLI)	++	+	++	++	++	+	3+	Pseudomonal infections, often combined with aminoglycoside
Cephalosporins								
First: cephalothin, cefazolin, cephalexin	++	3+	++	0	+	++	–	Surgical chemoprophylaxis, skin/soft tissue infections, also combined with aminoglycosides
Second: cefuroxime, cefoxitin, cefotetan	3+	++	++	0	++	++	–	Mild-moderate mixed anaerobic-aerobic skin/soft tissue, respiratory and abdominal infections
Third: cefotaxime, ceftriaxone	++	+	++	0	3+	3+	+	Severe Gram-negative infections including meningitis
3/4: ceftazidime, cefepime	++	+	+	0	3+	3+	3+	Pseudomonal and other Gram-negative rod infections
Other beta-lactams								
Aztreonam	–	–	–	–	3+	3+	3+	Severe systemic Gram-negative infections
Imipenem, meropenem	3+	3+	3+	++	3+	3+	3+	Severe systemic infections (not MRSA)
Vancomycin, fusidic acid, linezolid, streptogramins	–	MRSA	++	3+	–	–	–	Serious staphylococcal infections, especially MRSA; enterococcal infections
Aminoglycosides								
Streptomycin	–	–	–	–	–	3+	–	Tuberculosis, Gram-negative zoonoses (brucellosis, plague, tularaemia)
Gentamicin	–	–	–	–	++	3+	3+	Severe systemic Gram-negative infections
Tobramycin	–	–	–	–	++	++	3+	Pseudomonal infections
Amikacin	–	–	–	–	++	3+	3+	Otherwise-resistant Gram-negative rod infections
Chloramphenicol	3+	MRSA	3+	++	3+	++	–	MRSA, rickettsial and rare infections
Lincosamides								
Clindamycin, lincomycin	3+	++	++	–	–	–	–	Anaerobic infection, toxoplasmosis
Macrolides								
Erythromycin	++	++	++	+	++	–	–	Chancroid, legionellosis, pertussis, Campylobacter infection
Roxithromycin	++	++	++	+	++	–	–	Erythromycin substitute
Azithromycin	3+	+	+	–	3+	–	–	*Chlamydia*, STDs, unusual infections
Clarithromycin	++	3+	3+	+	3+	–	–	*Chlamydia*, MAC, leprosy
Tetracyclines	+	+	+	+	+	+	–	Unusual bacteria: *Borrelia* spp., brucellae, mycoplasmata, rickettsiae, vibrios
Nitroimidazoles								
Metronidazole, tinidazole	3+	–	–	–	–	–	–	Anaerobic infections, amoebiasis, giardiasis
Quinolones								
Norfloxacin	–	–	–	–	–	++	–	Urinary infections (2nd line)
Ciprofloxacin	–	+	+	–	3+	3+	++	Serious Gram-negative infections (MRSA)
Moxi/gatifloxacin	++	++	++	++	3+	3+	++	Difficult atypical pneumonia
Rifamycins								
Rifampicin (rifabutin p. 231)	++	MRSA	3+	3+	3+	++	+	TB, MRSA, leprosy, prophylaxis in meningococcal and haemophilus meningitis
Trimethoprim and sulphonamides	–	+	+	–	+	++	–	Mild urinary and respiratory infections, nocardial infection, toxoplasmosis, PCP

Efficacy: 3+, usually effective (> 80% strains usually sensitive); ++, moderate efficacy (50–80% strains usually sensitive); +, poor efficacy (25–50% of strains usually sensitive); –, minimal or no efficacy; 0, no efficacy. Hint to students: highlight every 3+.

AnO, anaerobes (e.g. *Clostridia*, *Bacteroides* spp.); Sta, staphylococci; Str, streptococci; Enc, enterococci; GNC, Gram-negative cocci (e.g. *Neisseria*, *Haemophilus* spp.); GNR, Gram-negative rods, especially enteric (e.g. *E. coli*); Ps, pseudomonads; MAC, *Mycobacterium avium* complex; MRSA, meticillin- (and multi-) resistant *S. aureus*; PCP, *Pneumocystis jirovecii* pneumonia; STD, sexually transmitted diseases; BLI, beta lactamase inhibitor.

different side chains give the different cephalosporins, which are often classified into first, second, third and fourth 'generations' (Table 1) by their date of introduction; more logical classifications exist but are less used.

Pharmacokinetics. Cephalosporins behave like penicillins, although the later drugs have longer half-lives, especially ceftriaxone, and penetrate well to CSF and brain.

Spectrum. This changes somewhat with the generations, but all are broad-spectrum, active against many Gram-positive, Gram-negative and anaerobic bacteria. Enterococci are resistant to all. In general, first generation are best against Gram-positive bacteria, second generation best against anaerobes, and third generation best against Gram-negative rods. Major uses are given in Table 1.

Toxicity. Low toxicity is similar to the penicillins.

Cost. This varies, ascending with the generations.

Table 2 The CBA of antibiotics

Clinical syndrome	Bacterial causes	Antibiotic(s) of choice
Pharyngitis	*S. pyogenes*, *C. diphtheriae* (viruses)	Penicillin
Pneumonia		
Classical	*S. pneumoniae*	Penicillin*
'Atypical'	*Chlamydia*, *Legionella*, *Mycoplasma*, etc.	Erythromycin plus ceftriaxone
Cystitis	*E. coli* and other enteric Gram-negative rods	Amoxicillin ± clavulanate, or cephalexin
	S. saprophyticus	Trimethoprim, norfloxacin
Urethritis	*N. gonorrhoeae*	Ceftriaxone (PPNG) or ciprofloxacin
	C. trachomatis	Azithromycin

*Ceftriaxone if resistance.

PPNG, Penicillinase-producing *N. gonorrhoeae*.

Antimicrobials: specific antibacterials II

Other β-lactams

Aztreonam is a mono-bactam, i.e. a single β-lactam ring. Its action and pharmacokinetics are like an injectable cephalosporin, but its spectrum is like the aminoglycoside gentamicin, i.e., solely Gram negative, including many pseudomonads. Its use is restricted by its high cost.

Imipenem, meropenem and ertapenem are carbapenems, structurally like penicillin except that carbon replaces the sulphur atom in the five-member ring. Their actions and pharmacokinetics are like an injectable cephalosporin, but their spectrum is wonderfully wide (Table 1, p. 229), though they are inactive against MRSA, *E. faecium*, and some Gram-negative rods. Their use is restricted by policy and cost to serious systemic infections before precise microbial diagnosis.

Vancomycin and teicoplanin

Vancomycin and teicoplanin are glycopeptides and are bactericidal to Gram-positive bacteria.

Pharmacokinetics. Neither is absorbed from the gut, so vancomycin is given intravenously, by slow infusion to decrease the side effects of headache and flushing (the '**red man**' **syndrome**). Teicoplanin is also given intramuscularly. Distribution of both is wide into most fluids and tissues, but suboptimal into CSF and brain. Their half-lives are long, hence 12- or 24-hourly dosing. Excretion is renal and, because of toxicity, serum levels are usually monitored, though safe levels are not established!

Spectrum. Use is limited to severe Gram-positive (including MRSA) infections, and oral treatment of unresponsive *C. difficile*-associated colitis. **Linezolid** and **streptogramins** are active against most glycopeptide-resistant Gram-positive bacteria.

Toxicity. The main toxic effect is hearing loss, but phlebitis or neutropenia can also occur. Nephrotoxicity is uncommon with current preparations.

Cost is relatively high.

Protein synthesis inhibitors

All act on the 30S or 50S bacterial ribosome. Only aminoglycosides are bactericidal.

Table 1 Simplified antimicrobial sensitivities

	Anaerobes e.g. clostridia.	Streptococci	Staphylococci	GNR, enteric	GNR, pseudomonads
Penicillin G, V	3	3	3 or –	–	–
Cloxacillins/Vancomycin	2	2	3	–	–
Cephalosporin					
1st generation	2	2	3 or –	1	–
2nd generation	2	2	3 or –	2	–
3rd/4th generation	2	2	3 or –	3	1–2
Gentamicin	–	–	–	3	3
Tobramycin					
Nor/ciprofloxacin					
Aztreonam					

Key: 3 >, 80% strains sensitive; 2, 50–80% strains sensitive; 1 <, 50% strains sensitive; –, Not active.

Aminoglycosides

The aminoglycosides contain streptamine or a streptidine-containing aminocyclitol, with side chains that are modified to produce the individual drugs. **Gentamicin** is actually a mixture of three related molecules.

Pharmacokinetics. Aminoglycosides are not absorbed from the gut, so must be injected for systemic use. They are not metabolised significantly and have a relatively long half-life, about 3 hours, so usually are given once- or twice-daily. Excretion is renal. Penetration is relatively poor into bone, lung and sputum, and non-existent into CSF and brain.

Spectrum. Aminoglycosides are bactericidal with a broad Gram-negative spectrum (Table 1); however, their uptake into cells is prevented by anaerobiosis so they are ineffective against anaerobes. They are mainly used against enteric Gram-negative rods; **gentamicin**, **tobramycin** and **amikacin** are also active against pseudomonads. **Streptomycin** was used for tuberculosis but is now used mainly in Gram-negative zoonoses including brucellosis, plague and tularaemia.

Toxicity. Aminoglycosides have both renal and ototoxicity, related mainly to total dose. This is reflected later in peak than in trough levels, which should be monitored carefully, especially in the old, the underweight and those with renal or auditory impairment.

Cost. This is minimal for gentamicin (including monitoring), higher with tobramycin and very high with amikacin.

Chloramphenicol

Chloramphenicol is a natural product that is now chemically synthesised. Action is on bacterial protein synthesis at the 50S ribosome, and is usually bacteriostatic only.

Pharmacokinetics. Chloramphenicol is lipophilic; it is orally absorbed and has wide penetration including into the interior of the eye, the CSF and brain. It is metabolised by the liver and excreted renally. It can also be given by injection.

Spectrum. Like its pharmacokinetics, the spectrum is also almost ideal, being extremely broad and including most bacteria, chlamydiae, rickettsiae and mycoplasmata. It is also cheap.

Toxicity. The use of this otherwise ideal antibiotic is limited by two toxicities. An unpredictable irreversible marrow aplasia causing aplastic anaemia occurs rarely (1 in 30000) and is fatal without marrow transplantation. If liver function is impaired, chloramphenicol levels rise above normal, and dose-related reversible marrow hypoplasia can occur; newborns who fail to metabolise chloramphenicol adequately die from toxic complications ('**grey baby syndrome**').

Lincosamides

Clindamycin and lincomycin are bacteriostatic, on bacterial protein synthesis at the 50S ribosome, like macrolides and chloramphenicol. They are orally absorbed, but are also injectable, and widely distributed apart from CSF and brain. They are metabolised by the liver and excreted renally.

Spectrum. They are mainly used against anaerobes or staphylococci. Clindamycin is a reserve drug in toxoplasmosis.

Toxicity. Toxic effects include allergy, a metallic taste, and initiation of pseudomembranous enterocolitis associated with *C. difficile* overgrowth (p. 159).

Cost as well as toxicity limits their use.

Macrolides

The macrolides have an unusual 14- or 15-member macrocyclic lactone ring with sugars attached. There are four macrolides in clinical use: **erythromycin**, **roxithromycin**, **azithromycin** and **clarithromycin**. Action is bacteriostatic, on bacterial protein synthesis at the 50S ribosome.

Pharmacokinetics. Erythromycin base is inactivated by gastric acid so is protected by enteric-coating or given as a salt or ester. Intravenous use often causes thrombophlebitis. The half-life is about 2 hours, and excretion is hepatic; as a result, care is needed in liver failure but dosage is unaltered in renal impairment.

Spectrum. Macrolides are mainly used against Gram-positive and unusual bacteria: chlamydiae, legionellae, mycoplasmata and non-tuberculous mycobacteria (Table 1, p. 229).

Toxicity. These are very safe antibiotics with low toxicity.

Cost is low for erythromycin, higher for the three newer drugs.

Tetracyclines

The tetracyclines have a basic structure of four fused rings (Fig. 1, p. 228) with, as usual, side-chain changes to produce different members of the family. Action is bacteriostatic, on bacterial protein synthesis at the 30S ribosome (like aminoglycosides, which however are bactericidal).

Pharmacokinetics. Tetracyclines are orally absorbed yet also injectable; they are widely distributed including CSF and brain. Metabolism occurs in the liver, and excretion is renal.

Spectrum. The spectrum of tetracyclines is very broad, including most pathogenic bacterial genera (except *Pseudomonas*), plus chlamydiae, mycoplasmata and rickettsiae, but is not deep, with many resistant bacterial strains. The use of tetracyclines as growth promoters added to livestock feed increased the numbers of resistant strains. Use is, therefore, chiefly for unusual bacteria.

Toxicity. This is low, apart from deposition in immature bone and teeth (causing discoloration), and the usual allergy or gut intolerance.

Cost is low.

Nucleic acid synthesis inhibitors

Nitroimidazoles

Metronidazole and **tinidazole** are nitroimidazoles, with a unique mode of bactericidal action, acting as electron acceptors and producing intermediate compounds toxic to bacterial DNA.

Pharmacokinetics. They are well absorbed, penetrate widely, are metabolised by the liver, and excreted by the kidney.

Spectrum. Their spectrum includes almost all pathogenic anaerobes (except some cocci), microaerophilic bacteria and some parasites. Their principal use is in prophylaxis and treatment of anaerobic bacterial infections, and in amoebiasis, giardiasis and trichomoniasis.

Toxicity is minimal, and cost is now low.

Quinolones

Structurally, the quinolones (e.g. **norfloxacin** and **ciprofloxacin**) are fluoroquinolone carboxylic acid derivatives with two six-member rings, and distinctive side chains. Action is bactericidal by inhibiting bacterial DNA gyrase, hence preventing supercoiling of DNA.

Pharmacokinetics. Quinolones are well absorbed and distributed, but serum concentrations are low. Their half-lives are relatively long, about 4 hours, and excretion is renal.

Spectrum. Older drugs mainly kill Gram-negative bacteria including pseudomonads, with poor activity against Gram-positive and anaerobic bacteria, now improved with broad-spectrum quinolones. Norfloxacin is used mainly in urinary and gut infections, while ciprofloxacin is used chiefly in serious systemic Gram-negative infections. Numerous other quinolones are available in different countries.

Toxicity can affect the CNS with headache, mood changes and fits.

Cost is moderate to high.

Trimethoprim and sulphonamides

Sulphonamides are derived from sulphanilamide, a single ring compound structurally similar to, and competing with, an intermediate in folic acid synthesis, para-aminobenzoic acid. They are commonly used in combination with trimethoprim, which inhibits the next step to tetrahydrofolic acid in folic acid synthesis. **Co-trimoxazole** is sulphamethoxazole plus trimethoprim.

Pharmacokinetics. All have good absorption, wide distribution, long half-lives (to 10 hours) and renal excretion.

Spectrum. Chiefly Gram-negative rods were sensitive, but resistance is now common. Uses are mild urinary or respiratory infections, and unusual infections including *P. jirovecii* pneumonia, nocardiosis, chancroid and typhoid fever.

Toxicity. This is mainly allergy with rash and fever. Megaloblastic anaemia is uncommon and reversed by folinic acid.

Cost is low.

Rifamycins

The rifamycins are red-coloured derivatives of a natural product, rifamycin B.

Pharmacokinetics. All are well absorbed orally, penetrate widely including the CNS, and are cleared by liver metabolism and excretion mainly in bile.

Spectrum. Because rifamycins enter cells they are used against intracellular organisms such as mycobacteria. **Rifampicin** is a first line drug for TB and leprosy, and also used for resistant (especially MRSA) staphylococcal infections (with fusidic acid) and as prophylaxis in contacts of meningococcal and *Haemophilus* meningitis. **Rifabutin** is used in combination with other drugs (e.g. ethambutol, clarithromycin) in the treatment and prophylaxis of atypical mycobacterial infections (e.g., MAC) in AIDS.

Toxicity. Rifampicin has few toxic side effects but numerous drug interactions. It colours body fluids blood-red.

> *Antimicrobials: specific antibacterials*
>
> - Spectrum determines use, which is modified by toxicity and cost.
> - Penicillins, cephalosporins and other beta-lactams are safe, effective bactericidal antibiotics of great use in a wide range of infections, limited by developing resistance.
> - Aminoglycosides, particularly gentamicin, are very effective against many Gram-negative infections but need careful dosing and monitoring because of toxicity. Resistance is a lesser problem.
> - Metronidazole is very useful against most anaerobes, while clindamycin is less reliable and more costly.
> - Older broad-spectrum bacteriostatic antibiotics including chloramphenicol, co-trimoxazole and tetracyclines are now mainly used for unusual bacteria, chlamydiae, mycoplasmata or rickettsiae.
> - Quinolones are costly and used mainly in special infections.
> - Vancomycin, teicoplanin and linezolid are reserved for serious resistant Gram-positive infections.

Antimicrobials: special antimicrobials

Antimycobacterial drugs

All mycobacterial infections need prolonged treatment with two or more drugs because:

- their cell-wall mycolic acids make them impermeable to many drugs
- mycobacteria grow slowly, requiring long-term treatment
- some mycobacteria are intracellular pathogens so drugs must enter human cells
- antibiotic resistance is common, and most infections contain some resistant bacteria
- incidence is rising in the immuno-deficient, whose natural defences are impaired or absent.

Tuberculosis

Isoniazid (INAH) is synthetic isonicotinic acid hydrazide which is bactericidal, probably by inhibiting mycolic acid synthesis. It is well absorbed orally and widely distributed, including the CNS. It is used only in mycobacterial infections, chiefly TB, and toxicity is neurological (prevented by routine pyridoxine) or hepatic.

Rifampicin. See p. 231.

Ethambutol is a synthetic mycobacteriostatic drug, probably inhibiting RNA synthesis. It is well absorbed and well distributed. It is used only in mycobacterial infections, chiefly TB. Toxicity includes optic neuritis, so dosage and regular vision/fundus reviews are critical.

Pyrazinamide is a synthetic tuberculocidal drug which is absorbed orally and penetrates both the CNS and cells, including macrophages. Hepatotoxicity was previously common with high doses, but safer, lower doses are effective and widely used.

Streptomycin is an aminoglycoside; it is bactericidal, causing abnormal proteins to be synthesised. It is not absorbed orally, penetrates the CNS poorly, is excreted by the kidney and has auditory toxicity. It is now little used as therapy is usually entirely oral.

Reserve drugs. Cycloserine, **ethionamide**, **prothionamide** and **viomycin** are used if resistance or intolerance exist to first-line drugs.

Leprosy

Dapsone is a synthetic sulphone, very similar to sulphonamides. It is cheap, given orally, usually well tolerated and was widely used alone for decades until widespread resistance forced the present combined therapy with rifampicin (p. 104). It is also used in toxoplasmosis, usually with pyrimethamine.

Clofazimine is unusual – it is a phenazine dye, weakly bactericidal, mode of action ill-understood and long-delayed, pharmacokinetics complex with unreliable absorption, wide distribution, accumulation in tissues and slow biliary excretion. It is used with rifampicin and dapsone in multi-bacillary leprosy, or in dapsone intolerance. Deep skin pigmentation is a troublesome side-effect.

Atypical mycobacteria

Rifabutin, ethambutol, clarithromycin and ciprofloxacin (for *M. avium* complex, MAC, p. 61, 133, 150) and co-trimoxazole (for *M. marinum*, p. 196, 231) are suppressive.

Antifungal drugs

Antifungals can be classified like antibacterials, by target site and chemical groups (Table 1).

Amphotericin B is a major parenteral drug for systemic fungal infections, acting on cell membrane function. It is poorly distributed, but low concentrations in blood, CSF and urine do not correlate with efficacy. Excretion is biliary, and slow; renal toxicity is considerable. Formulation, dosage and administration are specialised and debatable. It is also used in amoebic meningoencephalitis and leishmaniasis.

Nystatin is a polyene acting on fungal cell membrane function. It is not absorbed orally or parenterally so is only used locally on *Candida* spp. infections of skin, mouth, or vagina.

Allylamine. Terbinafine inhibits ergosterol synthesis in fungal cell membranes. It is well absorbed orally and locally. Being active against dermatophytes, moulds and yeasts, it is used for skin and nail infections.

Azoles include **clotrimazole**, **miconazole** and **econazole** (used locally), and **ketoconazole**, **fluconazole**, **itraconazole**, **voriconazole** and **posaconazole** (used systemically for systemic disease). All inhibit ergosterol synthesis in fungal cell membranes. All are well absorbed orally; fluconazole and voriconazole are also given intravenously. Ketoconazole is active against *Candida* spp., the four systemic mycotic fungi, but not *Cryptococcus*, *Aspergillus* or *Mucor* spp. Fluconazole is, in addition, active against *C. neoformans*, while itraconazole also has some activity against some *Aspergillus* and *Mucor* spp., exceeded by voriconazole with activity also against *Fusarium* spp. and *Scedosporium* spp. Toxicity is low, but drug interactions with warfarin, isoniazid, rifampicin, ciclosporin or phenytoin can be dangerous.

Echinocandins. Caspofungin inhibits the synthesis of glucan in fungal cell walls of *Candida* spp. and *Aspergillus* spp. It is only given i.v., penetrates tissues well, has few side effects, interacts only with ciclosporin, and renal impairment is not a contraindication.

Flucytosine is a pyrimidine, and its metabolite 5-fluorouracil inhibits fungal DNA synthesis. It is absorbed orally but

Table 1 Classes of antifungal drugs

Target	Chemical class	Mode of action	Drug	Spectrum
Cell membrane				
Function	Polyenes	Membrane leakage by ergosterol binding	Amphotericin B	Very wide
			Nystatin	Local candidiasis
Synthesis	Azoles	Inhibit ergosterol synthesis	Clotrimazole, miconazole	Medium, local
			Ketoconazole	Broad, systemic
			Fluconazole	Broader, systemic
			Itraconazole	Broader still, systemic
			Voriconazole	Broadest, systemic
	Allylamine	Inhibits ergosterol synthesis	Terbinafine	Skin & nail infections
Cell wall				
Synthesis	Echinocandins	Inhibit glucan synthesis	Caspofungin	*Candida* spp. & *Aspergillus* spp.
Nucleic acid synthesis				
	Pyrimidines	Metabolite 5-fluorouracil inhibits DNA synthesis	Flucytosine	Cryptococcosis; combined in systemic candidiasis
	Benzofurans	Inhibit DNA synthesis (may also inhibit cell-wall chitin synthesis)	Griseofulvin	Dermatophytes

Table 2 Major antiprotozoal drugs

Disease	Antiprotozoal drug
Amoebiasis	Metronidazole/tinidazole, diloxanide (emetine)
Giardiasis	Metronidazole/tinidazole, furazolidone, nitazoxanide
Trichomoniasis	Metronidazole/tinidazole
Amoebic meningoencephalitis	Amphotericin B
Cryptosporidiosis	Nitazoxanide, paromomycin
Malaria	Artemesinins-lumefantrine, atovaquone-proguanil, chloroquine, doxycycline, mefloquine, primaquin, quinine
Toxoplasmosis	Pyrimethamine, sulphadiazine, clindamycin
Pneumocystosis	Pentamidine, co-trimoxazole, atovaquone, dapsone
Leishmaniasis	Pentamidine, antimony compounds,[a] amphotericin B
Trypanosomiasis	
African	Pentamidine, antimony compounds[a]
American	Benznidazole, nifurtimox

[a] Includes suramin, melarsoprol and tryparsamide.

Table 3 Major anthelminthic drugs

Disease	Anthelmintic drugs[a]
Ascariasis (roundworm), threadworms, hookworms	Mebendazole, albendazole, flubendazole, pyrantel pamoate
Trichuriasis	Mebendazole, albendazole, flubendazole
Strongyloidiasis	Ivermectin
Cutaneous larva migrans, toxocariasis, trichinosis	Albendazole, flubendazole, ivermectin
Filariasis	Diethylcarbamazine, ivermectin
Hydatids, taeniasis and other cestodes	Albendazole, flubendazole, praziquantel, niclosamide
Schistosomiasis or gut flukes	Praziquantel, oxamniquine
Liver or lung flukes	Praziquantel, bithionol

[a]Mebendazole, albendazole, flubendazole, thiabendazole and pyrantel pamoate should not be used in pregnancy.

also given parenterally. It is widely distributed, and largely excreted unchanged by the kidney. Activity is mainly against *Cryptococcus* and *Candida* spp. Dose-related toxicity includes gut intolerance, hepatotoxicity and marrow suppression, especially in AIDS and/or renal impairment.

Antiparasitic drugs

Parasites are eucaryotes so it is harder to find drugs selectively toxic to them. Table 2 lists the major antiprotozoal drugs.

Antimalarials

Artemisinin derivatives. Artemether and **artesunate** are the most rapidly parasiticidal antimalarials, especially combined with **lumefantrine**. Oral treatment is safe, effective and short, replacing quinine for uncomplicated falciparum malaria.

Chloroquine is a 4-aminoquinoline, well absorbed orally and also given intravenously. It concentrates so much in liver, spleen and CNS that loading doses are unnecessary. Resistance in *P. falciparum* is now so widespread that it is only useful in Central America and parts of the Middle East. It does not eradicate the pre-erythrocytic liver stage (p. 78).

Mefloquine is a quinolinemethanol, well absorbed orally, concentrated in the liver and slowly excreted in the faeces, with a very long half-life of 17 days. Resistance is uncommon but increasing in South East Asia. It has troublesome neu-

rological and cardiac toxicity, so requires careful use.

Primaquine is an 8-aminoquinoline which is well absorbed orally, widely distributed (including the liver) and rapidly metabolised, being undetectable in 24 hours. It is used in a 14-day course for radical cure of *P. vivax* and *P. ovale* malaria. Haemolysis is common, especially in glucose 6-phosphate dehydrogenase deficiency.

Quinine, used for over 400 years, is a natural alkaloid. It is given orally or intravenously (<u>not</u> intramuscularly) and is metabolised in the liver, with some renal excretion and a half-life of 18 hours. It is schizontocidal only, so must be used with another drug such as doxycycline. Dosage is critical, and ECG and blood pressure should be monitored for cardiotoxicity.

Other antiprotozoal drugs

Antimonials. These include **suramin** (for prophylaxis and early treatment) and **melarsoprol** (for meningoencephalitis, 'sleeping sickness') in trypanosomiasis, and pentavalent compounds such as

sodium antimony gluconate used in leishmaniasis. All are given by slow intravenous injection, are toxic and require special care and knowledge.

Metronidazole, tinidazole. See p. 231.

Nitazoxanide is a new oral drug used against cryptosporidiosis and giardiasis.

Pentamidine is a diamidine which binds to DNA. It is given intramuscularly or intravenously to treat Gambian trypanosomiasis and *P. jirovecii* pneumonia (PCP), or by inhalation for PCP prophylaxis. As it does not enter the CNS, it is useless for the neurologic stage of trypanosomiasis. Common toxic effects include hypoglycaemia, hypotension, renal impairment and rashes.

Anthelminthics

Benzimidazoles. Mebendazole is little absorbed so used against intestinal nematodes. **Albendazole** and **flubendazole** are well absorbed, well tolerated and widely effective against most intestinal and tissue nematodes (not filariae) (Table 3). **Thiabendazole** is an unpleasant emetic drug, superseded by ivermectin for strongyloidiasis, and by mebendazole, albendazole and flubendazole for helminths.

Diethyl carbamazine (DEC) is a piperazine derivative, well absorbed orally, well distributed, and metabolised in 48 hours before renal excretion. It kills all human microfilariae but is less active against adult worms, especially *O. volvulus*. Repeat courses are often needed. Minor side effects are common, including allergic itchy rash and transient worsening of symptoms.

Ivermectin is a macrolide antibiotic, orally well absorbed and particularly active against *O. volvulus* microfilariae. It has minimal side effects and almost abolishes infectivity for 6–12 months after one dose. Its effect on adult worms is less well established.

Praziquantel is a prazino-isoquinoline stereoisomer mixture! It is an important drug, active against all three species of schistosomes, most other cestodes and also most flukes. It is well absorbed and well tolerated.

Antimicrobials: special antimicrobials

- The major anti-tuberculous drugs are isoniazid, rifampicin, ethambutol and pyrazinamide: treatment usually begins with three drugs (four if resistance is likely), then decreases to two for many months. Resistance is an increasing problem.
- Leprosy is now usually treated with dapsone, rifampicin and clofazimine.
- Superficial mycoses are treated with nystatin or an azole, while invasive, systemic or disseminated mycoses need amphotericin B, and/or a newer azole.
- A wide range of drugs is needed for protozoal and helminthic diseases, and treatment remains unsatisfactory for many.

Antimicrobials: antiviral drugs

The steps in viral replication (p. 16–17, 149, 200) are the basis for antiviral drug action, and should be reviewed. In summary, they are:

1. **Early stage** of Recognition, Attachment, Penetration (entry) and Uncoating.
2. **Central stage** of (reverse transcription and integration in retroviruses), mRNA Synthesis, Protein synthesis and Genome (nucleic acid) replication. Enzymes involved include DNA polymerase (reverse transcriptase, then integrase in retroviruses).
3. **Final stage** of Assembly (with proteases in retroviruses) and Release (with or without Enveloping).

Attachment

Enfuvirtide is the first fusion inhibitor for HIV infection, a peptide that binds to part of gp41 envelope glycoprotein, inhibiting viral entry. It is only given by injection, and local reactions can be a problem.

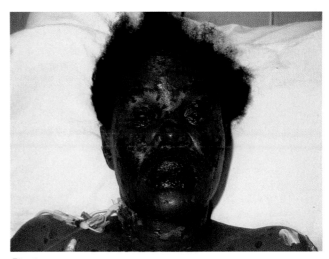

Fig. 1 **Tenofovir toxic epidermal necrosis.**

Uncoating

Amantadine and **rimantadine** block the M2 protein ion channel of the influenza virus envelope, preventing uncoating. As they only act on Influenza A, have considerable cerebral side-effects, and resistance emerges rapidly, they are little used.

DNA polymerase inhibitors of nucleic acid synthesis

Nucleoside reverse transcriptase inhibitors (NRTIs), retroviruses

These include **abacavir** (ABC), **didanosine** (ddI), **emtricitabine** (FTC), **lamivudine** (3TC), **tenofovir** (TDF, actually a nucleotide), and **zidovudine** (ZDV, formerly AZT). Zalcitabine (ddC) and Stavudine (d4T) are discontinued. All inhibit DNA synthesis by inhibiting reverse transcriptase, causing <u>chain termination</u> and so blocking DNA provirus production. Emtricitabine and lamivudine are also used against Hepatitis B. All are used in **HAART** (<u>Highly Active Anti-Retroviral Therapy</u>) which uses three (or more) drugs, commonly two NRTIs with either an NNRTI or a PI (Protease Inhibitor, see below). Dosage, combinations, side-effects, resistance development and interactions with other drugs are complex and common – seek specialist advice. Toxic epidermal necrosis from tenofovir is a fearsome side-effect (Fig. 1).

Non-nucleoside reverse transcriptase inhibitors (NNRTIs), retroviruses

Nevirapine, **delavirdine** and **efavirenz** inhibit viral DNA synthesis not by chain termination but by binding near the active site of reverse transcriptase of HIV-1 (not HIV-2). They are only used in combination with NRTIs, otherwise resistance and cross-resistance rapidly develop. Delavirdine is little used due to inconvenient dosage. The other two are useful and enter CSF well, but have CNS, liver and skin (rash) side-effects.

Integrase inhibitors logically act next in retroviruses, but are described below for convenience.

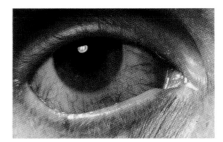

Fig. 2 **Cidofovir iritis.**

Nucleoside inhibitors, herpesviruses

Aciclovir (prodrug **famciclovir**) and **penciclovir** (prodrug **valaciclovir**) are guanosine nucleoside analogues with a 3-carbon acyclic carbon fragment instead of the cyclic ribose. They are phosphorylated by viral thymidine kinase then cellular enzymes to triphosphate forms which selectively inhibit viral DNA polymerase rather than host (human) DNA polymerase. They have good activity against HSV-1 and -2, lesser activity (so need higher dose and concentrations) against Varicella-zoster virus, and no activity against CMV. All are available for oral use, but aciclovir has poorest absorption and shortest half-life, so now is not used orally. However only aciclovir is given intravenously. They are used to treat acute attacks, and at times prophylactically for frequent relapses or in immunocompromised patients. Side-effects are rare.

Ganciclovir and **valganciclovir** are also guanosine analogues, with a 4-carbon fragment instead of ribose. They are activated by CMV-encoded and host phosphokinases, and then inhibit CMV DNA polymerase, so are used to treat CMV infections including retinitis, coli-tis, oesophagitis, pneumonitis and CNS infections, especially in AIDS and other immunocompromised patients. Ganciclovir is usually given initially, intravenously, then oral valganciclovir. They may also be used prophylactically before immunosuppression. Side-effects include bone marrow suppression with thrombocytopenia and/or leucopenia.

Cidofovir is a nucleotide cytidine analogue lacking ribose. Although active against most herpesviruses, it is mainly used as a reserve drug against CMV infections. It is given weekly, but is commonly nephrotoxic, and also causes iritis (Fig. 2). It can also be used in severe papillomavirus and poxvirus infections such as molluscum contagiosum or vaccinia in immunocompromised patients or smallpox.

Trifluorothymidine (trifluridine) is a thymidine nucleoside analogue with three fluorine atoms instead of hydrogen in the methyl group. It is too toxic for systemic use, but sometimes used for herpes simplex kerato-conjunctivitis. The similar drug **iododeoxyuridine** with iodine instead of the methyl group is now superseded.

Vidarabine with arabinose instead of ribose was used in HSV-1 encephalitis, but is less effective and more toxic than aciclovir, so now not used.

Non-nucleoside inhibitors, herpesviruses

Foscarnet is not a nucleoside analogue but a pyrophosphate analogue which inhibits herpesvirus DNA polymerases directly, without activation by intracellular kinases like the nucleoside analogues. It is used in HSV or CMV infections with resistance or intolerance to the aciclovir group or ganciclovir respectively.

Nucleoside inhibitors, other viruses

Ribavirin is a guanosine nucleoside analogue which after phosphorylation inhibits synthesis of mRNA and early transcription in both DNA and RNA viruses. It is now available for aerosol, oral and i.v. use. It is used in severe RSV pneumonitis, some viral haemorrhagic fevers, and with interferon in Hepatitis C. Its many troublesome side-effects include bronchospasm, hypotension, rash, fits and haemolytic anaemia.

Adefovir is a nucleotide analogue of AMP which is used in chronic active hepatitis B as it inhibits the DNA polymerase.

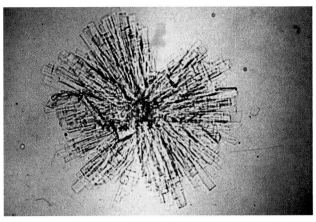
Fig. 3 **Indinavir crystal.**

Integrase inhibitors, preventing integration of viral into cell DNA

This new class of anti-retroviral drugs act after reverse transcriptase produces viral DNA from viral RNA, preventing its integration into human DNA (p. 149). Two drugs in clinical trial in 2007 include MK 0518 given orally, and GS 9137 boosted with ritonavir (see below).

Protein synthesis inhibitors

Interferon-alpha (and the longer-acting **pegylated** interferon conjugated with **p**olyethyleneglycol) block both viral RNA transcription and protein synthesis in many viruses. They are used in acute or chronic hepatitis B with lamivudine, in chronic hepatitis C with ribavirin, and at times in papillomavirus infections or Kaposi's sarcoma from HHV8 in AIDS.

Side-effects are common and unpleasant, and response is not universal, relapse common and cure rare.

Fomiversen is the first anti-sense drug, i.e. a single-strand DNA with base sequence complementary to viral mRNA. It therefore binds to mRNA and blocks translation to viral protein. It is used to treat CMV retinitis.

Methisazone inhibits the protein synthesis of pox viruses by blocking translation of late mRNA. It has been used to treat smallpox, or disseminated vaccinia from smallpox vaccine.

Protease inhibitors (PIs), preventing structural protein formation

These include **saquinavir, indinavir, ritonavir, nelfinavir, fosamprenavir, atazanavir** and **lopinavir** (with ritonavir). They act by inhibiting the proteases which normally cleave polyproteins to produce retroviral nucleocapsid proteins. Proviral DNA remains integrated so the cell is still infected, but infectious virus is not released. They are only used in combination with NRTIs ± an NNRTI to delay resistance developing. Low-dose ritonavir is also used to boost the levels of a second co-administered PI by inhibiting its metabolism by hepatic cytochrome P450 enzymes. Side-effects are seldom severe, but include gut and liver enzyme disturbance, possibly lipodystrophy, and urinary crystalluria (Fig. 3) and kidney stones from indinavir.

Viral release inhibitors

Zanamivir and **oseltamivir** (developed by Australians) inhibit the viral neuraminidase and hence the release of influenza A or B virus from infected cells, thus limiting spread to other cells and other people. Zanamivir is given by aerosol and may cause bronchospasm, while oral oseltamivir may cause nausea, diminished by food. If given early for therapy they reduce the severity and duration of illness by about 30%, and also the frequency of complications. They can also be used in short-term prophylaxis of contacts (80% effective) or longer term for 4–6 weeks during epidemic peaks. They appear effective against early strains of avian influenza, but further mutations may cause resistance.

Antiviral drugs

1. **These can act at any stage of the viral replication cycle:**
   - **Early stage** of Recognition, Attachment, Penetration and Uncoating
     - **Attachment (Fusion) Inhibitor** for HIV is enfuvirtide.
     - **Uncoating** of influenza virus is inhibited by amantadine and rimantadine.
   - **Central stage** of (reverse transcription and integration in retroviruses), mRNA synthesis, Protein synthesis by translation and Genome (nucleic acid) replication. Enzymes involved include DNA polymerase (reverse transcriptase = RT, then integrase in retroviruses), and the drugs are:
     - **Nucleoside RT inhibitors (NRTIs)** for HIV including abacavir, didanosine, emtricitabine, lamivudine, tenofovir and zidovudine
     - **Non-nucleoside RT inhibitors (NNRTIs)** for HIV including nevirapine, delavirdine and efavirenz
     - **Integrase inhibitors (IIs)** for HIV are becoming available
     - **Nucleoside inhibitors** for herpes viruses include the aciclovir group for HSV, plus ganciclovir, valganciclovir and cidofovir for CMV
     - **Non-nucleoside inhibitor** for herpes viruses is foscarnet
     - **Nucleoside inhibitors** for other viruses are ribavirin and adefovir
     - **Protein synthesis inhibitors** are interferons for Hepatitis B and C and papillomaviruses or HHV8, fomiversen for CMV and methisazone for pox viruses.
   - **Final stage** of Assembly (with proteases in retroviruses) and Release (with or without Enveloping). Drugs are:
     - **Protease inhibitors (PIs)** for HIV are saquinavir, indinavir, ritonavir, nelfinavir, fosamprenavir, atazanavir, lopinavir. All are usually boosted with ritonavir.
     - **Viral release inhibitors** for influenza are zanamivir and oseltamivir.
2. **Highly active anti-retroviral therapy** (HAART) is with 3 or more drugs, often 2 NRTIs with an NNRTI or a boosted PI.
3. Many viral infections still lack effective antiviral drugs.

Vaccines and immunisation

Boring immunisation schedules obscure exciting stories including Jenner's popularisation of vaccination to prevent smallpox, Pasteur's courageous production of rabies and anthrax vaccines, the dedicated sub-culture for 10 years of the **b**acillus *M. bovis* by **C**almette and **G**uérin to produce BCG, the conquest of polio by the Salk and Sabin teams, and today's genetic engineering of safe, specific, effective vaccines.

Definitions

Immunisation is the artificial production of immunity to an infection:

- **active** immunisation by stimulating the host to produce protective antibody and/or cell-mediated immunity
- **passive** immunisation by administering preformed antibody.
- **Simultaneous** and **combined** immunisation are described below.

Vaccination is a specific form of immunisation using vaccinia (the virus causing mild cowpox) to protect against variola (causing virulent smallpox). **Vaccine** is now a general term for any preparation containing one or more **immunogens**, i.e. substances stimulating active immunity. These are usually antigens of the microbe itself or, rarely, a closely related microbe (e.g. vaccinia for variola).

Immunogenicity is the ability to produce immunity, usually qualified as poor, good or excellent.

Adjuvants are substances enhancing the immune response, including:

- aluminium (widely used) and other salts
- bacterial products: killed *B. pertussis* in DPT is both an adjuvant to the toxoids and an immunogen itself
- cytokines (interleukins 1 and 2): experimental
- special delivery systems: antigen on small spheres such as phospholipid liposomes (experimental).

Active immunisation

Traditional types of vaccine (Table 1) are as follows.

Live attenuated bacteria or viruses

BCG, Measles-Mumps-Rubella (MMR) and oral polio vaccines are examples. Production is by the selection of mutants.

Advantages usually include high, long-lasting immunity and few side-effects. Disadvantages include potential risks from inadequate attenuation, reversion to virulent wild type, contamination by other viruses, and persistent infection especially if unknowingly given to an immunocompromised patient. However, genetic engineering of deletion mutants lacking specific virulence genes is now possible and will remove most risks.

Inactivated ('killed') bacteria or viruses

Production is by chemical inactivation, often with formaldehyde. Advantages include safety because of non-infectivity, stability, and relative ease of production. Disadvantages include lower immunogenicity and hence repeated doses.

Microbial components

Viral proteins or bacterial polysaccharides or proteins ('acellular' pertussis) are used as antigens. Production is by extraction of pneumococcal, meningococcal or *H. influenzae* type b (Hib) capsular polysaccharides (the latter conjugated to carrier protein to increase immunogenicity); by purification of plasma from hepatitis B surface-antigen chronic carriers; or by recombinant DNA technology in yeasts (hepatitis B). Advantages include production of serotype-specific (Hib) or multivalent vaccines. Disadvantages include the exacting safety measures to remove live infectious material.

Inactivated toxin (toxoid)

Production is by inactivation, usually by formaldehyde, of the bacterial toxin.

Advantages include long-lasting immunogenicity and the ability to **c**ombine several immunogens, e.g. **d**iphtheria and **t**etanus toxoids as CDT (plus killed or acellular *B. pertussis* in 'DPT', 'triple antigen'). Disadvantage is the restriction to toxin-mediated disease.

Heterologous vaccines

These use immunisation across species, i.e. using vaccinia, an animal virus sharing antigens with smallpox, to immunise humans.

Experimental vaccines

Cloned or synthetic peptides. Cloning genes into *E. coli*, yeast, insect or mammalian vectors produces a range of potentially immunogenic peptides (or glycosylated proteins). These are tested for potent T-cell and B-cell 'epitopes' to trigger T- and B-cell responses. Advantages are the wide range of microbes potentially suitable, the specificity and the safety. Disadvantages are the complex technology, wide-ranging testing, unsuitability for carbohydrate or glycolipid antigens and, often, the need to increase immunogenicity. The latter can be achieved by attachment to larger carriers such as tetanus toxoid or polylysine to which eight antigen peptides have been attached: the 'octopus' molecule.

Microbial vectors for cloned genes. Production is by using an existing vaccine as the expression vector (e.g. BCG) with the inserted gene(s) as a polyvaccine, which in the patient multiplies to deliver immunising protein or peptide. Advantages are the potential for polyvaccines, even a one-shot vaccine. As BCG induces cell-mediated immunity, it could

Table 1 **Major current vaccine types and usage**			
Type	**General use**	**Specific use**	**Developmental**
Live attenuated bacteria	BCG	Typhoid (oral), tularaemia	Cholera, shigellosis
Live attenuated virus	Measles, mumps, rubella, polio (oral), influenza (rare), varicella	Yellow fever, smallpox, adenovirus	RSV, CMV, HSV, rotavirus
Inactivated bacteria	Pertussis (outmoded)	Cholera, plague, Q fever, typhus	Gonorrhoea
Inactivated virus	Polio (injectable)	Hepatitis A, rabies, Japanese encephalitis	
Microbial components	*H. influenzae* b,[a] influenza, meningococcal,[a] pertussis (acellular)	Hepatitis B, anthrax, pneumococcal,[a] typhoid (inj)	Lyme disease
Toxoid	Diphtheria, tetanus		Cholera, botulism
Protozoal			Malaria

[a]Polysaccharide.

in theory carry antigens for other persistent intracellular organisms including *Brucella, Listeria, Rickettsia, Chlamydia, Histoplasma, Leishmania, Toxoplasma* spp., malaria and many viruses! Disadvantages are the complex technology and the unsuitability for carbohydrate or glycolipid antigens.

Anti-idiotype vaccines
Production of anti-idiotype vaccines is by making a first antibody to the antigen, then making numerous second antibodies to the first and testing to find a second antibody (anti-idiotype) resembling the antigen. This protein second antibody can be used as a surrogate antigen. Advantages are safety, specificity and the ability to make an immunogen from carbohydrate or glycolipid antigens, which cannot be cloned or synthesised as above. Disadvantages are the complex technology and the wide-ranging search required to find suitable anti-idiotypes.

Passive immunisation

Passive immunity is produced by giving pre-formed specific or non-specific immunoglobulin. The effect is therefore immediate but temporary.

Specific immunoglobulin is from convalescent or immunised donors or, sometimes, from immunised horses (e.g. against gas gangrene or diphtheria). It is used post-exposure in the non-immunised for botulism, gas gangrene, hepatitis B, rabies, snake or scorpion bite and tetanus; in varicella-zoster exposure in the immunocompromised; and in treatment of diphtheria, gas gangrene and tetanus.

Non-specific immunoglobulin is from pooled normal plasma from blood donors. It was used in normal hosts before travel (against hepatitis A when vaccine unavailable) or post-exposure (measles), or monthly in antibody immunodeficiencies, such as agammaglobulinaemia, or in bone marrow transplants (for CMV protection).

Combined active and passive immunisation is used in post-exposure prophylaxis in the unvaccinated for rabies or tetanus (Table 2) or at birth to babies of hepatitis B carrier mothers.

Simultaneous immunisation with several vaccines by different syringes at different sites is usually satisfactory, except for yellow fever and cholera vaccines, which reduce antibody response to each other.

When and who to vaccinate

Immunisation is a life-long commitment:

- immunisation schedules for childhood and adolescence are published for each country; schedules vary depending on disease incidence and vaccine costs
- adults should have ADT (adult diphtheria/tetanus) and oral polio vaccine (OPV) every 10 years from 15 to 65 years, pneumococcal vaccine at age 65, and influenza vaccine yearly thereafter, particularly with pulmonary or cardiac disease
- specific occupations need specific vaccines, including hepatitis B (health workers), anthrax, plague, Q fever, rabies, and tularaemia

- special-risk groups needing specialised protection are the armed forces, college students, the homeless, prisoners and pregnant mothers
- travellers need **R**outine, **R**equired and **R**ecommended vaccines, such as hepatitis A, meningococcal, typhoid, cholera and yellow fever vaccines, depending on the area (p. 216).

Contraindications to vaccination
Contraindications and adverse reactions vary with each vaccine, but there are three general rules:

1. Live vaccines should not be given in pregnancy or to immunocompromised patients, except measles vaccine to HIV-positive children.
2. Conversely, inactivated or component vaccines are safe. Splenectomised patients should have pneumococcal and meningococcal vaccines, before splenectomy if possible for best antibody response.
3. The adverse effects of all available vaccines are many times less than their benefit.

Future needs

Major infections with no satisfactory vaccine include hepatitis C, sexually transmitted diseases (especially gonorrhoea, HIV and syphilis), malaria, schistosomiasis, trypanosomiasis and other parasitic diseases, and viral infections including CMV, HSV and RSV. In all, antigenic variation, poor immunity even after natural infection, and the threat of reversion or latency with living attenuated vaccines are obstacles slowly being overcome.

Table 2 **Tetanus prophylaxis in managing wounds**
1. The wound itself must be cleaned, debrided and managed appropriately
2. Toxoid alone is dependable up to 10 years after full immunisation
3. Immunoglobulin is added for tetanus-prone wounds

Tetanus immunisation history	Minor, clean wounds		All other wounds	
	Tet toxoid, CDT[a] or ADT[a]	Tetanus immunoglobulin	Tet toxoid, CDT[a] or ADT[a]	Tetanus immunoglobulin
3 doses or more, and < 5 years from last dose	No	No	No	No[b]
3 doses or more but 5–10 years from the last	No	No	Yes	No[b]
3 doses or more but > 10 years from the last	Yes	No	Yes	Yes[c]
Less than 3 doses or uncertain	Yes	No	Yes	Yes

[a] CDT or ADT is preferred to tetanus toxoid, to boost immunity to diphtheria also.
[b] In some countries, immunoglobulin is advised for tetanus-prone wounds (penetrating, necrotic or neglected) in this category.
[c] TPW, tetanus prone wounds only, in some countries.

Vaccines and immunisation

- Immunisation is a safe, cost-effective way of preventing many severe health- or life-threatening diseases and should be used in childhood and adolescence, in adult life and in special groups including health workers and travellers.
- The adverse effects of all available vaccines are many times less than their benefit.
- Mild upper respiratory tract infection is not a contraindication to immunisation: more serious disease with fever above 38°C should only defer immunisation by 10 days.
- Every medical consultation is an opportunity to consider immunisation.

Clinician and laboratory: microbial detection and identification

Microbiology laboratories help clinicians directly in four ways:

A. Detecting and identifying the microbes causing infections
B. Measuring host antibody response when microbes aren't easily detected
C. Guiding therapy
D. Assisting infection control.

Laboratories also help indirectly by teaching and research.

The laboratory, the clinician and the patient are all helped when the clinician provides written notes about the specimen, the sufferer and the suspected pathogen(s). This means:

- specimens correctly collected, legibly labelled and swiftly sent to the laboratory, so pathogens survive
- clinical conditions, differential diagnoses and administered antimicrobials noted on the request slip
- possible peculiar pathogens noted, so relevant special techniques are used.

DETECTING AND IDENTIFYING THE MICROBES

Detecting and identifying the microbes causing infections usually requires four steps:

1. specimen collection, transport and processing
2. direct detection methods
3. culture
4. identification.

1. Specimen collection, transport and processing

Specimens should be collected from the site of infection and any spread. Specimens include swabs (good), fluids (better) or tissue (best).

Swabs. Eye, ear, nose, throat, wound, ulcer and genital swabs are easily obtained but provide small volumes which dry easily, so stains may be poor and cultures negative.

Fluids. Samples of pus, urine, sputum, bile, CSF and blood are better, as volumes are greater and organisms survive transport better; stains or cultures are more likely to be positive.

Tissue. Samples of tissue are best as organisms are usually most concentrated and most viable, though tissue is most difficult to collect.

Processing specimens. While specimens are sometimes processed beside the patient (blood films for malaria, fungal scrapings, genital discharges), most are transported to the laboratory for processing, as quickly as possible to preserve pathogens. Transport media can be used if delay is unavoidable but may interfere with microscopy and stains. *When in doubt about specimen collection, transport or processing, ask the laboratory.*

2. Direct detection methods

Direct methods include microscopy, stains, and detection of antigen, nucleic acid or metabolic products. These take minutes or a few hours and can provide a microbe-specific diagnosis for many fungi and parasites, and for viruses or bacteria with distinctive morphology, staining, antigens or metabolic products.

Direct microscopy

Direct microscopy is used for larger organisms with distinctive shapes. Techniques include:

- **wet mount** in saline for genital and gut parasites
- **KOH** for fungi in skin scrapings
- **Indian ink** to highlight cryptococci in fluids (Fig. 1)
- **dark field (dark ground) microscopy** (DGM) for syphilis.

Stains

Stains are used to show and differentiate microbes:

- **Gram's stain** is the quick, easy, usual stain for common bacteria, showing their shape and cell wall type (p. 3).
- **Acid-fast stains** (Ziehl-Neelsen, Auramine-rhodamine) are used for mycobacteria (Fig. 2), *Nocardia* and *Cryptosporidium* spp.
- **Special stains** for organisms not staining with the above:
  - toluidine blue or PAS for fungi and *P. jirovecii*
  - silver stains for fungi, legionellae, *P. jirovecii*, rickettsiae and treponemes

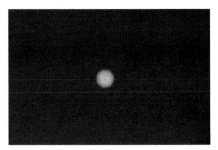

Fig. 1 *C. neoformans* (Indian ink).

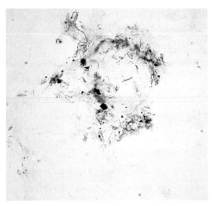

Fig. 2 *M. tuberculosis* (ZN stain).

  - Giemsa or Wright's stains for malaria; overwhelming bacteraemia may rarely be seen in blood films
  - acridine orange for staining DNA, even in damaged microbes
  - methylene blue for faecal leucocytes.
- **Special viral techniques** include light microscopy for inclusion bodies or giant cells, and electron microscopy for viral size and morphology.

Antigen detection

Antigen detection (= immunodetection) uses specific antibody to detect a microbial antigen:

- **Agglutination** uses antibody coupled to latex particles or RBC which visibly agglutinate with antigen (e.g. capsular polysaccharide, protein), detecting *N. meningitidis*, *H. influenzae*, *S. pneumoniae*, *S. pyogenes*, *Cryptococcus neoformans* (Fig. 3) and viruses.
- **Co-agglutination** uses protein A of *S. aureus* to attach to the Fc part of an antibody and thus orientate the antigen-specific Fab fragment outward to agglutinate with antigen.
- **Direct immunofluorescence** (DIF) uses fluorescein-tagged antibody, detecting, e.g., viruses.

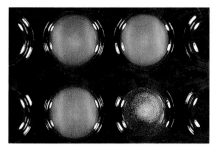

Fig. 3 **Antigen detection (latex agglutination) of _C. neoformans_.**

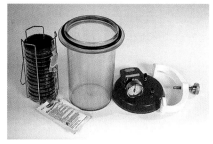

Fig. 4 **Anaerobic jar components.**

- **ELISA** (enzyme linked immunosorbent assay, an **EIA**, Enzyme Immuno-Assay) has almost replaced **radioimmunoassay** (RIA). Both use a solid phase such as a microtitre plate with antibody which binds antigen. This is then measured by the binding of a second ligand either labelled by radioactivity (RIA) or an enzyme detected by colour change (ELISA/EIA).
- **Immunocytochemistry** uses specific antibody on tissue sections.
- **Monoclonal antibody** is being increasingly used.

Nucleic acid detection

This is achieved in several ways:

- **Polymerase chain reaction** (PCR) multiplies even one segment of DNA a million times in a few hours. It is very specific and so sensitive that contamination is a problem without fastidious technique. It is now the standard method for many pathogens.
- **Nucleic acid probes** use labelled DNA or RNA to probe for target nucleic acid. They are very specific, being used (± PCR) to quantify 'viral load' in HIV.
- **Plasmid fingerprinting** separates plasmids by agarose gel electro-phoresis and is used epidemiologically.
- **Restriction enzyme** analysis shows defined DNA nucleotide sequences; it is also used epidemiologically.

Metabolic product detection

This includes gas liquid chromatography (GLC), detecting the different fatty acids produced by different anaerobic bacteria, helping rapid identification.

3. Culture

Culture of microbes in specimens takes at least some hours, more usually one or more days; it can be more specific than non-cultural methods and gives live organisms for full identification and sensitivity testing. Each specimen type is cultured in several particular media chosen to grow the likely pathogens. Media may be enriched, selective, indicator, specific or a combination. Media may be liquid to give maximum growth (e.g. from swabs), solid to separate different organisms, or tissue culture, particularly for viruses and small bacteria.

Enriched media. Enriching substances to encourage growth include blood agar (BA) or chocolate agar (CA), which is blood agar heated to 60°C, releasing nutrients for fastidious bacteria.

Selective media. These use inhibitory substances to inhibit growth of some bacteria. They may be combined with indicator and/or enrichment substances. They include:

- MacConkey agar (Mac) or deoxycholate citrate agar (DCA), which contain bile as an inhibitor that enteric bacteria survive, plus lactose and an indicator to differentiate between lactose and non-lactose fermenters (p. 46)
- Sabouraud's dextrose agar, with low pH to grow fungi but inhibit other organisms
- Lowenstein-Jensen agar, with glycerol to grow mycobacteria, and malachite green to inhibit other bacteria.

Indicator media. These use pH indicators in Mac and DCA, or can use anti-serum (e.g. Hayward's medium for the Nagler test for clostridia).

Special media. Fastidious organisms require special media, including Robertson's cooked meat medium (RCM or CMM) for growing anaerobes, or special media for _Chlamydia_, _Mycoplasma_, or _Rickettsia_. Tissue culture for viruses uses cytopathogenic effect (CPE, ± haemadsorption, interference, and neutralisation), Complement Fixation, Haemagglutination-Inhibition, Fluorescent Antibody Assay, ImmuneElectronMicroscopy, RIA, and ELISA.

Incubation. Cultures may be incubated in special atmospheres: CO_2 for _Haemophilus_ and _Neisseria_ spp., anaerobic for clostridia and Gram-negative anaerobes, or microaerophilic for _Campylobacter_ spp. (Fig. 4). Special temperatures are also sometimes required (e.g. 42°C for _Campylobacter_ spp. or 30°C for _M. ulcerans_).

4. Identification

Provisional identification is often possible, except for viruses, through:

- Gram (or other) stain
- organism's shape (coccus or rod), pattern (chains, pairs) and characters (capsule, spores, intracellular position, ova, cysts, conidia)
- growth requirements (aerobic, anaerobic, fastidious, bile resistance).

Definitive identification is usually then either by serological methods, including antigen detection as above, or biochemical methods.
Biochemical methods include:

- enzyme detection including coagulase, catalase, oxidase
- substrate utilisation, especially sugars including lactose, sucrose, glucose
- metabolism of sugars oxidatively (aerobically) or fermentatively (anaerobically).

Microbial detection and identification

- Clinicians must provide **c**orrectly **c**ollected and **l**egibly **l**abelled specimens for proper processing.
- Clinicians must notify **c**linical **c**onditions, **d**ifferential **d**iagnoses and **a**ntimicrobials **a**dministered for reliable results.
- Direct detection depends on microscopy, stains, antigen detection (immunodetection), nucleic acid detection or metabolic product detection.
- Culture on enriched, selective, indicator and/or specific media gives further information plus live organisms for full identification and antimicrobial sensitivity tests.
- Identification if not definitive from the above information is made by biochemical and serological tests.

Clinician and laboratory: antibody response and guiding therapy

Measuring host antibody response

Measuring host antibody levels (called 'titres') using a specific antigen is the converse of microbial antigen detection (p. 238–239), often adapting the same methods, including agglutination (Fig. 1), flocculation, precipitation, particle- and haem-agglutination and its inhibition (HAI), complement fixation tests (CFT), enzyme immunoassays (EIA) including ELISA, fluorescent antibody and neutralisation tests. These major analyses are part of serology.

Antibody analysis is used only when the microbe or an antigen cannot easily or safely be found (e.g. *Brucella, Mycoplasma, Rickettsia* infections, systemic mycoses, many viruses) for it has three major disadvantages: firstly, a specific antigen must be used, so the specific disease must be suspected; secondly, 2–4 weeks pass before IgM antibodies are detectable; and, thirdly, IgG may be present already from previous infection or immunisation, hence the need usually to show an antibody rise (see below).

Clinical uses are:

- diagnosis of acute infection, usually by antibody rise in two 'paired' sera, one acute and one convalescent; sometimes an elevated IgM in a single acute serum sample is used, or a single elevated convalescent antibody if a response is short-lived, e.g. legionellosis
- determining the immune status, either before immunisation (e.g. rubella) or after exposure ('needlesticks', hepatitis B and C, HIV).

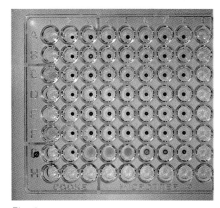

Fig. 1 **Antibody detection by particle agglutination.**

Guiding therapy

Sensitivity testing

There are two steps in antibiotic sensitivity testing.

First, a precise laboratory method measures whether the organism is affected by ('susceptible' to) chosen concentration(s) of the test antibiotic. A single concentration in disc methods gives only an approximate susceptibility, while dilution tests with a series of concentrations give an exact MIC (minimum inhibitory concentration: the lowest concentration inhibiting microbial growth) and can be continued to give the MBC (minimum bactericidal concentration: kills the microbe).

Secondly, with rules based on experience, an imprecise prediction of the likely clinical response is given:

S: susceptible or sensitive, i.e. likely to respond
R: resistant, i.e. unlikely to respond
I: intermediate, may respond to very high dose or where antibiotic is concentrated, e.g. in urine.

Methods use known amounts of antibiotic and include the following.

Diffusion tests (6–18 hours)

Disc diffusion uses antibiotic in paper discs placed on a lawn of organism on special agar (Fig. 2). The antibiotic diffuses outwards giving a gradient of decreasing concentration, so zone size is related to degree of susceptibility. The test is cheap, easy and accurate if standardised.

Stokes' adaptation of disc diffusion uses a sensitive control organism, either on half the plate or concentrically around the periphery (Fig. 3). It helps control disc quality.

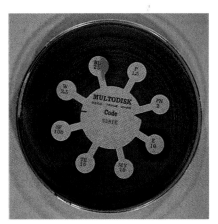

Fig. 2 **Sensitivity test: disc method.**

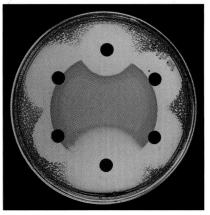

Fig. 3 **Sensitivity test: J Stokes method.**

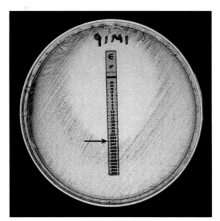

Fig. 4 **Sensitivity test: E-test strip: *Nocardia* sp./imipenem.**

E-test uses a graded concentration on a strip, so the MIC is read where the junction of growth–no growth intersects the strip (Fig. 4). It is exact, useful for unusual organisms or antibiotics, but relatively expensive.

Dilution tests (4–18 hours)

Agar dilution uses antibiotic diluted uniformly through special agar, testing about 30 different organisms per plate (Fig. 5). It is exact and economic when testing at least 25 organisms daily but usually takes 16–18 hours.

Broth dilution uses antibiotic diluted in broth in tubes or microtitre plates. It also is exact and economic in larger laboratories; it is the basis of several common *automated systems*, taking 4–6 hours.

Killing curves (6–18 hours)

Some automated methods use broth and measure killing curves over time instead of the simple 'growth–no growth at one point in time' information provided by the diffusion or dilution methods above.

Synergy tests (usually overnight)

Tests to measure whether two antibiotics show synergy (at least four times greater effect than expected by addition), indifference (no effect on each other) or antagonism (decreased effect) usually use a chequer-board of broth dilutions in microtitre plates, with one antibiotic in doubling dilutions across and the other down.

Enzyme detection

Beta-lactamase is easily detected (e.g. in *H. influenzae* and many enteric Gram-negative rods) by a special cephalosporin, nitrocefin, which changes colour in a few hours when the lactam ring is broken by beta-lactamase (Fig. 6).

Extended-spectrum beta-lactamases (**ESBLs**) destroy third-generation cephalosporins and are now found in numerous enteric pathogens in hospitals. They

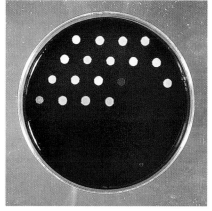

Fig. 5 **Agar dilution, control.**

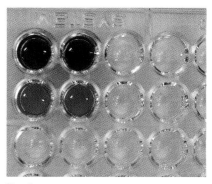

Fig. 6 **β-lactamase test (nitrocefin).**

are easily shown in 12–18 hours in the laboratory when the clavulanate in an amoxicillin-clavulanate disc inactivates the ESBL and, thus, causes expansion of the zone around a nearby cefotaxime (or other third generation cephalosporin) disc (Fig. 7). Antibiotic-induced cephalosporinases in **ESCAPPMs** (p. 218) and **metallo-betalactamases** are shown by related techniques.

Antibiotic and other assays

Antibiotic levels can be measured overnight by bio-assay, measuring zones around four wells in agar, three containing known concentrations of the antibiotic and one with the patient's serum. This is cheap, slow and inexact.

Chemical methods are now common, exact, quick (20–60 minutes) and affordable. 'Peak' levels taken 10–30 minutes post-dose, and 'trough' levels taken pre-dose have been the usual samples for aminoglycosides and vancomycin. Efficacy of aminoglycosides is related to the peak level and the **a**rea **u**nder the (level-time) **c**urve (AUC), while toxicity is more related to the trough.

Serum bactericidal titre is the killing power of the patient's serum against the organism causing their endocarditis or other serious infection. Cure is believed

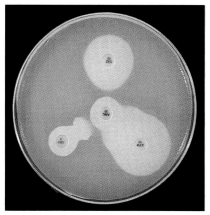

Fig. 7 **Extended spectrum β-lactamase test (ESBL).** Note deformed zone around third-generation cephalosporin induced by adjacent clavulanic acid disc.

more likely if serum diluted 1:8 kills their organism, but this view is challenged so this overnight test is now uncommon.

Giving advice

Giving advice on appropriate tests to do, and the meaning of particular test results is an important function of medical microbiologists and of senior scientists. They can also give advice on appropriate therapy, especially if infectious disease physicians are not available.

Assisting infection control

This is detailed on page 219.

Antibody response and guiding therapy

■ Host antibody response is used to diagnose infection only when the causative microbe is not easily or safely detected by microscopy, culture, antigen or nucleic acid detection. Inherent disadvantages are the need for specific antigens, the slowness of antibody response, and the possible presence of IgG antibody from previous infection or immunisation, so paired acute and convalescent sera and IgM tests are preferred.
■ Antibody tests are also used to find the person's immune status before or after immunisation, or after exposure.

■ Antimicrobial sensitivity tests attempt to predict a patient's response from a laboratory test without reference to the host defence mechanisms so cannot be 100% reliable.
■ Antimicrobial levels, usually in serum, rarely in CSF, can be used to estimate both likely efficacy and possible toxicity. There cannot be a single level which separates safety from toxicity.
■ Giving advice on appropriate tests, the meaning of results, appropriate therapy and infection control are important functions of clinical microbiologists and infectious disease physicians.

Further reading

Medical microbiology

- Medical Microbiology. Mims C, Playfair JHL et al. Mosby, 3rd edn, 2005. *Established British book with excellent illustrations.*
- Medical Microbiology. Greenwood D et al. Churchill Livingstone, 16th edn, 2003. *Very established British book, updated and detailed.*
- Notes on Medical Microbiology. Timbury M, McCartney AC, Thakker B, Ward KN. Churchill Livingstone, 1st edn, 2002. *Amalgam of two Notebooks, succinct and clear.*
- Medical Microbiology. Murray PR, Rosenthal KS, Pfaller MA. Wolfe, 5th edn, 2005. *US book with clear text and beautiful diagrams.*
- Medical Microbiology and Immunology. Levinson WE. Lange, 2004. *US book, clear but dull presentation; strong in virology and immunology.*

Virology

- Principles and Practice of Clinical Virology. Zuckerman AJ, Banatvala JE, Pattison JR, Griffiths PD, Schoub BD (eds). Wiley, 5th edn, 2004. *Large, detailed book with over 50 international authors.*

Infectious diseases

- Mandell, Douglas and Bennett's Principles and Practice of Infectious Diseases. Mandell GL, Bennett JE, Dolin R. Churchill Livingstone, 6th edn, 2004. *Encyclopaedic 2-volume reference text.*
- Infectious Diseases – A Clinical Approach. Yung A, Spelman DW et al. IP Communications, 2nd edn, 2005. *Entirely different approach, by patient presentation rather than by disease or organisms.*

Antimicrobial use

- Antibiotic and Chemotherapy. Finch R, Greenwood D, Norrby S R, Whitley R. Churchill Livingstone, 8th edn, 2003. *The standard British text.*
- The Use of Antibiotics. Kucers A, Crowe SM, Grayson ML, Hoy JF. Butterworth Heinemann, 5th edn, 1997. *Encyclopaedic, comprehensive, extensive text and references.*
- Antibiotic Guidelines. Spicer WJ and Writing Group. Therapeutic Guidelines, 13th edn, 2006. *Concise pocket book, also available on CD with several updates each year.*
- Sanford Guide to Antimicrobial Therapy. Gilbert DN et al. 36th edn, 2006. *Concise pocket book, also available on CD.*

Sexually transmitted diseases and HIV/AIDS

- Sexual Health Medicine. Russell D, Bradford D, Fairley C (eds). IP Communications, 1st edn, 2005. *Not only sexually transmitted disease, but also reproductive health, control, sexuality issues.*
- Sanford Guide to HIV/AIDS. 14th edn, 2005. *Authoritative US text; tiny print in pocket version.*

Tropical/travel medicine

- Manson's Tropical Diseases. Cook G, Zumla A (eds). Saunders, 21st edn, 2002 (1st edn 1898). *Classic text for over a century, continues to be relevant.*
- Tropical Infectious Diseases. Guerrant RL, Walker DH, Weller PF. Churchill Livingstone, 2nd edn, 2006. *Two-volume reference book.*
- Lecture Notes on Tropical Medicine. Beeching N, Gill G, Bell D. Blackwell Science, 5th edn, 2004. *Nice small book, clearly set out, very good tables.*
- Travel Medicine. Yung A, Ruff T, Torresi J, Leder K, O'Brien D. IP Communications, 2nd edn, 2004. *Pre-travel guide of principles, immunisation, major syndromes, special problems.*

Index

Pages 34–93 cover SPECIFIC PATHOGENS. Pages 94–223 cover CLINICAL INFECTIONS.

A

Abacavir, 234
Abdominal infections
  abscess, 164–5
  tropical, 173
Abscess, 34, 35
  brain, 102–3
  breast, 214
  Brodie's, 206
  central nervous system, 102
  dental, 115
  extradural, 103
  intra-abdominal, 164–5
  intrarenal, 176, 177
  liver
    amoebic, 168
    pyogenic, 168–9
  lung, 130–1
  orbital, 109
  pelvic, 185
  perinephric, 176
  periodontal, 115
  psoas, 157
  subdural, 103
  subperiosteal, 109
  tubo-ovarian, 185
  vulval, 187
Absidia spp., 195
Absidia corymbifera, 76
Acanthamoeba spp., 80
  keratitis, 108
Aciclovir, 102, 234
Acinetobacter spp., 43
Acinetobacter calcoaceticus var
    anitratus, 2
Acquired immune response, 28
Actinomadura spp., 202
Actinomyces spp., 62
  brain abscess, 102–3
  canaliculitis, 109
  focal CNS infections, 102
  gingivitis, 115
  lung abscess, 130
  meningitis, 94
  mycetoma, 202
  periapical/alveolar abscess, 115
  salpingitis, 184
Actinomyces israelii, 134
Actinomycosis, 122, 134, 209
Acute disseminated
    encephalomyelitis, 96–7
Acute phase proteins, 27
Acute phase reactants, 32
Adefovir, 235
Adenovirus diarrhoea, 161
Adherence, 31
Adhesins, 21
Adhesion, 26
Adjuvants, 236
Aerococcus viridans, 55
Aeromonas spp., 51

Aeromonas hydrophila, 51, 195
  wound infections, 196
Aeromonas liquefaciens, 51
Aerophobia, 96
Aflatoxins, 8
African eye worm, 77, 86, 111
Aggressive pathogens, 23
AIDS, 149-51
  causative virus, 149
  chemoprophylaxis, 151
  chemotherapy, 151, 234-5
  cholangiopathy, 166–7
  clinical stages, 149
  confirmatory tests, 151
  control and prevention, 151
  dementia, 151
  malignancies, 150-1,
  opportunistic infections, 150
  wasting syndrome, 151
  see also HIV/AIDS
Airborne transmission, 24
Albendazole, 85, 102, 169, 213, 233
Allylamine, 232
Alternaria alternata, 75
Alternative pathway, 27
Amantadine, 234
Amastigote, 83
Amikacin, 229, 230
Amino acids, 5
Aminoglycosides, 229, 230
Amoebae, 80–81
Amoebiasis, cutaneous, 204
Amoebic dysentery, 162
Amoebic liver abscess, 168
Amoebic meningoencephalitis, 80
Amphotericin B, 70, 71, 75, 76, 94,
    102, 232
Ampicillin, 94
Anaerobic bacteria,
  Gram positive, 39, 41
  Gram negative, 54-55
Anaphylaxis, 30
Ancylostoma braziliense, 204
Ancylostoma duodenale, 85, 162
  diarrhoeal disease, 163
Angiostrongylus cantonensis, 98, 99
Animal bite infections, 196–7
Anthelminthics, 233
Anthrax, cutaneous, 194
Antibacterials, 226–7, 228–9, 230-1
  activity, 227
  aminoglycosides, 229, 230
  aztreonam, 230
  beta-lactams, 229, 230
  cell membrane function
    inhibitors, 227
  cell wall synthesis inhibitors, 226,
    228–9
  chloramphenicol, 230
  classification, 226
  clinical use, 227
  lincosamides, 229, 230

macrolides, 229, 231
mechanisms of resistance, 227
nitroimidazoles, 229, 231
nucleic acid synthesis inhibitors,
    227, 231
pharmacokinetics, 227
physicochemical properties, 227
protein synthesis inhibitors,
    226–7
quinolones, 231
rifamycins, 229, 231
side effects and toxicity, 227
tetracyclines, 231
vancomycin and teicoplanin, 230
Antibodies, 19, 28–9
  classes of, 28–9
  mode of action, 28
Antibody defects, 220–1
Antibody response, 240
Antibody-dependent cell-mediated
    cytotoxicity, 19
Antibody-dependent cytotoxicity,
    30
Antifungal drugs, 232–3
Antigenic variation, 31
Antimalarial drugs, 233
Antimycobacterial drugs, 232
Antiparasitic drugs, 233
Antiprotozoal drugs, 233
Antisepsis, 224
Antiviral drugs, 234–5
  DNA polymerase inhibitors,
    234–5
  fusion inhibitors, 234
  integrase inhibitors, 235
  protease inhibitors, 235
  protein synthesis inhibitors, 235
  release inhibitors, 235
  uncoating inhibitors, 234
ANUG, 114, 115
Aphthous stomatitis, 113
Apicomplexa, 10
Apolipoprotein B, 19
Arachnida, 12
  infections, 13
Arboviruses, 77, 146
  encephalitis, 96
Artemether, 233
Artemisinin derivatives, 233
Artesunate, 233
Arthritis, 145
  infective, 210–11
  with rash, 146
Arthropoda, 12, 77
Ascaris lumbricoides, 12, 85, 162
  cholangitis, 166
  diarrhoeal disease, 163
  eggs, 13
Ascomycotina, 6
Asepsis, 224
Aspergilloma, 134
Aspergillosis, 68, 102, 134, 157

Aspergillus spp., 9, 68, 195
  canaliculitis, 109
  characteristics, 68
  endophthalmitis, 112
  stomatitis, 113
Aspergillus flavus, 8, 68, 134
Aspergillus fumigatus, 68, 134
Aspergillus niger, 134
  diagnosis, 7
Astrovirus diarrhoea, 158, 161
Atazanavir, 235
Atypical viral-like agents, 14–15
Autoclaving, 225
Autotrophs, 4
Auxotrophy, 4
Azithromycin, 64, 229, 231
Aztreonam, 229, 230

B

B-cells, 28
Bacillus spp., 39
  keratitis, 108
Bacillus anthracis, 39, 56
  lymphadenitis, 137
  toxin, 21
Bacillus cereus, 39, 195
  diarrhoea, 158, 160
  endophthalmitis, 112
Bacteraemia, 34, 39, 142–3
  Salmonella spp., 48
Bacteria, 2–5
  capsule, 31, 34
  cell wall, 3, 31
  see also individual genera and
    organisms.
Bacterial overgrowth syndromes,
    159
Bacterial vaginosis, 187
Bacteriuria, 175
Bacteroides spp., 22, 54
  bite infections, 197
  brain abscess, 102
  crepitant anaerobic cellulitis, 194
  empyaema, 131
  periapical/alveolar abscess, 115
Bacteroides fragilis, 54
  cholecystitis, 166
  lung abscess, 130
Bacteroides gingivalis, 115
Bacteroides intermedius, gingivitis,
    115
Bairnsdale (Buruli) ulcer, 202–3
Balamuthia mandrillaris, 80
Balanitis, 186
Balantidium coli, 10, 11, 81
  diarrhoeal disease, 162
Barcoo rot, 38
Bartonella spp., 67
Bartonella bacilliformis, 67
Bartonella henselae, 67
Bartonella quintana, 67, 77

Basidiomycotina, 6
Beef tapeworm, 88,162
Bejel, 203
Beta-lactams, 229, 230
Beta-lactamase, 241
Bifidobacterium spp., 62
Biliary infections, 166–7
  AIDS cholangiopathy, 166–7
  cholangitis, 166
  cholecystitis, 166
  portal pylephlebitis, 167
Biovars, 57
Black death, 57
Black piedra, 74, 198
Blastomyces dermatitidis, 9, 72, 135
  chemotherapy, 72
  clinical syndromes and
    management, 72
  confirmatory tests, 72
Blastomycosis, 135
Blepharitis, 108
Bone infections (Osteomyelitis),
    206–209
Bordetella bronchiseptica, 45
Bordetella parapertussis, 45, 123
Bordetella pertussis, 44–5, 123
  clinical syndrome and
    management, 44–5
  confirmatory tests, 44
  virulence factors, 45
Borrelia spp., 59
  relapsing fever, 154–5
Borrelia afzelii, 59
Borrelia burgdorferi, 56, 59, 77
  Lyme disease, 57, 77, 99
  meningitis, 94
Borrelia garinii, 59
Borrelia recurrentis, 59, 77
Botulism, 104
  infant, 41
  wound, 41
Boutonneuse fever, 66
Bovine spongiform
encephalopathy, 100
Brain abscesses, 102–3
Branhamella spp., 43
Breast infections, postnatal, 214
Brill-Zinsser disease, 67
Brodie's abscess, 206
Bronchial infections, 124–5
Bronchiectasis, 125
Bronchiolitis, 116
Bronchiolitis obliterans, 116
Bronchitis, acute, 124
Brucella spp., 56
  lymphadenitis, 137
  meningitis, 94
  uveitis, 112
Brucella abortus, 212
  granulomatous hepatitis, 173
Brucella canis, 212
Brucella melitensis, 212
Brucella suis, 212
Brucellosis, 99, 209, 212
Brugia malayi, 86
  filariasis, 205
Brugia timori, filariasis, 205
Bruton's agammaglobulinaemia, 221
Bubonic plague, 213
Bullous impetigo, 192
Burkholderia spp., 52
Burkholderia cepacia, 52
  in cystic fibrosis, 125

Burkholderia mallei, 52
Burkholderia pseudomallei, 52, 134
  lymphadenitis, 137
Burkitt's lymphoma, 145
Burns, infected, 197
Burst size, 16

C

Calabar swellings, 111
Cladosporium carrionii, 75
Calicivirus, diarrhoea, 158, 161
*Calymmatobacterium (Klebsiella)
    granulomatis*, 49, 188.
Campylobacter spp., 50–1
  clinical syndromes and
    management, 50–1
  confirmatory tests, 50
  control, 51
  diarrhoea, 160
Campylobacter coli, 50
Campylobacter fetus, 31
Campylobacter foetus, 50
Campylobacter jejuni, 50
  diarrhoea, 158
Campylobacter lari, 50
Canaliculitis, 109
Cancrum oris, 113, 122
Candida spp., 6, 9, 23, 68–9
  canaliculitis, 109
  characteristics, 68–9
  chorioretinitis, 112
  endophthalmitis, 112
  infective arthritis, 210
  stomatitis, 113
Candida albicans, 7, 9, 22, 68–69
  balanitis, 186
  suppurative thrombophlebitis,
    136
Candida glabrata, 68
Candida parapsilosis, 68
Candida tropicalis, 68
Candidiasis, 25, 102, 157, 187
  cutaneous, 199
  macronodular, 199
  mucocutaneous, 221
Capnocytophaga canimorsus, 197
Capsules, 31, 34
Carbuncles, 192
Carcinogens, sources of, 23
Cardiobacterium hominis, 53, 140
Caries, 114
Caspofungin, 232
Cat scratch disease, 197
Ceftriaxone, 94, 102
Cefuroxime, 35
Cell-mediated hypersensitivity, 30
Cell-mediated immunity, 9, 19, 29
  defects in, 221
Cellulitis, 191, 192–3
  crepitant anaerobic, 194
  synergistic necrotic, 195
Central nervous system
  abscesses, 102
  ADEM, 96
  cysts, 103
  diffuse non-viral infections,
    98–99
  encephalitis,
    acute, 95-6
    chronic, 100-101
  focal lesions, 102
  meningitis, 39, 94–5

rabies, 96
  viral and prion diseases, 100–1
Cephalexin, 35
Cephalosporins, 228–9
Cephalothin, 35
Cerebritis, 94
Cervical infections, 182–3
  cervicitis, 182–3
  human papillomavirus, 182
Cervical lymphadenitis, 122
Cervicitis, 182–3
  causative organisms, 182
  chemotherapy, 183
  clinical features, 182–3
  confirmatory tests, 183
  control and prevention, 183
Cestodes (Tapeworms), 12–13,
    88–89
Chagas' disease, 77, 110, 138
Chalazion, 108
Chancriform ulcers, 194
Chancroid, 188
Chemical humoral mediators, 27
Chemical peritonitis, 164
Chemotaxis, 26
Chemotrophy, 4
Chicken-pox, 146
Chiclero's ear, 205
Children, viral infections, 144–6
Chinese liver flukes, 90, 173
Chitin, 6
Chlamydia spp., 64–5
Chlamydia pneumoniae
  bronchitis, 124
  laryngitis, 123
  tonsillitis, 118
Chlamydia trachomatis, 64–5
  cervicitis, 172
  characteristics, 64-5
  conjunctivitis, 108
  Fitz-Hugh Curtis syndrome, 173
  lymphadenitis, 137
  pathogenesis, 64
  pneumonia, 126
  portals of entry, 25
  prostatitis, 177
  salpingitis, 184
  urethritis, 180
Chlamydophila spp., 64–5
Chlamydophila pneumoniae, 65
Chlamydophila psittaci, 65
Chloramphenicol, 229, 230
Chloroquine, 233
Cholangitis, 166
Cholecystitis, 166
Cholera, 159
Chorioretinitis, 112
Chromobacterium spp., 53
Chromoblastomycosis, 75, 204
Chronic Muco-cutaneous
Candidiasis (CMC), 221
Chronic granulomatous disease, 220
Chronic obstructive pulmonary
  disease, 124–5
Chryseobacterium spp., 53
Chryseobacterium meningosepticum,
    53
Cidofovir, 234
Ciliates, 10, 81
Ciliophora, 10
Ciprofloxacin, 229, 231
Citrobacter spp., 47
  antibiotic sensitivity, 46

Citrobacter freundii, 47
Clarithromycin, 229, 231
Classical complement pathway, 29
Claviceps purpurea, 8
Clindamycin, 130, 229, 230
Clofazimine, 232
Clonorchis sinensis, 173
  cholangitis, 166
Clostridium spp., 22, 40–1
Clostridium botulinum, 41, 104
  clinical syndromes and
    management, 41
  confirmatory tests, 41
  diarrhoea, 158, 160
  pathogenesis and virulence, 41
  toxin, 21
Clostridium difficile, 41
  clinical syndrome and
    management, 41
  confirmatory tests, 41
  pathogenesis and virulence, 41
  toxin, 21
Clostridium diphtheriae, 137
Clostridium novyi, 41
Clostridium perfringens, 2, 40–1
  cholecystitis, 166
  clinical syndromes, 40–1
  confirmatory tests, 40
  crepitant anaerobic cellulitis, 194
  diarrhoea, 158, 160
  gas gangrene, 41
  management, 41
  pathogenesis and virulence, 40
  puerperal sepsis, 214
  salpingitis, 184
  toxin, 21
Clostridium septicum, 41
Clostridium tertium, 41
Clostridium tetani, 41, 105
  clinical syndrome and
    management, 41, 105
  confirmatory tests, 41
  pathogenesis and virulence, 41
  portals of entry, 25
Clotrimazole, 232
Clue cells, 187
Coagulase-negative staphylococci,
    34, 140, 208, 218
Coagulation, 27
Coccidioides immitis, 9, 72–3, 135
  chemotherapy, 73
  clinical syndromes, 73
  confirmatory tests, 73
Coccidioidomycosis, 135
Colitis,
  amoebic, 162
  haemorrhagic (*E. coli*), 160
Colonisation, 20
Comamonas spp., 52
Common cold, 116
Common Variable
  Immunodeficiency, 220
Common vehicle transmission, 24
Complement, 27
Complement defects, 220
Congenital herpes, 201
Conidiobolus coronatus, 75
Conjugation, 5
Conjunctivitis, 108, 222
Contact, 24
Contamination, 20
Corneal ulcers, 108–9
Coronavirus diarrhoea, 161

Corynebacterium spp., 38
Corynebacterium diphtheriae, 38
  portals of entry, 25
  tonsillitis, 118
  toxin, 21
Corynebacterium haemolyticum, 38
Corynebacterium jeikeium, 38
Corynebacterium minutissimum, 38, 74
Corynebacterium pseudodiphtheriticum, 38
Corynebacterium xerosis, 38
Cotrimoxazole, 94, 231
Coxiella spp., 66
Coxiella burnetii, 67
Crepitant anaerobic cellulitis, 194
Creutzfeldt-Jakob disease, 100–1
  variant, 100, 101
Croup, 116–17
Crustacea, 12
  infections, 13
Cryptococcoma, 129
Cryptococcosis, 102, 135
Cryptococcus spp., 6, 7
  endophthalmitis, 112
Cryptococcus neoformans, 6, 9, 23, 70, 72, 135, 195
  chemotherapy, 70
  chorioretinitis, 112
  clinical syndromes, 70
  CNS infection, 98
  confirmatory tests, 70
  control, 70
  meningitis, 94
Cryptosporidium spp., 10, 11, 79
  cholangitis, 166
Cryptosporidium parvum, 23
  diarrhoeal disease, 162
Curvularia geniculata, 75
Cutaneous larva migrans, 204
Cycloserine, 229, 232
Cyclospora cayetanensis, 79, 162
Cyst
  central nervous system, 103
  hydatid, 103, 169, 205
  phaeomycotic, 204
Cystic fibrosis, 125
Cysticercosis, 102
Cystitis, 174–5
Cytokines, 29, 32
Cytokine decoys, 19
Cytomegalovirus, 144
  congenital, 144
  infant, child, adult, 144
  ventriculitis, 96
Cytosol, 6
Cytotoxic T-cells, 29

D

Dacryoadenitis, 109
Dacryocystitis, 109
Dapsone, 232
Defensins, 19
Delavirdine, 234
Delayed-type hypersensitivity, 30
Dengue fever, 77, 146–7
Dental/periodontal infections, 114–15
Dento-alveolar infections, 114
Dermatology *see* Skin and soft tissue infections
Dermatophytoses, 198–9
Dermonecrotic toxin, 38

Diabetic foot infections, 195
Diarrhoeal disease, 158–63
  antibiotic-associated, 159
  bacterial, 160–1
  causative organisms, 158–9
  clinical syndromes, 158
  confirmatory tests, 158
  intestinal helminths, 163
  pathogenesis, 158
  protozoa, 162
  sources of infection, 158
  special syndromes, 159
  travellers and immigrants, 217
  viral, 161
  see also individual pathogens
Didanosine, 234
Dientamoeba fragilis, 11, 81, 84
  diarrhoeal disease, 162
Diethyl carbamazine, 233
DiGeorge syndrome, 221
Dikaryomycota, 6
Dilution tests, 241
Dimorphic fungi, 7
Diphtheria, 118, 120–1, 138
  bronchial, 120
  cutaneous, 120–1
  naso-pharyngeal, 120
  pharyngeal, 120
Diphtheria exotoxin, 38
Diphyllobothrium latum, 89, 162
  diarrhoeal disease, 163
Disinfectants, 225
Disinfection, 224–5
  chemicals, 225
  heat, 225
  pasteurisation, 225
  washing, 225
Disseminated intravascular coagulation, 33
Diverticulitis, 165
DNA polymerase inhibitors, 234–5
Donovanosis, 188
Doubling time, 4
Doxycycline, 94
Dracunculus medinensis, 86–7, 204–5
Dwarf tapeworm, 89, 162-3
Dysentery, 158

E

Echinocandins, 232
Echinococcus spp., 89
Echinococcus granulosus, 89, 134
  hydatid cyst, 103, 169
Echinococcus multilocularis, 89, 134
  hydatid cyst, 103, 169
Ecthyma gangrenosum, 195
Econazole, 232
Efavirenz, 234
Effector cells, 28
Ehrlichia spp., 66
Ehrlichia chaffeensis, 66
Ehrlichia phagocytophila, 66
Ehrlichia sennetsu, 66
Ehrlichiosis, 66
Eikenella corrodens, 53, 140
  bite infections, 197
Elderly patients, 223
Elementary bodies, 64
Elephantiasis, 86
ELISA, 239
Empyaema, 131

Emtricitabine, 234
Encephalitis, 200
  acute, 96
  chronic, 100
Encephalomyelitis, postinfectious, 105
Encystment, 81
Endocarditis, infective, 34, 39, 140–1
Endogenous infection, 25
Endolimax nana, 80
Endometritis, 184
Endophthalmitis, 112
Endoplasmic reticulum, 6
Endotoxins, 32
Enfuvirtide, 234
Entamoeba coli, 80
Entamoeba hartmanni, 80
Entamoeba histolytica, 10, 11, 23, 80
  cutaneous infection, 204
  diarrhoeal disease, 158, 162
  focal CNS infections, 102
Enteric fever, 48,155
Enterobacter spp., 49
  antibiotic sensitivity, 46
  cystitis, 174
  suppurative thrombophlebitis, 136
Enterobacter aerogenes, 49
Enterobacter cloacae, 49
Enterobacter sakazakii, 49
Enterobacteriaceae, 46–9
  see also individual species
Enterobius vermicularis, 81, 84, 162
  characteristics, 84
  diarrhoeal disease, 163
  eggs, 13
  life cycle and pathogenesis, 84
Enterococcus spp., 22, 36–7
Enterococcus faecalis, 36
Enterocolitis, 158
Enterocytozoon spp., 162
Enterovirus, 200
Entner-Doudoroff anaerobic pathway, 4
Enzymes, 35
Eosinophilic meningitis, 99
Epidemic myalgia, 200
Epidemic typhus, 66
Epidermolysis bullosa atrophica, 220
Epidermophyton spp., 6, 74
Epidermophyton floccosum, 75, 108
Epididymitis, 186
Epiglottitis, 120
Epimastigote, 83
Epstein-Barr virus, 144–5
Ergot alkaloids, 8
Erysipelas, 190–1
Erysipeloid, 39, 196
Erysipelothrix rhusiopathiae, 39
  wound infections, 196
Erythema infectiosum, 145
Erythema marginata, 191
Erythema multiforme, 127
Erythema nodosum, 191
Erythrasma, 74, 202
Erythromycin, 35, 229, 231
ESBL (Extended Spectrum Beta-Lactamase producing) bacteria, 218, 241
ESCAPPM bacteria, 219, 241
Escherichia coli, 4, 22, 46–7
  characteristics, 46-47
  crepitant anaerobic cellulitis, 194

  diarrhoea, 158, 160
  EAEC, EIEC, EHEC, EPEC, ETEC, 160
  epididymitis, 186
  hospital-acquired infections, 218
  intrarenal abscess, 176
  lung abscess, 130
  portals of entry, 25
  toxin, 21
Espundia, 205
Ethambutol, 232
Ethionamide, 232
Ethylene oxide, 224
Eubacterium spp., 62
Eukaryotes, 2
Eumycotic mycetoma, 75, 204
Exogenous infection, 25
Exophiala werneckii, 74, 198
Extradural abscesses, 103

F

Famciclovir, 234
Fascial space infections, 119
Fasciola hepatica, 90
  cholangitis, 166
Fasciolopsiasis, 173
Fasciolopsis buski, 90–1, 162, 173
Fatal familial insomnia, 100, 101
Fetal infections, 214–15
Fever, 32
  haemorrhagic, 147
  with myalgia, 147
  pyrexia of unknown origin, 156–7
  in travellers, 216
Fibrinolysin, 27
Filamentous fungi, 7
Filarial worms, 86
Filariasis, 77, 205
Filobasidiella neoformans, 6
Filtration, 224
Fish tank granuloma, 196, 203
Fish tapeworm, 89, 162-3
Fitz-Hugh Curtis syndrome, 173
Flagella, 3
Flagellates, 10
  blood and tissue, 82–3
  intestinal, 81
Flaviviruses, 146–7
Flinders Island SF, 66
Flubendazole, 233
Flucloxacillin, 94, 102
Fluconazole, 70, 94, 232
Flucytosine, 70, 94, 102, 232–3
Flukes (Trematodes), 12-13, 90–1, 173
Fomivirsen, 235
Fonsecaea compacta, 75
Fonsecaea pedrosoi, 75
Food poisoning, 158
Formaldehyde, 224
Formalin, 224
Fosamprenavir, 235
Foscarnet, 235
Fournier's gangrene, 194, 195
Francisella tularensis, 56, 57, 77, 213
  lymphadenitis, 137
  ocular manifestations, 110
Fungaemia, 142–3
Fungi, 6–9
  characteristics, 6–9
  dimorphic, 7
  filamentous, 7

Fungi (cont'd)
  invasive zygomycosis, 76
  opportunistic *Aspergillus* and
      Candida spp., 68-69
  skin and adjacent tissues, 74–5
  systemic mycoses, 70-73
  yeasts, 7
*see also individual genera and
organisms*
Furuncle, 192
Furunculosis, 192
Fusarium solani, 75
Fusidic acid, 229
Fusobacterium spp., 22, 54
  bite infections, 197
  canaliculitis, 109
  periapical/alveolar abscess, 115
  tonsillitis, 118
Fusobacterium necrophorum, 130
Fusobacterium nucleatum, 54
  empyaema, 131

G

Ganciclovir, 102, 234
Gangrene
  diabetic foot, 195
  Fournier's, 194, 195
  gas, 195
  infected vascular, 195
  Meleney's, 194
  synergistic, 194
Gangrenous stomatitis, 113, 122
Gardnerella vaginalis, 180
Gas gangrene, 195
  Clostridium perfringens, 41
Gas-forming infections, 194–5
Gastroenteritis, 48, 158
Gastrointestinal tract
  ciliates, 81
  diarrhoeal disease, 158–63
  flagellates, 81
  nematodes, 84–5
Gay bowel syndrome, 159
Gene therapy, 18
General paresis of the insane, 99
General practice patients, 222
  common infections, 222
Generation time, 4
Genetics, 5
Genital herpes, 187, 200–1
Genital tract
  balanitis, 186
  cervical infections, 182–3
  epididymitis, 186
  orchitis, 186
  salpingitis and pelvic
      inflammatory disease, 184–5
  vaginitis, 187
  vulvo-vaginitis, 187
Genome, 5
Gentamicin, 229, 230
Gerstmann-Straussler-Scheinker
      syndrome, 100, 101
Giant intestinal fluke, 90-1, 162, 173
Giardia spp., 10
Giardia lamblia, 11, 81
  diarrhoeal disease, 162
Giardiasis, 81
Gingivitis, 114
Gingivo-stomatitis, 200
Glandular fever, 144
Glomerulonephritis, acute, 178

Glutaraldehyde, 224
Golgi apparatus, 6
Gonorrhoea
  cervical, 182-3
  conjunctival, 108
  of joints, 210
  pelvic (PID), 184-5
  pharyngeal, 118
  urethral, 180-1
Gram stain, 2
Gram-negative bacteria, 3
Gram-positive bacteria, 3
Gram-positive rods, 38–9, 52–3
Gram's stain, 238
Granuloma inguinale, 188
Granuloma venereum, 188, 189
Granulomatosis infantiseptica, 39
Granulomatous hepatitis, 173
Granulomatous meningo-
      encephalitis, 80
Grey Baby Syndrome, 230
Guiding therapy, 240–1
  antibiotic levels, 241
  dilution tests, 241
  enzyme detection, 241
  killing curves, 241
  sensitivity testing, 240–1
  synergy tests, 241
Guinea worm, 86–7, 204–5
Gumma, 99

H

HAART therapy, 151
HACEK group, 140
Haemoflagellates, 82–3
Haemolytic Uraemic Syndrome
      (HUS), 160
Haemophilus spp., 22
  conjunctivitis, 108
*Haemophilus
      actinomycetemcomitans*,
      53, 140
  periodontitis, 115
Haemophilus aphrophilus, 44, 140
Haemophilus ducreyi, 44
  lymphadenitis, 137
Haemophilus haemolyticus, 44
Haemophilus influenzae, 44
  blepharitis, 108
  bronchitis, 124
  chemotherapy, 44
  clinical syndromes, 44
  confirmatory tests, 44
  control, 44
  in cystic fibrosis, 125
  epididymitis, 186
  epiglottitis, 120
  infective arthritis, 210
  laryngitis, 123
  meningitis, 94
  orbital infections, 109
  osteomyelitis, 206
  otitis media, 106
  septicaemia, 142
  sinusitis, 107
  tracheitis, 123
Haemophilus parainfluenzae, 44
Haemorrhagic conjunctivitis, 200
Haemorrhagic fevers, 147, 148
  with pulmonary syndrome, 147
  with renal syndrome, 148
Hafnia spp., 49

Hairy leukoplakia, 145
Hand, foot and mouth disease, 200
Hansen's disease *see* Leprosy
Hantavirus pulmonary syndrome,
      117
Heat
  disinfection, 225
  sterilisation, 224
Helicobacter pylori, 51
  characteristics, 51
Helminths, 12
  eggs, 13
Helper/inducer T-cells, 29
Hendra virus, 117
Hepatitis, 201
  granulomatous, 173
  viral *see individual types*
Hepatitis A, 170
Hepatitis B, 170–1
  portals of entry, 25
Hepatitis C, 171–2
  portals of entry, 25
Hepatitis D, 14–15, 172
Hepatitis E, 172
Hepatitis F, 172
Hepatitis G, 172
Herpangina, 200
Herpes labialis, 200
Herpes simplex virus, 200–1
  encephalitis, 96
  mucosal and skin infections, 200
  systemic infections, 200
Herpes zoster, 19, 146
Herpetic whitlow, 200
Heterophyes spp., 90
Heterophyes heterophyes, 162, 163
Heterotrophs, 4
Hidradenitis suppurativa, 192
Histoplasma capsulatum, 9, 23,
      70–1, 72, 135
  chemotherapy, 71
  chorioretinitis, 112
  characteristics, 71
  host interaction, 71
  infection, 71
  lymphadenitis, 137
Histoplasmosis, 70, 135
HIV/AIDS, 149–51
  causative agent, 149
  classification, 149
  clinical features, 149–51
      AIDS, 150
      asymptomatic, 149
      dementia/HIV encephalopathy,
          151
      malignancy, 150–1
      opportunistic infections (OIs),
          150
      persistent generalised
          lymphadenopathy (PGL), 149
      seroconversion illness, 149
      wasting syndrome, 151
  confirmatory tests, 151
  control and prevention, 151
  management, 151, 234–5
Hookworm, 85, 162–3
Hordeolum (Stye), 108
Hospital-acquired infections, 218–19
  characteristics, 219
  infection control, 219
Host defence, 20–21, 24–33
Host response, 32–3
  fever, 32

  malnutrition, 33
  metabolic changes, 33
  shock, 32–3
Host-microbial relationship, 20–1
  contamination, colonisation and
      infection, 20
  disease and microbial species, 21
  microbial attack and host
      defence, 20
  pathogenicity, virulence and
      invasiveness, 20–1
Human bite infections, 196–7
Human papillomavirus, 182
Human T-cell lymphotropic virus-1,
      100
Hyalohyphomycosis, 75, 204
Hydatid cyst, 103, 169, 205
Hydatid disease, 102, 134, 178
Hydatid worms (*Echinococcus* spp.)
      88-9
Hydrogen peroxide, 224
Hymenolepis diminuta, 162
Hymenolepis nana, 89, 162
  diarrhoeal disease, 163
Hypersensitivity, 8, 30
Hypopyon, 108

I

IgA, 28
IgD, 29
IgE, 29
IgG, 28
IgM, 28
Imipenem, 229, 230
Immigrants, 216–17
Immune disorders, 30–1
  diagnosis, 31
  evasion of host defences, 31
  hypersensitivity, 30
  immunodeficiency, 30–1
Immune evasion, 19
Immune response, 26
Immune-complex mediated
      hypersensitivity, 30
Immunisation, 28, 236–7
  active, 236–7
  contraindications, 237
  passive, 237
  timing of, 237
Immunocompromised patients
  infections, 220–1
  necrotising infections, 195
  pneumonia, 129
  stomatitis, 113
  see also HIV/AIDS, 149-151
Immunodeficiency, 30–1
Immunogenicity, 236
Impedins, 21
Impetigo, 190
  bullous, 192
Incidence rates, 24
Indinavir, 235
Infection, 20-33
  endogenous, 25
  exogenous, 25
  general responses, 32–3
  host-microbial factors, 20–23
  initiation, 24-5
  reservoirs and sources of, 24
  routes of transmission, 24–5
  ruptured host defences, 25-31
  see also individual infections

Infection control, 219
Infective dose, 21
Infective peritonitis, 164
Influenza, 117
Ingestion, 26
Innate immunity, 26
Insecta, 12
    infections, 13
Integrase inhibitors, 234, 235
Interferon-alpha, 235
Intermediary metabolism, 4–5
Intertrigo, 199
Intervertebral disc infections, 211
Intra-abdominal abscess, 164–5
Intrarenal abscess, 176, 177
Invasiveness, 20–1
Iodamoeba butschlii, 80
Ionising radiation, 224
Iridocyclitis, 112
Iritis, 222
    cidofovir-induced, 234
Iritis pearls, 110
Irradiation, 224
Isoniazid, 232
Isospora belli, 79, 162
Itraconazole, 71, 72, 102, 232
Ivermectin, 85, 233
Ixodes, 25, 59

J

Joint infections, 210–11

K

Kala-azar, 152, 168
Kallikrein, 27
Kaposi's sarcoma, 19
Kawasaki disease, 154
Keratitis, 108–9
Kerato-conjunctivitis, 200
Kerion, 199
Ketoconazole, 69, 232
Killing curves, 241
Kingella spp., 43
Kingella kingae, 140
Klebsiella spp., 22, 48–9, 53, 195
    characteristics, 46-9
    crepitant anaerobic cellulitis, 194
    cystitis, 174
    epididymitis, 186
    intrarenal abscess, 176
    suppurative thrombophlebitis, 136
Klebsiella granulomatis, 49, 53, 188
Klebsiella oxytoca, 48
Klebsiella ozaenae, 49
Klebsiella pneumoniae, 31, 48
    lung abscess, 130
Klebsiella rhinoscleromatis, 49, 122
Koplik's spots, 145
Kuru, 100, 101

L

Laboratory methods, 238–241
    antibiotic assays, 241
    antibody measurements, 240
    clinical advice, 241
    cultures, 239
    direct detection methods, 238
    identification, 239
    sensitivity testing, 240-1
    specimen handling, 238

Lactobacillus spp., 62
Lamivudine, 234
Larva migrans, 87
    cutaneous, 204
Laryngitis, 123
Laryngo-tracheo-bronchitis, 116–17
Latent pathogens, 23
Lectin pathway, 27
Legionella spp.
    lung abscess, 130
    pneumonia, 127
Legionella pneumophila, 45
    clinical syndromes and
        management, 45
    confirmatory tests, 45
    control, 45
Legionnaires' disease, 45
Leishmania spp., 11, 82
    characteristics, 82
Leishmania braziliensis, 82, 152, 205
Leishmania donovani, 31, 82, 152
    lymphadenitis, 137
Leishmania major, 205
Leishmania mexicana, 82, 152, 205
Leishmania tropica, 82, 152, 205
Leishmaniasis, 205
Lemierre's disease, 119
Leprosy, 104, 105, 202
    classification, 104
    congenital, 214
    ocular manifestations, 110
    skin manifestations, 202
    treatment, 232
Leptospira spp.
    lymphadenitis, 137
    meningitis, 94
Leptospira biflexa, 56, 59
Leptospira interrogans, 56, 59, 212
Leptospirosis, 212
Lincomycin, 229, 230
Lincosamides, 229, 230
Linezolid, 229, 230
Lipopolysaccharide, 3
Listeria monocytogenes, 38–9, 154
    congenital infection, 214
    lymphadenitis, 137
    meningitis, 94
Listeriosis, 154
    congenital, 214
Lithotrophy, 4
Liver abscess
    amoebic, 168
    pyogenic, 168–9
Liver infections, 168
Loa loa, 77, 86
    ocular manifestations, 111
Loboa loboi, 75, 204
Lobomycosis, 75, 204
Loiasis, 77
Lopinavir, 235
Ludwig's angina, 121
Lumbar puncture, 95
Lumefantrine, 233
Lung abscess, 130
Lung fluke, 91, 105, 135
Lupus vulgaris, 202
Lyme disease, 57, 77, 99, 138, 154
Lymphadenitis, 137
Lymphangitis, 136–7, 191
Lymphogranuloma venereum,
    188–9
Lymphokines, 29
Lysogeny, 17

Lysosomes, 6
Lysozyme, 27

M

Macrolides, 229, 231
Madura foot, 75, 202
Madurella spp., eumycotic
    mycetoma, 202
Madurella grisea, 75
Madurella mycetomatis, 75
Major histocompatibility complex,
    29
Malaria, 77, 104, 105, 152–3, 168, 217
    prophylaxis, 216
Malassezia furfur, 74
Malnutrition, 33
Mannan Binding Lectin, 26
Mastoiditis, 106–7
Maternal infections, 214
Measles, 145
Mebendazole, 84, 233
Mefloquine, 233
Melarsoprol, 233
Meleney's gangrene, 194
Melioidosis, 134
Memory cells, 28
Meningitis, 39, 222
    acute, 94–5
    aseptic, 95, 201
        causative organisms, 94
    chronic, 98-99
    eosinophilic, 99
    postnatal, 215
Meropenem, 229, 230
Metabolism, 4
Metagonimus spp., 90
Metagonimus yokogawai, 162
    diarrhoeal disease, 163
Metapneumovirus, 116
Metazoa, 12
Metronidazole, 23, 80, 94, 102, 130,
    229, 231
Miconazole, 232
Microbial attack, 22–29
    aggressive pathogens, 23
    defences, skin and mucous
        membranes, 25
    definition, 22
    entry, 25
    latent pathogens, 23
    non-specific defences, 26–7
    normal flora, 22–3
    opportunist pathogens, 23
    reservoirs and sources, 24
    route of transmission, 24–5
    second-line defences, 26–7
    specific defences, 28–9
Microbial detection/identification,
    238–9
Micrococcus spp., 34
Microsporidia spp., 162
Microsporum audouinii, 75
Microsporum canis, 74, 75, 198
Microsporum equinum, 74, 75
Microsporum ferrugineum, 75
Microsporum fulvum, 75
Microsporum gallinae, 75
Microsporum gypseum, 74, 75
Microsporum nanum, 75
Microtubules, 6
Microvesicles, 6
Milkers' nodes, 148, 201

Mitochondria, 6
Mollaret's meningitis, 201
Molluscum contagiosum,
    148, 201
Monkey pox, 148
Monkeypox, 201
Monokines, 29
Moraxella spp., 22, 43
    clinical syndromes and
        chemotherapy, 43
    confirmatory tests, 43
Moraxella catarrhalis
    bronchitis, 124
    laryngitis, 123
    otitis media, 106
Morganella spp., 49
    antibiotic sensitivity, 46
MRSA (Methicillin Resistant
        Staphylococcus aureus), 218
Mucocutaneous candidiasis, 221
Mucor spp., 6, 195
Mucorales, 76
    characteristics, 76
Mucormycosis, 76
Multicellular parasites, 12–13
    characteristics, 12–13
    *see also individual genera and
        species*
Multiple serotypes, 19
Mumps, 145
Murine typhus, 66
Mutations, 18
Mycetoma, 75, 202
    actinomycotic, 202
    eumycotic, 75, 202, 204
Mycobacteria, 3
    atypical infections, 133
Mycobacterium spp., 22, 31, 60–1
    tonsillitis, 118
Mycobacterium avium, 23
Mycobacterium avium-intracellulare,
    61
    granulomatous hepatitis, 173
Mycobacterium chelonae, 61
Mycobacterium fortuitum, 61
Mycobacterium kansasii, 61
Mycobacterium leprae, 60–1, 104
    chemotherapy and control, 51
    chorioretinitis, 112
    clinical syndromes, 51
    confirmatory tests, 51
    congenital, 214
    granulomatous hepatitis, 173
    uveitis, 112
Mycobacterium marinum, 61, 203
    wound infecions, 196
Mycobacterium scrofulaceum, 61
Mycobacterium tuberculosis, 60
    chemotherapy, 60
    chorioretinitis, 112
    clinical syndromes, 60
    CNS infection, 99
    confirmatory tests, 60
    focal CNS infections, 102
    granulomatous hepatitis, 173
    intervertebral disc infections, 211
    lymphadenitis, 137
    meningitis, 94
    virulence and pathogenesis, 60
    see also Tuberculosis
Mycobacterium ulcerans, 61
Mycoplasma spp., 6, 22, 63
    pneumonia, 127

Mycoplasma genitalium, urethritis, 180
Mycoplasma hominis, 63
  salpingitis, 184
Mycoplasma pneumoniae, 63
  bronchiolitis, 116
  bronchitis, 124
  croup, 116
  laryngitis, 123
  meningitis, 94
Mycoses
  cutaneous, 74–5
  subcutaneous, 75, 204
  superficial, 74
  systemic, 135
Mycotoxicosis, 68
Mycotoxins, 8
Myocarditis, 138, 200
Myonecrosis
  clostridial, 195
  non-clostridial, 195
Myositis,
  anaerobic streptococcal, 195

Naegleria fowleri, 11, 80
Nagler plates, 40
Necator americanus, 85, 162
  diarrhoeal disease, 163
Necrotising fasciitis, 191, 195
Neisseria spp., 22
  otitis media, 106
Neisseria gonorrhoeae, 2, 31, 42
  cervicitis, 172
  characteristics, 42
  Fitz-Hugh Curtis syndrome, 173
  pathogenesis and virulence, 42
  portals of entry, 25
  prostatitis, 177
  salpingitis, 184
  tonsillitis, 118
  urethritis, 180
Neisseria meningitidis, 2, 42–3
  characteristics, 42-43
  epididymitis, 186
  meningitis, 94
  septicaemia, 142
Nelfinavir, 235
Nematodes, 12
  infections, 13
  intestinal, 84–5
  tissue, 86–7
Neonatal herpes, 201
Neonatal infections, 144, 214–15
  non-viral, 214-15
  viral, 144
Nevirapine, 234
Nikolsky's sign, 192
Niridazole, 87
Nitazoxanide, 79, 233
Nitroimidazoles, 229, 231
Nocardia spp., 62, 195
  brain abscess, 102–3
  characteristics, 62
  focal CNS infections, 102
  lung abscess, 130
  meningitis, 94
  mycetoma, 202
Nocardia asteroides, 134
Nocardiosis, 134–5
Noma, 113, 122

Non-antibody-dependent cell-mediated cytotoxicity, 19
Non-nucleoside reverse transcriptase inhibitors, 234, 235
Norfloxacin, 229, 231
Normal flora, 22–3
Norwalk virus diarrhoea, 158, 161
Nucleic acid probes, 239
Nucleoside inhibitors, 234
Nystatin, 69, 232

O

Ocular infections, 108–9
  deep, 112
  tropical, 110–11
Onchocerca volvulus, 86
  endophthalmitis, 112
  ocular manifestations, 111
Onchocerciasis, 111
Onychomycosis, 199
Opisthorchis sinensis, 90
Opisthorchis viverrini, 173
Opisthotonos, 105
Opportunist pathogens, 23
Opsonins, 26
Orbital cellulitis, 109
Orchitis, 186
Orf, 148, 201
Organotrophy, 4
Orientia spp., 66
Ornithodorus, 59
  relapsing fever, 154
Oro-facial infections, 122–3
Ortho-phthalyl-aldehyde, 224
Orthomyxovirus, 117
Oseltamivir, 235
Osteomyelitis, 206–7, 208–9
  acute contiguous-focus, 207
  acute haematogenous, 206
  acute ischaemic-neuropathic, 207
  chronic (pyogenic), 207, 209
  fungal, 208–9
  subacute, 208
  vertebral body, 208
Otitis externa, 106
Otitis media, 106
Oxygen-dependent killing, 26
Oxygen-independent killing, 26

P

Paecilomyces lilacinus, 74
Pancreatitis, 165
Pandoraea spp., 52
Paracoccidioides brasiliensis, 9, 72–73, 135
  chemotherapy, 73
  clinical syndromes and management, 73
  confirmatory tests, 73
  lymphadenitis, 137
  paracoccidioidomycosis, 122
Paracoccidioidomycosis, 62, 135
Paragonimiasis, 105, 135
Paragonimus westermani, 91, 105, 135
Paratrophy, 4
Paronychia, 192, 199
Parotitis, 122
Parvovirus B19, 145

Pasteurella multocida, 56, 57
  bite infections, 197
  osteomyelitis, 207
Pasteurisation, 224, 225
Pathogenicity, 20–1
  fungi, 8
  protozoa, 10
Pediculus humanus, 59, 77
  relapsing fever, 154–5
Pelvic abscess, 185
Pelvic inflammatory disease, 184–5
Pemphigus neonatorum, 193
Penciclovir, 234
Penicillin, 23, 94, 102, 228, 229
Penicillinase resistance, 35
Penicillium marneffii, 75, 151
Pentamidine, 233
Pentose phosphate cycle, 4
Peptidoglycan, 3, 32
Peptococcus spp., 22, 54–5
Peptococcus anaerobius, 55
Peptostreptococcus spp., 22, 54–5
  crepitant anaerobic cellulitis, 194
  periapical/alveolar abscess, 115
Peracetic acid, 224
Pericarditis, 138–9, 200
  tuberculous, 138–9
  viral, 139
Pericoronitis, 115
Perinatal infections, 215
Perinephric abscess, 176
Period of infectivity, 21
Periodontal infections, 114–15
Periodontitis, 115
Periplasmic space, 3
Peritonitis, 164, 185
Peritonsillar abscess (quinsy), 119
Peritonsillitis, 119
Pertussis, 123
Phaeohyphomycosis, 75, 204
Phagocyte defects, 220
Phagocytosis, 21, 26
Phagosomes, 31
Pharyngitis, 118–19
Phialophora verrucosa, 75
Phosphoketolase pathway, 5
Phototrophy, 4
Phthirus pubis, 77
Picornavirus diarrhoea, 161
Piedraia hortae, 74, 198
Pig threadworm, 87, 213
Pili, 3
Pinta, 203
Pinworm, 81, 84, 162
Pityriasis versicolor, 74, 198
Pityrosporum orbiculare, 74
Pityrosporum ovale, 9
Plague, 25, 56-7, 77, 213
  bubonic, 137, 213
  pneumonic, 213
  septicaemic, 213
Plasmalemma, 6
Plasmid fingerprinting, 239
Plasmodium spp., 10, 11, 77, 78
  acute glomerulonephritis, 178
Plasmodium falciparum, 78, 104, 152
Plasmodium malariae, 78, 152
Plasmodium ovale, 78, 152
Plasmodium vivax, 78, 152
Platyhelminthes, 12
Plesiomonas shigelloides, 51
Pneumocystis jirovecii, 23

Pneumonia
  abnormal host, 128–9
  aspiration, 128, 129
  hospital-acquired, 128–9
  immunocompromised patients, 129
  neonatal, 126
  normal host, 126–7
  postnatal, 215
  previously healthy patients, 126–7
  with underlying pulmonary disease, 128
  see also individual pathogens
Poliomyelitis, acute, 97
Polymerase chain reaction, 239
Pontiac fever, 45
Pork tapeworm, 88, 112, 162
Porphyromonas asaccharolytica, 54, 55
Porphyromonas gingivalis, 54
Portal pylephlebitis, 167
Portals of entry, 25
Post-anginal septicaemia, 119
Post-gonococcal cervicitis (PGC), 182
Post-gonococcal urethritis (PGU), 180
Post-polio syndrome, 97
Postnatal infections, 215
Pott's disease of spine, 209
Pott's puffy tumour, 107
Poxvirus, 148, 201
Praziquantel, 91, 102, 153, 233
Pregnancy, viral infections, 144
Preseptal (periorbital) cellulitis, 108
Prevalence rates, 24
Prevotella bivia, 54
Prevotella disiens, 54
Prevotella intermedia, 54
Prevotella melaninogenica, 54
Primaquine, 233
Primary response, 28
Prions, 15, 93
Prion disease, CNS, 100–1
Proctocolitis, 159
Progressive multifocal leucoencephalopathy, 100
Propionibacterium spp., 62
Prostatitis, 174, 176–7
Protein A, 34
Proteus spp., 49
  antibiotic sensitivity, 46
  cystitis, 174
Proteus mirabilis, 49
Proteus vulgaris, 49
Prothionamide, 232
Protozoa, 10–11
  characteristics, 10-11
  diarrhoeal disease, 162
  See also individual genera and organisms
Providentia spp., 49
  antibiotic sensitivity, 46
Pseudallescheria spp., 68
  eumycotic mycetoma, 202
Pseudallescheria boydii, 75
Pseudo-diphtheria, 121
Pseudomonas spp., 52
  antibiotic sensitivity, 46
  keratitis, 108
Pseudomonas aeruginosa, 52
  Characteristics, 52
  cystitis, 174

Pseudomonas aeruginosa (cont'd)
  hospital-acquired infections, 218
  in cystic fibrosis, 125
  osteomyelitis, 207
  otitis externa, 106
  septicaemia, 142
Pseudomonas pseudomallei, 130
Pseudovirions, 15
Psoas abscess, 157
Psychotropics, 8
Puerperal sepsis, 214
Purines, 5
Purpura fulminans, 191
Pyelitis, 174
Pyelonephritis, 174, 175
Pyoderma gangrenosum, 194
Pyogenic liver abscess, 168–9
Pyomyositis, tropical, 203
Pyonephrosis, 175
Pyrantel pamoate, 84
Pyrazinamide, 232
Pyrexia of unknown origin, 156–7
  causes, 156
  investigation, 156–7
  management, 157
  types of, 156
Pyrimethamine, 79, 94, 102
Pyrimidines, 5
Pyrogens
  endogenous, 32
  exogenous, 32
Pyruvate metabolism, 5

Q

Queensland tick typhus, 66
Quinine, 233
Quinolones, 231

R

Rabies, 96
Ralstonia spp., 52
Rat bite fever, 197
Red Man Syndrome, 230
Reiter's syndrome, 112, 180
Relapsing fever, 77, 154–5
Reservoirs, 9, 11, 13, 24, 218
Respiratory tract infections
  bronchial, 124–5
  elderly patients, 223
  empyaema, 131
  lung abscess, 130
  pneumonia, 126–9, 215
  throat, 118–19
  tropical/rare, 134–5
  viral, 116–17
Restriction enzyme analysis, 239
Retroviruses, 149
  see also HIV/AIDS 149–151
Rheumatic fever, 139
Rhinocerebral zygomycosis, 76, 103
Rhinoscleroma, 122
Rhinosporidiosis, 75, 122, 204
Rhinosporidium seeberi, 75, 122
Rhizopus spp., 6, 195
Rhizopus arrhizus, 76
Ribavirin, 116, 235
Rickettsia spp., 66–7
  meningitis, 94
Rickettsia akari, 66
  lymphadenitis, 137
Rickettsia australis, 66

Rickettsia conorii, 66
Rickettsia honei, 66
Rickettsia prowazeckii, 66–7, 77
Rickettsia rickettsii, 66, 67
Rickettsia tsutsugamushi,
  lymphadenitis, 137
Rickettsia typhi, 66, 67
Rifabutin, 231
Rifampicin, 94, 229, 231
Rifamycins, 229, 231
Rimantadine, 234
Risus sardonicus, 105
Ritonavir, 235
Ritter's disease, 193
River blindness, 86
Rocky Mountain spotted fever, 67, 77
Romana's sign, 110
Rotavirus, diarrhoea, 158, 161
Roundworm, 12-13, 85, 162-3, 166
Roxithromycin, 229, 231
Rubella, 145–6
  congenital rubella syndrome, 145

S

Salivary gland calculi, 122
Salivary gland infections, 122
Salmonella spp., 48, 56
  antibiotic sensitivity, 46
  characteristics, 48
  diarrhoea, 158, 160–1
  portals of entry, 25
Salmonella cholerae-suis, 48
Salmonella dublin, 48
Salmonella enteritidis, 48
Salmonella paratyphi, 48
Salmonella typhi, 23, 48
Salpingitis, 184–5
Salpingo-oophoritis, 184
Sarcocystis hominis, 11
Sarcomastigophora, 10
Sarcoptes scabiei, 77
SARS, 117
Scabies, 77
Scalded skin syndrome, 193
Scarlet fever, 191
  staphylococcal, 193
Scedosporium spp., 68
Schistosoma spp., 91, 153
Schistosoma haematobium, 91
Schistosoma japonicum, 91
Schistosoma mansoni, 91
Schistosomiasis, 153, 168,
  178–9
Scrapie, 100
Scrofuloderma, 202
Scrub typhus, 66
Second-line defences, 26–7
  complement, 27
  natural killer cells, 26
  phagocytosis, 26
SEN-virus, 172
Sennetsu fever, 66
Sensitivity testing, 240–1
Septic jugular vein
    thrombophlebitis, 119
Septic shock, 142
Septicaemia, 142–3
  postnatal, 215
Serratia spp., 49
  antibiotic sensitivity, 46
  cystitis, 174
Serratia marcescens, 49

Severe acute respiratory syndrome
    (SARS), 117
Severe combined
    immunodeficiency, 221
Sexually transmitted diseases,
    188–9, 216–217
  see also individual diseases
Sheep liver fluke, 90, 166
Shigella spp., 47
  antibiotic sensitivity, 46
  chemotherapy, 47
  clinical syndromes, 47
  confirmatory tests, 47
  control, 47
  diarrhoea, 158, 161
Shigella boydii, 47
Shigella dysenteriae, 47
Shigella flexneri, 31, 47
Shigella sonnei, 47, 51
Shigella toxin, 21
Shingles, 146
Shock, 32–3
Sialadenitis, 122
Sin Nombre, 117, 147
Sinusitis
  acute, 107
  chronic, 107
Skin and soft tissue infections
  bacterial, 202–3
  cutaneous candidiasis, 199
  cutaneous mycoses, 198–9
  elderly patients, 223
  fungal and parasitic, 204–5
  pre-existing conditions, 197
  staphylococcal, 192–3
  streptococcal, 190–1
  subcutaneous mycoses, 199
  superficial mycoses, 198
  travellers, 217
  tropical, 202–3
  viral, 200–1
Sleeping sickness, 77, 105
Slime layers, 34
Smallpox, 148, 201
Sodium antimony gluconate, 233
Sources of infection, 24
South American blastomycosis, 62
Spirillum minor, 53
Spirochaetal infections, 203
Spontaneous Bacterial Peritonitis
    (SBP), 164
Spores, 3
Sporothrix schenckii, 9, 75
Sporotrichosis, 75, 204
Staphylococcus spp., 34–5
  brain abscess, 102
  characteristics, 34–5
  see also individual species
Staphylococcus albus, 34
Staphylococcus aureus, 22, 34-5
  blepharitis, 108
  characteristics, 34-5
  clinical syndromes, 35
  conjunctivitis, 108
  in cystic fibrosis, 125
  diarrhoea, 158, 161
  hospital-acquired infections, 218
  identification, 35
  infective arthritis, 210
  intervertebral disc infections, 211
  keratitis, 108
  lung abscess, 130
  orbital infections, 109

osteomyelitis, 206, 207
otitis media, 106
portals of entry, 25
sepsis, 32
stye/chalazion, 108
suppurative thrombophlebitis,
    136
tracheitis, 123
wound infections, 196
Staphylococcus epidermidis, 22, 34
  clinical syndromes, 35
  identification, 35
Staphylococcus saprophyticus, 34
  clinical syndromes, 35
  cystitis, 174
  identification, 35
Stenotrophomonas spp., 52
Stenotrophomonas maltophilia, 52
Sterilisation, 224–5
  chemicals, 224
  filtration, 224
  heat, 224–5
  irradiation, 224
Stibogluconate, 82
Stimulatory hypersensitivity, 30
Stomatitis, 113
  aphthous, 113
  gangrenous, 113, 122
  immunocompromised patients,
    113
Stomatococcus spp., 34
Strawberry cervix, 187
Streptobacillus moniliformis, 53
Streptococcus spp., 22, 36–7
  chemotherapy, 37
  clinical syndromes, 37
  confirmatory tests, 36
  control, 37
  pathogenesis and virulence, 36–7
  see also individual species
Streptococcus agalactiae
  classification and habitat, 36
  clinical syndromes, 37
  pneumonia, 126
Streptococcus bovis, equinus, 36
Streptococcus milleri, 36
Streptococcus minor, 137
Streptococcus mitis, 36
Streptococcus moniliformis, 137
Streptococcus mutans, 114
  classification and habitat, 36
Streptococcus pneumoniae, 2, 21,
    36-7
  bronchitis, 124
  characteristics, 36
  clinical syndromes, 37
  conjunctivitis, 108
  meningitis, 94
  orbital infections, 109
  otitis media, 106
  portals of entry, 25
  sepsis, 32
  septicaemia, 142
  virulence factors, 37
Streptococcus pyogenes, 2, 21, 36
  acute glomerulonephritis, 178
  blepharitis, 108
  characteristics, 36
  clinical syndromes, 37
  conjunctivitis, 108
  laryngitis, 123
  lymphadenitis, 137
  orbital infections, 109

Streptococcus pyogenes (cont'd)
  puerperal sepsis, 214
  septicaemia, 142
  tracheitis, 123
  virulence factors, 37
  wound infections, 196
Streptococcus salivarius, 36
Streptococcus sanguis, 36
Streptococcus viridans, 37
Streptogramins, 229, 230
Streptomycin, 229-230, 232
Strongyloides stercoralis, 23, 85, 162
  chemotherapy, 85
  characteristics, 85
  clinical syndromes, 85
  diarrhoeal disease, 163
  larva, 23
  life cycle and pathogenesis, 85
Stye, 108, 192
Subacute sclerosing
        panencephalitis, 100
Subdural abscesses, 103
Sulphadiazine, 79
Sulphonamides, 229, 231
Suppressor T-cells, 29
Suppurative thrombophlebitis, 136
Suramin, 83, 153, 233
Surgical site infections, 196
Sycosis barbae, 192
Synergy tests, 241
Syphilis, 58-9, 189, 203
  brain abscess, 103
  CNS infection, 98
  congenital, 214
  endemic (bejel), 203
Systemic infections
  mycoses, 135
  tropical, 152-3
  viral, 144-8

T

T-cells, 28, 29
Tabes dorsalis, 99
Taenia saginata, 88, 162
Taenia solium, 88, 162
  endophthalmitis, 112
Tanapox, 148, 201
Tapeworms, 12, 13, 88-9
  eggs, 13
  infections, 13
Tapir nose, 205
Teichoic acids, 34
Teicoplanin, 230
Tenofovir, 234
Tetanospasmin, 41
Tetanus, 105
Tetracyclines, 94, 229, 231
Thiabendazole, 233
Third- and fourth-line defences, 28-9
Threadworm, 13, 81, 84, 162-3
Throat infections, 118-19
Tinea barbae, 74, 198-9
Tinea capitis, 74, 198-9
Tinea corporis, 74
Tinea cruris, 74
Tinea nigra, 74, 198
Tinea pedis, 74, 198
Tinea unguium, 74, 199
Tinea versicolor, 74, 198
Tinidazole, 229, 231
Tobramycin, 229, 230
Toll-like receptors, 26, 29

Tonsillitis, 118-19
Torulopsis spp., 6
Toxic shock syndrome, 193
Toxins, 21, 35
Toxocara spp.
  chorioretinitis, 112
  endophthalmitis, 112
Toxocara canis, 87, 155
  ocular manifestations, 110
Toxocara cati, 87, 155
  ocular manifestations, 110
Toxocariasis, 155
Toxoplasma spp., 10
Toxoplasma gondii, 11, 31, 78-9
  chemotherapy, 79
  chorioretinitis, 112
  characteristics, 78-9
  endophthalmitis, 112
  lymphadenitis, 137
  meningitis, 94
  ocular manifestations, 110
Toxoplasmosis, 23, 102
  congenital, 214-15
Tracheitis, 123
Trachoma, 64-5, 111
Transduction, 5
Transformation, 5
Transfusion transmissible virus, 172
Transmissible spongiform
        encephalopathies, 100
Transposons, 227
Travellers, 216-17
  food and drink precautions, 216
  immunisation, 216
  malaria prophylaxis, 216
  personal medical kit, 216
  sexually transmitted diseases, 216
Traveller's diarrhoea, 158
Trematodes, 12, 13, 90-1, 173
  eggs, 13
  infections, 13
Trench fever, 77
Treponema carateum, 59
Treponema pallidum, 58
  chemotherapy, 58
  chorioretinitis, 112
  clinical syndromes, 58
  CNS infection, 98
  confirmatory tests, 58
  control, 58
  focal CNS infections, 102
  granulomatous hepatitis, 173
  lymphadenitis, 137
  meningitis, 94
  portals of entry, 25
  virulence and pathogenesis, 58
  yaws, 110-11, 155, 203
Treponema pertenue, 59, 110-11,
        155, 203
Tricarboxylic acid (Krebs) cycle, 4
Trichinella spiralis, 87, 213
Trichinosis, 213
Trichomonas vaginalis, 81
  portals of entry, 25
  urethritis, 180
Trichomoniasis, 187
Trichophyton concentricum, 75
Trichophyton equinum, 75
Trichophyton mentagrophytes, 74, 198
Trichophyton mentagrophytes var
        interdigitale, 75
Trichophyton mentagrophytes var
        mentagrophytes, 75

Trichophyton rubrum, 74, 198
Trichophyton schoenleinii, 74
Trichophyton verrucosum, 75
Trichophyton violaceum, 75
Trichosporon beigelii, 74, 198
Trichuris trichiura, 84-5, 162
  diarrhoeal disease, 163
Trifluorothymidine, 234
Trigonitis, 174
Trimethoprim, 229, 231
Tropheryma whippelii, 62
Trophozoite, 10, 81
Tropical infections
  abdominal, 173
  bone, 208-9
  nervous system, 104-5
  ocular, 110-11
  oro-facial, 122
  respiratory tract, 134-5
  sexually transmitted, 188-9
  skin and soft tissue
    bacterial, 202-3
    fungal and parasitic, 204-5
  systemic, 152-3
  urinary, 178-9
Tropical spastic paraparesis, 100
Tropical sprue, 159
Tropical ulcer, 203, 217
Trypanosoma spp., 10, 82-3
  characteristics, 83
  lymphadenitis, 137
Trypanosoma brucei, 31, 77, 82, 83, 105
Trypanosoma brucei rhodesiense, 82,
        105
Trypanosoma cruzi, 11, 77, 82, 138
  ocular manifestations, 110
Trypanosoma gambiense, 11, 77, 82,
        105
Trypanosoma rhodesiense, 11, 82
Trypanosomiasis, 153
  African, 105, 153
  South American, 77, 83, 110, 138
Trypomastigote, 83
Tuberculides, 202
Tuberculosis, 132-3
  bone, 209
  brain abscess, 103
  chemotherapy, 133
  clinical syndromes, 132-3
  confirmatory tests, 133
  control and prevention, 133
  cutaneous, 202
  latent, 132
  post-primary, 132
  primary, 132
  treatment, 232
  urinary tract, 179
  see also Mycobacterium tuberculosis
Tuberculosis verrucosa cutis, 202
Tubo-ovarian abscess, 185
Tularaemia, 77, 213
Typhoid fever, 48, 155
Typhus, 66-7, 77
  murine, 66

U

Ulcer
  Bairnsdale (Buruli), 202-3
  chancriform, 194
  corneal, 108-9
  tropical, 203, 217
Ultraviolet light, 224

Umbilical stump infections, 215
Universal precautions, 219
Urea urealyticum, 63
Ureaplasma spp., 63
  salpingitis, 184
Ureaplasma urealyticum, 180
Ureteritis, 174
Urethral syndrome, 174
Urethritis, 174, 180-1, 184
  characteristics, 180-1
  confusing conditions, 181
Urinary tract infections, 174-5
  cystitis, 174-5
  elderly patients, 223
  pyelonephritis, 175
  tropical, 178-9
Uveitis
  anterior, 112
  posterior, 112

V

Vaccination, 236
Vaccines, 236-7
Vaccinia virus, 201
Vaginitis, 187
Valaciclovir, 234
Valganciclovir, 234
Vancomycin, 35, 229, 230
Vancomycin Intermediate S. aureus
        (VISA), 218
Vancomycin Resistant Enterococci
        (VRE), 218
Varicella zoster, 146
Vector-borne transmission, 24
Veillonella spp., 22, 55
Veldt sore, 38
Ventilator Associated Pneumonia
        (VAP), 218
Vibrio spp., 50
  characteristics, 50
Vibrio alginolyticus, 50
Vibrio cholerae, 50
  diarrhoea, 158, 161
  portals of entry, 25
  toxin, 21
Vibrio parahaemolyticus, 50
  diarrhoea, 158, 161
Vibrio vulnificus, 50
Vidarabine, 235
Vincent's angina, 118
Vincent's infection, 115
Viomycin, 232
Viral disease, CNS, 100-1
Viral envelopes, 14
Viral enzymes, 14
Viral infections
  respiratory tract, 116-17
  nervous system, 94-7, 100-101
  skin and soft tissues, 200-1
  systemic, 144-8
Viral nucleic acids, 14
Viral proteins, 14
Viral release inhibitors, 235
Virion, 14
Viroids, 15
Virokines, 19
Virulence factors, 20-1
  Bordetella pertussis, 45
  Clostridium spp., 40
  Pseudomonads, 52
  staphylococci, 35
  streptococci/enterococci, 36

Virus particle, 14–15
  characteristics, 14-15
  See also groups and individual viruses
Viruses, 14–19, 92–3
  classification, 92–3
  DNA, 92
  genetics, 18
  host cell interaction, 15–18
    assembly and release, 16
    attachment, 16
    genome replication, 17
    mRNA synthesis, 16, 17
    penetration, 16
    protein synthesis, 16
    recognition, 16
    uncoating, 16
  human hosts, 18–19
  infected cell, 15
  replication, 16–17

  RNA, 93
  See groups and individual viruses
VISA (Vancomycin Intermediate S. aureus), 218
Visna, 100
Vitamin A deficiency, 33
Voriconazole, 68, 71, 75, 102, 232
VRE (Vancomycin Resistant Enterococci), 218
Vulva abscess, 187
Vulval warts, 189
Vulvo-vaginitis, 187

Wangiella dermatitidis, 75
Warts, 201
  vulval, 189
Weil's disease, 212
Whipple's disease, 62

Whipworm, 64-5, 162-3
White piedra, 74, 198
Whooping cough, 123
Wound infections, 196
Wuchereria bancrofti, 77, 86
  filariasis, 205
  lymphadenitis, 137

X-linked lymphoproliferative disease, 145

Yaws, 110–11, 155, 203
Yeasts, 7
Yellow fever, 148
Yersinia enterocolitica, 56, 173
  diarrhoea, 158, 161

Yersinia pestis, 25, 56, 57, 77, 213
  lymphadenitis, 137
  portals of entry, 25
Yersinia pseudotuberculosis, 56–7, 173
Yersinosis, 173

Zanamivir, 235
Zidovudine, 234
Zoonoses, 212–13
Zoonotic bacteria, 56–7
Zygomycetes
  endophthalmitis, 112
  stomatitis, 113
Zygomycosis, 75
  invasive, 76
Zygomycota, 6